The History of the U.S. Army Medical Service Corps

Tom O. Mathews
Col. Ret.

The History of the U.S. Army Medical Service Corps

by

Richard V.N. Ginn

OFFICE OF THE SURGEON GENERAL
AND
CENTER OF MILITARY HISTORY
UNITED STATES ARMY
WASHINGTON, D.C., 1997

Library of Congress Cataloging-in-Publication Data

Ginn, Richard V.N., 1943–
The history of the U.S. Army Medical Service Corps / by Richard V.N. Ginn.
p. cm.
Includes bibliographical references and index.
1. United States. Army. Medical Service Corps—History.
I. Title
UA223.G546 1996
355.3'45'0973—dc20 96–19473
CIP

CMH Pub 30–19–1

First Printing

Foreword

The United States Army Medical Service Corps is an important national resource with a long and distinguished history. Many thousands of officers have proudly served in its ranks, selflessly prosecuting the nation's defense missions in peace and war throughout the world. With varied academic backgrounds and disciplines, these officers have been widely recognized and highly regarded leaders in their respective fields. They represent the growth in medical science and military medical operations and administration over two centuries.

This work documents the history of the Medical Service Corps through the work of an active duty MSC officer who began researching and writing in 1983 when the corps assumed this task as its own project. The account is the story of the corps, told by the corps for its members, the Army, its sister services, and the nation it serves. The lessons of its history are rooted in America's wartime experiences, and they are intended for those who will follow in the hope that our future leaders will learn from the past. It is also important that progress documented by this account continue, for the officers of the Medical Service Corps have by no means achieved their highest goals.

MACK C. HILL
Brigadier General
Chief, Medical Service Corps

JOHN W. MOUNTCASTLE
Brigadier General
Chief of Military History

The Author

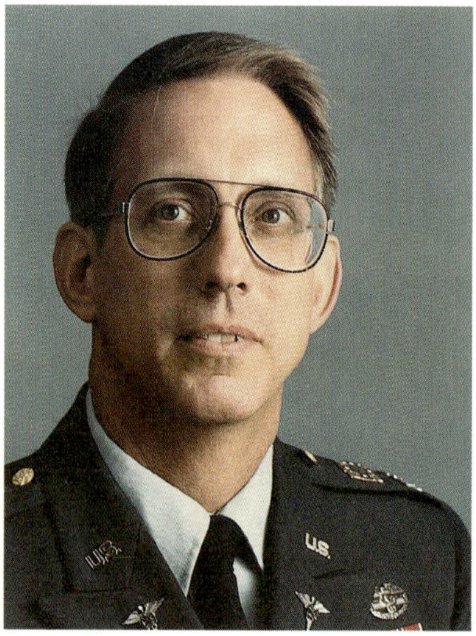

Col. Richard Van Ness Ginn is a native of Miami, Florida. He was commissioned from ROTC as a Distinguished Military Graduate in 1965 upon graduation with a BA from Stetson University and entered active duty in 1966 after graduate study. He has an MA from Duke University and an MHA from Baylor University. Completion of the U.S. Army–Baylor University Program in Healthcare Administration in 1977 as the Distinguished Honor Graduate was followed by a residency in the Office of the Assistant Secretary of Defense for Health Affairs. In 1981 he was an honor graduate of the U.S. Army Command and General Staff College, where he also served as a student instructor. He is a 1990 graduate of the U.S. Army War College. His decorations include the Legion of Merit, the Combat Medical Badge, and the Senior Parachutist Badge.

His principal assignments have included tours at medical platoon and company levels of airborne infantry units in Panama and Vietnam; Aide-de-Camp to the Commander, and Chief, Force Development Branch, U.S. Army Medical Research and Development Command (USAMRDC), Washington, D.C.; Professional Services Administrator, Brooke Army Medical Center, Fort Sam Houston, Texas; Personnel Policy Officer, Office of the Surgeon General (OTSG) and Special Assistant to the Chief, Medical Service Corps, the Pentagon; Deputy Commander for Administration, 196th Station Hospital, Supreme Headquarters Allied Powers Europe, Belgium; Inspector General, 7th Medical Command, Heidelberg, Germany; Chief of Staff, USAMRDC, Fort Detrick, Maryland; Chief of Education and Training, OTSG, Falls Church, Virginia; and Chief, Health Services Division, Officer Personnel Management Directorate, U.S. Total Army Personnel Command, Alexandria, Virginia.

Colonel Ginn is a fellow of the American College of Healthcare Executives and is listed in *Who's Who in America*. In 1977 he became the first Army Medical Service Corps officer to win the Sir Henry Wellcome Medal, the oldest award of the Association of Military Surgeons of the United States, and in 1982 he was the first recipient of the association's Young Federal Health Care Administrator Award. He is a member of the Order of Military Medical Merit. He wrote this book while stationed in Washington, Belgium, Germany, Maryland, and Virginia. Colonel Ginn retired in December 1995 and is currently Senior Vice President, Capital Health Services, Fairfax, Virginia.

Preface

The purpose of this volume is to present a history of the U.S. Army Medical Service Corps (MSC) from its origins during the American Revolution to its status in 1994. With this objective in mind, it addresses several audiences.

First are the young MSC officers who may be unfamiliar with the historical underpinnings of their corps. For them, the evolution of the corps' past reveals insights into its future since the types of problems met and solved in the past are the ones most likely to recur in the years ahead. I am told that colonels are supposed to read what captains write. This time a colonel wrote something for captains to read.

A second audience is the scholarly community of historians. For these professionals, the work adheres to established rules of historical research and serves as a tool for further analysis of the often baffling bureaucratic structure of our armed services. The third audience consists of those who served in the MSC or its precursors, as well as other members of the Army Medical Department and the public at large. For that group the book endeavors to elucidate the principal themes in this administrative history in which evolution rather than revolution has been an enduring characteristic.

The book belongs to the Medical Service Corps, especially to those who will carry its legacy into the future. It also belongs to all the people of the Army Medical Department and the other branches of the Army. It should be of assistance to anyone interested in how the Army provides medical support to soldiers and their families. Above all it belongs to American soldiers, those splendid, noble patriots whose support is the *raison d'etre* of the MSC. I have attempted to provide enough Medical Department history, doctrine, and principal debates to illuminate how the MSC emerged from more than two centuries of American history. I hope that the book and its documentation of sources will serve those who will labor to understand how that process occurred so as to prevent repeating previous mistakes and to capitalize on earlier successes. The text ends in 1995, but appendixes have been updated to the time of printing.

One editorial note is in order. As a rule, the rank of an individual is cited as held at that point in the narrative. Generally, no attempt is made to document the final grade upon separation from the military.

This work would not have been undertaken without the strong determination of two officers who decided to prosecute and underwrite the initiative and served as successive chiefs of the Medical Service Corps: Brig. Gens. France F. Jordan and Walter F. Johnson. Their successors as chiefs of the corps maintained support for the project. It stands on the shoulders of many individuals who worked on earlier attempts at writing the history of the corps, beginning in 1953. Their accumulation of files and documents was of invaluable assistance, as was their foresight in pursuing the goal of documenting the MSC story. All chapters of the first draft were reviewed by former chiefs of the corps as well as by many others from varied backgrounds. Twelve of that group served as active readers during the initial drafting of the volume: Mr. Frank Boccia; Mary C. Gillett, Ph.D.; Brig. Gen. William A. Hamrick, FACHE, USA, Ret.; Brig. Gen. France Jordan, USA, Ret.; Col. John T. Leddy, O.D., USA, Ret.; Col. Roy D. Maxwell, Ph.D., USA, Ret.; Col. Douglas E. Moore, USA, Ret.; Brig. Gen. Manley C. Morrison, USA, Ret.; Brig. Gen. Andre J. Ognibene, M.D., USA, Ret.; Col. James E. Spiker, USA, Ret.; Mrs. Emily Ginn Van Orden; and Lt. Col. Joseph W.A. Whitehorne, USA, Ret. Their candid criticism kept the author in check and compelled a wider range of view.

Mary F. Loughlin was the first editor. She helped shape the early drafts, but her participation was ended by her untimely death in 1992. Susan Carroll replaced her as editor in 1994. She was superbly professional, and did yeoman work in straightening out the manuscript and later in creating the index. Helen Wadsworth took the corps to heart and was faithful and patient as a talented photo researcher whose contributions continued into the printing of the book. Col. Timothy Jackman, MSC, was appointed assistant to the corps chief in the fall of 1989 and became a treasured help as my Washington connection while I was in Europe. Tim also served as a member of the U.S. Army Center of Military History (CMH) panel for the book. Ann Martens, the secretary to the chief during the time I was in Europe, was always helpful.

I leaned heavily on the CMH staff from the beginning. Although the book had been dropped from the center's projects, its staff continued to provide me with assistance at every step of the way. Brig. Gen. William A. Stofft, and later Brig. Gen. Harold W. Nelson, as CMH commanders, were supportive and encouraging. Jeffrey J. Clarke, Ph.D., CMH chief historian, became a guiding light as the head of the CMH panel that reviewed the manuscript. The members of his panel were most helpful, particularly Col. Robert J. T. Joy, M.D., USA, Ret., a long-standing mentor to whom I had turned for coaching when I was first tapped for this task. I am also grateful to Dr. Clarke and Albert E. Cowdrey, Ph.D., of the CMH staff, for coaching me during the final drafts of the manuscript. Jeff's support was unflagging, and Bert was enormously giving of his time and considerable talent in shaping the text. My appreciation also goes to John Elsberg, CMH editor in chief, who oversaw the production of the volume, and to Steve Hardyman, Beth MacKenzie, and Catherine Heerin of CMH who shepherded the manuscript through its printing, adopting the book as their own.

Special commendation is also due to Donna Griffitts, for twelve years, until her untimely death in 1986, the head of the Joint Medical Library of the Army and Air Force Surgeons General. Donna had an abiding faith in the Medical Department and a genuine love of its history. Her assistance was treasured by me and countless others over those years. She was a great help during the initial research phase of the book from 1983 to 1986. Donna symbolizes the many people who gave of themselves to this project and who made it possible.

Finally, computers were with me from the beginning as automation swept through the military, government, and industry. The solitary author in his study is about the right picture, electronically enhanced. But the cast of helpers would not be complete without saluting my wife, Angélica, and our two children, Angie Ann and Rick. I cannot repay them for their forbearance and love, especially since the task of writing and research occupied my evenings and weekends for much of over eleven years.

The Army and our nation have a great deal to be thankful for in the contributions of the men and women of the magnificent U.S. Army Medical Service Corps. I have always been proud to wear the silver caduceus. The privilege of writing this book has reinforced that pride. Yet, as always in these things, any errors of fact or interpretation are the author's responsibility alone.

Springfield, Virginia
November 1996

Richard V.N. Ginn
Colonel, MSC (Ret.)

Contents

Tables

Charts

Illustrations

The History of the U.S. Army Medical Service Corps

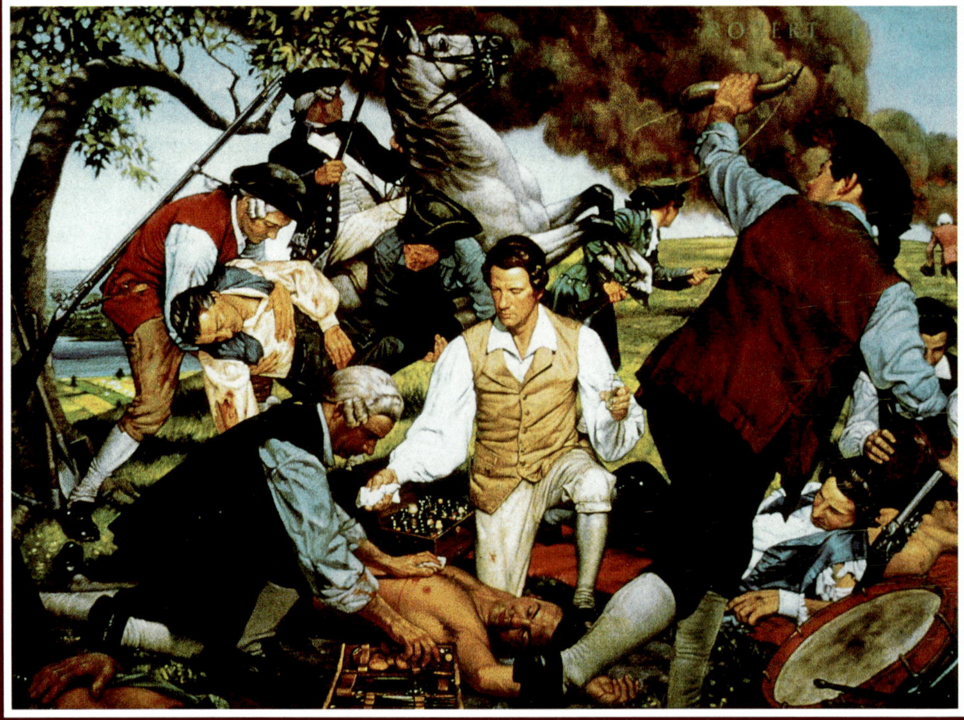

Robert A. Thom's painting, America's First Apothecary General, *depicts Andrew Craigie.*

1

Early Military Medicine

The U.S. Army Medical Service Corps (MSC) traces its roots to the American Revolution. Today, MSC officers in twenty-six specialties (*see Appendix M*) are valued members of the Army's medical team. They provide administrative skills ranging from health care administration to aeromedical evacuation, scientific expertise in fields as diverse as optometry and microbiology, and administrative services at all levels of the United States military medical establishment. Their corps, along with the Medical Corps (physicians), Army Nurse Corps (nurses), Dental Corps (dentists), Veterinary Corps (veterinarians), and Army Medical Specialist Corps (dietitians, physical therapists, occupational therapists, and physician assistants), constitute the officer corps of the Army Medical Department. Those officers are joined by enlisted soldiers, noncommissioned officers, and civilians to form the complete team.

The evolution of the Medical Service Corps as part of that team occurred as the United States Army learned that military medical support was impossible without officers specifically dedicated to a wide variety of duties that someone other than physicians, nurses, dentists, or veterinarians should perform. Oftentimes those responsibilities involved health care specialties that emerged only gradually from developments in medical technology. In other cases they were functions that became necessary for the operation of an increasingly complex military medical support system that demanded professionalism and specialization.

The origins of the MSC predate the founding of the United States. On 30 April 1775, the Provincial Congress of Massachusetts Bay appointed Andrew Craigie, a graduate of the Boston Latin School, as apothecary of the Massachusetts Army. Congress referred to Craigie as the "commissary of medicinal stores" and charged him with providing beds, linen, and other supplies necessary for patient care to the troops gathering around Boston.[1] On 27 July 1775, the Continental Congress created "an hospital" (the forerunner of the Army Medical Department) for its army of 20,000 soldiers.[2] An apothecary was among the personnel specified in the resolution, and in time Craigie assumed that duty. His duties were similar to those performed by present-day MSC pharmacists and medical logistics officers. His legacy is commemorated by the Association of Military Surgeons of the United States, which recognizes a federal government pharmacist each year with the Andrew Craigie Award.[3]

The evolution from apothecary to pharmacist, and the development of the other medical administrative and scientific specialties of the present-day Medical

Service Corps, accompanied progress in medical technology. Revolutionary Army apothecaries, physicians, and surgeons did the best they could, but they practiced medicine before the invention of the stethoscope and general acceptance of the concept that living organisms, such as bacteria, cause disease. Sulfa drugs, antibiotics, x-ray, and the understanding that insects and animals can serve as vectors for disease were more than a century away. Bleeding was often the therapy of choice, and anesthetics had not yet muted the agony of patients in surgery.[4]

Progress in medical technology—along with public awareness that practitioners could actually do something for those in their care—produced new specialties and organizational requirements necessitating greater variety and sophistication of staff. The need for military officers in emerging health care specialties became evident in varying degrees during the period from the Revolution to World War I. Medical logistics, for example, increasingly became a vital element in the support of combat operations, and repeated failures illustrated all too clearly the need for individuals trained in management and business practices. The preparation and dispensing of medications became the province of pharmacists and, eventually, a specialty in military medicine. The need for a coherent medical evacuation and treatment doctrine became painfully apparent during the Civil War, and an effective response required the creation of a new commissioned officer specialty, the ambulance corps officer. Increased sophistication of organizations also required officers specializing in administration. And, as preventive medicine became a reality, the medical advances that made this possible spawned scientific specialties beyond the imagination of anyone in George Washington's army.

From Revolution to Reform

Deficiencies in the Army's medical support capability during the Revolution, 1775–1783, demonstrated a need for specialists in medical logistics and for a rational system of supply. The Army had no coordinated medical supply system; each colony raised its own regiments, and regimental surgeons relied on their home colonies for medical supplies. The chaotic system was made worse by inflation and problems in communication and transportation. Some commanders complained of severe shortages. There was great pressure on Andrew Craigie, who found in one hospital that there was not only a shortage of drugs but also of the most basic items such as bandages, needles, and blankets. The Massachusetts Bay Congress appointed a committee to study the medical supply problems, but the actions of one provincial body could not resolve the larger issues. The Continental Congress attempted a solution in August 1775 when it designated a druggist, Dr. William Smith, as purveyor for medical supply. Later, Congress reorganized the Army into three districts and provided each district with an apothecary general whose duty it was "to receive, prepare, and deliver medicines, and other articles of his department to the hospitals and army." Craigie's efforts contributed to an improved situation by the summer of 1778, the same year in which the first Army formulary appeared.[5]

The Regular Army nearly ceased to exist after the Revolution and was retained principally for Indian fighting. In 1784 Congress reduced it to eighty enlisted soldiers, a few officers, and no medical personnel. Congress authorized an Army of 718 in 1789, one of about four thousand in 1794, and a medical department in 1799, but did little to organize the central medical establishment. Medical support for soldiers continued to remain primarily the responsibility of state militia regiments that remained under the control of the state legislatures. Control of medical logistics was held by those outside the Medical Department, and weaknesses that had surfaced during the Revolution were not corrected.

In 1809 Dr. William Upshaw, surgeon of the 5th Infantry near New Orleans, denounced the failings of the system, which were compounded by the corruption of his commander, Brig. Gen. James Wilkinson. An unfortunate force of about two thousand soldiers was decimated by disease as it deployed to defend the newly acquired lower Mississippi territories. Over one thousand soldiers fell ill, and most died. Upshaw bitterly complained of caring for sick soldiers, only to see them die for lack of food or medicine, declaring, "Humanity mourns such a sight."[6]

In addition to the need for a functional medical supply system, the necessity for basic management practices and for the relief of physicians from nonclinical duties contributed to the evolution of medical administrative specialties. In 1808 Dr. Edward Cutbush, medical director of the Pennsylvania militia during the Whiskey Rebellion, published the first manual on hospital administration. In it he defined the hospital steward, the forerunner of Army medical noncommissioned officers, in terms recognizable today as similar to those describing a hospital administrator.[7]

Cutbush's hospital steward was necessarily an individual "of strict integrity and sobriety," whose duties included discipline of staff and patients, personnel management, patient administration, food service operations, medical supply, cost accounting, procurement of supplies and equipment, subsistence, property accountability, and supervision of the ward master. The steward enforced hospital rules, seeing to it that "no one should spit on the floors or walls."[8] Cutbush's hospital staff also included a purveyor, "not a *medical man*, but one conversant with business," whose duty it was to purchase the items necessary for patient care.[9] Pharmacy operations were provided by apothecaries who compounded medications for the patients from prescriptions written by the physicians and surgeons.

The War of 1812 resulted from increasingly tense relations between the United States and England over a variety of matters unresolved by the War of Independence. At the time a somewhat strengthened U.S. Army numbered just over sixty-five hundred soldiers.[10] While inconclusive, the conflict increased national pride and produced a national anthem.[11] But military medicine differed little from that practiced during the Revolution, except that it was less organized—there was still no medical department. Its burdens were increased by poor military leadership, unpreparedness, and an amateurishness and confusion in organization and command that cost the nation many defeats in the field. The need for expansion of health care specialties was voiced in the reports of Dr. James Mann, medical director for the Northern Department. Mann complained that the press of his various administrative duties as hospital surgeon, including sanitation inspections, kept him from fulfilling all of his clinical tasks.[12]

Deficiencies in medical logistics again surfaced, and campaigns along the Canadian border were routinely marked by breakdowns in the medical supply system. Medical personnel were criticized for their part in the "great mortality" in 1813 at French Mills, a militia post just west of Plattsburg, New York. Dr. Mann argued that the absence of dedicated medical transportation assets was at fault. Medical supplies had been loaded wherever there was room on the boats and "were either consumed by the troops, damaged, or lost." In other instances, medical supplies destined for Mann's area had been diverted by higher authority outside the surgeon's control.[13] A 12th Infantry inspector noted that "the Surgeon complains he is without drugs, hospital stores, or surgical instruments."[14]

Establishment of a Permanent Medical Department

The many failures in delivery of medical services during the war helped to provoke a strong movement for reform and organization after it was over. American military medicine took a great step forward on 14 May 1818, when Congress created a permanent chief of the Medical Department, an act which gave permanency to the department itself. Joseph Lovell, appointed as the surgeon general, set up his new office and, in accordance with the wishes of Congress, accounted for his actions in annual reports. He quickly moved to consolidate the authority of the Medical Department and to establish administrative procedures.[15]

The new department included an apothecary general and two assistants. They were responsible for purchasing medical supplies and equipment, compounding and preparing medicines, accounting for the distribution of supplies and equipment, and reporting expenditures annually. Surgeon General Lovell was confident that those medical administrative and scientific functions would be well executed by his apothecary general, Francis LeBaron, who was qualified "both from his knowledge of medicines and habits of business."[16]

Medical logistics support for the Army was high among Lovell's priorities. He feared the department would be handicapped by the low pay allotted to the assistant apothecaries general and by the difficulty this posed in recruiting from urban areas such as New York and Philadelphia. He was also concerned about control over medical logistics, believing that his greatest problem would be preventing interference in medical procurement by commanders outside the Medical Department who were subject to influence by private contractors and were often overcharged. Lovell's fears were realized when the position of apothecary general was abolished even though the surgeon general was not released from responsibility for medical logistics.[17]

The small size and slender resources of the Medical Department were all the more noticeable by contrast with developments then going on in Europe. The time of the Napoleonic Wars and after was marked by great advances in military medical organization. Napoleon's chief surgeon, Baron Dominique Jean Larrey, had in 1793 created a "flying ambulance," a mobile field hospital with surgeons, stretchers, and supplies carried in horse-drawn conveyances that could be rapidly moved to the points of greatest need on the battlefield. Larrey had so refined his flying ambulance that in 1799, at Aboukir, Egypt, he reported that no casualties were left more than fifteen minutes without being properly treated.[18]

By 1831 French military medical doctrine encompassed Larrey's mobile field hospitals and an ambulance corps. Manning tables for the medical evacuation and treatment system of French divisions included five administrative officers and three pharmacy officers.[19] However, removal of the wounded was still performed by a soldier's comrades, who would then return only reluctantly to the battlefield. The ambulance corps was thus a rudimentary organization that depended for litter bearers and other manual labor upon soldiers detailed from combat units.[20]

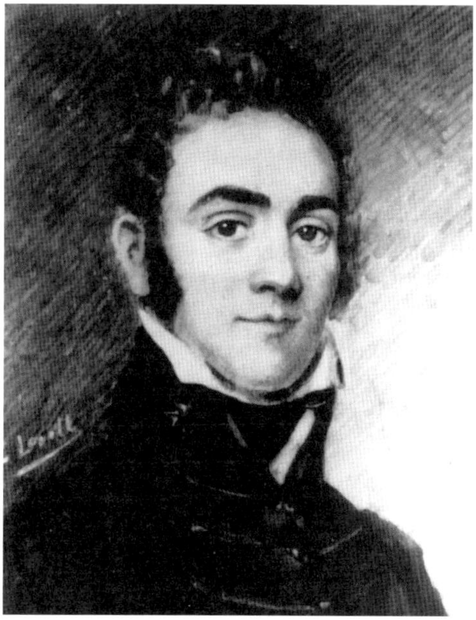

Surgeon General Lovell

A generation later Americans were also witness to the British experience in the Crimean War.[21] Between April 1854 and June 1856 England sent some eighty-three thousand soldiers to fight in Russia; nearly twenty thousand died, over four-fifths of them from disease. The fate of the wounded within the evacuation and treatment system was precarious. Lifted from the mud of the field hospitals for transport by sea back to Turkey, many died from the rigors of the trip. Wounded soldiers were laid on the decks of ships, some of which foundered in the winter sea. Once in the British hospital at Scutari, the patients were placed in two rows, feet to feet, in wards where the dead could not be removed as fast as the sick came in. It was a "vista of woe."[22] Descriptions of suffering and the shortcomings of the British medical system caused a public outcry that catalyzed formation of a politically influential sanitary commission. This led to pressures in England and in other countries to improve the administrative and scientific capabilities of military medicine so as to prevent repetition of the catastrophes in the Crimea.

The more fortunate wounded and sick were taken to the improved British hospitals of Florence Nightingale. Nightingale had arrived in Constantinople in 1854 as the nursing superintendent of the English military hospitals in Turkey. Justly regarded as a pioneer in hospital administration as well as nursing education, Nightingale forcefully improved the sanitation of British hospitals at a time when filth was the standard. She proved politically astute and in time became a fixture in British national life. She personified a growing demand for public oversight of military medicine.[23]

Nightingale's observations on military hospitals demonstrated her understanding of them as complex enterprises requiring specialized management skills. She believed the head of a general hospital should be selected "for his fitness alone, i.e., his capacity for administration, and not upon grounds of professional eminence."[24] She also advocated an organization that would free physicians to practice medicine. The staff should include a registrar for maintenance of records and reports and a hospital treasurer, who would make payments, keep accounts of receipts and expenditures, and audit the steward's account.[25] Finally, she vigorously supported creation of a statistical capability, calling it "the most important science in the world," because it provided a mathematical distillation of clinical experience.[26] Nightingale's grasp of the need for specialists in hospital administration, medical records and reports, medical financial management, and statistics shows that the need for a corps of officers for those specialties was recognized long before such organizations were ever created.

Such progressive thinking, unfortunately, was absent from the United States Army. Brig. Gen. Thomas Lawson, surgeon general for the twenty-five years from 1836 to 1861, served the longest of any surgeon general, but he led the department without imagination. His failure to undertake planning for large-scale hostilities resulted in a department incapable of handling the casualties from the early battles of the Civil War.[27]

Yet he achieved some small victories, one of which was his success in obtaining permanent authority for appointing hospital stewards. He wrote Secretary of War Jefferson Davis that the important duties of the stewards required the selection of "steady, sober and intelligent men," something that did not happen when line commanders had to detail personnel for those jobs. He recommended their appointment with the rank and pay of first sergeant.[28] The War Department provided for a competitive selection process and restricted their number to one at each post.[29] Lawson also recognized, though he did not succeed in establishing, the need for Medical Department control over medical logistics. He observed that medical items were liable to be stolen, damaged, or destroyed by storekeepers, teamsters, or muleteers who "handle a box containing the choicest medicines as roughly as if they were boxes of camp-kettles and mess pans."[30]

In the War with Mexico, 1846–1848, Maj. Gen. Winfield Scott commanded an expeditionary force that fought outside the United States, away from its support base. Disease continued to dominate the medical battlefront. Over one hundred thousand soldiers served in the conflict; 12,896 died, but of them only 1,629 were killed in action or died from wounds, a distressing ratio.[31] There was no ambulance corps or hospital corps to provide a systematic evacuation and treatment system. Wounded soldiers were gathered up by soldiers detailed for that purpose and taken to hospitals, which were set up in the nearest convenient buildings. Wagons were used to evacuate casualties, but there were no vehicles designed expressly for that purpose. At least the agony of surgery was now diminished for some patients by the first use of anesthesia in wartime.[32]

The remaining years before the Civil War were dominated by the Indian campaigns, which required small, mobile units stationed at widely separated posts. A progressive measure was the inclusion of ambulances in the force structure and the restriction of their use to movement of the sick and wounded. Medical Department regulations specified a leaner medical support for the Indian campaigns than that provided for fighting "a civilized enemy."[33] Commands smaller than five companies were allotted just one two-wheeled ambulance.

The last years of General Lawson's administration witnessed some efforts at planning for medical support. The surgeon general convened a board of medical officers in 1858 that examined "ambulance wagons" and recommended Medical Department control over all its vehicles. Another board of medical officers was convened the following year to examine revised supply tables and to select a field ambulance, although it failed to adopt a standard design. That board also recommended a casualty evacuation doctrine, but no plan was adopted.[34] On the whole, the Medical Department between the time of Lowell and the Civil War failed to keep up with progressive developments abroad. Instead, progress would come through the shock of war.

At War With Ourselves

The Civil War brought misery to the Republic and extraordinary challenges to the Army Medical Department. It produced a casualty evacuation and treatment doctrine that continues today, and it drew the tapestry of evolving medical specialties into sharper relief. The fields of medical logistics, pharmacy, hospital administration, records administration, and statistical reporting grew as they contributed to the effectiveness of the department. Technology in such matters as instruments and ambulances advanced. And the work of sanitary commissions reflected a climate for change highlighted by politically charged public oversight of military medical activities.

The revolution in organization was all the more striking because the state of medical art had not changed that much from earlier days. Clinicians made increasing forays into a scientific understanding of health and disease, but the causes of disease were maddeningly perplexing. Fingers were not yet pointed at such things as germs and mosquitoes.[35] Both sides, Blue and Gray, shared a common military medical heritage. Sick call for Confederate soldiers in the Army of the Tennessee was held immediately after reveille, and their treatment depended upon whatever the medical officer happened to have. Dr. William H. Taylor, a Southern surgeon, said his medical practice became very simplified in the field. "In one pocket of my trousers I had a ball of blue mass, in another a ball of opium. All complainants were asked the same question: 'How are your bowels?' If they were open I administered a plug of opium, if they were shut I gave a plug of blue mass [a commonly used medication whose principal ingredient was mercury]."[36] The use of anesthesia, typically chloroform, was common, but surgeons were in a quandary between the desire to use techniques made possible by anesthesia and the threat of infection that would follow if they did. Certainly their surgical techniques were not elegant: "We groped for bullets with roughened porcelain-tipped probes, the mark of lead on the probe recording the locality of the ball."[37] Field hospitals were marked by piles of amputated limbs.[38]

The opening of the war gave little hint that progress of any sort lay ahead. The Army numbered only some twenty thousand soldiers when fighting began at Fort Sumter in April 1861, and the Medical Department was also very small—only

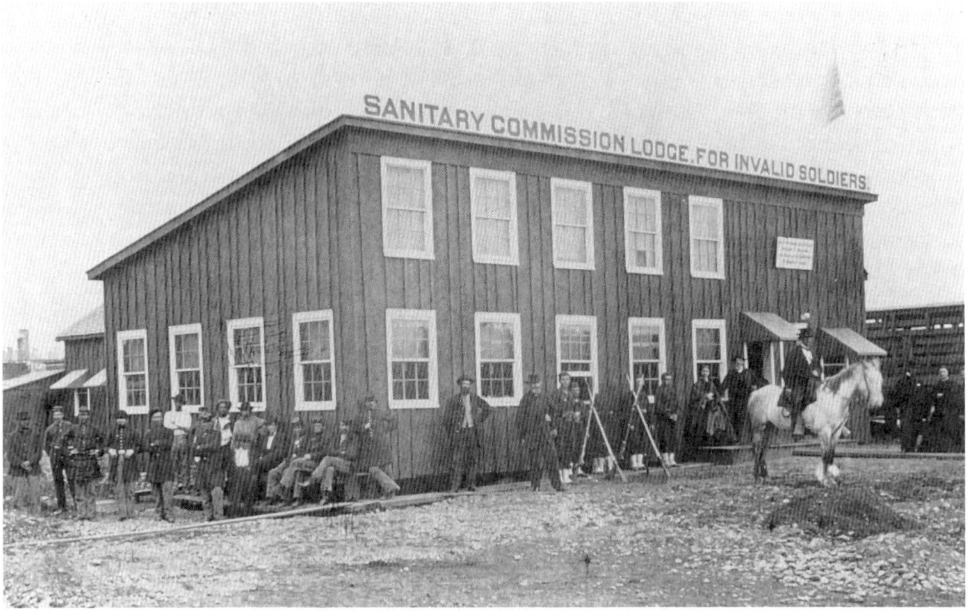

U.S. Sanitary Commission Lodge for Invalid Soldiers, Alexandria, Virginia

113 uniformed physicians, of whom 24 resigned to join the Confederacy. But the number of medical officers mushroomed to 3,000 as the department expanded to 204 general hospitals operating 136,894 beds.[39]

Care of the wounded became an early preoccupation of the public. The pioneering efforts of Florence Nightingale and French and English sanitary commissions did not go unnoticed. Women formed soldiers' aid societies throughout the United States to provide organized help to the Union effort. One of those groups, the Woman's Central Association of Relief for the Sick and Wounded of the Army, combined with other groups to form the United States Sanitary Commission, which soon won a presidential mandate to conduct its inquiries. Like its Crimean War predecessors, the Sanitary Commission served as an external catalyst for change, becoming known as Lincoln's "fifth wheel" and acting as a gadfly to the War Department. It furnished supplies and volunteer assistance to the Medical Department and brought public opinion to bear on its operations. Its special investigators included experts in emerging disciplines related to medicine such as chemistry, physiology, and statistics, scientific specialties that would eventually be incorporated into the Medical Service Corps.[40]

Members of the commission presented charges of Medical Department mismanagement on their first visit to the surgeon general, and from then on the commission and the department routinely clashed. The commission pushed for well-stocked medical depots, a large ambulance corps under direct medical control, and the construction of hospitals using the latest European innovations. In pursuing those aims it influenced the dismissal of one surgeon general, Brig. Gen. Clement A. Finley, and the selection of his replacement, Brig. Gen. William A.

Hammond. The commission also earned the unrelenting animosity of perhaps the most powerful man in Washington next to President Abraham Lincoln, Secretary of War Edwin M. Stanton.[41] In the West, the Western Sanitary Commission also kept pressure on the Medical Department, forcing changes to the Army's medical supply table over the objections of the Western Department's medical director.[42]

Medical support deficiencies, while perhaps not discernible in peacetime, became deadly in war. In 1862 the department's inadequacies came under scathing attack in the Congress where there were charges of the "grossest mismanagement" of Army hospitals, demands for the employment of medical inspectors, and calls for General Finley's removal. Army physicians were called self-satisfied old men (Surgeon General Lawson had been seventy-two and in bad health when Fort Sumter fell) who had removed themselves from the practice of medicine and were out of touch with contemporary practice.[43] What was reported in Congress was experienced firsthand by the writer Louisa May Alcott (she later would publish *Little Women*). Alcott volunteered for duty as a nurse at an Army hospital in Washington, D.C., in 1862. There she worked in "famine and filth" among "violent odors that assaulted the human nose."[44] It was, said one soldier who also worked in a Union hospital, "our terrible Hospital Service."[45]

Yet, while Stanton accused the Medical Department of "general imbecility," it would not be fair to ascribe all medical support failures solely to the department's ineptitude.[46] After all, Army doctrine at the time was designed for fielding small detachments in the Indian campaigns, and the military buildup for the Civil War was dependent upon the formation of volunteer regiments (roughly equivalent to today's battalions). Regiments provided for their own medical support, so medical officers quite naturally were concerned primarily with their own units, not others. The medical system in support of the regiments was sketchy, and there was no overall plan for evacuation and hospitalization of casualties in successive steps back to the general hospitals. There was no doctrine to unite people, equipment, and facilities into an integrated system of support.

The impact of this structural disarray was compounded by the lethality of Civil War battlefields. Though most individual weapons were muzzle-loading muskets, barrels had been rifled to increase the accuracy of fire and amplify its range. Rifled muskets fired the so-called minié ball—not a ball at all, but a heavy, conical bullet that did great damage when it smashed into flesh and bone. Late in the war breech-loading rifles completed the revolution in weapons by giving a greater rate of fire. Yet tactics failed to keep pace with technological progress, and soldiers attacking in tight formations across open fields were simply mowed down. The resulting carnage ruthlessly exposed the inadequacy of the evacuation and hospital systems.

Toward an Ambulance Corps

Soldiers wounded in July 1861 at First Bull Run had to fend for themselves because there was a "pitiful absence of provision for the wounded."[47] Ambulance drivers were generally either impressed soldiers or wagon and hack drivers pulled from the streets of Washington, and rumors of forthcoming roundups sent drivers fleeing from the city. Surgeons reported drivers who were insubordinate or drunk or who appropriated space inside the ambulances intended for blankets and food. As to the vehicles themselves, the Army had been forced to round up commercial wagons and hacks to serve as ambulances.[48]

Second Bull Run, the following summer, demonstrated that little had improved after a year of combat operations. Army surgeons at Centreville, Virginia, operated on casualties who lay without blankets on the bare earth. Surgeon Thomas A. McParlin, medical director of the Federal Army of Virginia, wrote that Americans should follow the lead of the Europeans. "A well-organized regularly established ambulance corps would have been a blessing."[49] The need was felt in other theaters as well. In Missouri, Surgeon John H. Brinton reported that the lack of adequate evacuation capability had caused abandonment of the wounded. Those who were able crawled to whatever cover they could reach; many were captured.[50]

The absence of personnel dedicated to the evacuation mission required commanders to use combat soldiers to remove the wounded from the battlefield, further reducing the Army's fighting strength. Not surprisingly, the speedy return of soldiers who left the battlefield to assist the wounded was problematic. A Confederate report echoed the universal complaint of line commanders: "If any from the ranks are drawn from the fight to carry off the wounded, they never return until the fight is over, and thus three are lost to the company instead of one wounded."[51]

Confederate Army medical organization mirrored the Union's, as leadership of the Southern medical department was in the hands of former Union medical officers, including Confederate Surgeon General Samuel Preston Moore. While the Confederate medical manual was based on U.S. Army regulations, its field medical doctrine included the European concept of a sanitary corps with officers and soldiers designated for evacuating the wounded. Those soldiers would serve in the front lines, where "not infrequently they lose their lives in accomplishing their benevolent tasks."[52]

A variety of ideas for an ambulance system surfaced in the Union Army. One was for an ambulance company of two lieutenants and sixty-seven soldiers for each corps, with the entire ambulance organization under command of a medical officer. A variation of that idea was an ambulance company for each division. The Sanitary Commission proposed an ambulance regiment for the Army of the Potomac.[53] Some medical officers adopted partial remedies. The Army of the Potomac published an order written by Surgeon Charles S. Tripler, the medical director, detailing twenty-five soldiers per regiment as an ambulance corps under the supervision of the brigade surgeon. Tripler required the medical officers to train the medical soldiers on a daily basis and sent his medical inspectors out to check on the instruction. The inspectors also checked the number and kind of ambulances, their condition, and whether the soldiers and vehicles were employed solely in medical evacuation.[54] In the West, Surgeon Brinton organized the regimental ambulances into ambulance trains, each under a noncommissioned officer "whose business it was to see that a continuous line of wagons should ply between the scene of conflict and the general hospitals."[55]

Brig. Gen. William A. Hammond, a 34-year-old officer, replaced General Finley as surgeon general in April 1862. Hammond, at six feet, two inches in height, 250 pounds, possessing a booming voice and an aggressive and abrasive personality, was by no means a shrinking violet. Backed by the Sanitary Commission, he had been appointed by President Lincoln over Secretary of War Stanton's objections and immediately incurred the wrath of that powerful man.[56] But at first inertia rather than hostility was Hammond's chief problem. Hammond quickly focused on the need for a coordinated evacuation and treatment capability and recommended establishment of an ambulance corps. However, Maj. Gen. Henry W. Halleck, the Army's general-in-chief, rejected the proposal, declaring that ambulances would add to the problem of large combat trains, the ever-present "tooth-to-tail" argument. Halleck also feared that the presence of medical personnel on the battlefield would spread panic among soldiers who might view them as harbingers of suffering and death. Hammond tried again in September, pleading: "I only ask that some system may be adopted." He lamented that 600 wounded soldiers still lay unattended on the battlefield of Second Bull Run, dying of starvation and neglect. His pleas were again rejected.[57]

The surgeon general persisted, making the establishment of a permanent hospital and ambulance corps the highest priority in his annual report for 1862.[58] He argued that it would enable the Medical Department to enlist soldiers specifically for hospital nursing duties and for the operation of field ambulances, rather than having to depend on the unreliable practice of detailing soldiers from other branches. However, he was unable to get War Department support for his proposal that year.

The Letterman Plan

That same year, however, Hammond selected Maj. Jonathan Letterman as medical director for the Army of the Potomac. What the surgeon general was blocked from doing for the Army, the 38-year-old Major Letterman was able to do for the Army's largest combat formation by putting together an ambulance corps as part of a unitary medical support system. Letterman, a veteran officer with thirteen years in the Army and field medical experience in the campaigns against the Seminole, Navajo, Apache, and Ute Nations, reported on 1 July 1862 to Maj. Gen. George McClellan in Virginia at Harrison's Landing on the James River. Here the Seven Days Battle was in progress and casualties were mounting. Letterman inherited what McClellan described as a collapsed situation: "Supplies had been almost exhausted or necessarily abandoned or destroyed, and the medical officers [were] deficient in numbers or broken down by fatigue."[59]

Letterman, a man of "remarkable energy and ability,"[60] moved quickly to establish an integrated medical capability based on three principal elements: a coordinated system of casualty evacuation from the point of wounding back through the division rear; organization of medical logistics, including supply tables and transportation; and establishment of division field hospitals as part of the evacuation chain. Supported by his commander, he set forth his plan in Army of the Potomac General Orders 147, 2 August 1862, which placed all ambulances

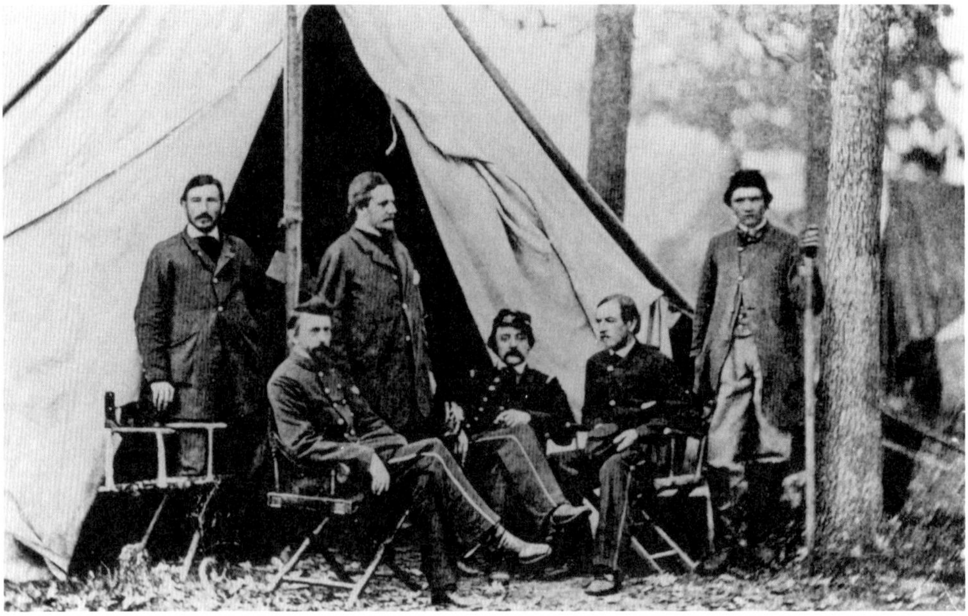

Major Letterman (second from left) *with his staff*

under the control of the medical director. Captains commanded the corps-level ambulance organization, first lieutenants commanded at the division level, second lieutenants led at the brigade level, and sergeants at the regimental level. Those ambulance officers were progenitors of present-day Medical Service Corps ground and air ambulance officers.[61]

Letterman's use of nonphysician officers to command ambulance units represented a significant shift in Army Medical Department policy. He intended to relieve the physicians from duties that distracted them from their primary mission of patient care, especially in combat. Letterman knew that at such times the needs of the wounded "prevented any supervision [of ambulances], when supervision was, more than at any other time, required."[62]

Another important feature of Letterman's plan was the assignment of vehicles to the direct control of the medical director. Two-patient ambulances, each with two privates and a driver, were allocated on the basis of three for each infantry regiment, two for each cavalry regiment, and one for each artillery battery. Two supply wagons were assigned to each division's ambulance corps. The use of those vehicles was strictly restricted to the Medical Department. Only medical personnel were permitted to accompany the sick and wounded to the rear, and only bona fide patients were allowed to ride in the ambulances.[63] A Union chaplain described Letterman as "virtually a medical dictator."[64]

Letterman implemented his plan later in the year as the Army of the Potomac fought in Virginia and then moved north into Maryland. It was only partially in place for the Battle of Antietam in September 1862, where, during twelve hours of combat, casualties from both sides rose to over 22,700. McClellan's casualties

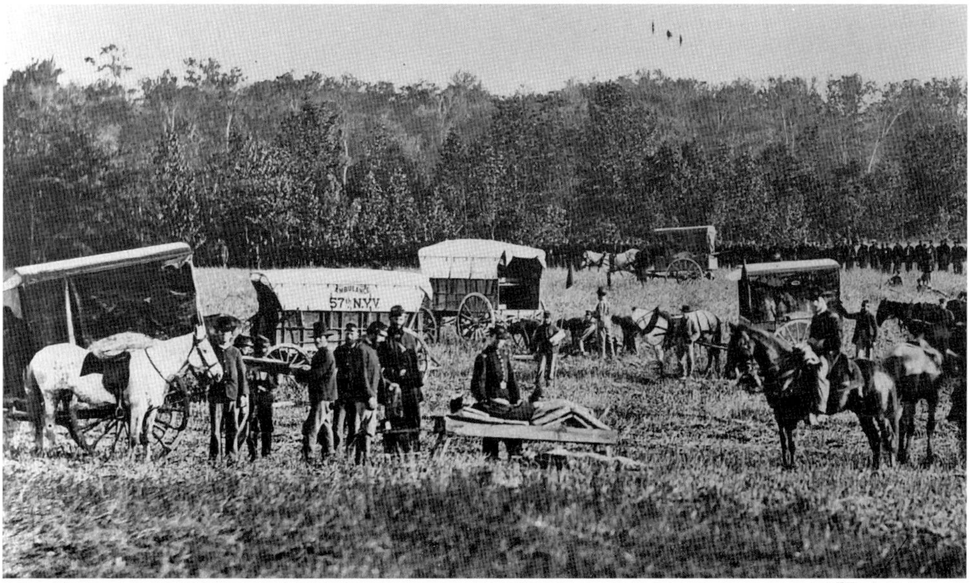

Wagons of the 57th New York's ambulance corps remove wounded from the field after the Battle of Fredericksburg.

mounted to 25 percent of the soldiers who went into action. On the Union right wing, where Letterman's plan was in place, casualties were rapidly evacuated and all wounded within the Union lines were removed during the night. Casualties on the left, where the new evacuation plan was not in place, were not removed until the following night.[65]

Full implementation of Letterman's plan occurred three months later, at Fredericksburg. There, Letterman reported that the ambulance corps had begun to evacuate the wounded after dark on 13 December and by daylight had removed all the casualties except some twenty soldiers who were within the Confederate lines. Surgeon General Hammond, visiting the Army of the Potomac, was pleased with the results;[66] even more important, commanders began to recognize the advantages of a system that reduced straggling as it saved the wounded.

General McClellan wrote that Letterman's ambulance corps decreased the number of combat soldiers pulled from the battlefield, "one of the great desiderata for our armies."[67] The Army of the Potomac continued to benefit from its unified medical support capability in battles after Antietam.[68] There were 14,193 wounded Union soldiers at Gettysburg, 1–3 July 1863, yet there were no wounded left on the battlefield within Union lines by early morning the day after the battle. Letterman reported: "I know of no battlefield from which wounded men have been so speedily and so carefully removed."[69] By the summer of 1864 the Army of the Potomac's ambulance corps numbered 800 ambulances with 66 officers and 2,600 enlisted soldiers. The medical director's central control provided the flexibility necessary to tailor the medical system to meet changing requirements. Capt. J. G. Pelton, chief of II Corps ambulances, said he could easily shift vehicles and medical soldiers throughout his corps area of operations so as to place the evacuation capability where it was most needed.[70]

Union Army units that failed to adopt Letterman's innovations continued to experience difficulty in battlefield evacuation. Surgeon Glover Perin, upon becoming medical director of the Army of the Cumberland in February 1863, found an inefficient ambulance service. He attributed this to the absence of commissioned ambulance corps officers, the lack of attendants, and the control of ambulances by the Quartermaster Department. He adopted a modified Letterman plan, but even with that in place the Army of the Cumberland left behind an estimated twenty-five hundred of its wounded at Chickamauga in September 1863.[71] Surgeon Thomas A. McParlin, then medical director of the Army of Virginia, received a copy of Letterman's plan and submitted it to his commander, Brig. Gen. John Pope, but there was not enough time to implement it before Second Manassas. McParlin believed that Pope's army would greatly benefit from an ambulance corps. "The lessons of experience should not be disregarded, especially in matters of such transcendant importance. At such a time, a well organized, regularly established ambulance corps would have been a blessing."[72]

Other armies agreed. The South was never able to field an evacuation and treatment system as sophisticated as the North's, but in Europe, French Army surgeons applauded the American innovation of placing the treatment and evacuation systems under complete medical control. As knowledge of Letterman's innovation spread, European armies proceeded to adopt his system.[73]

A by-product of these innovations was the emergence of a small cadre of junior officers who understood the problems of medical evacuation. Those ambulance corps officers were often recognized for their achievements and valor. Letterman cited Capt. J. M. Garland for outstanding service in equipping the II Corps ambulance organization and for the care and diligence with which his soldiers removed the wounded at Antietam. Surgeon Henry S. Hewitt recognized Capt. S. Windecker, 103d Ohio Volunteers, for managing the Army of the Ohio evacuation system "in the most systematic and praiseworthy manner." Windecker's leadership had enabled Hewitt to keep just one physician with each regiment, while moving the others to the field hospitals where their medical talents could be pooled.[74]

Lt. Henry Knight was cited for his courage under fire during the Union Army's disastrous assault at Fredericksburg in 1862. Capts. W. F. Drum, B. W. Baldwin, and J. G. Pelton of the Army of the Potomac won commendations for ambulance operations that were "well and gallantly performed."[75] Lt. Joseph C. Ayer, chief of the 1st Division ambulances, estimated that his unit evacuated nearly six hundred soldiers during Fredericksburg, and in 1863 he reported that his ambulances evacuated 1,157 casualties in the Battle of Gettysburg.[76] Letterman commended the ambulance corps for performing in a "commendable and efficient manner" at Gettysburg, on a day in which one ambulance corps officer and four privates were killed.[77]

On 11 March 1864, Hammond's efforts and the success of Letterman's plan, backed by petitions and lobbying efforts, resulted in congressional action that established a permanent ambulance corps. The law authorized corps commanders to detail officers and enlisted soldiers to form their ambulance organizations and provided for the examination of candidates by boards of medical officers. As one citizens' committee put it, the Army should carefully screen the officer candidates because of the special trust it placed in them, and they should "at least equal the best of the fighting-men in gallantry."[78] The War Department implemented the law in General Orders No. 106, 16 March 1864, a directive that also gave commanders the authority to create a distinctive uniform for members of the Ambulance Corps.[79]

Despite his success, Letterman had grown tired. In December 1863 he asked for relief from "18 months of arduous and eventful duty." He was reassigned as Medical Inspector of Hospitals, Department of the Susquehanna.[80] General Hammond, while successful in obtaining the Ambulance Corps legislation, had become further alienated from Secretary of War Stanton. In May 1864 he was dismissed from the service by a court-martial on charges trumped up by Stanton.[81] Letterman resigned from the service at the end of the same year. The achievements of both lived on after them.

Other Emerging Specialties

Outside the Union's Ambulance Corps, other specialists appeared during the Civil War. A remarkable example of hospital administration could be found on the Confederate side of the line. In Richmond, Sally Louisa Tompkins headed Robertson Hospital, which, staffed with Confederate Army physicians, had a mortality rate lower than any other in the city. Abuses by some private hospitals caused the Confederacy to pass a law restricting the treatment of Confederate soldiers to hospitals commanded by commissioned officers. Jefferson Davis desired to retain Tompkins' hospital, and thus Captain Tompkins became the only woman commissioned in the Confederate Army.[82]

Such specialists were needed. Administrative requirements bedeviled medical officers of both sides, a situation aggravated by the rapid expansion from a small regular army to a very large, mostly volunteer, military. "Army doctors in administrative positions apparently were quite at a loss in performing the duties incident to them."[83] They were assisted by enlisted hospital stewards, who were responsible for general administration and were superior to all other hospital noncommissioned officers, enlisted soldiers, and nurses.[84] But seldom was there the guiding hand of an officer who understood administration and was devoted to that function alone.

Pharmacy was emerging as the accepted specialty for the compounding and dispensing of drugs. Schools of pharmacy had been established in the 1820s and the American Pharmaceutical Association formed in 1852. Civilian pharmacists were employed in the larger Army hospitals in the Civil War because, unlike the French, the Americans provided no commissions for pharmacists. The *American Journal of Pharmacy* criticized the lack, but there was no movement in that direction, and the argument over commissioning pharmacists would continue well into the next century.[85]

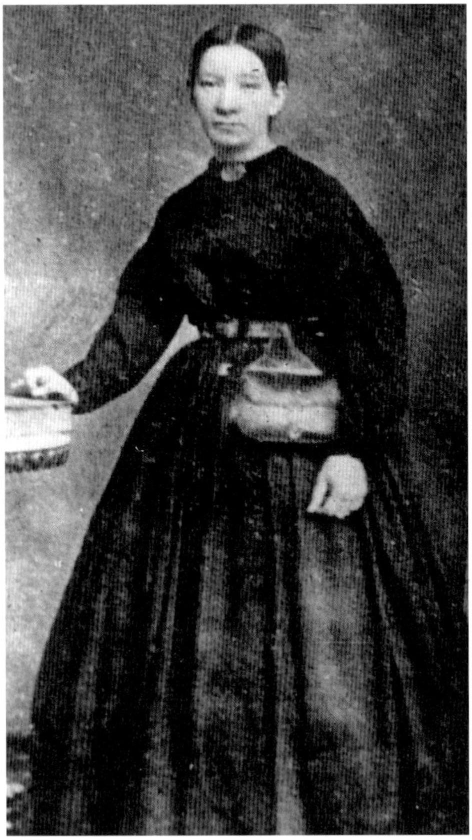

Captain Tompkins

Chiropody, performed by civilians under contract to the Army, would be incorporated into the Medical Service Corps in the next century. Isachar Zacharie, a skilled chiropodist and political opportunist, received publicity as the favored bunion cutter for Lincoln, Secretary of War Stanton, and General McClellan. Lincoln credited Zacharie as the specialist who "put me on my feet," and his fame led to calls for the creation of a chiropody corps.[86]

The need for a medical supply system operated by members of the Medical Department was a lesson learned over and over again. Supply problems generated frequent complaints, but line officers continued to relegate medical logistics to the status of "least important in the Army."[87] Letterman, as he had done with the ambulances, worked out an arrangement with the Army of the Potomac's quartermaster that gave him exclusive control of medical wagons. He said that it was very important to place this capability within the medical organization so as to make the medical system self-sustaining and largely independent.[88]

Congress improved the situation on 20 May 1862, when it authorized the Medical Department to commission U.S. Army Medical Storekeepers (USAMS), a precursor of Medical Service Corps medical logistics officers. General Hammond, while pleased with the congressional action, said the number allotted was too small. The War Department appointed a selection board, limited appointments to apothecaries or druggists, and required applicants to post a $40,000 bond before entering active duty—an extraordinary sum for the day.[89]

Hammond called the medical storekeepers "a most useful class of officers,"[90] and he expanded their duties to include medical purveying, thereby releasing physicians in those assignments to medical duties. Four of the six successful candidates were later given additional appointments as acting medical purveyors. Medical storekeepers were paid $1,750 a year, including the quarters and allowances of a first lieutenant, but no rank was assigned and by custom they were addressed variously as "captain" or "mister." Their abridged military status meant that neither they nor their families were eligible for pensions or death benefits. Congress rectified the oversight in 1867 by giving them the rank and pay of cavalry captains.[91]

Henry N. Rittenhouse, USAMS, described his position as "one of considerable magnitude." Hennell Stevens, USAMS, said accountability was "right and thorough."[92] George Taylor Beall, USAMS, was commissioned as a medical storekeeper in 1866 and assigned to the medical purveyor's office in Santa Fe, New Mexico. In 1875 he transferred to the St. Louis Medical Depot where he was responsible for purchasing over $1 million in medical supplies and equipment before his retirement in 1894.[93] The duties of Rittenhouse, Stevens, and Beall required a knowledge of pharmaceuticals, but Rittenhouse insisted that the major prerequisite was general management skills. "Scientific knowledge is not much called into play; what is required is a thorough business knowledge, a familiarity with the various customs of ordinary business transactions, sound judgment, and intimate acquaintance with the regulations, laws, orders, and circulars of the Medical Department."[94]

Overall, Civil War advances in the care of the sick and wounded had resulted less from improvements in medical science than from improved organization for medical support and the addition of new specialists to the Medical Department, such as the officers of the Ambulance Corps and the U.S. Army Medical Storekeepers. The war had seen the emergence of a genuine chain of evacuation, the appearance of large numbers of female nurses in the military hospitals, and the creation of the largest, most complex, best integrated military medical system the United States was to know until the twentieth century.

From Appomattox to Havana

The period that followed was a contradictory time for military medicine. The Medical Department, like the rest of the Army, declined in numbers. The special laws that had been passed for the prosecution of the Civil War expired when the war ended, and along with them the wartime structure of the Ambulance Corps, the general hospitals, and the hospital transports and trains disappeared. The Medical Department forfeited the progress it had made toward establishing commissioned officers in medical administrative specialties. The law that created the Ambulance Corps expired in 1866. There were two commissioned U.S. Army Medical Storekeepers in 1888, but there were none ten years later when the United States went to war with Spain.[95]

There were efforts to counter those unfortunate events. In 1885 the surgeon general, Brig. Gen. Robert Murray, said the department had plans for the reestablishment of an ambulance system in the event of war. General Murray also argued that the department needed soldiers trained to provide medical care and treatment in the hospitals, and his efforts led to the creation of an enlisted hospital corps in 1887. Those medical soldiers were charged with performing "all necessary hospital services in garrison, camp, or field."[96] Some militia organizations began to experiment with dedicated medical units that would continue to exist during peacetime as well as during wars. Massachusetts established an ambulance corps for its militia in 1885, but without the provision of ambulance corps officers.[97]

Above all, the period that followed the Civil War was the time when the revolution began that transformed medicine into a science. The germ theory of disease was gradually worked out by European researchers and slowly (and in some cases reluctantly) adopted by American doctors. Army medical officers provided some leadership in the new science, notably Brig. Gen. George Miller Sternberg, who served as surgeon general from 1893 to 1902.[98] Maj. Walter Reed studied the new science and began training others at the Army Medical School, established in 1893.[99] Treatment modalities had also improved. The clinical thermometer, hypodermic syringe, and ophthalmoscope were in common use, as was the "Roentgen Ray," the x-ray, which permitted noninvasive viewing within the body. This new technology was used by the Medical Department in Cuba. Both anesthesia and aseptic surgery were accepted practices, and orthopedic surgery beyond amputation was possible.

The war against Spain in 1898 demonstrated the difficulties facing a fledgling world power as it quickly raised and moved ground forces in its first overseas deployment. Public support for Cuban independence and growing sentiment against Spanish influence in the Western Hemisphere turned to passion when the U.S. battleship *Maine* sank at anchor in Havana harbor on 15 February 1898. The United States declared war on the twenty-fifth, and the "splendid little war" was on. A hastily assembled expeditionary force arrived off Santiago, Cuba, on 21 June with seventy-one medical officers and eighty-nine reporters, "the former to experience many troubles, the latter to cause many."[100] Santiago surrendered on 17 July, and Spain signed the Treaty of Paris in December, withdrawing from Cuba and ceding Guam, Puerto Rico, and the Philippines to the United States.

The mobilization was anything but efficient, but national policy dictated speed, and that policy was effective even though the war was over before the logistic support was fully organized. The weaknesses included medical support, and, as Major Reed put it, the Medical Department got a "black eye."[101]

After declaring war with Spain, Congress acted to increase the Regular Army and to create a volunteer force, and the Army grew from 28,000 to nearly 275,000 personnel. Despite this dramatic growth, Congress did not increase the hospital corps, which numbered 791.[102] General Sternberg, unable to expand the corps, did obtain authority to transfer soldiers from the line. But, as one chief surgeon complained, "they palmed off on the Medical Department the most undesirable element in the companies, men whom the captains wanted to get rid of."[103] On the brighter side, hospital corps volunteers included medical students, pharmacists, and recent medical school graduates, an infusion of talent embraced as a welcome asset.[104]

Lessons From the War With Spain

The war with Spain brought into sharper focus some of America's inadequacies in providing medical support to its military forces, part of the larger difficulty in projecting military power. The irony of organizational problems in the U.S. military at a time when the nation prided itself on its talent for business was not lost on those who sought to learn from the conflict. It moved Theodore Roosevelt to reflect that "it was curious that when war came we should have broken down precisely on the business and administrative side, while the fighting edge of the

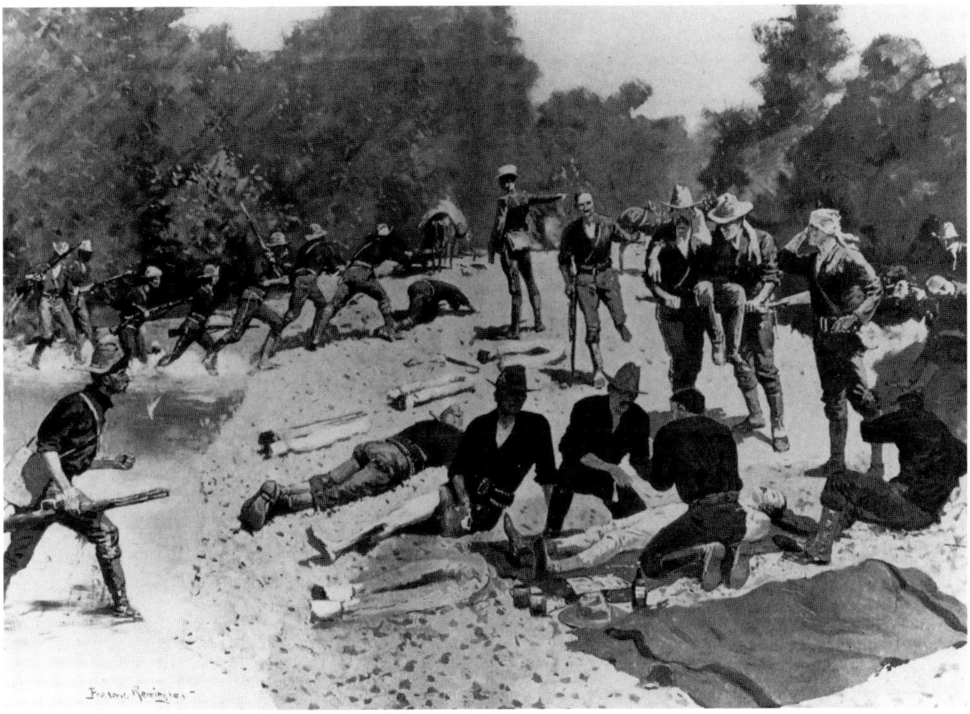

Frederic Remington's drawing, Field Hospital at the "Bloody Ford" of San Juan Creek

troops left little to be desired."[105] In most cases, the cure for the Medical Department's deficiencies required the addition of commissioned officers in administrative and scientific specialties necessary for a modernized military force.

The Medical Department's problems were thrashed out by a presidential panel. Called the Dodge Commission for its head, Grenville M. Dodge, it began hearings in September 1898. President William McKinley asked the panel to investigate charges of "criminal neglect of the soldiers in camp and field and hospital and in transports."[106]

Medical logistics was a major source of complaint. Theodore Roosevelt, who would parlay his wartime exploits into the governorship of New York, testified that medical supplies were insufficient at the front. There had been no cots for the wounded and no ambulances at San Juan Hill. He later wrote that "the condition of the wounded in the big field hospitals in the rear was so horrible, from the lack of attendants as well as of medicine, that we kept all the men we possibly could at the front."[107] One field hospital in Cuba consisted of little more than a few tents without cots, mattresses, or clothing for the patients. When Clara Barton of the American Red Cross visited the hospital at Siboney, she found wounded lying on the ground. Brig. Gen. William R. Shafter, who complained that the surgeon general "does not seem to appreciate the situation," had halted because his force could no longer handle the casualties.[108] Stateside camps also had problems. Col.

William A. Pew, Jr., commander of the 8th Massachusetts Infantry at Chickamauga Park, Georgia, pointed out that his surgeon had requisitioned drugs but never received any.[109]

General Sternberg testified that shipping of medical supplies and equipment to Cuba had been outside the Medical Department's control. Much was late and much was lost, including an entire 200-bed hospital. Seventeen ambulances had been loaded at Tampa for Shafter's corps; three landed in Cuba. Other medical vehicles, supplies, equipment, and even animals loaded at Tampa were never seen again. The ambulance service, such as it existed, had been decimated by an ineffectual supply system.[110]

In some cases medical logistics difficulties had been ameliorated by detailing line officers to serve as quartermasters and commissary officers for medical units. But problems remained. At the heart of the situation was the structural weakness of the Medical Department in its lack of a dedicated medical logistics organization and specially trained officers, and this deficiency had inevitably led to shortages in needed supplies and equipment where they were needed most. The surgeon general's lack of executive power underlay the failures, a point made by one of General Sternberg's defenders. "Our experience has taught us in a most forcible way that the Medical Department should have charge of everything pertaining to the sick and wounded."[111]

Closely related to the lack of medical logistics officers was the absence of officers dedicated to medical administration, a subject that received attention by the Dodge Commission. Certainly the unfamiliarity of military physicians with Army procedures had complicated matters, but the administrative duties expected of physicians were counterproductive. Physicians assigned to field hospitals were saddled with numerous tasks ranging from the maintenance of patient records to the supervision of food service operations. Physicians commanded ambulance units because the Medical Department had lost its ambulance corps officers.[112]

Sternberg recommended simplification of administrative procedures so that physicians could concentrate on their professional duties, but the problem went further than that. Witnesses repeatedly observed that many medical officers were good physicians but incompetent administrators. The situation had become so muddled in the II Corps that the chief surgeon, frustrated with the volunteer medical officers, had taken direct action in selecting commanders of the hospital enlisted detachments.

> The inability of medical officers to grasp the company organization and its papers and lack of mental force or training to control the men led finally to my requesting authority to place one of the officers of the line, who are allowed as quartermasters in the division hospitals, in command of the Hospital Corps companies, and gradually matters became systematized.[113]

That solution went to the heart of the matter by attempting to include in the structure of medical units officers dedicated to specific administrative functions.

The need for management expertise was also evident in the administration of Army hospitals. The commander of the hospital at Camp Wikoff, a rest camp hurriedly constructed at Montauk Point, Long Island, for soldiers returning from

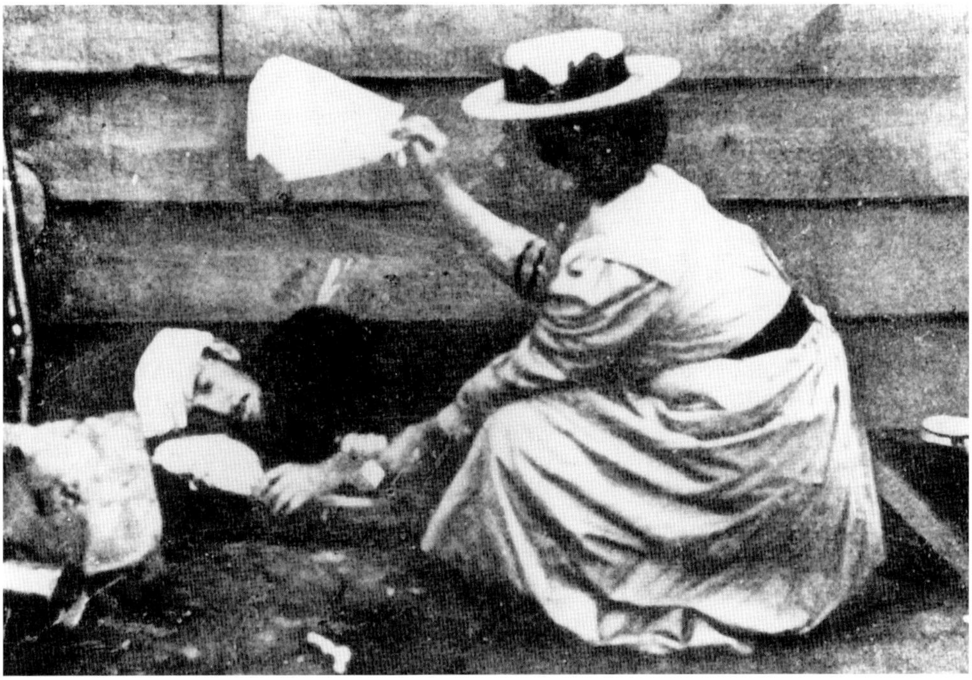

Red Cross nurse helps a sick soldier at the railroad station at Camp Wikoff, Montauk Point, New York.

Cuba, was battered by his experience. He said one of the lessons he learned was the need for "experienced executive men" on the hospital staff.[114] Maj. Jefferson R. Kean, commander of the 2d Division hospital at Camp Cuba Libre, Florida, believed that the lack of hospital administrative staff was the principal deficiency during the war. He suggested two administrative officers for hospitals under 300 beds, three for those over that size: "Without such staff assistance it is impossible for the commanding officer of a large hospital to keep his property and money secure, and, what is even more important, to carefully supervise the medical administration and see to it that the patients are properly cared for."[115]

Another witness proposed two surgeons for every headquarters, one for administrative duties, the other for clinical responsibilities. More than one military surgeon suggested that since good physicians were not necessarily good administrators, the administrative part of the work could and should be handled by a line officer detailed for that purpose. Brig. Gen. Joseph P. Sanger, a former inspector general of the Army and a division commander in Cuba, included the duty of hospital commander in that category.[116]

General Sternberg also came under fire for shortcomings in preventive medicine and sanitation. Line commanders were responsible for the state of sanitation in their units, while the surgeon general was responsible for the setting of standards and policy. Sternberg had acted upon his responsibilities by issuing a circular directing medical officers to undertake a series of sanitation measures, as well as "buck-up" circulars when the first directive failed to make a dent in the ubiquitous sanitation problems. Unfortunately, a small regular army might be expected to respond to directives, but not so with a hastily formed army of volunteer officers and recently enlisted conscripts, and Army camps remained smelly pestholes. Sternberg was a distinguished scientist with an international reputation as a bacteriologist.[117] Nevertheless, preventive medicine measures were ignored while he "rested on the power of his circular."[118]

The results were unfortunate: 932 soldiers were killed in action or died from wounds, yet 5,438 died of disease. In some cases, as with typhoid, the mechanics of transmission were known; in others, such as yellow fever and malaria, they were not. In any event, disease took its toll of lives and affected national strategy. Fear of disease, particularly yellow fever, was intense. A round-robin letter, signed by all but one of Shafter's commanders after the fall of Cuba, was sent to President McKinley demanding the withdrawal of American forces before yellow fever killed them.[119] Part of the remedy lay with better application of existing preventive medicine doctrine. However, part of the remedy resided in medical advances that would increasingly provide medical officers with effective tools.

Emerging Themes

Some basic factors leading toward the creation of the Medical Service Corps had emerged by the late nineteenth century. One was the impact of outside influences upon the Medical Department. Examples included the influence of the U.S. Sanitary Commission during the Civil War, the Dodge Commission after the war with Spain, and the national press during both emergencies. Problems that the Medical Department could avoid addressing in peacetime it inevitably had to confront in war, when shortcomings in military medical support were discovered by families of casualties and the politicians who represented them. The formation of a casualty evacuation doctrine and a corps of ambulance officers was catalyzed by such outside intervention.

At the same time the evolution of the Army itself repeatedly demonstrated the need for new officer administrative specialties, particularly in medical logistics, casualty evacuation, and—for lack of a better word—paperwork. The creation of the Ambulance Corps, the institution of U.S. Army Medical Storekeepers, the detailing of line officers to medical units, and the desire for "executive men" in hospitals were all evidence of this movement. All of these needs resurfaced in 1916 during the Punitive Expedition in Mexico, led by General John J. Pershing. The surgeon of the Southern Department reported that administrative duties were a burden for his physicians, especially those called up from the National Guard "to whom the paperwork of the Medical Department is utterly unfamiliar."[120] But Medical Department administrative functions would continue to be performed by physicians as long as other officers were unavailable.

Technology and doctrine advanced with the introduction of ground ambulance units into the force structure. The Medical Department bought its first motor ambulance, a White Steamer, in 1906. In 1911 the department established an organization for an ambulance company of 5 medical officers, 9 noncommis-

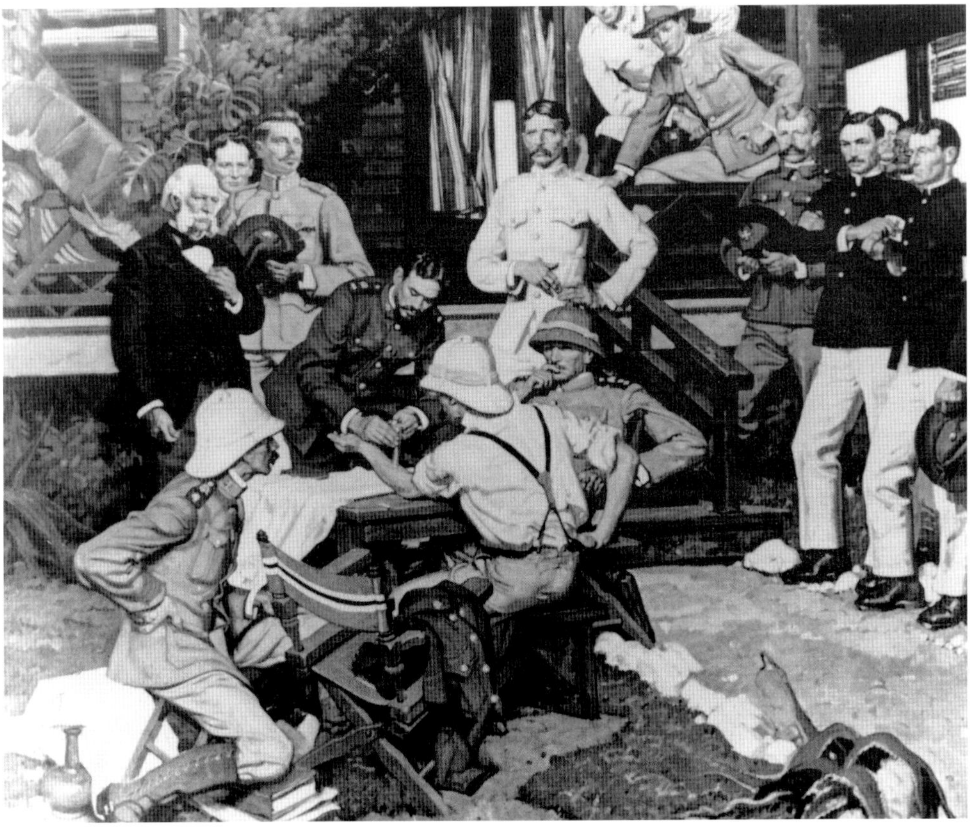

Dean Cornwell's painting, Conquerors of Yellow Fever

sioned officers, and 69 privates. Each ambulance company had the capability of establishing a dressing station, providing ambulance support with twelve ambulances, and attaching litter squads and runners to battalion aid stations. Motorized ambulances were used for the first time in 1916 during the Mexican Punitive Expedition, and Pershing's surgeon recommended replacing animal-drawn ambulances with motorized vehicles.[121]

As the Army changed, grew, and professionalized, so did medicine, creating a need for experts in new scientific specialties. During the early 1900s American medicine continued to expand its horizons. Synthetic drugs became a possibility, and in 1910 Paul Ehrlich developed an arsenic compound, salvarsan, to combat syphilis. Major orthopedic surgery and increasingly sophisticated laboratory tests were more widely available. X-ray diagnosis, sanitation, preventive medicine, and the general use of vaccines enhanced military medical capabilities while creating the need for new expertise.[122] And a future surgeon general, Col. William M. Gorgas, learned to work with an expanded medical team during this period.

During the war with Spain the country had witnessed the devastating impact of disease upon its Army, especially the effects of yellow fever, typhoid, and

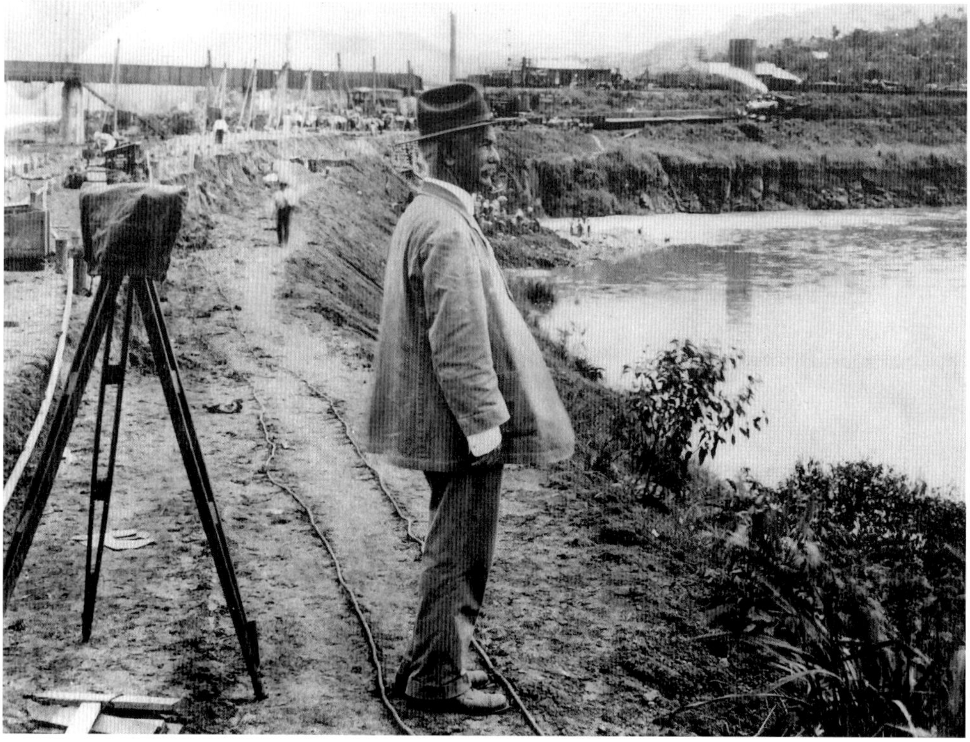

Colonel Gorgas in Panama during construction of the canal

malaria. The result was to add impetus to scientific investigations into diseases of military significance. General Sternberg supported research after the war, sponsoring Maj. Walter Reed's work in Cuba, which identified the method of yellow fever transmission. Convincing proof of the mosquito's role in the spread of yellow fever and malaria meant that those diseases could be prevented by controlling the insects.

Building on those findings, William Gorgas, then a major, waged a strenuous preventive medicine campaign beginning in 1898 in Havana and continued in pioneering work during construction of the Panama Canal. France's futile attempt to build a transisthmian canal had made Panama synonymous with pestilence and disease. Indeed, fear of yellow fever was so intense that arriving Americans sometimes brought their own coffins. Gorgas and his wife, Marie, rendered immune because of earlier bouts with the disease, arrived in Panama in the summer of 1904.[123] By 1906 his medical team had eliminated yellow fever there by waging war on the *Stegomyia* mosquito and had greatly reduced malaria by attacking the *Anopheles*. Gorgas estimated that his team saved over seventy-one thousand lives in the course of the canal project, a figure he based on the mortality rates from the French experience.[124]

An important member of Gorgas' team in Cuba and Panama was Joseph L. LePrince, a sanitary engineer who had trained at Columbia University. LePrince,

Gorgas' assistant in Havana beginning in 1900 and chief sanitary inspector of the Isthmian Canal Commission from 1904 to 1914, was regarded by Marie Gorgas as one of her husband's most effective aides. Another member of Gorgas' team in Panama was his son-in-law, William D. Wrightson, a sanitary engineer who had served on a team in 1916 headed by Gorgas that traveled throughout Central and South America on behalf of the International Health Board.[125] Gorgas' experience in capitalizing on the talents of LePrince and Wrightson exemplified a new reliance on nonphysician medical scientists.[126]

The Medical Department's experience through the end of the nineteenth century thus pointed to the need for new doctrine, organization, equipment, and personnel. Fortunately, many of the lessons learned were acted upon during the period leading up to World War I. The department improved its doctrine and training, prepared new supply tables, distributed improved field equipment, and in 1908 established a Medical Reserve Corps for physicians, a forerunner of the Army Reserve.[127] It also set the stage for important steps in the evolution of the Medical Service Corps.

Notes

[1] Craigie: William O. Owen, *The Medical Department of the United States Army: Legislative and Administrative History During the Period of the Revolution (1776–1786)* (New York: Paul Hoeber, 1920), pp. 19, 24, hereafter cited as Owen, *Medical Department*; Lyman F. Kebler, "Andrew Craigie, the First Apothecary General of the United States," *Journal of the American Pharmaceutical Association* 17 (January 1928): 63, 65. Apothecary: Lines were not firmly drawn in colonial times. The English pattern was that physicians were a learned elite who did no work with their hands. Surgeons were a lower order and practiced a craft. Apothecaries, one of whom was the English poet John Keats, compounded and dispensed drugs and also saw and treated patients. John Morgan, *A Discourse upon the Institution of Medical Schools in America* (Philadelphia: William Bradford, 1765), pp. iii, v; Paul Starr, *The Social Transformation of American Medicine* (New York: Basic Books, 1982), pp. 37–40; Joseph M. Toner, *Contributions to the Annals of Medical Progress and Medical Education in the United States Before and During the War of Independence* (Washington, D.C.: Government Printing Office, 1874), pp. 58, 105–06; Herbert Clarke, *The Apothecary in Eighteenth Century Williamsburg* (Williamsburg, Va.: Colonial Williamsburg Foundation, 1965), pp. 4, 5, 7, hereafter cited as Clarke, *Williamsburg Apothecary*; Edward Kremers and George Urdang, *History of Pharmacy*, 3d ed. (Philadelphia: J.B. Lippincott, 1963), pp. 145–49; Owen, *Medical Department*, p. 140; Philip Cash, *Medical Men at the Siege of Boston* (Philadelphia: American Philosophical Society, 1973), p. 3.

[2] Department: Owen, *Medical Department*, pp. 28–30, 32; Harvey E. Brown, *The Medical Department of the United States Army from 1775–1873* (Washington, D.C.: Surgeon General's Office, 1873), pp. 6–7, 10.

[3] AMSUS award: "Annual Awards," *Military Medicine* 150 (December 1985): 708. The award was established in 1959. AMSUS, the Society of the Federal Health Agencies, was founded in 1891 and incorporated by Congress in 1903.

[4] Medical capability: M.A. Reasoner, "The Development of the Medical Supply Service," *Military Surgeon* 63 (July 1928): 4–8, a good summary of medical progress, hereafter cited as Reasoner, "Development of Medical Supply"; Mary C. Gillett, *The Army Medical Department, 1775–1818* (Washington, D.C.: U.S. Army Center of Military History, 1981), pp. 129–49; Richard H. Shryock, *Medicine and Society in America, 1660–1860* (New York: New York University Press, 1960), p. 52.

[5] Medical supply: Cash, *Medical Men at the Siege of Boston*, p. 134; George B. Griffenhagen, "Drug Supplies in the American Revolution," *U.S. National Museum Bulletin* 225 (1961, Contributions from the Museum of Science and Technology, Paper 16), pp. 110–15, 129–30. Reorganization: Owen, *Medical Department*, pp. 12, 59–60. Smith: Brown, *Medical Department*, p. 24. Quoted words: Law of 7–8 April 1777, cited in Gillett, *Army Medical Department*, p. 201. First formulary: William Brown, M.D., is credited as the author of the *Lititz Pharmacopoeia*, the first edition of which was printed on 12 March 1778. Edward Kremers, "The Lititz Pharmacopoeia," *Badger Pharmacist* (June–December 1938): 5–6.

[6] Quoted words: Reasoner, "Development of Medical Supply," p. 12.Wilkinson: Gillett, *Army Medical Department*, pp. 140–42; Russell F. Weigley, *History of the United States Army* (New York: Macmillan, 1967), p. 107, 113–14; David A. Clary and Joseph W.A. Whitehorne, *The Inspectors General of the United States Army, 1777–1903* (Washington, D.C.: Office of the Inspector General and Center of Military History, U.S. Army, 1987), pp. 86–88. Wilkinson rented swampland as a campsite for his army.

[7] Stewards: Edward Cutbush, *Observations on the Means of Preserving the Health of Soldiers and Sailors and on the Duties of the Medical Department of the Army and the Navy*, including "Some Remarks on Hospitals and Their Internal Arrangement," pp. 160–210 (Philadelphia: Thomas Dobson, 1808), pp. 198–201. Some observers cite Florence Nightingale's *Notes on Hospitals* (London: John W. Parker & Sons, 1859) as the first manual; others point to Joseph J. Woodward's *The Hospital Steward's Manual* (Philadelphia: J.B. Lippincott, 1862).

[8] Quoted words: Cutbush, *Observations*, p. 208.

[9] Quoted words: Ibid., p. 166.

[10] Rebuilding: Ibid., pp. 80–81; Gillett, *Army Medical Department*, pp. 129–49.

[11] War of 1812: See Weigley, *History of the United States Army*, pp. 117–33. It ended with the Treaty of Ghent, signed in Belgium on Christmas Eve, 1814.

[12] Need for administrative support: James Mann, *Medical Sketches of the Campaigns of 1812, 1813, and 1814* (Dedham, Mass.: H. Mann and Co., 1816), p. vi.

[13] Failures: Ibid., pp. 120, 257, 259.

[14] Quoted words: Cited in Reasoner, "Development of Medical Supply," p. 12.

[15] Lovell: Brown, *Medical Department*, pp. 107–08; *U.S. War Department, Surgeon General's Office, Annual Report of the Surgeon General*, 1 May 1819, hereafter cited as *SG Report*, followed by date and page, when given.

[16] Apothecary general: Brown, *Medical Department*, p. 112; *SG Report*, 1 May 1819, p. 22. Quoted words: *SG Report*, 1 November 1819, p. 16.

[17] Apothecary general: Congress abolished the Medical Department apothecary general and assistant apothecary general positions in 1820. Brown, *Medical Department*, p. 145.

[18] Larrey: In time the vehicle used for moving patients became known as the ambulance, but in the beginning "ambulance" meant the entire evacuation and treatment unit. See: Dominique Jean Larrey, *Memoirs of Military Surgery and Campaigns of the French Army*, trans. Richard W. Hall (Baltimore: Joseph Cushing, 1814), pp. v–ix, 28–29, 78, 223–24; Leon Legouest, *Chirurgie D'Armee* (Paris: J.B. Bailliere, 1863), p. 984; M. Boudin, *Systeme des Ambulances des Armees Francais et Anglais* (Paris: J.B. Bailliere, 1855), p. 5; Julie M. DiGioia et al., "Baron Larrey: Modern Military Surgeon," *American Surgeon* 49 (May 1983): 226–30; Lyman A. Brewer, "Baron Dominique Jean Larrey (1766–1842)," *Journal of Thoracic and Cardiovascular Surgery* 92 (December 1986): 1096–97; Thomas Longmore, *A Manual of Ambulance Transport*, ed. William A. Morris (London: Harrison and Sons, 1893), pp. 2, 7–10, 21–26, 39; Unpublished paper, James Warren Wengert, M.D., "The Military Ambulance," September 1981, in Office of the Chief, Medical Service Corps, Office of the Surgeon General (DASG-MS); Mann, *Medical Sketches*, p. 247; Cutbush, *Observations*, p. 164; Gillett, *Army Medical Department*, pp. 85–87.

[19] French doctrine: Larrey, *Memoirs of Military Surgery*, p. 223.

[20] Doctrinal weakness: Legouest, *Chirurgie D'Armee*, p. 984; Bennett A. Clements, "Memoir of Jonathan Letterman, M.D.," *Journal of the Military Service Institution* 4 (September 1883): 5–6. Solferino: The weaknesses inherent to the incomplete system caused a debacle at Solferino, Italy, in June 1859. The suffering so distressed a Swiss banker, Henry Dunant, that he organized the Geneva Conventions for the sick and wounded and later formed the Red Cross. J. Henry Dunant, *A Memory of Solferino*, trans. District of Columbia Chapter of the American Red Cross (published 1862 as *Un Souvenir de Solferino*; reprinted Washington, D.C.: American Red Cross, 1939), pp. 39–46; Carol Z. Rothkopp, *Jean Henri Dunant* (New York: Franklin Watts, 1969), pp. 6, 40–48.

[21] Crimean War: Louis C. Duncan, "The Comparative Mortality of Disease and Battle Casualties in the Historic Wars of the World" (hereafter cited as Duncan, "Comparative Mortality"), in Duncan, *The Medical Department of the United States Army in the Civil War*, one volume printed in sections (Washington, D.C.: Office of the Surgeon General, 1910), pp. 25–26, volume hereafter cited as Duncan, *Medical Department in the Civil War*. England and France fought with Turkey and Sardinia against Russia, mostly on the Russian Crimea peninsula, to successfully block Russian designs on Turkish territories.

[22] Evacuation: Louis Baudens, *On Military and Camp Hospitals and the Health of Troops in the Field*, trans. Franklin B. Hough (New York: Baillaire Brothers, 1862), p. 182; Edward Bruce Hamley, *The War in the Crimea* (reprint, Westport, Conn.: Greenwood Press, 1971), pp. 167–73, 179. Quoted words: Hamley, p. 173.

[23] Nightingale: Zachary Cope, *Florence Nightingale and the Doctors* (Philadelphia: J.B. Lippincott, 1958), pp. 14–16, 61–62, 99.

[24] Quoted words: Florence Nightingale, *Notes on Matters Affecting the Health, Efficiency and Hospital Administration of the British Army* (London: Harrison and Sons, 1858), p. 220.

[25] Staff: Ibid., pp. 220–28, 288.

[26] Quoted words: Ibid., p. 107.

[27] Lawson: Mary C. Gillett, "Thomas Lawson, Second Surgeon General of the U.S. Army: A Character Sketch," *Prologue* 14 (Spring 1982): 23–24.

[28] Quoted words: *SG Report*, 1855, p. 13.

[29] Stewards: War Department, *Regulations for the Medical Department of the Army* (1861; reprint Knoxville, Tenn.: Bohemian Brigade Bookshop, 1989), pp. 10, 16, hereafter cited as *Regulations for the Medical Department.*

[30] Quoted words: Ibid., p. 5.

[31] War with Mexico: Weigley, *History of the United States Army*, pp. 173–96; Richard H. Coolidge, *Statistical Report on the Sickness and Mortality in the Army of the United States, January, 1839, to January, 1855* (Washington, D.C.: A.O.P. Nicholson, 1856), pp. 606, 610; Leonard Wood, *Our Military History, Its Facts and Fallacies* (Chicago: Reilly and Britton Co., 1916), p. 147.

[32] Military medicine: Louis C. Duncan, "A Medical History of General Zachary Taylor's Army of Occupation in Texas and Mexico, 1845–47," *Military Surgeon* 48 (1921): 79; Duncan, *Medical Department in the Civil War*, pt. 6, p. 37; Duncan, "Medical History of General Scott's Campaign to the City of Mexico in 1847," *Military Surgeon* 47 (1920): 604–07; Fielding H. Garrison, *Notes on the History of Military Medicine* (Washington, D.C.: Association of Military Surgeons of the United States, 1922), p. 170; J. Antonio Aldrete, "The First Administration of Anesthesia in Military Surgery: On Occasion of the Mexican-American War," *Anesthesiology* 61 (November 1984): 585.

[33] Indian Wars: *Regulations for the Medical Department*, pp. 17, 18.

[34] Planning efforts: U.S. War Department, Surgeon General's Office, *The Medical and Surgical History of the War of the Rebellion*, 2 vols., vol. 2, 2d ed., *Surgical History* (Washington, D.C.: Government Printing Office, 1883), p. 933, series hereafter cited as War Department, *Medical and Surgical History*; Brown, *Medical Department*, p. 212. Ambulances: Arnold G. Fisch, Jr., and Robert K. Wright, Jr., *The Story of the Noncommissioned Officer Corps: The Backbone of the Army* (Washington, D.C.: U.S. Army Center of Military History, 1989), p. 76, hereafter cited as Fisch and Wright, *Noncommissioned Officer Corps.*

[35] Medical progress: Shryock, *Medicine and Society*, p. 150.

[36] Quoted words: Horace H. Cunningham, *Doctors in Gray: The Confederate Medical Service* (Baton Rouge: Louisiana State University, 1958), p. 111. Also see George W. Adams, *Doctors in Blue: The Medical History of the Union Army in the Civil War* (New York: H. Schuman, 1952), p. 112; William M. Straight, "Medical Logistics of the Confederate Army," *Bulletin of the University of Miami School of Medicine* 15 (Spring 1961): 60. Blue mass: Also called mercury mass and blue pills, a combination of several ingredients, of which approximately 35 percent was mercury. If the illness didn't kill you the cure would.

[37] Quoted words: Silas Weir Mitchell, *The Medical Department in the Civil War* (Chicago: American Medical Association, 1914), p. 11, hereafter cited as Mitchell, *The Medical Department.*

[38] Hospitals: For an eyewitness account see Rice Bull, *Soldiering: The Civil War Diary of Rice C. Bull, 123rd New York Volunteer Infantry*, ed. K. Jack Bauer (Novato, Calif.: Presidio Press, 1977), pp. 73–74.

[39] Medical Department: Speech, Henry W. Bellows, President, U.S. Sanitary Commission, at the Academy of Music, Philadelphia, 24 Feb 1863 (Philadelphia: C. Sherman, Son, 1863), pp. 8–9, in archives of the American Hospital Association, Chicago, Ill., hereafter cited as Bellows, 1863 Speech; Mitchell, *The Medical Department*, p. 5; *SG Report*, 1865, p. 3.

[40] Sanitary Commission: William Q. Maxwell, *Lincoln's Fifth Wheel* (New York: Longmans, Green, 1956), pp. 1–2; Charles J. Stille, *History of the United States Sanitary Commission* (Philadelphia: J.B. Lippincott, 1866), pp. 166, 551; Bellows, 1863 speech. The Sanitary Commission's investigators included John W. Draper, professor of chemistry; Edward Jarvis, statistician; and H.A. Johnson, professor of physiology and histology. For an insider's description of the commission's activities, including the role of women, see Katharine Prescott Wormeley, *The United States Sanitary Commission: A Sketch of Its Purposes and Work* (Boston: Little, Brown, 1863). "Never before in the history of the world have women had such an opportunity to use themselves for great purpose" (ibid., p. 41).

[41] Commission influence: Stille, *Sanitary Commission*, p. 48; Maxwell, *Lincoln's Fifth Wheel*, p. 94. Finley's dismissal: Maxwell, *Lincoln's Fifth Wheel*, p. 118; James M. Phalen, *Chiefs of the Medical Department* (Carlisle Barracks, Pa.: Medical Field Service School, 1940), p. 40; A. Howard Meneely, *The War Department, 1861* (New York: Columbia University Press, 1928), pp. 227, 355. Frederick Law Olmsted, the Sanitary Commission's outspoken secretary general, called Finley "a self-satisfied, supercilious, bigoted block-head" (Meneely, *The War Department*, p. 227).

[42] West: Jacob G. Forman, *The Western Sanitary Commission* (St. Louis: R.P. Studley, 1864), pp. 16–17.

[43] Congress: "Management of Government Hospitals," Francis P. Blair and John C. Rives, eds., *Congressional Globe* (Washington, D.C.: Blair and Rives, 1862), 37th Cong., 2d sess., 30 Jan 1862, pp. 557–59; quoted words, p. 557. The *Globe* was the predecessor to the *Congressional Record.* Lawson: Phalen, *Chiefs of the Medical Department*, p. 36.

[44] Quoted words: Louisa May Alcott, *Hospital Sketches* (New York: Saganore Press, 1863), pp. 16, 57.

[45] "Terrible": Bull, *Soldiering*, p. 25. See his account of nursing a fellow soldier, pp. 23–25.

[46] Quoted words: Allan Nevins and Milton H. Thomas, eds., *The Diary of George Templeton Strong*, 4 vols. (New York: Macmillan, 1952), 3: 218.

[47] Quoted words: Duncan, *Medical Department in the Civil War*, pt. 1, p. 6.

[48] First Bull Run: Maxwell, *Lincoln's Fifth Wheel*, p. 167; Duncan, *Medical Department in the Civil War*, pt. 3, pp. 43, 54. See also Stewart Brooks, *Civil War Medicine* (Springfield, Ill.: Charles C. Thomas, 1966), p. 13.

[49] Quoted words: War Department, *Medical and Surgical History*, app., pt. 1, vol. 1, p. 117.

[50] Brinton's report: Ibid., p. 19.

[51] Evacuation: See Clements, "Memoir of Jonathan Letterman," pp. 5–6; War Department, *Medical and Surgical History*, app., pt. 1, vol. 1, p. 23.Quoted words: J. Julian Chisholm, *A Manual of Military Surgery for the Use of Surgeons in the Confederate Army* (Richmond: West and Johnston, 1861), p. 92, hereafter cited as Chisholm, *Confederate Manual.*

[52] Confederate doctrine: Cunningham, *Doctors in Gray*, pp. 27–28; Chisholm, *Confederate Manual*, pp. 92–93, 438–40, 443–47; Alvin R. Sunseri, "The Organization and Administration of the Medical Department of the Confederate Army of Tennessee," *Journal of the Tennessee State Medical Association* 53 (April 1960): 168, hereafter cited as Sunseri, "Confederate Army of Tennessee." Also see Frank R. Freeman, "Administration of the Medical Department of the Confederate States Army, 1861–5," *Southern Medical Journal* 80 (May 1987): 637. Quoted words: Chisholm, *Confederate Manual*, pp. 92–93. System: For a wounded Union prisoner's account of the Confederate medical support system see Bull, *Soldiering*, pp. 57–82.

[53] Proposals: War Department, *Medical and Surgical History*, app., pt. 1, vol. 1, p. 50, and pt. 3, vol. 2, p. 932; Stille, *Sanitary Commission*, p. 103.

[54] Tripler's plan: War Department, *Medical and Surgical History*, app., pt. 1, vol. 1, p. 59.

[55] Doctrine: Duncan, *Medical Department in the Civil War*, pt. 2, p. 21; John H. Brinton, *Personal Memoirs of John H. Brinton* (New York: Neale Publishing Co., 1914), pp. 124–25. Quoted words: Ibid., p. 27.

[56] Hammond: Phalen, *Chiefs of the Medical Department*, pp. 42–46; Maxwell, *Lincoln's Fifth Wheel*, pp. 169, 194; Louis C. Duncan, "The Strange Case of Surgeon General Hammond," *Military Surgeon* 64 (January 1929): 102, 104, hereafter cited as Duncan, "Surgeon General Hammond." Stanton was bitter: "I'm not used to being beaten, and don't like it" (quoted in Nevins and Thomas, eds., *Diary of George Strong*, 3: 314).

[57] Hammond's pleas: Reprints of correspondence, Stanton to Hammond, 21 Aug and 7 Sep 1862, and Stanton to McClellan, 25 Oct 1862, in "Notes on the Recent Civil War," *Historical Magazine* (April 1867): 231–32; Maxwell, *Lincoln's Fifth Wheel*, p. 194; Duncan, "Surgeon General Hammond," p. 110; War Department, *Medical and Surgical History*, app., pt. 3, vol. 2, pp. 933–34. After the war was over, the official Medical Department history concluded that "notwithstanding the opinion of General H.W. Halleck, no panics or stampedes were reported as having been caused by the presence of non-combatants of the Ambulance Corps" (ibid., p. 943).

[58] Hammond persists: *SG Report*, 10 Nov 1862. Also see Henry I. Bowditch, *A Brief Plea for an Ambulance System*, pamphlet (Boston: Ticknor and Fields, 1863), p. 25.

[59] Letterman: James M. Phalen, "The Life of Jonathan Letterman," *Military Surgeon* 84 (January 1939): 62; Clements, "Memoir of Jonathan Letterman," pp. 2–4. Quoted words: U.S. Congress, House, *Report of George B. McClellan, Army of the Potomac*, H. Exec. Doc. 15, 38th Cong., 1st sess., 22 Dec 1863, p. 26.

[60] Quoted words: George B. McClellan, *McClellan's Own Story* (New York: Charles L. Webster, 1887), p. 127, hereafter cited as McClellan, *Own Story.*

[61] Letterman's plan: Later amended and reissued as War Department General Orders (WDGO) 85, 24 Aug 1863. War Department, *Medical and Surgical History*, app., pt. 3, vol. 2, pp. 933, 938–41; Jonathan Letterman, *Medical Recollections of the Army of the Potomac* (New York: D. Appleton, 1866), p. 20; McClellan, *Own Story*, p. 127; Duncan, *Medical Department in the Civil War*, pt. 4, p. 22; Edward Lymon Munson, *The Principles of Sanitary Tactics; A Handbook on the Use of Medical Department Detachments and Organizations in Campaign* (Menasha, Wisc.: Press of Bonta Publishing Co., 1911), pp. 18–19, hereafter cited as Munson, *Sanitary Tactics*; Clements, "Memoir of Jonathan Letterman," p. 10; George H. Lyman, *Some Aspects of the Medical Service in the Armies of the United States During the War of the Rebellion* (Boston: S.J. Parkhill, 1891), p. 22, hereafter cited as Lyman, *Medical Service During the War of the Rebellion.*

[62] Quoted words: Letterman, *Medical Recollections*, p. 23.

[63] Ambulances: For a harrowing description of an ambulance ride see Bull, *Soldiering*, pp 83–85.

[64] Control: War Department, *Medical and Surgical History*, pt. 3, vol. 2, pp. 938–41. Quoted words: Duncan, *Medical Department, Civil War*, pt. 6, p. 39.

[65] Antietam: Letterman, *Medical Recollections*, pp. 42–43, 80; Stephen W. Sears, *Landscape Turned Red* (New York: Ticknor and Fields, 1983), pp. 295–96; Livermore, *Numbers and Losses in the Civil War in America, 1861–1865* (New York: Houghton Mifflin, 1900), pp. 92–93; War Department, *Medical and Surgical History*, pt. 3, vol. 2, p. 937; John W. Schildt, *Antietem Hospitals*, (Chewsville, Md.: Antietem Publications, 1987), pp. 10–11.

[66] Fredericksburg: War Department, *Medical and Surgical History*, app., pt. 1, vol. 1, p. 131; Brinton, *Personal Memoirs*, p. 222.

[67] "Desiderata": Bowditch, *A Brief Plea*, pp. 27–28.

[68] Successes: War Department, *Medical and Surgical History*, app., pt. 1, vol. 1, pp. 141–42, 148, 205.

[69] Gettysburg: Ibid., pp. 141–42. Quoted words: Ibid., p. 142.

[70] Pelton's report: Ibid., p. 219.

[71] Chickamauga: Ibid., pp. 265–66.

[72] Quoted words: Brinton, *Personal Memoirs*, pp. 111–12.

[73] South: Sunseri, "Confederate Army of Tennessee," p. 168. European status: Jean Larrey, *Memoirs of Military Surgery*, pp. v–ix, 28–29, 78, 223–24. Legouest's views: Leon Legouest, *Le Service de Sante des Armees Americaines*, (Paris: J.B. Bailliere, 1863), p. 4.

[74] Garland and Windecker: War Department, *Medical and Surgical History*, app., pt. 1, vol. 1, p. 98; Letterman, *Medical Recollections*, pp. 42–43, 313.

[75] Quoted words: War Department, *Medical and Surgical History*, app., pt. 1, vol. 1, p. 167.

[76] Ayer: Duncan, *Medical Department in the Civil War*, pt. 6, p. 15, and pt. 7, p. 16.

[77] Killed in action and quoted words: War Department, *Medical and Surgical History*, app., pt. 1, vol. 1, p. 142.

[78] Quoted words: *The Ambulance System: Reprinted from the North American Review, January 1864, and Published, for Gratuitous Distribution, by the Committee of Citizens Who Have in Charge the Sending of Petitions to Congress for the Establishment of a Thorough and Uniform Ambulance System in the Armies of the Republic* (Boston: Crosby and Nichols, 1864), p. 15.

[79] Ambulance Corps legislation: 13 Stat. 20–22, 11 Mar 1864; William O. Owen, *A Chronological Arrangement of Congressional Legislation Relating to the Medical Corps of the U.S. Army from 1785–1917* (Chicago: American Medical Association, 1920), p. 24, hereafter cited as Owen, *Legislation, 1785–1917*; WDGO 106, 16 Mar 1864, Pentagon Library, The Pentagon, Washington, D.C. (PL).

[80] Letterman: Maxwell, *Lincoln's Fifth Wheel*, p. 179, 185; Clements, "Memoir of Jonathan Letterman," p. 20; Phalen, "The Life of Jonathan Letterman," pp. 63–64. Letterman's daughter believed he was frustrated by the Army's slowness in adopting his plan. Catherine Letterman to Wilber M. Brucker, Secretary of the Army (Sec Army), 4 Oct 1957, Medical Service Corps history files, U.S. Army Center of Military History, Washington, D.C. (MSC-USACMH). Quoted words: Letterman, *Medical Recollections*, p. 185.

[81] Court-martial: War Department Special Orders (WDSO) 3, 3 Sep 1863, PL; Phalen, *Chiefs of the Medical Department*, pp. 44–45; Maxwell, *Lincoln's Fifth Wheel*, pp. 233–47; Brown, *Medical Department*, p. 235; Brinton, *Personal Memoirs*, p. 256. President Hayes exonerated Hammond in

1878, belatedly restoring the reputation of a man who had pushed the Medical Department into action. Congressional action on 15 March restored Hammond to the Army and placed him on the retired list in the grade of brigadier general. In his brief tenure Hammond had organized a medical museum, a Medical Department school, and a military medical history program that would make major contributions to medical literature. He had pressed for the creation of permanent hospital and ambulance corps and for departmental autonomy in its facilities, construction, supply, and transportation.

[82] Tompkins: Robert S. Holzman, "Sally Tompkins: Captain, Confederate Army," *American Mercury* 88 (March 1959): 127–30; *Dictionary of American Biography*, "Sally Louisa Tompkins"; David B. Sabine, "Captain Sally Tompkins," *Civil War Times Illustrated* 4, no. 7 (1965): 36–39. Tompkins was buried with full military honors in 1916. Her hospital had 73 deaths for 1,333 admissions from August 1861 to April 1865. Brooks, *Civil War Medicine*, p. 57.

[83] Physicians and administration: Cunningham, *Doctors in Gray*, pp. 126, 249; Sunseri, "Confederate Army of Tennessee," p. 18. Quoted words: Charles Lynch, Frank W. Weed, and Loy McAfee, *The Surgeon General's Office*, vol. 1 of the series The Medical Department of the United States Army in the World War (Washington, D.C.: Government Printing Office, 1925), p. 47, hereafter cited as Lynch, *Surgeon General's Office*.

[84] Stewards: War Department, *Regulations for the Medical Department*, p. 8; Joseph J. Woodward, *The Hospital Steward's Manual* (Philadelphia: J.B. Lippincott, 1862), pp. 43–45, 313. See also George R. Wren, "The First Trained U.S. Hospital Administrator and His Textbook," *Hospital & Health Services Administration* 26 (Winter 1981): 56; Joseph P. Peters, "How the Civil War Changed Hospital Care," *Modern Hospital* 98 (May 1962): 114, 172; Brooks, *Civil War Medicine*, pp. 34, 50; Joseph Israeloff, "The Emerging Role of the Medical Service Corps Officer in the Evolution of the Army Medical Service," *Military Medicine* 125 (April 1960): 269.

[85] Pharmacists: Shryock, *The Development of Modern Medicine* (New York: Alfred A. Knopf, 1947), p. 152; Edward R. Fell, "The Pharmaceutical Department of a U.S.A. Hospital," *American Journal of Pharmacy* 37 (1865): 107–10; Editorial, "Military Pharmaceutists," *American Journal of Pharmacy* 34 (1862): 94. For example, the 3,600-bed Army General Hospital at Chestnut Hill, Pennsylvania, had twelve contract pharmacists.

[86] Zacharie: "The Head and Foot of the Nation," *New York Herald*, 3 October 1862; Charles M. Segal, "Isachar Zacharie: Lincoln's Chiropodist," *American Jewish Historical Quarterly* 43 (December 1953): 78–79, 81. Quoted words: Segal, p. 71.

[87] Quoted words: Letterman, *Medical Recollections*, p. 32.

[88] Medical logistics: *SG Report*, 1855, p. 5; Duncan, *Medical Department in the Civil War*, pt. 5., p. 21; Maxwell, *Lincoln's Fifth Wheel*, p. 171. For complaints see: Surgeon Charles B. Tripler to Surgeon General William A. Hammond, 9 May 1862; Brigade Surgeon J.H. Thompson to Brig. Gen. J.G. Foster, USA, 1 Mar 1862, and subsequent correspondence ending in Maj. J. Belga, Quartermaster Corps (QM), to Thompson, 21 Mar 1862, Record Group (RG) 112, Series 12, Box 99, National Archives, National Archives and Records Administration, Washington, D.C. (NARA-NA). Letterman's view: Letterman, *Medical Recollections*, pp. 178–79; War Department, *Medical and Surgical History*, app., pt. 1, vol. 1, pp. 133–34.

[89] USAMS: 12 Stat. 403, 20 May 1862; Owen, *Legislation, 1785–1917*, pp. 21, 28, and 29; WDGO 55, 24 May 1862, PL; Brown, *Medical Department*, pp. 224–25, 253; Henry N. Rittenhouse, "U.S. Army Medical Storekeepers," *American Journal of Pharmacy* 37 (1865): 88–89; Caswell A. Mayo, "Why the Pharmaceutical Corps Should Be Established," *American Druggist* 66 (April 1918): 25.

[90] Quoted words: *SG Report*, 10 Nov 1862, p.7.

[91] Rank: 14 Stat. 423, 2 Mar 1867. Congress abolished the USAMS in 1876, but grandfathered those on active duty. 19 Stat. 61, 26 Jun 1876.

[92] Quoted words: Rittenhouse, "U.S. Army Medical Storekeepers," p. 89; Hennell Stevens, "The Medical Purveying Department of the United States Army," *American Journal of Pharmacy* 37 (1865): 98.

[93] Beall: Biographical note, Charles Ellsworth, U.S. Army Center of Military History (USACMH), 2 Sep 1967, drawn from RG 94, Records of the Adjutant General's Office (AGO), Appointments, Commissions and Personnel Branch, DASG-MS.

[94] Rittenhouse: Rittenhouse, "U.S. Army Medical Storekeepers," p. 90.

[95] Dismantling: Surgeon General Joseph K. Barnes summarized the process in *SG Report*, 1866, p. 2. For numbers, see *SG Report*, 1888, p. 145, and 1898, pp. 1154–56. Also see Lyman, *Medical Service During the War of the Rebellion*, p. 40; James A. Tobey, *The Medical Department of the Army* (Baltimore: Johns Hopkins, 1927), pp. 20–24. General Hammond's successor, Brig. Gen. Joseph K. Barnes, bemoaned the loss of Medical Department capability. "Congress followed the usual plan of reducing the Army and throwing into the discard everything learned in the meanwhile" (Reasoner, "Medical Supply Service," p. 19).

[96] Murray: *SG Report*, 1885, p. 39. Quoted words: *Statutes at Large of the United States of America, December 1885–March 1887* (Washington, D.C.: Government Printing Office, 1887), 24: 435–36.

[97] Massachusetts: Fisch and Wright, *Noncommissioned Officer Corps*, pp. 76–78.

[98] Sternberg: See James S. Simmons, "Military Preventive Medicine: The Keystone of Military Strength," in *Military Medicine Notes*, 3 vols. (Washington, D.C.: Army Medical Service Graduate School, 1951), 1: 4–5, copy in the Joint Medical Library of the Army and Air Force Surgeons General, Washington, D.C. (JML).

[99] Reed: *SG Report*, 1896, p. 23. Reed, professor of clinical and sanitary microscopy, trained medical officers in pathogenic bacteria and the microscopic study of sputum, urine, blood, and tumors.

[100] Quoted words: Percy M. Ashburn, *A History of the Medical Department of the United States Army* (Boston: Houghton Mifflin, 1929), p. 185.

[101] Mobilization: David F. Trask, *The War with Spain in 1898* (New York: Macmillan, 1981), pp. 192–93; Weigley, *History of the United States Army*, pp. 308–09. Quoted words: Maj Walter Reed, MC, to Maj William C. Gorgas, MC, 29 Jul 1901, cited in William C. Gorgas, *Sanitation in Panama* (New York: D. Appleton, 1915), p. 89. For discussion see: Lynch, *Surgeon General's Office*, p. 32; James Johnston, "Army Medical Service in the Spanish War," *New York Medical Journal* 82 (5 August 1905): 301–05.

[102] Expansion: Weigley, *History of the United States Army*, p. 297; *SG Report*, 1898, pp. 102, 148. The Regular Army strength was 2,143 officers and 26,040 enlisted. U.S. Congress, Senate, *Report of the Commission Appointed by the President To Investigate the Conduct of the War Department in the War with Spain*, 56th Cong., 1st sess., S. Doc. 221, 1: 113, hereafter cited as *Dodge Commission Report*. Hospital Corps: *SG Report*, 1899, p. 24.

[103] Quoted words: Rpt of Lt Col A.C. Girard, Chief Surgeon, II Corps, *SG Report*, 1898, p. 157.

[104] Volunteers: *SG Report*, 1891, p. 10.

[105] Quoted words: Theodore Roosevelt, *The Rough Riders* (New York: Charles Scribner's Sons, 1920), p. 185.

[106] Quoted words: *Dodge Commission Report*, 1: 6–7.

[107] Quoted words: Roosevelt, *The Rough Riders*, p. 119. Roosevelt's testimony: *Dodge Commission Report*, 5: 2267–69.

[108] Quoted words: Shafter to Adjutant General, War Department (WD), 29 Jul 1898, in War Department, *Correspondence Relating to the War with Spain* (Washington, D.C.: Government Printing Office, 1902), p. 186. "I will not quietly submit to having the onus laid on me for the lack of these hospital facilities" (ibid., 3 Aug, p. 187).

[109] Colonel Pew: *Dodge Commission Report*, 4: 1011.

[110] Medical deployment: *SG Report*, 1898, pp. 103, 116; Weigley, *History of the United States Army*, p. 302; Margaret Leech, *In the Days of McKinley* (New York: Harper and Brothers, 1959), pp. 261–62.

[111] Quoted words: Nicholas Senn, *Medico-Surgical Aspects of the Spanish American War* (Chicago: American Medical Association, 1900), p. 182, hereafter cited as Senn, *Medico-Surgical Aspects*.

[112] Shortcomings: *SG Report*, 1898, pp. 115–42, 158; *SG Report*, 1899, pp. 60–65; *Dodge Commission Report*, 1: 188–89, 571, 574, 686–87, and 5: 2107.

[113] Quoted words: Lt. Col. A.C. Girard in *SG Report*, 1898, p. 158.

[114] Quoted words: Maj. Frank J. Ives in *Dodge Commission Report*, 4: 2107. Camp Wikoff: "The strongest survivors of Shafter's campaign were not fit for a tramp of several miles . . . the regulars shambled into line like a retinue of ghosts with skeleton faces and blank unseeing eyes." Leech, *In the Days of McKinley*, p. 308.

[115] Quoted words: Ltr, Maj J.R. Kean, 18 Oct 1898, cited in Col E.M. Wones, MSC, Ret., draft section, sub: Introduction and Early Requirements, 1961, in 1958 MSC History Project, folder 239, box 15/18, MSC-USACMH. Also see report by Lt. Col. Louis M. Maus, Chief Surgeon, VII Corps, Fort Hamilton, New York, on the difficulty of converting civilian physicians into military medical officers. *SG Report*, 1899, p. 72.

[116] Proposals: *Dodge Commission Report*, 7: 325, and 4: 1121, 1146–47, 1413.

[117] Sternberg: He was called the father of American bacteriology. See Simmons, "Military Preventive Medicine," 1: 4–5.

[118] Sternberg's circular: Surgeon General's Office (SGO) Circular (Cir) 1, 25 Apr 1898; Cir 5, 8 Aug 1898; Cir 7, 5 Sep 1898, in Sternberg, *Sanitary Lessons of the War* (Washington, D.C.: privately published by Byron J. Adams, 1912), pp. 9–12. Criticism of Sternberg: Leech, *In the Days of McKinley*, pp. 300–308; Weigley, *History of the United States Army*, pp. 304–05. Sternberg defended himself (including criticism by Theodore Roosevelt) in his *Sanitary Lessons of the War*, pp. 8, 26. Other defenders include John M. Gibson, *Soldier in White* (Durham, N.C.: Duke University, 1958), pp. 199–209; Senn, *Medico-Surgical Aspects*, pp. 73–78, 182; Martha L. Sternberg, *George Miller Sternberg* (Chicago: American Medical Association, 1920). Sternberg did admit disappointment over the mortality rates (ibid., p. 188). Quoted words: Leech, *In the Days of McKinley*, p. 301.

[119] Disease: Duncan, "Comparative Mortality," p. 32. Round-robin letter: Leech, *In the Days of McKinley*, pp. 274–77; Roosevelt, *The Rough Riders*, pp. 209–12, 280–83.

[120] Quoted words: *SG Report*, 1917, p. 172. That sentiment was echoed by the 11th Division (Provisional). See ibid., p. 144.

[121] First ambulance: Rpt, George A. Scheier, Managing Editor, *Bulletin of the U.S. Army Medical Department*, Office of The Surgeon General (OTSG), sub: Army Medical Department Chronology, 1775–1947, 1 Oct 1947, pp. 35, 37, 46, copy in DASG-MS. Doctrine: James L. Bevans, "The Ambulance Company," in Sanitary Field Service School for Medical Officers (SFSS), *Sanitary Field Service* (Fort Leavenworth, Kans., 1912), pp. 4–9, 34, hereafter cited as FS Schools, *Sanitary Field Service*. First use: *SG Report*, 1917, p. 158.

[122] Advances: Louis H. Roddis, "Ten Greatest Advances in Medicine," *Military Surgeon* 115 (December 1954): 449; M.A. Reasoner, "The Development of the Medical Supply Service," *Military Surgeon* 63 (July 1928): 4; David McCullough, *The Path Between the Seas* (New York: Simon and Schuster, 1977), p. 416.

[123] Gorgas: *SG Report*, 1883, p. 12.

[124] Yellow fever: Marie D. Gorgas and Burton J. Hendrick, *William Crawford Gorgas: His Life and Work* (New York: Doubleday, Page and Company, 1924), pp. 8–11, 174, 187–88. Gorgas' estimate: William C. Gorgas, *Sanitation in Panama* (New York: D. Appleton and Company, 1915), pp. 182–204, 230–31, 283. Black workers found Panama four times as deadly as did whites. See McCullough, *The Path Between the Seas*, pp. 581–85.

[125]125. Wrightson: Biographical Sketch, The Historical Unit (THU), OTSG, in MSC-USACMH; 1st Lt R.W. Bamberg, MSC, citing memo, The Surgeon General (TSG) for Wrightson, in draft rpt, sub: History of the Medical Service Corps, 20 Sep 1954, THU, OTSG, folder 260, box 16\18, MSC-USACMH; Gorgas and Hendrick, *William Crawford Gorgas*, pp. 297–301.

[126] LePrince: Gorgas and Hendrick, *William Crawford Gorgas*, pp. 104, 150, 172, 254; McCullough, *The Path Between the Seas*, pp. 419, 449; Gorgas, *Sanitation in Panama*, pp. 182–204, 230–31; Gordon Harrison, *Mosquitos, Malaria and Man* (New York: E.P. Dutton, 1978), p. 164; Joseph A. LePrince and A.J. Orenstein, *Mosquito Control in Panama* (New York: G.P. Putnam's Sons, 1916), p. 303. LePrince became a commissioned officer of the U.S. Public Health Service in 1915 and served as its senior sanitary engineer from 1917 to 1935. He headed the antimalarial activities at Army and Navy training camps in the United States during the war, a program that reduced the malaria sick rate to less than one-half of one percent of that which occurred on Army bases in the South during the Spanish-American War.

[127] Reserves: Richard B. Crossland and James T. Currie, *Twice the Citizen: A History of the United States Army Reserve, 1908–1983* (Washington, D.C.: Office of the Chief, Army Reserve, 1984), pp. 17–20.

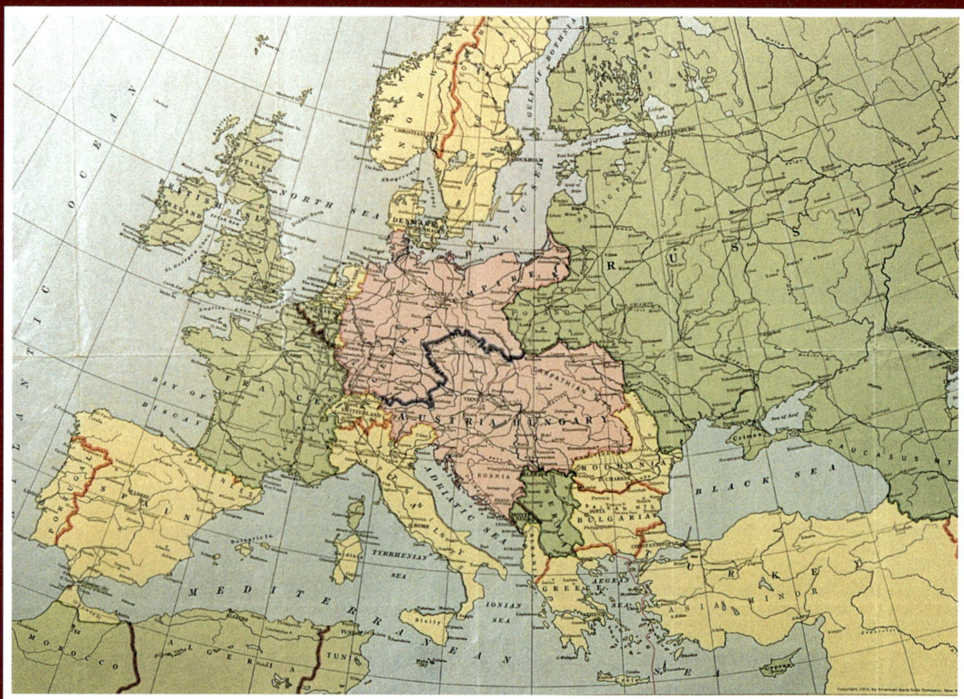

Map of Europe, 1914

2

World War I
The Ambulance Service

In April 1917 the United States entered World War I on the side of the Allies—France, Russia, Great Britain, and Italy. The British and French asked for immediate medical support because their medical systems were severely taxed. Their war against the Central Powers (Austria-Hungary, Germany, Turkey, and Bulgaria) was in its third year. While mobile war characterized the Eastern Front, barbed wire, machine guns, and the increased accuracy and rate of fire of weapons had created a static front in the west. "The two lines sat opposite each other and did nothing but hammer at each other."[1] Everywhere the war was bloody, and casualties were high. The combatants would suffer over 34 million casualties, including nearly 8 million deaths from wounds and disease.[2] Though a latecomer to the fighting, the United States mobilized over 4 million soldiers and deployed over 2 million to Europe; 106,378 would die before peace returned.[3]

The need for medical support was staggering. Great battles used up manpower at an incredible rate. During the 1916 Battle of the Somme, in seven days British artillery threw 1.5 million explosive and chlorine gas shells at the well-dug-in Germans. Yet when the British attacked, surviving Germans manned their machine guns and inflicted 60,000 casualties on the attackers during the first day alone. The battle lasted five months, during which there were some 420,000 British, 200,000 French, and 650,000 German casualties. British artillery preparation for the Third Battle of Ypres the following summer devoured the entire production of 55,000 British ammunition workers for a year, and a victory of very limited value cost them 8,222 casualties per square mile.[4]

To meet the needs of war, the U.S. Army's surgeon general, Maj. Gen. William M. Gorgas, presided over an enormous expansion of the Army Medical Department. When the United States entered the war his department consisted of less than 1,000 personnel, but it numbered over 350,000 when peace returned in November 1918. The Surgeon General's Office mushroomed from a staff of 153 at the beginning of the war to over 2,100 at its end. The Medical Department was authorized 444 physicians at the beginning of World War I, but it had 31,530 when the war ended. Nearly 24 percent of all American physicians served in the Army.[5]

Increases in the other specialties were also dramatic. By war's end the department had 4,620 dentists, 21,480 nurses, and 2,234 veterinarians. In addition, there were two new precursors of the Medical Service Corps. The U.S. Army Ambulance Service, formed in 1917, had 209 officers, and the Sanitary Corps, formed the same year, had 2,919. The department was rounded out with 281,341 enlisted soldiers and 10,695 civilian employees.[6]

Military medicine benefited from medical advances, but severe limitations remained. Sulfa drugs and antibiotics were yet to come, and some medical problems remained intractable. Measles and influenza were the most significant diseases for the Army in World War I because of respiratory complications, principally the scourge of the pneumonia which followed. The influenza epidemic of 1917–18 killed over 24,500 soldiers. Massachusetts Institute of Technology's "Roll of Honor" lists those alumni who died in World War I. Of the 123 listed, 41 died of pneumonia.[7] However, the addition of new organizations to the Medical Department enabled it to expand its medical team to accommodate the most advanced technology of its time and to post the best record yet for the medical support of an American army in the field.[8]

Volunteer Ambulance Officers

Put on your old gray bonnet
With the strap ahangin' on it,
And we'll go thru shrapnel & thru shell—
Then on roads of desolation
We will cure your constipation
With a wild night ride in hell![9]

As popular support for American participation in the war increased, volunteer organizations capitalized on that spirit, enrolling many young Americans who served as ambulance drivers in France and Italy. Until there was an opportunity for overseas service in the Army, the volunteers provided person-to-person proof of America's willingness to support its allies. They received short orientation courses and wore uniforms patterned after those of the U.S. Army. When deployed, they served under the command of the French or Italian Army units to which they were attached. Volunteer ambulance organizations preceded U.S. Army ambulance units in Europe, and their officers were predecessors of Medical Department commissioned ambulance officers.

The American Red Cross Ambulance Service actively recruited through its headquarters in New York and established units in France and Italy. By the spring of 1917 it had forty-six ambulance units supporting the Allies.[10] One who joined was eighteen-year-old Ernest Hemingway, who as a Red Cross second lieutenant became the first American wounded in Italy.[11] Hemingway received over two hundred artillery fragment wounds in his legs during a night attack in July 1918 and was further wounded by machine-gun fire when he carried a wounded Italian soldier to safety. He likened his left leg to the hide of an old horse that had been branded and rebranded by fifty owners.[12]

Another group, the Norton-Harjes Ambulance Service, was formed in 1914 by Richard Norton, an American archaeologist who served as its director, and A. Herman Harjes, a French banker. Norton-Harjes affiliated with the American Red Cross, and its members incurred a six-month obligation with the Red Cross when they joined. By July 1917 Norton-Harjes units had over six hundred

American ambulance drivers and three hundred ambulances.[13]

The largest of the volunteer ambulance groups was the American Field Service. The organization dated from the earliest days of the war, when the American colony in Paris outfitted a rudimentary ambulance service to support the French Army. In May of 1915 the American Field Service was operating 60 ambulances organized in 3 sections; by late 1917 it had 1,220 ambulances in 31 sections supporting 66 French divisions. Inspector General A. Piatt Andrew, former director of the mint and a future congressman, served as its director. Andrew was honored by France for his contributions with the Legion d'Honneur and by the United States with the Distinguished Service Medal.[14]

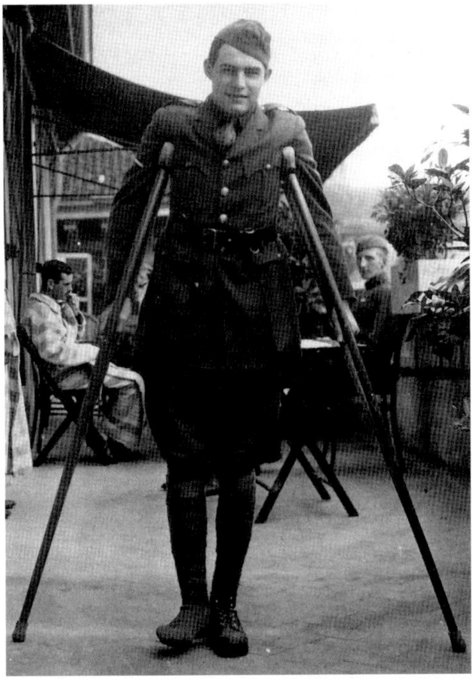

Ernest Hemingway convalescing at a hospital in Italy, April 1919; below, *Inspector General Andrew*

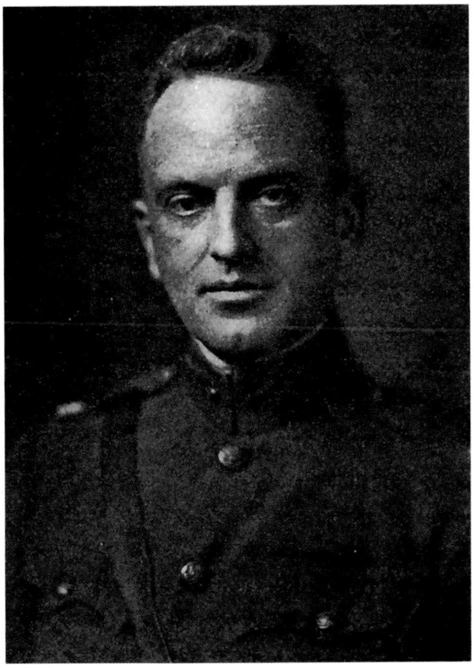

Although neither the Red Cross nor the American Field Service paid the volunteers, the French government insisted on reimbursing them at five cents a day, equivalent to the pay of a French soldier. The volunteers paid for their own transportation, clothing, uniforms, and personal equipment. As one put it, "the Americans not only had to be willing to risk their lives, they also had to pay to do it."[15]

The volunteer ambulance units refined motorized evacuation techniques that were later adopted by the U.S. Army when it entered the war. They incorporated Jonathan Letterman's ambulance corps officer, a specialty that had been lost to the U.S. Army for thirty years. Inspector General Andrew noted the similarity of his organization's doctrine with that of the French, who also used nonphysician officers to command the evacuation system. "From the French point of view, it was as illogical to

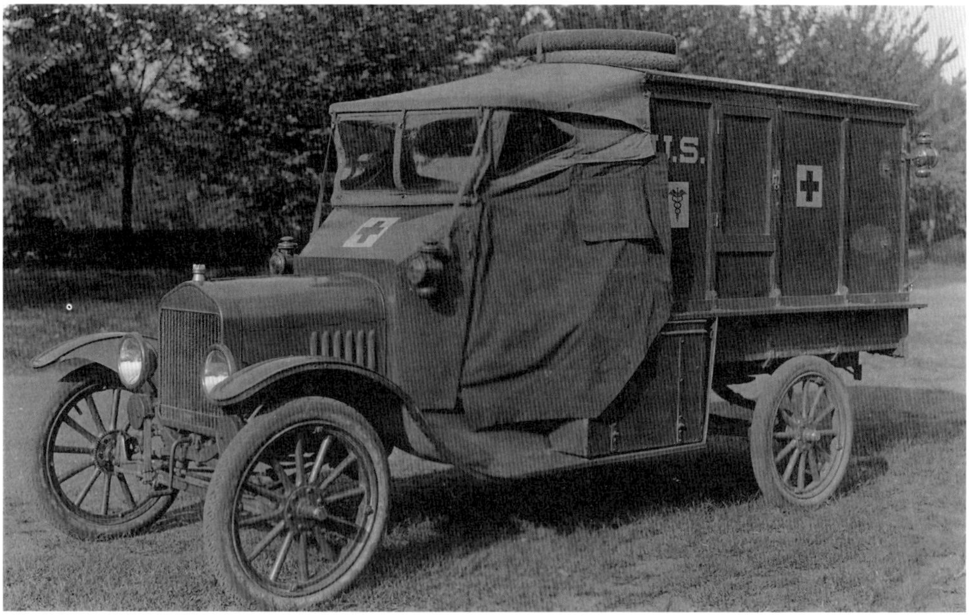

Standard Ford ambulance with storm curtains

expect doctors and surgeons to accomplish this work successfully as it would be to ask automobile experts to do surgical and medical work in the dressing stations and hospitals."[16]

Ford, Fiat, Peugeot, and General Motors Company ambulances were severely tested under combat conditions that demonstrated their advantages in speed and patient comfort. The Ford Model "T" could climb narrow mountain roads where patient movement previously was possible only on mules or in horse-drawn carts. The Ford put new meaning in "fording." It sat high and could get through flooded roads not accessible by lower vehicles. Indeed, French soldiers accused the Americans of painting water lines on their vehicles as depth gauges, and some calls for evacuation would request the ambulance "boats." If a road was blocked, the "T" could go cross-country. It was light enough that three or four soldiers could pick it up and move it if it stuck in a ditch or shell hole.[17]

Nevertheless, the motorized ambulances were primitive vehicles. The Ford's idiosyncrasies made mountain driving dicey. Its gravity gasoline feed did not work on steep grades, compelling drivers to back their vehicles up the hills. Another problem was that prolonged driving in low gear caused excessive and uneven wear on the transmission bands. To equalize the wear, drivers in mountainous terrain used the low-speed band during climbs, the reverse band to assist in controlling descents, and the foot brake on corners and the steepest parts of hills. Transmission bands would last ten to fourteen days with this technique. Mountain driving was further complicated by brakes that could not handle the steep grades. Drivers kept an eye peeled for strategically placed trees that could stop them if necessary. Sometimes patients had unforgettable rides.[18]

Unfortunately, automobile driving was not yet a universal skill, and the inexperienced drivers were further bedeviled by problems such as horseshoe nails in the roads. The nails raised havoc with the tires, which, in turn, raised havoc with the drivers, since this was before demountable rims. The crews were further tested by the hazardous conditions of the combat zone. At Verdun they navigated roads named for the risk of artillery fire—Dip of Death, Hell's Half Acre, and Dead Man's Turn. William Seabrook, an American Field Service volunteer, described how it was. "Those of us who used to laugh at danger have stopped laughing. . . . We don't come back any longer and tell each other with excited interest how close to our car this or that shell burst—it is sufficient that we came back."[19]

Medical Department Organization and Doctrine

While volunteers toiled in Europe, the Medical Department readied itself for war. Its doctrine for wartime medical support, built on the lessons learned in previous wars, rested upon the work of the staff of the Field Service School for Medical Officers at Fort Leavenworth, Kansas. Setting forth medical doctrine in landmark field manuals, Maj. Edward L. Munson, MC, and other officers at the school formed a vibrant group of medical planners whose foresight during the years of peace paid dividends when the United States again went to war.[20]

First to go in May 1917 were six base hospitals; some of their personnel were the first U.S. soldiers killed in action.[21] The Medical Department deployed an astonishing array of skilled personnel over the next year and a half to support Maj. Gen. John J. Pershing's American Expeditionary Forces (AEF). At the time of the Armistice 145,000 American soldiers were hospitalized in 152 base hospitals and 101 camp hospitals in France and England, backed up by 7 medical laboratories and 28 medical supply bases, depots, and stations. In addition, the Medical Department operated 147,636 beds in 92 hospitals in the United States.[22]

Army hospitals in Europe also served the field medical units of the 43 American divisions deployed to France, the 2 regiments sent to Russia and Italy, and the 19 divisions that remained in the United States. Each Army division contained 40,000 soldiers—28,000 combat soldiers and 12,000 support troops. General Pershing insisted on extensive training of the divisions prior to their commitment to battle, and the first committed did not go into combat until the latter part of April 1918, a year after the United States had entered the war.[23]

The Medical Department's doctrine for combat operations was built upon an evacuation scheme configured within three levels of medical support (*see Chart 1*). The zone of the advance was the first echelon. It extended from the front lines through the division area of operations. The second echelon, the line of communications, was the area of the field armies that supported divisions. The third echelon, the service of the interior, constituted the continental United States support base for overseas operations. Under wartime conditions Medical Department doctrine was adapted to the exigencies of combat, and the structure and procedures employed varied with the type of combat (trench or open warfare), the intensity of the fighting, and such other factors as terrain and weather.

CHART 1—WORLD WAR I ECHELONS OF MEDICAL SUPPORT

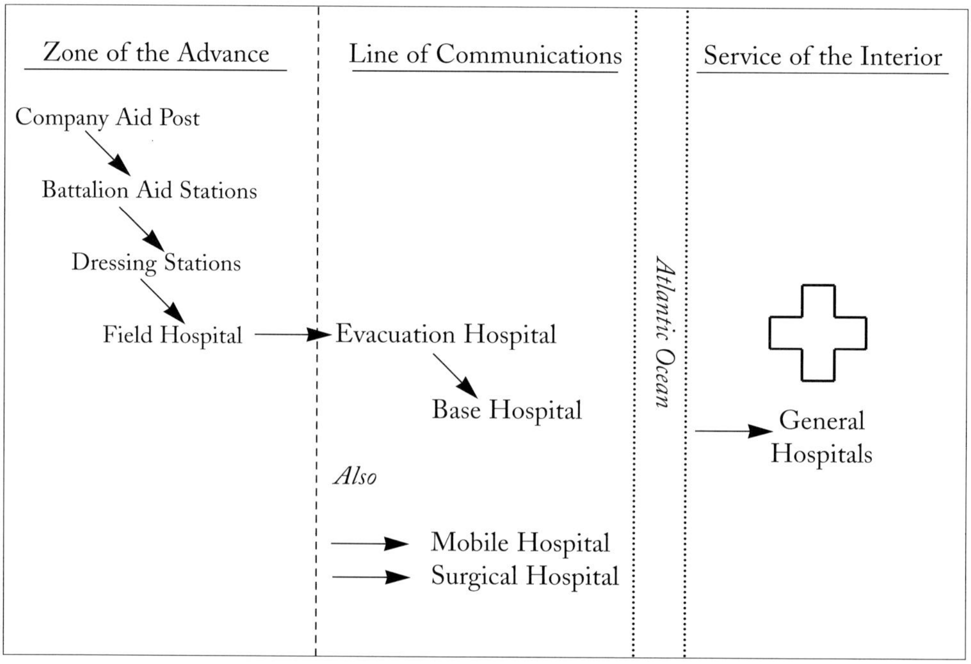

Source: Charles Lynch, Joseph H. Ford, and Frank W. Weed, *The Medical Department of the United States Army in the World War*, vol. 8 (Washington, D.C.: Government Printing Office, 1925), p. 1041.

Treatment of combat casualties was based on triage, a French term for sorting patients in mass casualty situations into categories: those who would die no matter what treatment was provided ("expectant"); those who would live if treatment were immediately rendered ("immediate"); and those whose treatment could safely be delayed ("delayed"). Initial medical attention was concentrated on the immediate group, and the evacuation system was based on the movement of serious cases to the rear for definitive treatment. Medical personnel, equipment, and supplies were under Medical Department control. Army regulations restricted ambulances to the Medical Department's use for movement of the sick and wounded and emergency transportation of medical supplies.[24]

Medical support in the zone of the advance was the responsibility of the medical elements within the divisions, including the medical support organic to the maneuver units and the division sanitary train. Two enlisted medical soldiers were customarily attached to each rifle company where they established a company aid post. Wounded soldiers were brought there for first aid treatment, carried from the front line by company bearers. Most divisions detailed soldiers from the line companies to supplement the number of litter bearers.

The battalion aid station was normally 250 to 500 yards to the rear of the front line, close enough to be able to render prompt treatment. It was staffed by

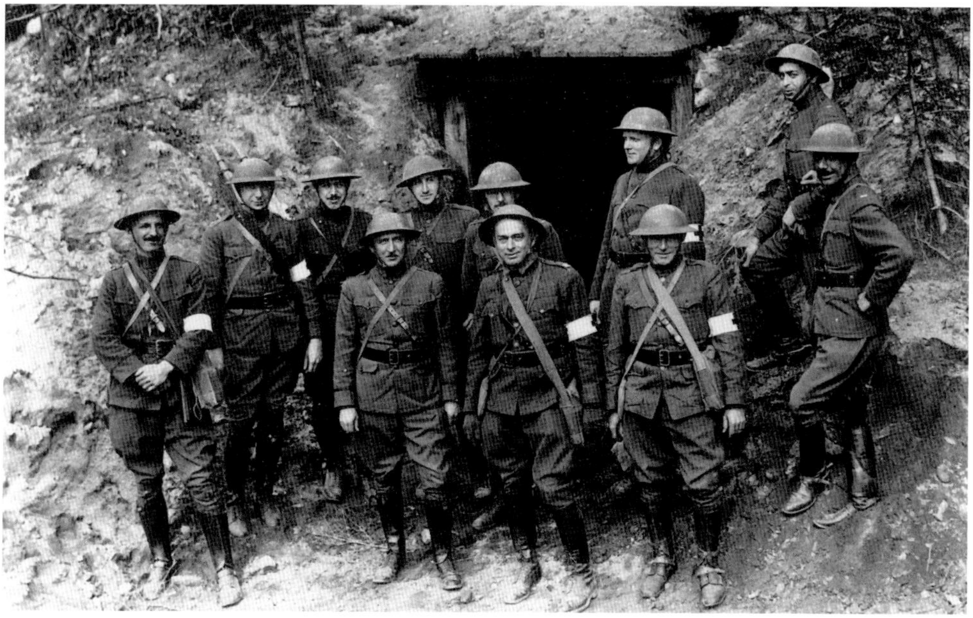

Officers of the 117th Sanitary Train in Bertricamp, France, April 1918

one or two physicians, a dentist (if available), four to six medics, plus two runners and one or more litter squads supplied by the supporting ambulance company. Battalion aid stations with two medical officers could split into two sections that leapfrogged to keep pace. Litter squads consisted of four bearers. It was found that 1,000 yards marked the limit of a squad's endurance, and distances greater than this were handled by squads in relay. The 305th Ambulance Company, supporting the 77th Division during the Meuse-Argonne offensive, had relays operating over routes as long as three and a half miles.[25]

Each division had a sanitary train (today's medical battalion), which consisted of an ambulance section, a field hospital section, and a medical supply unit. This organization had been made a part of the force structure in 1911 and formed an integrated medical support capability under unitary medical control that was flexible enough to be task-organized to meet changing conditions.[26] It provided the division surgeon with centralized control of the division medical assets. If needed, all ambulance companies in a division could be consolidated. Depending on the combat situation, the litter bearers might be under the control of the ambulance companies or under the regimental or battalion surgeons. If a battalion surgeon became a casualty, an ambulance company medical officer could replace him. In all, a division's medical personnel totaled 1,331 officers and enlisted personnel. Of that number, 991 were in the sanitary train.[27]

The ambulance section of the division sanitary train was organized on the basis of four ambulance companies per division (two per cavalry division). Each company provided twelve ambulances to evacuate casualties from the battalion aid stations to the company's dressing stations, 3,000 to 6,000 yards from the front, and farther

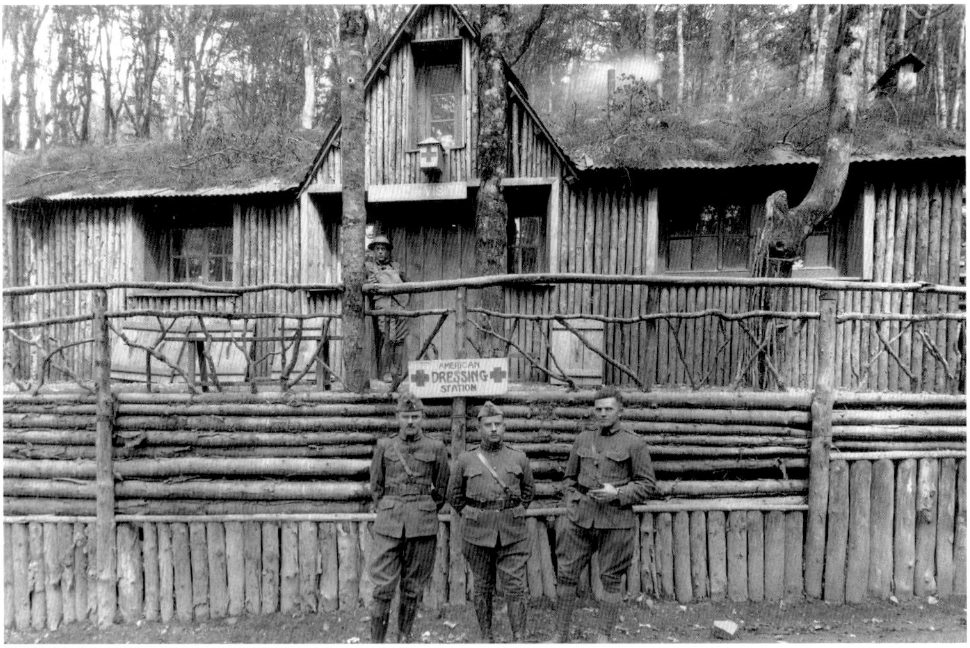

Officers at the dressing station of the 137th Ambulance Company in Amphersbach, Germany, August 1918

back to the field hospitals. The length of time required to transport wounded soldiers from the front lines to the field hospitals was affected by a variety of factors including road conditions, visibility, and traffic. The 3d Division, for example, averaged five hours' transit time during the Second Battle of the Marne and two and one-half hours during the Meuse-Argonne offensive. Overall, in the AEF the time from wounding until the arrival at the first triage point was five to six hours.[28]

The field hospital section of the division sanitary train operated four field hospitals set up six to eight miles from the front, rounding out the medical support in the zone of the advance. The field hospitals were on the order of more sophisticated dressing stations. Patients were stabilized there—as they were at earlier points in the evacuation chain—so that they could either be returned to their units or evacuated farther to the rear for more definitive care. Each hospital had a normal capacity of 108 beds, expandable to 162, thus providing a 432-bed (648-bed expanded) capability for a division in combat. In addition, this section operated eight dispensaries for routine medical care.[29] Patients evacuated from the field hospitals passed into the second echelon, the line of communications, where the evacuation hospital along with smaller mobile hospitals and surgical hospitals formed the principal early surgery capability in the theater of operations.[30] The evacuation hospital expanded from 340 to 1,000 beds during the war, but in some cases operated at higher capacities. Patients evacuated to the United States entered the third echelon of medical support, the service of the interior and its network of general hospitals and supporting facilities.

American doctrine was based on speed of evacuation, a basic philosophy that differed from that of the French.[31] The AEF evacuation system moved serious cases as quickly as possible to the rear after the patients had been appropriately stabilized for further movement. AEF evacuation hospitals essentially served as clearinghouses. Surgery was performed only as necessary to enable further evacuation of the casualties, and patients were held only until they could be safely moved.[32] The French, on the other hand, placed a more sophisticated capability farther forward than the Americans, and some of their hospitals had as many as 5,000 beds. The larger facilities provided definitive care for the wounded earlier in the evacuation chain. However, their large, immobile hospitals would be at a disadvantage if trench warfare turned into a war of movement.

Doctrinal differences between the Allies extended to the operation of the ambulance system. The Americans, based on their lessons learned from previous conflicts, kept ambulances under medical control and attempted to integrate treatment and resuscitation during evacuation. The French ambulance service was under the automobile service, divorced from medical control. Its focus was patient transport, and its personnel were not expected to have medical training. It depended for its success upon evacuation over shorter distances to a definitive treatment facility.[33]

The U.S. Army Ambulance Service

When the United States declared war against Germany, the status of American volunteers in Europe became uncertain because they now had a U.S. military obligation to fulfill. France, fearing the loss of ambulance volunteers, requested that the United States ensure the uninterrupted continuation of the vital service. U.S. leaders thus agreed to incorporate American volunteer ambulance units into the American Army and to continue their service at the front with the French.

The Army organized a new ambulance corps for that purpose. War Department General Orders No. 75, which established the U.S. Army Ambulance Service (USAAS), was issued on 23 June 1917—an important date in the evolution of the Medical Service Corps. Like the Sanitary Corps, which followed it by a week, it was a temporary expedient made possible through the special wartime powers given President Woodrow Wilson in the Act of 18 May 1917. The USAAS also afforded the Medical Department an expanded opportunity to commission individuals in specialties it needed. Its officer authorization was set at 203, and it was organized into 160 sections known as sanitary squad units. It soon increased to 214 officers in 169 sections. Sanitary squad units supported divisions on the basis of 1 per 10,000 combat soldiers.[34]

When the AEF deployed to France for its lengthy period of organization and training, General Pershing found that the volunteer organizations had set up a good ambulance system. The AEF worked to bring that system wholesale into the USAAS, and the volunteers were offered the opportunity to join the U.S. Army. The American Field Service was operating forty-seven sections in France at that point, and many of its 1,200 members enlisted in the USAAS or volunteered for other combat duties. Eighty-one volunteers were commissioned in the Army

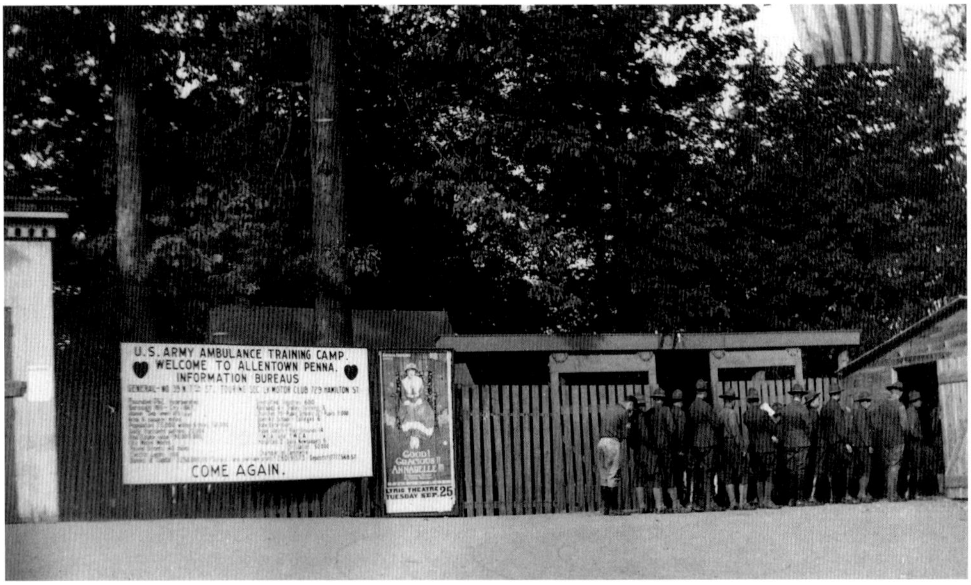
U.S. ARMY AMBULANCE TRAINING CAMP.
WELCOME TO ALLENTOWN PENNA.
INFORMATION BUREAUS
COME AGAIN.

Main gate to Camp Crane, Pennsylvania

Medical Department: sixty-nine in the USAAS and twelve in the Sanitary Corps, the other new Medical Department corps.[35]

Inspector General Andrew was commissioned a major in the USAAS and assigned as head of its Motor Transport Department. Andrew delivered to the AEF a valuable asset in his American Field Service, a mature organization with its own vehicle assembly and repair facility, supply depot, training camp, recreation facilities, and hospital. Perhaps most important, the American Field Service had three years' experience in combined operations with the French Army. Enough volunteers joined the USAAS to form an immediate nucleus of 28 sections, including 25 sections from the American Field Service and 3 sections from Red Cross units. These sections, when deployed with the Allied forces, were detached from the AEF and came under the direct command of the French or Italian units to which they were attached.[36]

Initially, USAAS officers were active duty Medical Corps physicians. Col. Percy L. Jones, MC, headed the USAAS, and Col. Elbert E. Persons, MC, assumed command of the training base. Eventually physicians were replaced by nonphysician USAAS commissioned officers. In August 1917, as Medical Corps officers were being ordered into clinical duties, Colonel Persons submitted to the surgeon general a list of noncommissioned officers he recommended for commissions in the USAAS. By the end of the war there were very few Medical Corps officers left in the Ambulance Service. One who commanded an ambulance company said that physicians viewed being posted to an ambulance company with "almost as much distaste as assignment as a battalion surgeon."[37]

The twentieth century ambulance corps officers performed well. General Gorgas said they made "an excellent record"[38] and "in every way justified their appointment."[39] By 30 June 1918, the USAAS had 173 officers, including 1 colonel, 2 lieutenant colonels, 3 majors, 30 captains, and 137 lieutenants. In all, 224 officers and 11,750 enlisted personnel served in the USAAS during the war. Three of its officers received the Distinguished Service Cross and sixty-six were awarded the French Croix de Guerre. Seventeen sections were cited in French Army orders. No officers were killed or wounded, but 182 enlisted soldiers were killed in action or died of wounds and another 320 were wounded or gassed.[40]

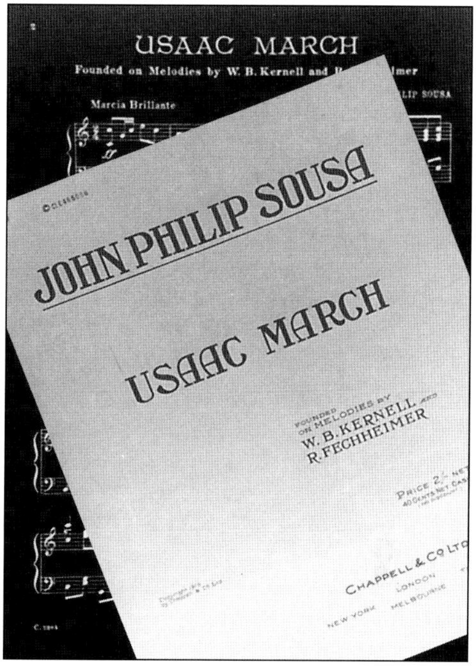

"USAAC March" sheet music

In the United States, USAAS recruits received their military training at Camp Crane, Allentown, Pennsylvania. Named for Brig. Gen. Charles H. Crane, surgeon general from 1882 to 1883, the camp occupied the Allentown fairgrounds, which also became the site of the USAAS headquarters. Recruits were billeted in available buildings, including horse barns, pig pens, and horse cooling sheds. Despite such makeshift quarters, the USAAS attracted the adventurous by offering the promise of quick and certain action in Europe. By 19 June 1917, over thirteen hundred volunteers were in training at Camp Crane; a week later, the number stood at thirty-three hundred. In all, 20,310 volunteers (2,085 officers and 18,225 enlisted) trained at Camp Crane between 1 June 1917 and 10 April 1919.[41]

Volunteers came from Army recruiting stations, predecessor volunteer ambulance units, and a variety of institutions and industrial organizations. Sponsors of USAAS sections included over forty universities and colleges. Harvard, which had led in the number of volunteers for the American Field Service, set another record by providing three USAAS sections. Other sponsors included corporations, cities, and sports groups.

The trainees were an exceptional group. Fifteen All-American football players among them became the nucleus of a team that played a winning season against a lineup that included Georgetown, Penn State, and Fordham. The camp band also attracted premier talent, and John Philip Sousa was among the guest conductors. Lt. Col. Clarence P. Franklin, MC, who succeeded Colonel Persons as the camp commander, convinced Sousa to write a march for the Army Ambulance "Corps," and the famous composer copyrighted the "USAAC March" in 1919.[42]

Not all the trainees had a grand time. To begin with, they found much to complain about with the food. Their arrival at Allentown "brought home to us for the first time the disturbing realization that we were in the army," with the moment of truth coming when they sat down to "one of the vilest suppers ever set before man since God made the world." The hungry soldiers were served a melange "on the same greasy tin pan, of salty corned beef and forlorn little prunes, mournfully swimming in their juice."[43]

Their transition into the life of a soldier was recorded in letters, diaries, and literature. In 1917 John Dos Passos returned from service in France with Norton-Harjes to find a draft notice awaiting him. Deciding to volunteer for the USAAS, he reported to Camp Crane. He later wrote of his "captivity" at "Syphilis Valley" where he said he had washed over a million windows.[44] His novel *Three Soldiers* was based on his experiences there and featured characters he encountered in training and later during his service in France.

Those who had volunteered to go "over there" were frustrated when the Army did not quickly ship them to Europe and became bored with repetitive tasks, such as marching day after day. Guth Station, a field training site complete with mud and trenches, was particularly vexsome. The grousing was reflected in the words to a marching ditty:

> Of course to drive an ambulance, you've got to learn to drill
> So every morning, afternoon they put us thru the mill,
> And when this war is over, you will find us at it still,
> For we never saw an ambulance and never, never will![45]

Over There

In time Camp Crane graduates did make it "over there." The first contingent arrived in France on 21 August 1917, commanded by Colonel Jones, who left Camp Crane to head up the USAAS in France from headquarters in Paris. There he had a strong deputy in A. Piatt Andrew, now a lieutenant colonel whose position as head of the Motor Transport Department placed him at the heart of the evacuation system. This, coupled with Andrew's experience in running the American Field Service organization, made him a central figure, and he served as the acting chief in Colonel Jones' absence. By July 1918 the USAAS had 77 sanitary squad units serving with the French Army; 49 units had been organized and trained at Camp Crane and added to the 28 units formed in Europe from the earlier volunteer organizations.[46]

The call of action in Europe also attracted Colonel Persons, who left Camp Crane to head up the USAAS units with the Italian Army. In June 1918 Persons took thirty units comprising 76 officers and 1,641 enlisted personnel to Italy where their arrival in Genoa was heralded by a parade with five marching bands. Colonel Franklin later left Camp Crane to join Persons as his deputy.[47] Not long after Persons' arrival in Italy, the AEF reassigned fifteen of his sections to American units in France as AEF losses mounted. Hard fighting during the St. Mihiel offensive had underscored the inadequacy of the AEF evacuation capability, which had less than 50 percent of its authorized ambulances, partly the result of shipping delays.[48]

USAAS officers and enlisted members continued in Europe the heritage of selfless dedication begun at Antietam. In France, Sanitary Squad Unit (SSU)

525, commanded by Lt. H. L. Biby, USAAS, received the French Croix de Guerre with Palm. Biby's unit had three soldiers killed and nineteen wounded or gassed in actions that included Verdun. SSU 503, commanded by Lt. Lars Potter, USAAS, received the Croix de Guerre with Silver Star for Bravery. SSU 585, an ambulance unit formed by Yale University, was commanded by Lt. John R. Abbot, USAAS, in its support of the French 128th Division. Abbot, praised by the members of his unit for "inspiring leadership"[49] and "guts,"[50] was wounded and decorated along with the other members of SSU 585 with the Croix de Guerre. One of the units that moved from Italy to France was the 649th Ambulance Section, which was attached to the U.S. 35th Division. Beginning 25 September 1918, the members of the 649th saw continuous action in the Meuse-Argonne where their twenty Ford ambulances evacuated over eight thousand wounded soldiers from the Argonne forest during a sixteen-day period, suffering eleven casualties in this action. Colonel Jones said the 649th reflected the USAAS spirit by "overcoming all obstacles in reaching the destination where the wounded are collected."[51]

The USAAS established a proud record. Pvt. George E. Shively, a member of SSU 585 who received the Distinguished Service Cross, said that their most fundamental principle was "the wounded *must* come in: difficulties and even impossibilities in the way form no excuse for failure. The impossible can be accomplished when men's lives are at stake." Their mission tested the courage of each ambulance driver. "If he chooses to shirk, there is no one to hinder; and if he himself falls, there is no one to help."[52] In Italy, USAAS crews were "often kept busy during day and night for long periods of time."[53] An example was SSU 526, whose commander, Capt. William A. Lackey, USAAS, was awarded the Italian Cross. Lackey's unit evacuated 29,852 patients during the Piave advance in June 1918.[54] Other USAAS crews met the challenges of combat in the rugged terrain of the Austrian front.

> The men would get three or four hours of sleep when we became completely exhausted and then would be right at it again. Driving the roads in wet or dry weather was a challenge in itself, with hairpin turns; but with a load of wounded and guns going off at their backs and in front of them, exhaustion would come upon them suddenly.[55]

As one participant put it: "An ambulance driver is nearly always in mortal danger."[56] Units operating on Mount Grappa would evacuate casualties to cable cars in which the patients were strapped and moved down the mountainside.

The USAAS benefited from lessons learned by the earlier volunteer organizations. For example, the ambulance bodies used by the American Field Service on the Ford chassis had evolved through trial and error. The USAAS eventually adopted that ambulance, but only after several thousand vehicles of inferior design were shipped to the AEF. One minor item that created a lot of difficulty for AEF units was the failure to adopt the American Field Service practice of adding oak tracks to the floor of the ambulances. Although standard U.S. Army litters had wooden legs, ambulance crews frequently encountered litters with iron legs, which tore up the vehicle floors unless they had been protected with the special tracks.[57]

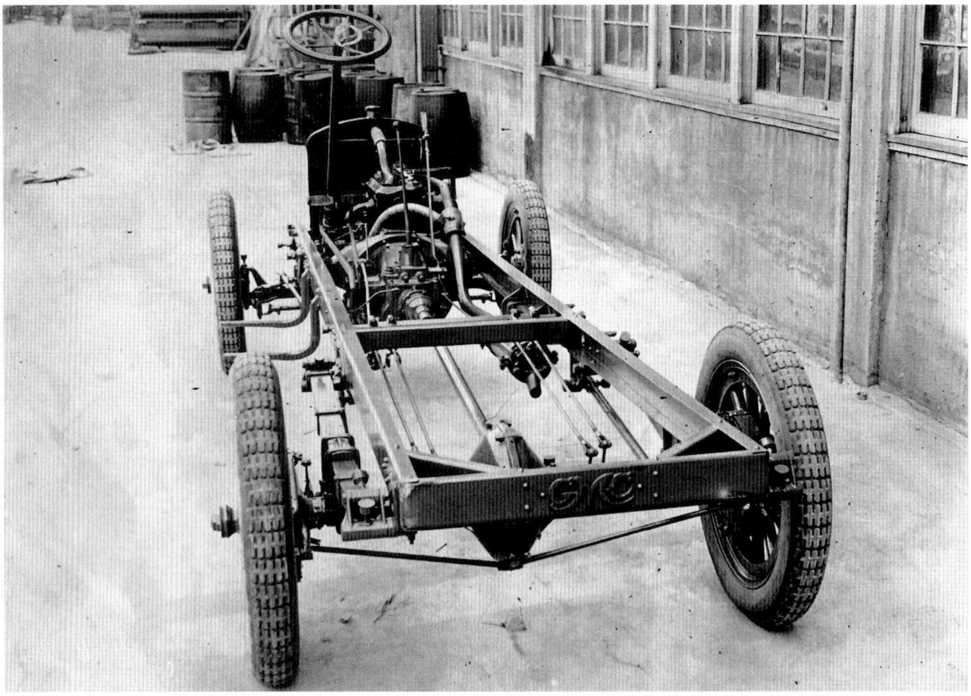

Standard General Motors ambulance chassis; below, *ambulance disassembled and boxed for shipment*

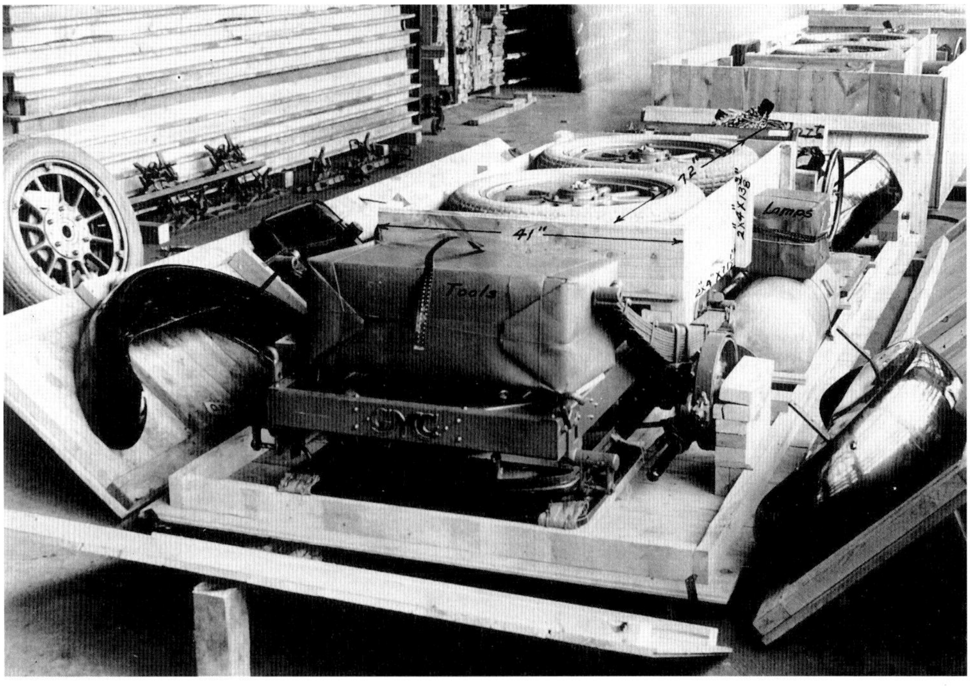

The requirement for a great number of vehicles caused the Medical Department to establish the Motor Ambulance Supply Depot in June 1917 at Louisville, Kentucky, to provide ambulance supply, repair, and salvage as well as a school for mechanics. Its staff included six Sanitary Corps officers. The department procured and shipped to Europe 3,070 GMC and 3,805 Ford ambulances. The vehicles were sent unassembled in two sections, the chassis and the body, because assembled vehicles were often damaged in transit. A motor ambulance assembly detachment of three Sanitary Corps officers and sixty technicians at St. Nazaire, France, prepared the ambulances for combat service. The detachment began assembling the vehicles at the rate of four per day in January 1918, a rate which later increased to fifteen per day.[58] In September 1918 the assembly functions and the Sanitary Corps officers involved with this mission were transferred to the Army's newly formed Motor Transportation Corps.[59]

The USAAS ambulance system settled into a mature operating capability that was fully integrated within the AEF organization. Its level of standardization as an operating system is reflected in guidelines used by the AEF inspector general for medical support operations in the combat zone. The condition of a medical unit's ambulances, the map-reading ability of enlisted and officer personnel, and the division surgeon's positioning of ambulance companies and field hospitals were all fair game for General Pershing's inspectors.[60]

Summary

American soldiers wounded in World War I enjoyed a much greater chance of surviving than had their predecessors in any previous war. Much of that was due to an improved evacuation system. By the time of the Armistice the Medical Department had evacuated 214,467 casualties in Europe and transported 14,000 sick and wounded to the United States.[61] It evacuated another 103,028 patients to the United States following the Armistice. This record was achieved through major Medical Department improvements, beginning with its doctrine for support of an army in the field. The medical support apparatus fielded by the American Expeditionary Forces was enormously improved in kind and amount from anything previously attempted in wartime.

The formation of the USAAS from predecessor volunteer ambulance organizations was a principal part of that improvement and was a significant step in the evolution of the Medical Service Corps. More important, it was a significant advance in the Medical Department's ability to perform its wartime mission through a functional adaptation to changing technology and warfare.

Notes

[1] Quoted words: Giulio Douhet, *Command of the Air*, trans. Dino Ferrari (New York: Coward-McCann, 1942), p. 157. C. S. Forester paints an indelible scene of the British commanding general at Verdun lighting his cigar at the moment the attack began: "As the tobacco flared a hundred and twenty thousand Englishmen were rising up from the shelter of their trenches and exposing their bodies to the lash of the German machine guns." Forester, *The General* (Boston: Little, Brown, 1936), p. 249.

[2] Statistics: Fielding H. Garrison, *Notes on the History of Military Medicine* (Washington, D.C.: Association of Military Surgeons of the United States, 1922), p. 199.

[3] Army figures: 50,510 battle deaths, 55,863 other deaths. Armed Forces Information Service, *Almanac, Defense 83* (Washington, D.C.: Government Printing Office, September 1983), p. 46. Casualty figures vary by source. For example, Col. Leonard P. Ayres, head of the Statistics Branch of the War Department General Staff, put Army and Marine deaths at 115,660: 57,460 disease; 50,280 battle; 7,920 other. *The War with Germany* (1919; reprint, New York: Arno Press, 1979), pp. 13, 123.

[4] Statistics: Theodore Ropp, *War in the Modern World* (New York: Collier Books, 1979), pp. 248, 250; John Keegan, *The Face of Battle* (New York: Penguin Books, 1978), pp. 235, 285. Keegan estimates one-third of the British soldiers killed or missing in action in the Battle of the Somme could possibly have survived if they had been evacuated within a few hours of wounding (ibid., p. 274).

[5] Gorgas: Gorgas had been appointed as the surgeon general and promoted to brigadier general in January 1914. In March 1915 he became the first chief of the Medical Department promoted to major general. George A. Scheirer, "Army Medical Department Chronology, 1775–1947," p. 45. Numbers: *SG Report*, 1919, 2: 1117. In 1918 there were 30,591 MC officers and 939 contract surgeons. SGO: Lynch, *The Surgeon General's Office*, p. 126; *Bulletin of the U.S. Army Medical Department* (October 1934): 4, a departmental journal known by various titles beginning in 1919 (see bibliographical note), hereafter cited as *Medical Bulletin* with date but without a volume number due to the number changes and restarts. The SGO numbered 2,103 at the peak: 265 officers, 30 nurses, 191 enlisted, and 1,617 civilian. U.S. physicians: "Medical Service in the World War," *Medical Bulletin* (31 May 1932): 2.

[6] Numbers: *SG Report*, 1919, 2: 1117.

[7] Disease: *SG Report*, 1918, pp. 172, 175; John H. Ruckman, ed., *Technology's War Record* (Cambridge: War Records Committee of the Alumni Association of the Massachusetts Institute of Technology, 1920), pp. 88–129; Garrison, *Notes on the History of Military Medicine*, p. 203; James S. Simmons, "The Division of Preventive Medicine, Office of the Surgeon General," *Medical Bulletin* (July 1941): 63–68; *Military Medical Manual*, 6th ed., rev. 1944 (Harrisburg, Pa.: Military Service Publishing Company, 1945), p. 346.

[8] Capability: Neuropsychiatry also posted advances. During the war the department developed a standard approach to shell shock—later called war neurosis—new names for the "depressed feeling" that Letterman had noted afflicted some soldiers. This consisted of treatment up front with a quick return to the soldier's unit after a brief period of rest, food, encouragement, and reassurance. Lynch, *The Surgeon General's Office*, p. 65; *SG Report*, 1917, p. 369; Letterman, *Medical Recollections*, p. 101. The World War I treatment would be relearned in subsequent wars as the best way of handling combat exhaustion, combat fatigue, combat stress reaction, or whatever term was in vogue at the moment.

[9] Quoted words: Edward E. Harding, "Norton-Harjes Section 60," in Virginia Spencer Carr, *Dos Passos: A Life* (New York: Doubleday, 1947), p. 133.

[10] Red Cross units: Lynch, *The Surgeon General's Office*, p. 546. Other American support included 1,100 American physicians called up for Army duty who were assigned to the British Expeditionary Force. See Bernard J. Gallagher, "A Yank in the B.E.F.," *American Heritage* 16 (June 1965): 18–26, 101–08.

[11] Hemingway: Carlos Baker, *Ernest Hemingway: A Life Story* (New York: Charles Scribner's Sons, 1919), pp. 36–50; Bernice Kert, *The Hemingway Women* (New York: W.W. Norton and Company, 1983), pp. 47–55, 218–19. Also see Michael S. Reynolds, *Hemingway's First War*

(Princeton, N.J.: Princeton University Press, 1976), pp. 147–49; and Reynolds, *The Young Hemingway* (London: Basil Blackwell, 1986), pp. 16–24, 55–57. Reynolds casts doubt upon Hemingway's commission.

[12] Hemingway: Hospitalized in Milan, he fell in love with Agnes Kurowsky, an American nurse who spurned his affections. In November he was promoted to first lieutenant; he returned to Chicago in January 1919 for recuperation. Hemingway's experience was the genesis of *A Farewell to Arms*. Ernest Hemingway, *A Farewell to Arms* (New York: Charles Scribner's Sons, 1929).

[13] Norton-Harjes: Carr, *Dos Passos*, pp. 117, 127, 138–39.

[14] American Field Service: Charles Lynch, Joseph H. Ford, and Frank W. Weed, *Field Operations*, vol. 8 of *The Medical Department of the United States Army in the World War* (Washington, D.C.: Government Printing Office, 1925), pp. 223–59, hereafter cited as Lynch, *Field Operations*; George Rock, *The History of the American Field Service, 1920–1955* (New York: American Field Service, 1956), pp. 7, 15, 24, hereafter cited as Rock, *History of the AFS*; Carr, *Dos Passos*, p. 127; American Field Service, *History of the American Field Service in France*, 3 vols. (New York: Houghton Mifflin, 1920), 1: 16, 23, hereafter cited as AFS, *AFS in France*; Edgar E. Hume, *The Medical Department Book of Merit* (Washington, D.C.: Association of Military Surgeons of the United States, 1925), p. 18.

[15] Quoted words: George C. Brown, ed., "With the Ambulance Service in France: The Wartime Letters of William Gorham Rice, Jr.," *Wisconsin Magazine of History* (Summer 1981): 279. Rice was an AFS volunteer whose father had been Grover Cleveland's private secretary when Cleveland was governor of New York. He wrote that Andrew "runs the service well," but never missed the chance to criticize the other volunteer ambulance units (p. 293).

[16] Quoted words: Andrew quoted in AFS, *AFS in France*, 1: 28–29.

[17] Vehicles: AFS, *AFS in France*, 1: 36, 391.

[18] Driving: Carr, *Dos Passos*, p. 132; AFS, *AFS in France*, 1: 511–12; John R. Smucker, Jr., *The History of the United States Army Ambulance Service with the French and Italian Armies, 1917, 1918, 1919* (Allentown, Pa.: USAAS Association, 1967), p. ix, hereafter cited as Smucker, *USAAS*.

[19] Escapades: Smucker, *USAAS*, p. xiv; Carr, *Dos Passos*, p. 132. Quoted words: AFS, *AFS in France*, 1: 449. They also learned from the courage of the French litter bearers, the "brancardiers." See Edward Weeks, *In Friendly Candor* (1946; reprint, Boston: Little, Brown, and Company, 1959), p. 6.

[20] Doctrine: The discussion of World War I doctrine is drawn from Lynch, *Field Operations*, pp. 105–259, 1021–67; FS School, *Sanitary Field Service*; Munson, *Sanitary Tactics*; and Frederick Paul Straub, *Medical Service in Campaign: A Handbook for Medical Officers in the Field* (Philadelphia: P. Blakiston's Sons, 1912).

[21] First killed in action: 1st Lt. William T. Fitzsimons, MC, and Pfcs. Rudolph Rubino, Jr., Oscar C. Tugo, and Leslie G. Woods were killed by aerial bombing at Base Hospital 5, 4 September 1917. *SG Report*, 1918, p. 261; American Battlefield Monuments Commission, *American Armies and Battlefields in Europe* (Washington, D.C.: Government Printing Office, 1938), p. 503.

[22] Medical capability: Lynch, *The Surgeon General's Office*, pp. 101, 327, 332; Frank Freidel, *Over There* (Boston: Little, Brown, 1964), p. 258; AEF Surg Gen to Commanding General (CG), Base Section #2, AEF, sub: Hospitalization Index of Medical Department Activities, 8th ed., 1 Dec 18, RG 120, Entry 588, File 321.6, NARA-NA.

[23] Training of AEF: Weigley, *History of the United States Army*, pp. 360, 385–86; John J. Pershing, *Final Report of Gen. John J. Pershing* (Washington, D.C.: Government Printing Office, 1919), pp. 5, 55, hereafter cited as Pershing, *Final Report*; Ayres, *War with Germany*, pp. 33–34.

[24] Ambulances: "All persons are prohibited from using them, or requiring or permitting them to be used for any other purpose." WD Reg 1437, WD, *War Department Regulations for the Army of the United States, 1913* (Washington, D.C.: Government Printing Office, 1913), with changes through 15 Apr 17, p. 289, PL.

[25] 305th Ambulance Company: Lynch, *Field Operations*, p. 563.

[26] 1911: Fisch and Wright, *Noncommissioned Officer Corps*, p. 78.

[27] Sanitary train: Pershing, *Final Report*, plate 15.

[28] Ambulance section: *SG Report*, 1917, p. 158; James L. Bevans, "The Ambulance Company," in FS School, *Sanitary Field Service*, pp. 4–9, 34. Advanced dressing stations were sometimes situated

1,500–2,000 yards from the front. 3d Division rate: Lynch, *Field Operations*, p. 109. Overall rate: Rpt, Maj Gen A.W. Brewster, AEF Inspector General (IG), sub: Report of Inspector General, American Expeditionary Forces, RG 120, E588, Box 115, File 525, Report of Inspector General, NARA-NA.

[29] Field hospital section: William N. Bispham, "The Field Hospital," in FS School, *Sanitary Field Service*, pp. 7–10; Lynch, *Field Operations*, p. 1034.

[30] Second echelon: Robert U. Patterson, "The Line of Communication Organization, Personnel, Materiel, Function and Administration," in FS School, *Sanitary Field Service*, p. 27; *SG Report*, 1919, 2: 1907.

[31] Doctrinal issue: There is fundamental doctrinal conflict between quickly clearing the battlefield versus conserving the fighting strength. The French gave primacy to the latter (and perhaps to a humanitarian impulse) by fielding a sophisticated surgical capability early in the evacuation chain. That option assumed greater survivability and faster return to duty through the earlier use of sophisticated treatment. However, it was elected at the expense of providing combat commanders a faster tempo of combat operations through a more quickly cleared battlefield and a smaller logistical tail in the forward area. The U.S. doctrine struck a good balance in World War I, handling the question with good sense and within the limits of the technology available at that time.The question remains an important one for the Army. For post-Vietnam discussion see Ronald F. Bellamy, "Contrasts in Combat Casualty Care," *Military Medicine* 150 (August 1985): 409–10, and Ltr, Bellamy to the ed., *Military Medicine* 151 (January 1986): 63–64; Karl D. Bzik and Bellamy, "A Note on Combat Casualty Statistics," *Military Medicine* 149 (April 1984): 229–31; Eran Dolev and Craig H. Llewellyn, "The Chain of Medical Responsibility in Battlefield Medicine," *Military Medicine* 150 (September 1985): 471–75. Bzik and Bellamy argue that "there are limits to what rapid evacuation can accomplish." Exceeding those limits in order to give first priority to clearing the battlefield leads to a policy of "scoop and run."

[32] Evacuation hospitals: Also see Gorgas, confidential report to Secretary of War (Sec War), *Inspection of Medical Services with American Expeditionary Forces* (Washington, D.C.: Government Printing Office, 1919), pp. 18–19, 46, hereafter cited as Gorgas, *Inspection of AEF Medical Services*.

[33] Evacuation: AFS, *AFS in France*, 1: 28–29.

[34] USAAS: AFS, *AFS in France*, 1: 10; Lynch, *The Surgeon General's Office*, p. 152; WDGOs 75 and 124, 23 Jun 17 and 20 Sep 17, PL; *SG Report*, 1918, pp. 268, 394; *SG Report*, 1919, 2: 1412.

[35] Integration into USAAS: AFS, *AFS in France*, pp. 1: 10, 30; Rock, *History of the AFS*, p. 22; *SG Report*, 1918, p. 268; Lynch, *Field Operations*, p. 238. A total of 784 were commissioned in various Army branches, including 578 in Infantry, Armor, Artillery, and Air Corps.

[36] Forming up: *SG Report*, 1918, p. 268; AFS, *AFS in France*, 3: 442.

[37] Substitution: Smucker, *USAAS*, pp. 12–20. Quoted words: Harry L. Smith, *Memoirs of an Ambulance Company Officer* (Rochester, Minn.: privately printed by Doomsday Press, 1940), p. 7.

[38] Quoted words: Gorgas, *Inspection of Medical Services*, p. 20. Gorgas inspected medical services in the AEF 8 September–16 October 1918.

[39] Quoted words: *SG Report*, 1919, 2: 1411–12.

[40] Numbers: *SG Report*, 1918, p. 394; *SG Report*, 1919, 2: llll; Smucker, *USAAS*, p. 77.

[41] Camp Crane: Smucker, *USAAS*, pp. xiv, 12, 33, 51, 79–148.

[42] Activities: Smucker, *USAAS*, pp. 25–27, 30–32. Some trainees formed an acting company, directed by Lt. Adolphe Menjou, and successfully toured the East Coast. Menjou became a movie star after the war. He costarred with Marlene Dietrich and Gary Cooper, among others, and appeared in such films as *A Star Is Born* and *A Farewell to Arms*. Sousa: Paul E. Bierley, Columbus, Ohio, to John Franklin, 12 Jun and 24 Jun 65; John R. Smucker, Wynnewood, Pa., to John Franklin, Philadelphia, Pa., 27 May 65 and 25 Jun 74; Mahlon H. Hellerich, Archivist, Lehigh County Historical Society, Allentown, Pa., to Smucker, 30 Aug 78, all in DASG-MS; John Philip Sousa, "USAAC March" (London: Chappell and Co., Ltd., 1919), photograph in Smucker, *USAAS*, p. 22.

[43] Quoted words: George J. Shively, ed., *Record of S.S.U. 585; Yale Ambulance Unit with the French Army, 1917–1919* (New York: E. L. Hildreth, 1920), p. 2, hereafter cited as Shively, *Record of S.S.U. 585*.

[44] Quoted words: Dos Passos to Arthur McComb, American Academy and Institute of Arts and Letters, 7 Oct 18, in Carr, *Dos Passos*, p. 156.

[45] Verse: Smucker, *USAAS*, p. 54.

[46] France: Lynch, *Field Operations*, p. 238; Smucker, *USAAS*, pp. 34–36, 44, 70, 112; *SG Report*, 1918, p. 268; *SG Report*, 1919, 2: 1419–23, 1485.

[47] Italy: Mrs. John Franklin, King of Prussia, Pa. (daughter-in-law of Clarence Franklin), to Ginn, 17 Jul 88, with encl, DASG-MS; Smucker, *USAAS*, pp. 57, 70–71.

[48] Redeployment: *SG Report*, 1919, 2: 1485; Smucker, *USAAS*, pp. 30–31, 50–51, 55–56; Inspector General (IG), Services of Supply (SOS), AEF, to IG, AEF, sub: Conditions in SOS, 26 Jul 18, DASG-MS. The units moved to France on 24 August 1918.

[49] Lt. Biby: Smucker, *USAAS*, p. 89; Lt. Potter, ibid., p. 81. Quoted words: Shively, *Record of S.S.U. 585*, p. 15. Abbot reported to the division surgeon ("médecin divisionnaire"), Lt. Col. Lejonne. Abbot's account of that relationship provides insight into the motivation of the American volunteers, as he complimented Lejonne for "dauntless energy," "unflinching devotion to duty," and for being a fearless officer whose "first thought was always for the comfort of his wounded." Ibid., p. 90.

[50] Quoted words: Guy Emerson Bowerman, Jr., *The Compensation of War: The Diary of an Ambulance Driver During the Great War*, ed. Mark C. Carnes (Austin: University of Texas Press, 1983), p. 122. SSU 585 was particularly well documented in having two accounts, Shively's and Bowerman's.

[51] Quoted words: *SG Report*, 1919, 2: 1419.

[52] Quoted words: Shively, *Record of S.S.U. 585*, p. 33.

[53] Quoted words: Smucker, *USAAS*, p. 56.

[54] Sanitary Squad Unit 526: Smucker, *USAAS*, p. 118.

[55] Quoted words: Smucker, *USAAS*, pp. 56–57.

[56] Quoted words: Smith, *Memoirs of an Ambulance Company Officer*, p. 47.

[57] Lessons learned: AFS, *AFS in France*, 1: 35–36.

[58] Ambulance depot: *SG Report*, 1918, p. 325. Assembly detachment: *SG Report*, 1919, 2: 1360–62. "Probably no organization ever arrived in France better equipped" (ibid., p. 1361).

[59] Transfer to Transportation Corps: *SG Report*, 1918, p. 325.

[60] IG: AEF IG to Inspectors, sub: Points for Consideration of Inspectors Concerning Operations of 4th Section, General Staff (checklist), 22 Jul 18, DASG-MS.

[61] Numbers: Pershing, *Final Report*, p. 77.

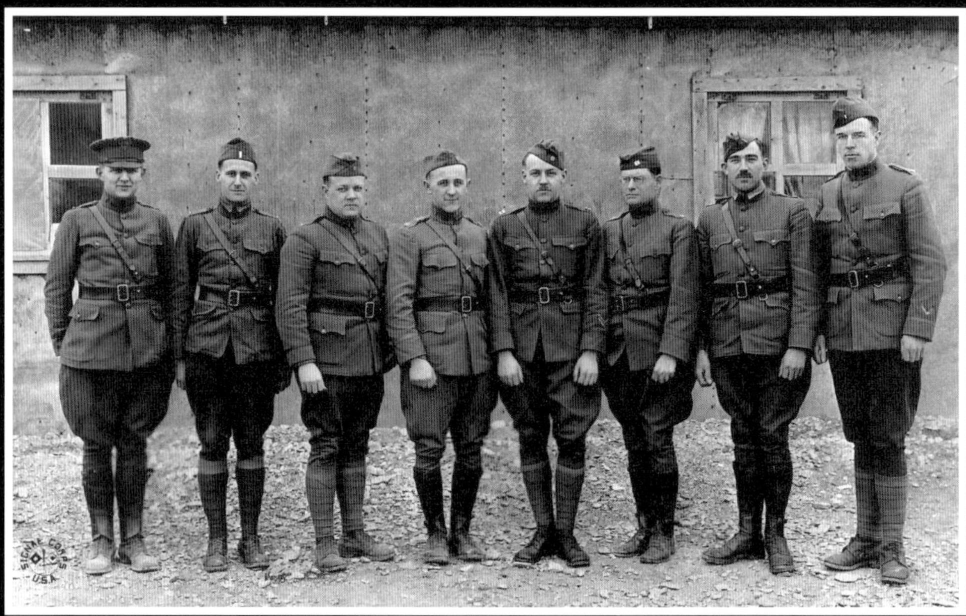

Sanitary Corps officers in Is-sur-Tille, France, February 1919

3

World War I
The Sanitary Corps

Upon assuming office in January 1914, Surgeon General William C. Gorgas initiated planning for what he believed would be the eventual U.S. participation in the war. His experiences in Cuba and Panama led him to support the establishment of a corps to provide the administrative and scientific specialists necessary for the military medical team. By spring 1916 Gorgas regularly testified before Congress, interspersing his testimony with excerpts from the proceedings of the French Chamber of Deputies on military medical lessons the French had learned. He noted the difficulty created by an insufficient number of military physicians and the burdening of that group with administrative responsibilities "which hamper and delay them in the performance of their regular tasks."[1] Gorgas described steps the French had taken to remove those responsibilities from military physicians, to the extent that in the first year of the war the French medical department had nearly twenty-five hundred administrative officers and twenty-five hundred apothecaries.[2]

Establishment of such a corps in the U.S. Army had to wait until entry of the United States into the war. Then General Gorgas' ability to put together an expanded medical support team for the Army was greatly advanced by War Department General Orders No. 80, 30 June 1917, which created an important precursor of the Medical Service Corps. Called the Sanitary Corps "for want of a better name,"[3] the organization enrolled newly commissioned officers with "special skills in sanitation, sanitary engineering, in bacteriology, or other sciences related to sanitation and preventive medicine, or who possess other knowledge of special advantage to the Medical Department."[4] The officer strength was set at a maximum of 1 per 1,000 total Army active duty strength, and the grades were initially capped at major. The order also provided for 3,905 enlisted personnel in grades from private to hospital sergeant.[5]

Just as the USAAS provided the Medical Department with nonphysician commissioned specialists for the benefit of the French and Italian armies, the Sanitary Corps did the same for the U.S. Army. This corps gave the department the capability to capitalize on new technology in a rich diversity of units with missions ranging from surgical instrument repair to cinematography. Maj. Gen. Merritte W. Ireland, Gorgas' successor as surgeon general, wrote that the corps "assisted notably" in the Medical Department's wartime performance.[6] In fact, the principal Medical Department wartime accomplishments cited in an account authorized by Secretary of War Newton D. Baker were those made possible by Sanitary Corps officers.[7]

TABLE 1—SANITARY CORPS OFFICERS BY SPECIALTY AREA AND GRADE ON ACTIVE DUTY 1 NOVEMBER 1918

	COL	LTC	MAJ	CPT	1LT	2LT	Total
Sanitation	1	2	9	79	81	41	213
Food and Nutrition		1	8	35	36	36	116
Laboratory			7	166	174	164	511
Venereal Disease			14	28	28		70
Psychology		1	17	31	31	28	108
Aviation (Psychology)			5	32	38	14	89
Finance and Supply			28	183	202	169	582
Reconstruction		1	14	29	54	52	150
X-Ray			1	1	23	3	28
Overseas			1	244	198	200	643
Hospitals			2	90	93	88	273
Miscellaneous			5	18	17	7	47
Total	1	5	111	936	975	802	2,830*

Based on Inclosures to Letter, The Surgeon General to The Adjutant General, sub.: Estimate of Department's Needs, 15 November 1918, MSC-USACMH.

*Peak strength of 2,919 was reached on 15 November 1918. *Surgeon General Report* 1919, II: 1112.

Growth of the corps was rapid. By 30 June 1917, there were 9 officers on active duty—2 majors, 4 captains, and 3 first lieutenants. A year later there were 1,345 officers—a number that included 3 lieutenant colonels and 42 majors—serving in such diverse roles as sanitary engineers, gas defense chemists, bacteriologists, psychologists, and medical supply officers. The corps reached its peak strength of 2,919 officers in November 1918 (*see Table 1 for a statistical summary*). By then it represented 7 percent of the officers in the AEF, and if the war had continued the department planned for 6,433 officers. Ranks remained relatively low. The corps included only two colonels and five lieutenant colonels, a parsimonious allotment that must have pleased the manpower planners.[8]

William D. Wrightson, the sanitary engineer who had served on Gorgas' staff in Panama, was commissioned as a major and assigned to the Surgeon General's Office on 31 July 1917. Wrightson was the first officer appointed in the Sanitary Corps, and he served as its de facto chief, signing correspondence as "the officer in charge of the Sanitary Corps."[9] Division chiefs in the Surgeon General's Office were responsible for the placement of officers in their specialty areas throughout the Army, but personnel matters affecting Sanitary Corps officers were coordinated with Wrightson.[10] He was promoted to lieutenant colonel in February 1918 and to colonel that August.[11]

One issue that came to his attention was General Gorgas' desire to commission qualified Hospital Corps sergeants in the Sanitary Corps. The surgeon general feared that the Medical Department would lose the expertise of its noncommissioned officers, who would seek appointments as line officers because they were blocked from serving as officers in the Medical Department.[12] Believing that the lack of opportunity demoralized them, he sought authority to commission them in the Sanitary Corps. The War Department granted his request and, at the same time, removed the grade limitation of major.[13]

In practice, one glitch remained. War Department policy required the transfer of newly commissioned officers to another unit. The effect of that rule was to dissuade hospital commanders from recommending their best soldiers since they knew they would lose them. One wrote the surgeon general that he had a shortage of qualified personnel to fill important administrative positions and was entirely dependent upon enlisted personnel with civilian experience. He was reluctant to recommend sergeants for appointment in the Sanitary Corps for fear of losing them. An example was his records administrator, an attorney in civilian life, who if commissioned would make an ideal registrar or personnel officer. But the transfer policy remained unchanged, despite entreaties by Gorgas.[14]

Administrative Specialty Officers

Because the Medical Department needed managers, Sanitary Corps officers were used in administrative roles to a much greater degree than suggested by the name of the corps. A shortage of physicians in combat units often caused the substitution of Sanitary Corps officers or, in some cases, line officers. As one report put it, physicians "had become too scarce to serve in drawing rations and clothing."[15] As in the scientific specialties, advances in the new science of management were producing demands for officer specialties in the Medical Department for which physicians were not prepared by their medical training. The Surgeon General's Office was determined to have enough managers at each hospital to free up physicians for the practice of medicine.[16] Consequently, Sanitary Corps officers filled a variety of positions formerly occupied by Medical Corps officers, such as registrar, adjutant, personnel officer, mess officer, medical property officer, and commanders of various medical units and patient detachments.

The process of substituting Sanitary Corps officers in administrative positions was not hasty. Quartermaster Corps officers were initially available for detail to the Medical Department, which lessened the urgency at the beginning. They performed duties in disbursing, medical supply, motor transport, laundry, and facilities management. Furthermore, the department's ability to draft physicians and its customary use of physicians in administrative roles mitigated against substitution. There was some debate over the proper utilization of Sanitary Corps officers, a reflection of underlying tension. Lt. Col. Alfred P. Upshur, MC, a hospital commander, wrote that Sanitary Corps officers could profitably serve in all the contemplated positions except adjutant. He said that that position, which was important for its broad managerial responsibilities, should be filled by a physician "for the same reasons that the commanding officer of a hospital is a medical officer."[17]

Indeed, as American involvement in the war began, the Medical Department increased the training of medical officers in administration. It began a special course in 1917 to train physicians for duty as adjutants.[18] However, that course was dropped in the spring of 1918 as the weight of converging events pushed the department into utilizing Sanitary Corps officers as adjutants and in other administrative duties. The situation became increasingly acute as more American forces entered combat and mounting casualty loads challenged the AEF medical treatment capability. The surgeon general's requests to increase the number of Sanitary Corps officers cited the need to release physicians for clinical duties.[19] In May 1918 the War Department authorized an increase of Sanitary Corps officers, stipulating that they would be used by the department in order to release physicians for "strictly professional work." The Medical Department accepted applicants for commissioning from all walks of life and also sought to commission sergeants with experience as chief clerk, mess sergeant, or registrar assistant. In short, change came about under the pressure of events and despite the misgivings of many medical officers. The pressure continued until the end of the war, which found a continuing shortage of physicians in both hospitals and divisional medical units, while the number of Sanitary Corps officers continued to expand.[20]

Among its members were experts in many arts. The success of Sanitary Corps officers in administrative positions was reflected in the Distinguished Service Medal awarded to Lt. Col. Robert A. Dickson, SnC.[21] Dickson, who entered the Navy in 1898, was a master hospital sergeant when he was commissioned in the Sanitary Corps. He was cited by the AEF for his work as head of the Chief Surgeon's Administrative Division. An especially irritating problem when the AEF first deployed to France was the absence of an effective postal service. All mail to Medical Department personnel was addressed to the chief surgeon, and Dickson had 10,000 letters on his hands by the time the matter was resolved.[22]

The characters in Joseph Heller's World War II novel *Catch 22* include Lt. Milo Minderbender, an engaging huckster who cornered the Egyptian cotton crop and, when the market collapsed, coated the cotton in chocolate and tried to sell it to the troops as cotton candy.[23] The Sanitary Corps had its own Milo Minderbender in Capt. Fred Pumphrey, SnC, who headed the Paris office of the postwar American Polish Typhus Relief Expedition as it set up operations in 1919.

Pumphrey funneled supplies and equipment to the expedition's Warsaw headquarters in a manner described as "scrambling, scrounging, cadging, wheedling, quarreling, and politicking." Pumphrey himself wrote that "with all my trickery around here I have spent endless hours in doing little favors for different parties that count in return favors being given." Pumphrey's spirited performance greatly pleased the expedition's commander, Col. Harry L. Gilchrist, MC, who said his "energetic action and hard work succeeded against colossal difficulties" in getting the humanitarian effort under way.[24]

Medical Logistics

Medical logistics was a major area of responsibility for Sanitary Corps officers. Gorgas had testified to Congress that providing medical logistics support for an army numbering in the millions would be "exceedingly difficult."[25] The AEF surgeon said a principal lesson learned from previous wars had been the necessity for "a well organized supply division in the Chief Surgeon's office, with single and absolute control."[26] Strong central supply organizations were established in the Surgeon General's Office and in the headquarters of the AEF. Sanitary Corps officers played important roles in their development.

Medical logistics quickly expanded in complexity and scope. Congress initially appropriated $1 million for medical supplies and equipment for fiscal year 1918, but by the end of the year it had appropriated nearly $174 million, and almost $300 million was appropriated in fiscal year 1919. A medical supply inventory of $1 million in 1916 increased a hundredfold by 1917.[27] This rapid expansion outpaced the department's staffing capability since it depended upon physicians to fill its key positions. The AEF chief surgeon reported a "great lack of personnel trained in Medical Department supply work,"[28] and in 1918 the surgeon general reported difficulty in fielding the necessary number of medical supply officers. The Sanitary Corps provided the department the means to meet the requirement—a challenging undertaking since those officers had to be recruited, commissioned, and posted at the various training camps before the medical supplies and equipment arrived. By the end of the war 331 Sanitary Corps officers were serving with the Medical Department's Supply Service, a number that included 288 former enlisted personnel. Only sixteen physicians were so employed at that point.[29]

The newly commissioned Sanitary Corps officers took charge. As might be expected, the medical supply buildup was not flawless. Both supplies and supply officers had to be in place before the troops arrived, but that did not always work out as planned, and frequently supplies were shipped to camps before buildings were ready for their storage. The medical supply officers improvised storage in farm buildings, in the open, or under canvas. Since they were the only Medical Department representatives on site, their responsibility for those precious items often meant they were on 24-hour duty until the camp became better established. They set up medical property accounts for issue and storage, medical supply issue for camps and divisions, and procedures for supply requisitions and accountability, and they undertook the supervision and training of supply personnel. Originally it was thought that one supply officer at a camp could serve as both the hospital property officer and the divisional supply officer, but this proved to be a poor system. The usual pattern became two medical supply officers, one for the base hospital and one for the division.[30]

At the beginning of the war the department's principal medical depots were in New York, St. Louis, San Antonio, Washington, D.C., and San Francisco. During the war depots were added at Atlanta, Philadelphia, Chicago, and Louisville. The expansion increased the need for officers competent in depot management. Experienced noncommissioned officers with medical supply experience were prime candidates and were selected for appointment in the Sanitary Corps on the basis of their performance at supply schools in Newport News, Virginia; Camp Meade, Maryland; and Camp Upton, New York. The Newport News school organized thirteen medical depot companies of three Sanitary Corps officers and forty-five enlisted soldiers each. Eight were shipped to France; one went to Liverpool, England; and another went to Vladivostok, Russia.[31]

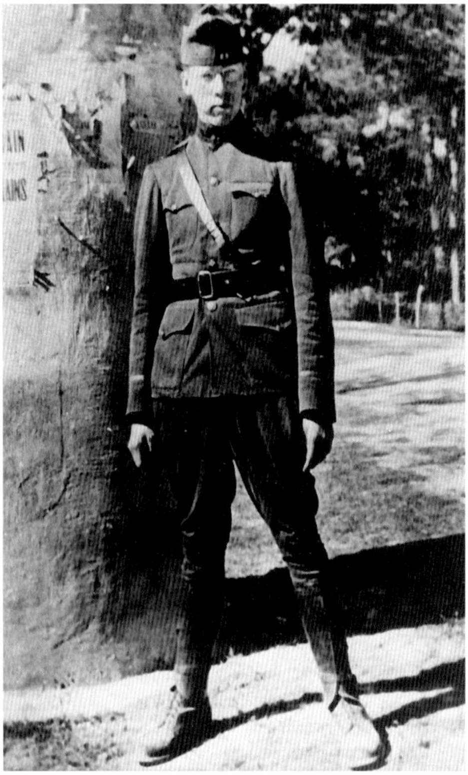

Captain Pilling

The Medical Department commissioned Sanitary Corps officers for medical logistics specialties from the best applicants it could find in manufacturing, jobbing, and wholesaling. Procurement was an area of particular emphasis, especially since Germany was dominant in the optical and surgical instrument industries. Fifty Sanitary Corps officers served as "expeditors" who assisted contractors in meeting their requirements. The department sought industrial assistance from experts—especially jewelers and toolmakers—in retooling for the manufacture of surgical instruments, and Sanitary Corps officers performed inspections of newly converted factories.[32] Hospital Corps sergeants commissioned in the Sanitary Corps as medical logistics officers provided special talents and experience. One was Capt. Oscar Burkard, SnC, who served as the medical supply officer at Camp Upton, New York. A veteran of long service, Burkard wore the last Medal of Honor awarded in the Indian Wars.[33]

Medical logistics specialties also included x-ray and medical equipment maintenance. The Surgical Instrument and Repair Service in Neuilly, France, headed by Capt. Henry N. Pilling, SnC, developed a fabrication capability for surgical instruments as well as the ability to fit artificial eyes and to repair typewriters. The shop assembled mobile field x-ray units by equipping Renault trucks with x-ray equipment and electrical generators. The equipment saw service in the Chateau-Thierry defense and the offense at St. Mihiel and in the final Argonne offensive.[34]

Medical maintenance soldiers played a starring role on the night of 11 November 1918, Armistice Day, when they drove one of the x-ray trucks, festooned with lights and a bevy of French ladies, down the full length of Paris' jam-packed Grand Boulevard des Italiens. (By one account, this was the only vehicle that made it all the way down the boulevard that night.) A threat of court-martial for the miscreants was later dropped, as was another for their subsequent feat of driving a five-ton Packard truck up the steps of the Paris Opera the next day.[35]

Resources Management

An Act of 26 September 1917 established new requirements for the auditing of military accounts. To meet them, the Surgeon General's Finance and Supply

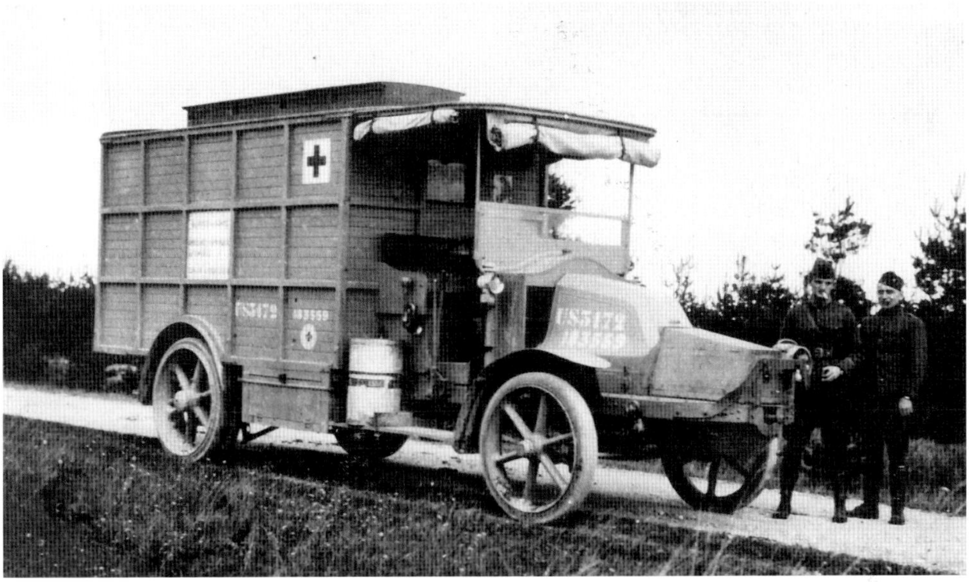

Renault truck outfitted with mobile x-ray equipment

Division initiated contacts with the banking industry as well as with insurance, railroad, and retail sales firms. It endeavored to identify executives for commissioning in the Sanitary Corps who had volunteered for military service or who had been drafted and were about to be inducted in the Army. The department had to work quickly because it was unable to transfer already-inducted soldiers from their assigned units.

A Medical Department finance contingent headed by Lt. Col. W. D. Whitcomb, SnC, arrived in France in January 1918 to form the AEF Surgeon's Accounting Division. Whitcomb's operation, which numbered 7 Sanitary Corps officers, 135 enlisted soldiers, and 15 French civilians, was responsible for auditing and disbursing funds for the purchase of medical supplies and equipment. By April 1919 the division had disbursed over $37 million since arriving in Europe. It was recognized for its wartime performance by the War Department's assistant auditor and the comptroller of the treasury.[36]

Hospital Administration

The expanding use of Sanitary Corps officers was also representative of changes occurring in hospital administration. The twentieth century saw the hospital become the central institution in American health care. There were an estimated 178 American hospitals in 1873; by 1914 there were 5,047. Advances in medical technology propelled a dramatic expansion in the ability of such institutions to treat and cure (rather than merely to house) their patients. At one time charitable institutions for strangers and the poor, hospitals became centers of community health catering to the middle class.[37]

Medicine—and the modern hospitals it required—was evolving into a prestigious field of endeavor, a transformation that was accompanied by an institutional revolution in American medical schools. Proprietary diploma mills closed all over the country in the early twentieth century, under attack from medical scientists housed in universities and the American Medical Association's Council on Medical Education. Ten schools closed in 1907 when the council began rating medical schools, and another ten closed in 1910 when the council issued its second report, at which point American medical schools were more advanced than they had ever been. The movement was given popular currency by the 1910 Flexner Report, which made instant headlines by describing the nation's medical schools, sometimes in scathing detail. By 1915 there were 96 medical schools, down from 160 in 1905, but those that survived were of much higher quality.[38]

Pressure for progressive medical education contributed to the demand for better hospitals. The American College of Surgeons (ACS) was formed in 1913 to advance the practice of surgery in the United States. The college desired to set standards for surgical training and practice, and it elected to survey American hospitals in order to identify those that could support good quality training programs. The ACS findings were distressing. Many hospitals, including some of the most prestigious American institutions, maintained no patient records and had no laboratory, x-ray, or other necessary diagnostic or treatment facilities. Only 13 percent of the 692 hospitals could meet the most simple requirements in 1918, the year of its first formal survey. The ACS leadership considered its list of approved hospitals so inflammatory that it was burned.[39]

The evolution of hospitals led to a requirement for their professional management. At that point the background of most American hospital administrators was principally medicine (nearly all male) and nursing and religious orders (predominantly female). The customary pattern in the United States was larger hospitals directed by physicians, middle-size facilities headed by members of the laity, and smaller hospitals headed by nurses. There were no formal training programs, and hospital administrators learned their profession on the job.[40] As one observer put it, most had been "pitch forked into their position without special training."[41]

The increasing complexity of hospitals and the influence of external pressures also affected the management of Army hospitals. During the war the administrative positions in Army hospitals, except that of commander, were filled by Sanitary Corps officers. The Medical Department wrote into its tables of organization a permanent requirement for five administrative officers in 500-bed hospitals—commanding officer, adjutant, registrar, quartermaster, and mess officer—along with a skeletal working organization that was added to as needed for expansion. The increasing sophistication of hospital design also led to the assignment of thirteen Sanitary Corps officers to the Hospital Construction Section of the Surgeon General's Office. Their responsibilities included design of hospitals, field design of building modifications, review of new requests, and administrative management of the projects.[42]

Patient Administration

In Army hospitals medical records maintenance and biostatistical reporting were performed by registrars. Emphasis by the American College of Surgeons on accurate medical records as a measure of quality of care catapulted the function to greater significance. In a similar fashion, biostatistics became increasingly important, and the Medical Department developed into a national resource in the compilation of epidemiological data.

Talented Sanitary Corps officers such as Maj. Charles B. Davenport made important contributions to patient administration. Davenport, a Harvard Ph.D. anthropologist and an internationally recognized statistician, had been the director of the Department of Genetics of the Carnegie Institute, Washington, D.C. He was instrumental in preparing the 1918 *Report of the Surgeon General*, a document of particular significance due to his analysis of disease conditions in the training camps. Another member of the Surgeon General's Medical Records Section, 2d Lt. Louis R. Sullivan, SnC, compiled the Medical Department's World War I data into 156 sections based upon twenty-two occupation and ethnic groups drawn from the 1910 census of the U.S. population. In Europe, 1st Lt. Robert H. Delafield, SnC, was assigned to the Office of the AEF Chief Surgeon where he provided medical records expertise for the expeditionary forces.[43]

Major Davenport also coauthored *Defects in Drafted Men*, which documented the results of the physical examinations of two million draftees plus another five hundred thousand men who were rejected by the draft boards. This study accounted for 60 percent of all men examined for the draft and was a significant sample of the United States male population between the ages of eighteen and thirty. Glendon H. Armstrong, SnC, a second lieutenant, was recognized for compiling the study data with electric sorting and tabulating machines; his work was part of the department's pioneering use of mechanical computing equipment. The report provided new if sometimes inexplicable insights into U.S. demographics. For example, the study found that 28 percent of those drafted were rejected because of physical impairment. As another example, epidemiologists were intrigued by its documentation of a low cancer rate in recruits from mountainous regions.[44]

Scientific Specialty Officers

Sanitary Corps scientific specialty officers were essential for the Medical Department's war against typhus and other communicable diseases. Officers who ran sanitation teams and rat extermination programs provided contributions that in their beneficial effects outpaced those of some of their more illustrious coworkers. The commissioning of these officers was another reflection of General Gorgas' keen interest in the prevention of disease and his understanding of the need for a complete team to achieve that goal.[45]

The deadly potential of communicable disease was clearly evident from the first days of the war. Although beginning in 1909 French and American biologists had identified the body louse as the vector for typhus, that knowledge by itself did not prevent the most intense epidemic of typhus in history from devastating

Serbia in 1915. Fear of the raging epidemic shut down Austria's opening attack against that country, and the Central Powers lost six months' initiative. Hans Zinsser concluded that "typhus may not have won the war but it certainly helped."[46] The American doughboys who later marched into Europe with the AEF were free from the threat of typhus. They went "over there" with the advantage of efforts by Sanitary Corps officers to systematically apply preventive medicine techniques across the range of militarily significant diseases.[47]

The Army's preventive medicine effort held the number of deaths from disease to 51,417 of the total 106,378 deaths during the war. The improvement was greatly attributable to Medical Department doctrine, which had moved preventive medicine to the forefront of its responsibilities. By 1912 the Army had said the military physician's first task was to instruct the command "in the elements of personal and camp hygiene."[48]

The lessons of the previous century, especially the preventive medicine failures of the Spanish-American War, were capitalized upon as the Army established a sanitation capability in training camps prior to the arrival of troops. This time the surgeon general did not "rest on his circular"; rather, the Medical Department was credited with being ubiquitous. General Gorgas set the example by personally inspecting all training camps to see that sanitation and hygiene standards were being enforced. He extended the same vigilance to Army hospitals; for example, he insisted that his medical inspectors eat unannounced at the hospitals they visited so as to sample the food served to patients.

Commanders at all levels were prodded by surgeons and inspectors general into paying attention to conditions that would affect the health of their commands. Preventive measures included establishment of water purification units and sewage treatment plants, construction of proper latrines and bathing facilities, removal of animal manure, regulation of kitchens and food preparation, fielding of rat extermination programs, and inspection of farms and dairies to ensure wholesome and disease-free food sources. There were systematic programs in malarious regions to drain and oil marshy areas near the training camps to prevent malaria, and soldiers returning from frontline duty in the trenches were subjected to delousing to prevent the spread of typhus. Preventive medicine efforts also included dramatic measures for the prevention of venereal disease.

Special efforts were also made to control flies and fly breeding. Indeed, a measure of the changed attitude was in the emphasis on eradication of the common fly, which was no longer viewed as a harmless plaything for children. In previous wars those insects had not been worthy of discussion, but in World War I "there was probably no other subject which received as much comment from sanitary inspectors of the Surgeon General's office as did the fly situation in our military stations at home." Sanitary Corps officers were important members of the medical team that prosecuted all of these initiatives that made such a difference in World War I.[49]

Sanitary Engineering

Sanitary engineers were a significant addition to the medical team. They augmented the department's capability with officers who were specialists in water purification, mosquito control, housing, ventilation, sewage and waste disposal, and control of flies. Competition for appointment as Sanitary Corps officers was keen because of the opportunity for commissioned status as well as the exercise of one's professional skills. Those who succeeded were assigned to the training camps to perform preventive medicine functions. The newly commissioned officers attended a one- to two-month course at the Medical Officers Training Camp, Camp Greenleaf, Chickamauga Park, Georgia.[50] Among them was 1st Lt. Joseph A. Tinsman, a sanitary engineer, who was the only Sanitary Corps officer to die from wounds in the war. Tinsman, a native of Harrisburg, Pennsylvania, had been an assistant engineer with the Pennsylvania Department of Health. Assigned to a water supply company, he was wounded on 4 November 1918 during the Meuse-Argonne offensive. He died six days after the Armistice.[51]

Efforts to establish sanitation capability at the training camps were initially hampered by camp design and construction policies that had been established before the Army had sanitary engineers to advise on those plans. Obtaining good waste disposal equipment was a problem raised to the attention of the secretary of war. Sanitary engineer officers found that failures in sewage disposal plants were caused by grease content much higher in camp sewage than in ordinary municipal sewage, and they led efforts to design new incinerators and treatment plants.[52]

In addition, sanitary engineers developed improved water supply operations. Although the Corps of Engineers was charged with the responsibility for water supply points, the Medical Department was responsible for the quality of water produced and the proper functioning of the purification systems that provided coagulation, sedimentation, and sterilization. This required special expertise for, as the surgeon general put it, "water purification plants and sewage plants were not simple mechanical efforts to be operated by men without professional skill."[53] By the end of the war approximately one hundred fifty AEF water plants were supervised by Sanitary Corps officers. Capt. A. Sidney Behrman, SnC, in July 1918 took a Sterilab mobile water purification unit to the front during the Chateau-Thierry offensive, the first such unit operated with American troops in an American sector.[54]

Sanitary engineering functions evolved to the point that in 1918 the surgeon general published a circular to formalize those duties. Sanitary engineers at large camps were charged with supervision of water purification and waste disposal systems, mosquito and fly control measures, consulting with camp surgeons on all engineering or structural aspects related to health and sanitation, and monthly reporting to the surgeon general. They served in sanitation detachments, division sanitary squads, survey parties, water tank trains, water supply companies, and overseas laboratories; as camp sanitary engineers; and as instructors at Camp Greenleaf, Georgia. The Medical Department was authorized 129 sanitary engineers by May 1918.[55]

The efforts to prevent disease through vigorous sanitation efforts in the stateside training camps were mirrored in the preventive medicine measures taken overseas, where the AEF encountered sanitation difficulties. French towns were afflicted with polluted water, and manure, the highly valued fertilizer of the French peasant, was "piled high in front of nearly every house." Pershing attached

2 sanitary squads to each division—each consisting of 1 officer, 4 noncommissioned officers, 20 privates, and 2 drivers—plus 1 mobile laboratory consisting of 1 officer and 5 enlisted personnel. Initially the squads were headed by physicians, but when possible they were replaced by Sanitary Corps sanitary engineers. One of those officers was 1st Lt. Ira V. Hisock, SnC. Hisock, an instructor in the Yale University School of Public Health, had enlisted in the Army. His division surgeon, discovering a talented private, got Hisock commissioned and placed in command of the 28th Sanitary Squad, then attached to his division.[56] The preventive medicine efforts of Lieutenant Hisock and his fellow officers paid off. "The manure was removed, the mud disappeared from the streets, water was chlorinated, prophylactic stations established, proper latrines made, kitchens regulated, baths established, in fact the machine was in motion, with errors of course, but moving and functioning well."[57]

Entomology

There was no provision for commissioning entomologists, and this was a handicap for the World War I medical team. Perez Simmons, an entomologist who enlisted for service with the Engineer Corps, wrote that the absence of this preventive medicine capability resulted in an epidemic of severe dysentery in his area of southwestern France during the summer of 1918. Simmons believed that the presence of commissioned entomologists would have prevented much of the suffering his unit endured.

Simmons was assigned to an engineer company engaged in 24-hour forestry operations to provide the AEF with lumber and railroad ties. The area was plagued by flies caused by the unit's poor sanitation practices; the soldiers had to eat with one hand while brushing away the flies with the other. Simmons' attempts to get action by the company commander were rejected, and although the regiment's leaders were periodically visited by inspectors, they "made hurried inspections, gave a little advice and usually praise, and departed." It was Simmons' conviction that commissioned entomologists would have been able to prod his command into doing something and possibly preventing the tragedy that ensued. In June nearly the entire company came down with dysentery, and the soldiers were still in a weakened condition when an influenza epidemic attacked several weeks later. Nine of Simmons' comrades died.[58]

X-Ray

Lt. Jerome Jeffrey, an x-ray equipment expert, was representative of the new scientific specialties provided by the Sanitary Corps. By the end of the war twenty-eight Sanitary Corps officers were serving in x-ray positions in the Surgeon General's Office, Medical Department schools and supply depots, and the AEF. Those officers directed technicians in installing, operating, and maintaining x-ray equipment; served with physicians as instructors in the x-ray schools; and provided the AEF's radiological capability in fixed and field locations.[59]

Maj. J. S. Schearer, SnC, a Cornell University professor of physics and electronics (radiology), established the Army x-ray school at Cornell, which trained physicians and technicians for the Medical Department. Experts in x-ray instal-

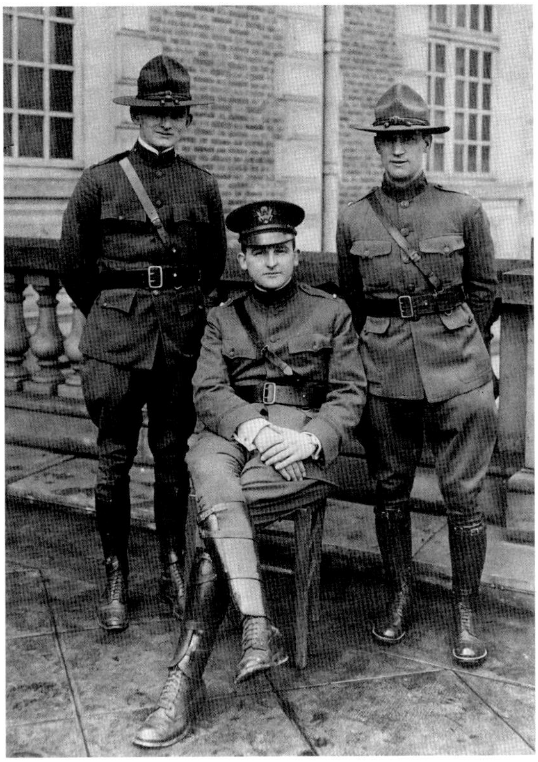

Lieutenant Jeffrey, standing at left; below, *technical staff and instructors at the Cornell School of Roentgenology in 1917. Major Shearer is seated; Lieutenant Jeffrey is at left; Lieutenant Noel is second from right.*

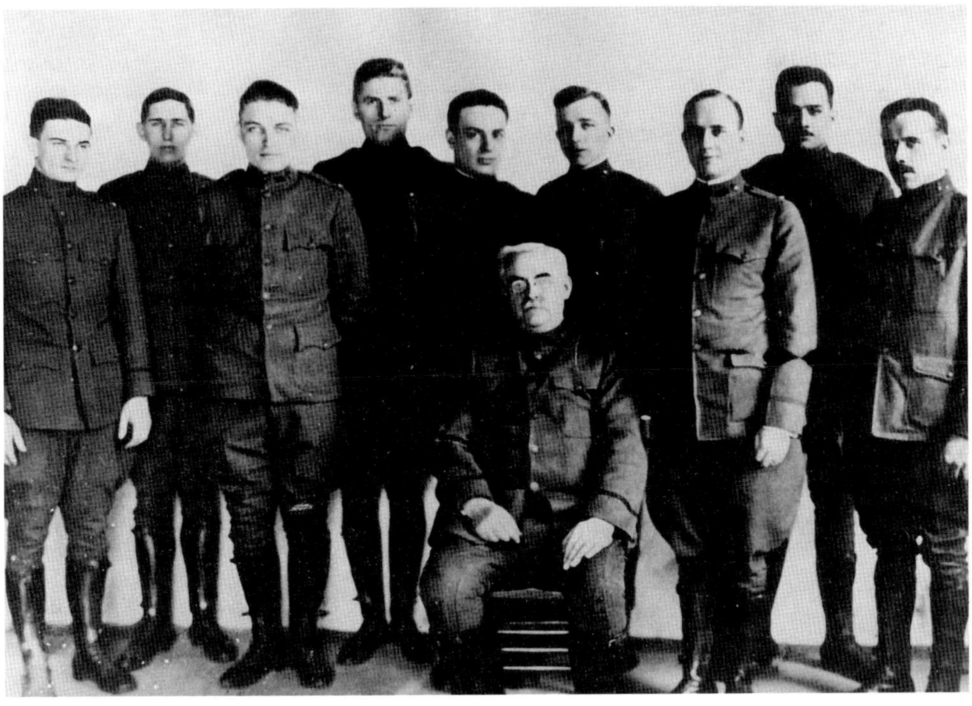

lation and repair were commissioned in the Sanitary Corps and provided a short course at the school prior to their utilization in the field. Officers at the school, with the advice and assistance of leading roentgenologists, developed an x-ray field apparatus as well as a visual scale for fluoroscopy radiation exposure that protected physicians and patients from severe radiation burns. Major Schearer developed a bedside x-ray unit that was used extensively during the war and for thousands of chest x-rays during the flu epidemic of 1918. One of his students, Lt. Victor A. Noel, SnC, became the medical equipment director for the Ritter Corporation after the war.[60]

Laboratory Specialties

Plans to draft physicians with medical laboratory qualifications proved unrealistic. The Medical Department discovered that even if it were able to identify those who were qualified, their number would be insufficient to its needs. Instead, the Sanitary Corps enabled the department to meet its requirement for laboratory specialties by commissioning scientists who were already trained in laboratory procedures or enlisted technicians who were qualified by experience and training.

Parasitologists, chemists, and bacteriologists from universities and state departments of health were offered direct commissions in the Sanitary Corps, where they performed a large number of laboratory procedures, including tests for meningoccus, diphtheria, pneumonia, meningitis, tuberculosis, and infection by hemolytic streptococcus as well as routine urinalysis, blood counts, malaria tests, blood cultures, and preparation of urethral smears for the diagnosis of venereal disease. Some operated rat extermination programs. The laboratory officers made significant contributions. For example, two parasitologists, Maj. Charles A. Kofoid, SnC, and Maj. Marshall A. Barber, SnC, developed a hookworm test considered more than twice as efficient as previous methods. Kofoid said that while 11 percent of the soldiers tested by the Army for hookworm were shown to be infected, he believed the rate would have been 25–50 percent if a better test had been used.[61]

The officers attended laboratory training courses at the Rockefeller Institute in New York City; Yale University, New Haven, Connecticut; the Army Medical School (later renamed the Walter Reed Army Institute of Research), Washington, D.C.; and the Sanitary Field Service School at Fort Leavenworth, Kansas. Sanitary Corps laboratory officers and Medical Corps physicians were paired together for the program at Fort Leavenworth. Some enlisted graduates of the training programs at those schools were also commissioned in the Sanitary Corps. Of the 413 enlisted graduates in 1918, 30 were commissioned under that program.[62]

Sanitary Corps officers served as instructors in the schools. For example, Capt. Donald D. Van Slyke, SnC, and Capt. C. S. Robinson, SnC, conducted a biochemistry training program at the Rockefeller Institute for chemistry graduate students and young faculty members from the various universities who were themselves candidates for Sanitary Corps commissions. Sanitary Corps officers also taught at the Yale University laboratory school, which trained 237 Sanitary Corps officers from 1 August 1918 to 1 January 1919, and at the Fort Leavenworth school, which trained a smaller number. Col. Michael Blew, SnC,

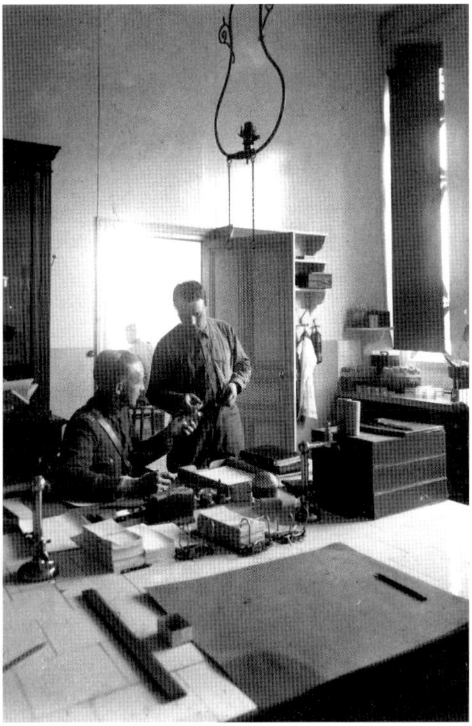

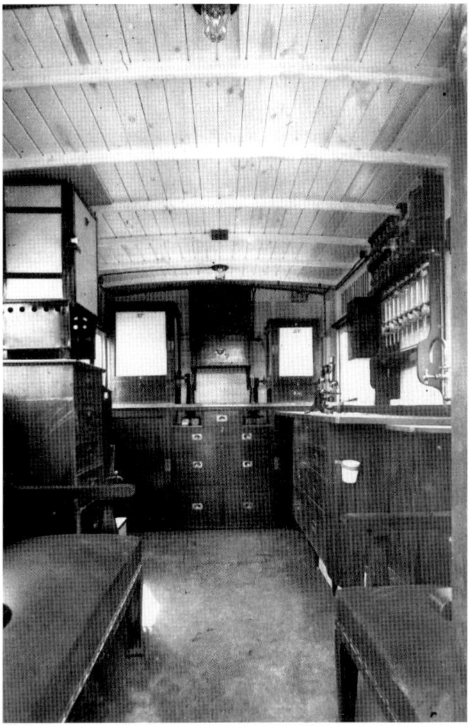

Bacteriological department in Dijon, France; right, *interior view of field laboratory car, with exterior shown below*

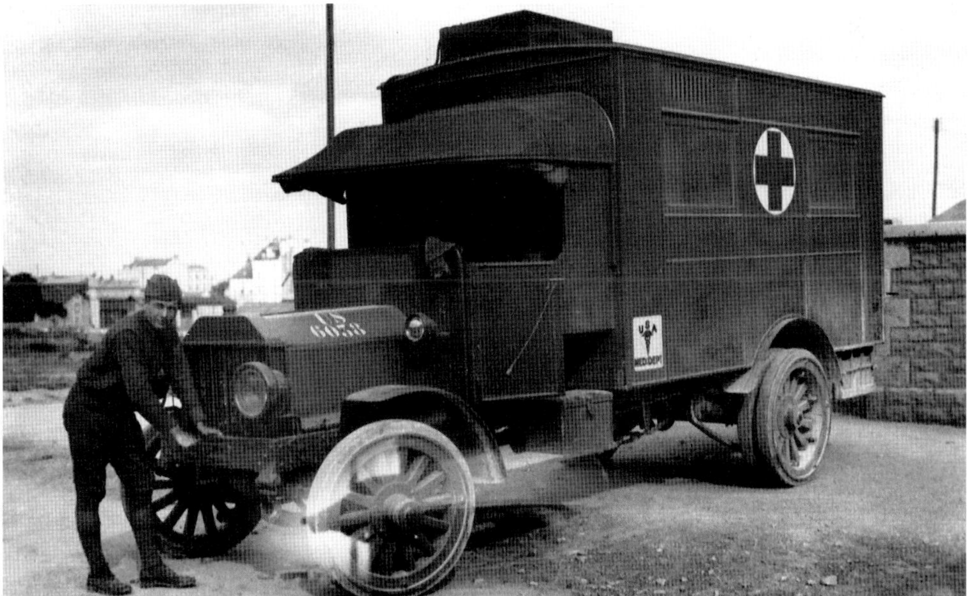

said his training at Fort Leavenworth included an hour daily for equitation, because horsemanship was considered essential for officers. Blew found it of little value in his wartime service. "I got to France, and the only thing I ever rode was a motorcycle sidecar in the mud, but we had to take equitation."[63]

The Fort Leavenworth school organized thirteen mobile laboratories, each headed by a Medical Corps officer whose staff included one Sanitary Corps officer and three to four enlisted soldiers. The mobile laboratories were innovations in medical support. Formed at the request of the AEF surgeon, they represented the first use of a laboratory capability as part of combat forces. They were part of the division-level medical support teams, where they provided an ability for chemical and bacteriological examination of water and urethral smears and the preparation of cultures for examination by fixed laboratories. Thirty-one mobile laboratories were operational by the end of the war and another nineteen were being organized.[64]

Physical Reconstruction

The war produced a distressingly large number of disabled soldiers. A Senate report estimated in January 1918 that there were thirteen million wounded and crippled soldiers among the European belligerents, including three million amputees, and Congress recognized that as United States forces entered combat they would incur a correspondingly high number of veterans who would need rehabilitation. However, no single U.S. government agency was tasked with the overall responsibility for the well-being of disabled veterans. Rather, there was a patchwork of veterans' benefits. As a solution, Congress tasked the Army and the Navy with providing medical care in cooperation with a newly formed Federal Board of Education, the forerunner of the Veterans Administration. The surgeon general organized a Division of Physical Reconstruction to direct vocational rehabilitation programs for disabled soldiers at twenty-seven Army hospitals. In May 1918 the War Department authorized 24 Sanitary Corps "educational officers" for this function, a number that increased to 119 in July. Those officers conducted special workshops, assisted in reconstruction therapy, instructed vocational courses, and assisted the mental and physical reconstruction efforts of the medical team.[65]

Maj. Bird T. Baldwin, SnC, was formerly a Harvard professor of educational psychology and an authority in child development and psychology. In April 1918 Baldwin was appointed as chief psychologist at Walter Reed General Hospital where he became the director of rehabilitation of disabled soldiers. There he developed a pioneering occupational therapy program in coordination with the psychological, medical, x-ray, and surgical services. It involved a variety of "curative shops" that enrolled one to three thousand patients monthly from October 1918 to March 1919. Baldwin published a monograph as a protocol for other hospitals to follow in developing their own programs.[66]

Nutrition

John R. Murlin, Ph.D., an assistant professor of physiology at Cornell University Medical School, unable to obtain an appointment in the Medical

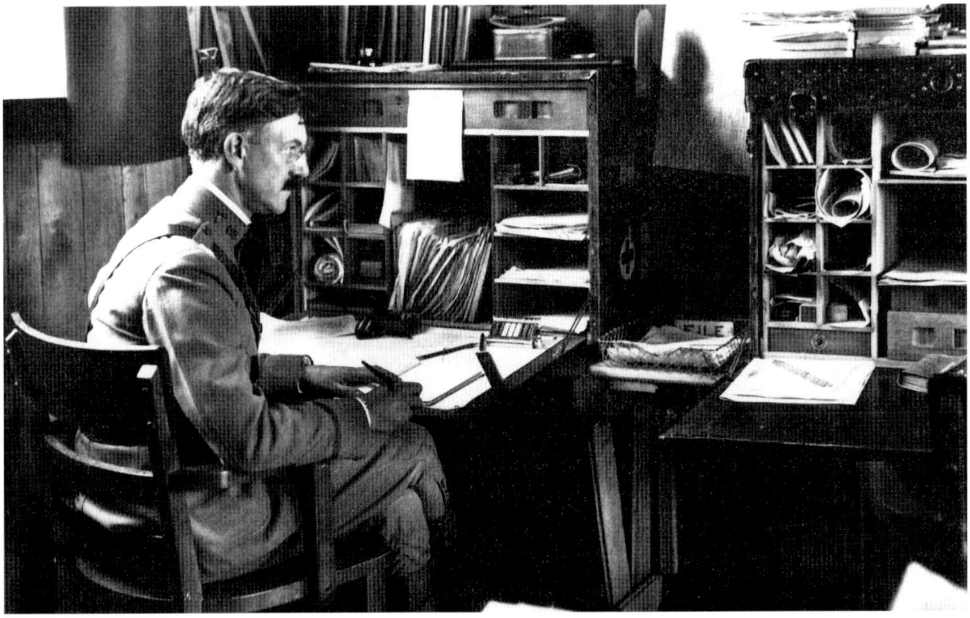

Sanitary Corps food expert in his office in Dijon, France

Department because he was not a physician, went to the Officers Training Camp at Plattsburg, New York, to be commissioned as a Quartermaster Corps officer. There he volunteered to assist the mess officer, an infantry officer inundated with complaints about the poor quality and wastage of food. Murlin's work convinced him of the need for nutritional surveys of Army camps, an idea which he recommended to Alonzo Taylor, Ph.D., the expert adviser to Herbert Hoover, the head of the U.S. Food Administration. Hoover saw Murlin's report and contacted General Gorgas, who, impressed with Murlin's work, offered him a commission as a major in the Sanitary Corps. Major Murlin was made head of the newly established Food and Nutrition Division in the Surgeon General's Office.

Murlin, Gorgas, Hoover, and other advisers hammered out a plan for teams of Sanitary Corps officers who would conduct nutritional surveys at Army camps. Murlin canvassed universities, medical schools, and agricultural stations for nutritionists, who were offered commissions in the Sanitary Corps. They conducted a pioneering program of surveys throughout the United States, beginning in October at Camp Crane, Allentown, Pennsylvania.[67] Murlin's program was particularly useful for the training his teams provided for cooks, mess sergeants, and mess officers as the Army moved toward a nutritionally sufficient ration for soldiers rather than just "filling the cavity."[68] Their efforts advanced the nutritional status of the Army even though some of the basic chemical and physiological processes were not understood.[69]

Maj. Samuel P. Prescott, SnC, a Massachusetts Institute of Technology (MIT) nutritionist, conducted a one-week course for nutrition officers at MIT in which the officers were instructed in the methods of preservation, handling, and inspection of various foods. The course later relocated to Camp Greenleaf, Georgia. In all, 116 Sanitary Corps officers served as nutrition officers. Their duties included advising commanders, quartermasters, and unit surgeons on the composition and nutritive value of foods, conducting nutritional surveys, inspecting food, assisting at the cooks and bakers schools, and assisting in coordinating mess requirements with subsistence supplies.[70]

One inspection of a nongovernmental source of food was considered newsworthy. The *Stars and Stripes* reported in 1918 that a raspberry drink sold to the troops as Bill's Bug Juice "was found to be all that its name implies."[71]

Psychology and Physiology

Sanitary Corps psychologists made important contributions in World War I. Robert M. Yerkes, Ph.D., professor of psychology at Harvard and president of the American Psychological Association, began to organize American psychologists to assist the War Department immediately upon the U.S. declaration of war. Under Yerkes' leadership they conducted demonstration trials in October and November 1917, using tests they developed in coordination with the American Psychological Association and the Psychology Committee of the National Research Council. With General Gorgas' support, Yerkes was commissioned as a major in the Sanitary Corps in August 1918 and was appointed chief of the newly formed Division of Psychology in the Surgeon General's Office. Yerkes and his assistant, Maj. Harold C. Bingham, SnC, recruited a talented team of officers. Capt. Edwin G. Boring, SnC, was one; he later became the Edgar Pierce Professor of Psychology at Harvard. Another was Maj. Louis M. Terman, SnC, who developed the Stanford version of the Binet-Simon intelligence test. The pioneering psychologists met resistance from the Army line as they introduced the use of psychological services in the Army. There was also resistance from within the Medical Department, even though Gorgas supported the initiatives.[72]

Yerkes' cause was not made easier by intelligence tests the Sanitary Corps psychologists conducted at four training camps. Those reports showed that physicians, dentists, and veterinarians had the lowest intelligence scores of 5,500 Army officers tested in the early trials. The alarming results reflected the still-evolving condition of U.S. medical training and the imperfect selection methods of the Medical Department. Col. Henry A. Shaw, MC, a medical inspector, at Gorgas' request gave a special report to the surgeon general on the test results. Shaw confirmed the findings as an accurate representation of the state of affairs and recommended immediate action to weed out undesirables from the Medical Corps.[73]

Using the early trials as their guide, beginning in the fall of 1917 Sanitary Corps psychologists conducted the first large-scale use of psychological testing as a method of screening Army inductees for mental ability. It was a watershed in the development and acceptance of intelligence testing in the United States. The department tested over 1.7 million inductees, including 41,000 officers. Based on those tests, the Army immediately discharged 7,800 soldiers, sent 10,014 to labor battalions, and placed 9,487 in development battalions. This was the first intelligence survey of a major portion of the American population. The Sanitary Corps officers discovered that draft boards had conscripted some soldiers with a mental age as low as four years. About 30 percent of the recruits were unable to read a newspaper or write a letter home.[74]

The department initially appointed sixteen psychologists as Sanitary Corps officers and provided temporary appointments in the civil service for another twenty-four; over one hundred officers were commissioned for this purpose during the war. They attended the School for Military Psychology at Camp Greenleaf, Georgia, headed by Capt. William S. Foster, SnC. There they received basic officer instruction in addition to training in psychological testing. The department established a psychology staff of four officers and six civilians at each of four installations: Camp Lee, Virginia; Camp Devens, Massachusetts; Camp Dix, New Jersey; and Camp Taylor, Kentucky.[75]

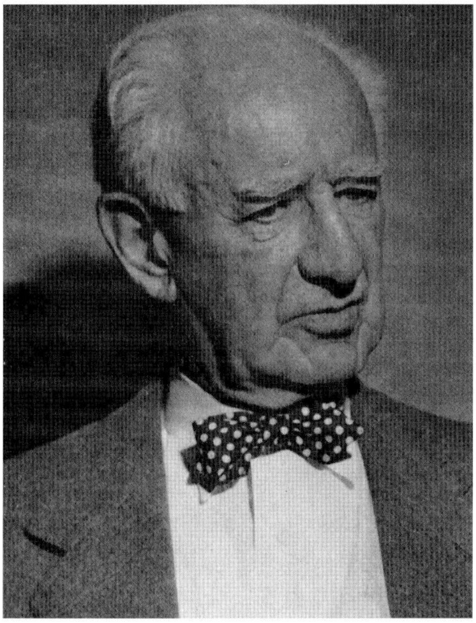

Professor Yerkes, later in life

The Army found the tests were useful in identifying the mentally incompetent, classifying recruits by mental capability, and selecting soldiers for specialties. The testing program refined its capability in order to identify soldiers with intellectual deficiencies for assignment to development battalions, to select soldiers for military and civilian schools, and to group training sections by ability. The psychology staffs at the Army training camps increased their proficiency to the point where they could test 2,000 soldiers a day and report the results within twenty-four hours. By July 1918, 79 Sanitary Corps officers were conducting screening tests at 28 camps and 3 general hospitals, a number which had increased by November to 97 officers at 33 camps.[76]

Sanitary Corps psychologists and physiologists also contributed to the development of Army aviation. Airships and airplanes were part of the new technology in World War I. Airplanes had become sufficiently sophisticated to perform aerial reconnaissance, close air support of ground forces, and bombing missions, and there were experiments during the war with "hospital ships," airplanes, typically JN–4 "Jennies," modified as air ambulances to carry one litter patient. Sanitary Corps officers and other Medical Department personnel assigned to the Medical Division of the Signal Corps Aviation Section headed *de facto* a separate medical department supporting Army aviation. There they contributed to the emerging field of aviation medicine.[77]

A desire to establish scientific methods of selecting aviation applicants resulted in the establishment of the Army's Medical Research Board. The board requested the immediate appointment of thirty-one Sanitary Corps physiologists and psychologists in 1917 to develop aviator classification standards and screen-

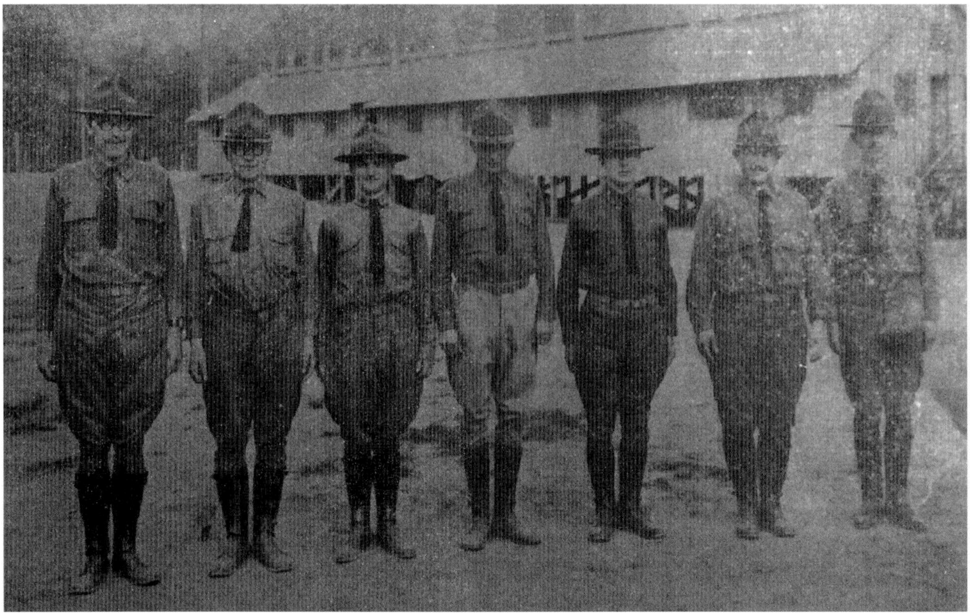

Staff of the School of Military Psychology, 1918. Captain Foster is at left.

ing tests. Maj. John B. Watson, SnC, organized the examining boards. The resulting program provided the Army with a means of selecting suitable candidates for flight training as well as for specialized training in pursuit bombers and night bombers and as artillery observers. The War Department used those tests to screen applicants at sixty-seven special examining stations around the country. Sadly, as much as the Army publicized its scientific methods, it never did fully dispel the notion that the examinations were actually a form of refined torture. One popular version had it that applicants were hit over the head with a mallet. Those who regained consciousness within fifteen seconds were considered "the stuff of which aviators are made" and accepted.[78]

The Medical Research Board established the Medical Research Laboratory at Hazlehurst Field, Mineola, Long Island, to investigate conditions affecting aviator performance. Maj. Edward C. Schneider, SnC, and Maj. Knight Dunlap, SnC, headed the physiology and psychology departments, respectively. Their first priority was to develop a test that would measure the ability of aviators to endure partial asphyxiation, an important question in a day of primitive oxygen breathing devices and before the advent of pressurized cabins. The investigators had little to go on initially, and their findings led to further research on general aviator performance and fatigue.[79]

In June 1918 the Medical Research Board asked for another 69 psychology and physiology officers. Colonel Wrightson supported that request and raised the ante to 140 officers, and later raised it to 199. Wrightson argued that the department had found it necessary to follow up initial screening with periodic examinations in order to detect "physical and temperamental deterioration" since 75 percent of aviation accidents were caused by pilots flying "when they are not in the pink of condition."[80]

Sanitary Corps physiologists and psychologists were members of the AEF Air Medical Research Laboratory, which went to France at the request of General Pershing in September 1918.[81] There, physiologists who had been instrumental in determining selection criteria for aviator training at the Mineola Laboratory were key figures in evaluating aviator performance once on active flying status. Edward Schneider, transferred from Mineola and promoted to lieutenant colonel, served as the physiology representative on the five-member medical research board that oversaw the aviation medicine research effort in the AEF. Schneider wrote the physiology chapter of the board's final report. Physiologists continued to concentrate on the effects of high altitude upon performance, using a rebreathing apparatus to test the ability of aviators to withstand oxygen deprivation. In addition, they evaluated a number of tests for physical efficiency as well as overall hygiene factors that would help flight surgeons determine aviator fatigue and general fitness. They devoted considerable attention to developing guidelines for the use of oxygen.[82] The work of the physiologists was complemented by psychologists who conducted psychometric tests to evaluate aviator performance. Capt. Floyd C. Dockeray, SnC, who earned his wings in France and the coveted rating of Reserve Military Aviator (RMA), authored the report's chapter on psychology. Together, those Sanitary Corps officers were valued members of the aviation medical team that reduced the number of accidents and increased the morale of aviators.[83]

Several issues had emerged by the end of the war that would form the basis for future trends. Both psychology and physiology had been demonstrated as disciplines necessary for the medical team. Yerkes proposed adding psychologists to infantry divisions, which would be the first use of psychologists in the forward combat area. He also proposed a mental health team concept of psychologists and psychiatrists. Both of those ideas would have to wait for their day to come. There was also a dispute brewing as the Medical Department resisted efforts by the line to transfer the psychological testing function (and the psychologists who did it) away from the Medical Department.[84]

Gas Defense

The first use of poison gas in World War I was by the Germans at Ypres in 1915. The Allies followed suit, and gas soon became a widely used weapon. The United States manufactured 10,000 tons of chemical weapons, much of which was sold to the French and British, but defensive measures by the combatants blunted much of the weapons' effectiveness. In the United States, initial disarray in offensive and defensive chemical warfare was resolved in a decision by the secretary of war in May 1917 directing the Medical Department to assume responsibility for the development and production of gas masks and goggles. The surgeon general established the Division of Gas Defense to carry out this mission, with an authorization for 154 Sanitary Corps officers, which was eventually headed by Lt. Col. Dewey Bradley, SnC. Maj. Knight Dunlap, SnC, developed a test for determining the effects of different types of masks on soldier performance as part of the division's efforts. Those responsibilities included development and acquisition of chemical sprayers for decontaminating trenches and oxygen apparatuses for resuscitation of gas victims.[85]

The Army's director of the Gas Service was charged with coordinating the multiple agencies—including the Medical Department—involved with chemical warfare, but without central authority. It was a confusing setup, which the director of the AEF Gas Service dismissed as "exceedingly embarrassing, cumbersome and inefficient." In a move contested by the Medical Department, the War Department transferred the Division of Gas Defense and its 294 Sanitary Corps officers to the reorganized Chemical Warfare Service in June 1918 as it placed all authority for chemical warfare under one head. There they performed the gas defense mission as members of the organization that was the forerunner to the Army Chemical Corps.[86]

The expertise of Sanitary Corps officers in decontamination made them natural candidates for another mission as the AEF went to war with the body louse. Some reports at the end of the war estimated that more than 90 percent of the soldiers were "lousy." The AEF Degassing Service was reorganized into the Bathing and Delousing Division, and its twenty Sanitary Corps officers set up a theater-wide organization. In all, 315 officers and over 3,000 soldiers operated delousing points within the divisions plus delousing plants at each embarkation point, which were capable of delousing 10,000 soldiers in twenty-four hours. The process consisted of bathing and disinfecting. The division used a variety of equipment including 6 large plant sterilizers, 68 stationary steam sterilizers, 283 horse-drawn sterilizers, and 583 improvised steam sterilizers. The division processed 11.3 million soldiers and 25 million articles of clothing.[87]

Venereal Disease Control

Sanitary Corps officers took part in an intensive venereal disease control program. Raymond B. Fosdick, assistant to the secretary of war, headed the Army's Commission on Training Camp Activities, whose programs included measures to provide recreation services for soldiers. The commission's Law Enforcement Division enforced provisions of the Military Draft Act that gave the president authority to establish prostitution-free zones around military installations. Forty Sanitary Corps officers, mostly lawyers commissioned as lieutenants, conducted those enforcement activities. Their efforts were complemented by commissioned officers of the U.S. Public Health Service who had targeted the cantonment areas as public health hazards.[88]

By November 1918 seventy Sanitary Corps officers were assigned to the venereal disease program. A magazine article that month proclaimed that the Army had reduced the venereal disease rate by 50 percent. It said American soldiers were "the cleanest set of fighting men in the world."[89] Unfortunately, the truth was that at that moment the AEF was experiencing the highest rate since deploying to Europe.[90]

After the Armistice Maj. Bascom Johnson, SnC, formerly counsel for the American Social Hygiene Association, and fifteen other Sanitary Corps officers went to France to serve as advisers to the AEF for its venereal disease control program. General Pershing had requested this assistance since the United States policy of total prohibition was at variance with the French policy of licensing houses of prostitution. All officers and enlisted soldiers were examined for venereal disease prior to their return to the United States. Those who were infected were restricted to "segregation camps" where detained officers and noncommissioned officers served as cadre. The large number held back required the AEF to organize a provisional regiment of six battalions. This in turn generated support requirements, and the Segregation Camp Hospital opened in June 1919 with a staff that included a Sanitary Corps officer as registrar.[91]

Photography

Photography, especially motion pictures, was another good example of new technologies provided to the Medical Department by the Sanitary Corps. In November 1917 Lt. Thomas L. W. Evans, SnC, formerly head of a New York photography firm, organized the Instruction Laboratory at the Army Medical Museum, Washington, D.C. His organization included a Motion Picture Section, initially headed by Lt. Robert Ross, SnC. Ross, as a major, took Museum Unit #1, a still and motion picture team, to France.[92]

Ross was replaced in Washington by Lt. Charles W. Wallach, SnC, who produced a thirty-minute film on venereal disease, *Fit To Fight*, which caused quite a stir at the Rotary International Convention in June 1918. The film was later a national source of controversy when local Rotary clubs sponsored showings, "usually for men and boys over 16."[93] (Sixty-five years later the Army Staff exhibited a nice touch of amnesia when it used the same title for an Army physical fitness program.)

Pharmacy, Chiropody, and Optometry

In 1916 the War Department had authorized the advancement of pharmacists to hospital sergeant and master hospital sergeant. Pharmacists continued to serve in the Army as enlisted soldiers in World War I. The absence of opportunity for commissioned status was galling to pharmacists who believed they should be used in their professional capacity as pharmacy officers as well as in administrative duties such as adjutant and medical supply officer in order to relieve physicians from nonclinical duties. Ironically, while pharmacists, as executives of pharmaceutical and medical supply companies, provided expert advice to the surgeon general through membership in advisory committees, they were ineligible for commissions in their area of expertise. Pharmacists argued that this prevented the Army from having access to officers with ability and talent in a specialized field it needed. They maintained that a corps of commissioned pharmacists would ensure the establishment of well-organized pharmacy operations throughout the Army and would prevent conditions such as those described in the sick call at one training camp. "The drugs were set out on an old pine board and the doctor put his hand into the tin cans and handed out pills or tablets into the grimy hands of the sick men, with verbal instructions as to their use."[94]

For the first time the department provided for foot care to soldiers. There was growing recognition that doughboys marching off to the transports taking them to France would benefit from "the promotion of foot efficiency," and the Surgeon General's Division of Orthopedic Surgery considered the promotion of foot care—and getting the Army to procure enough shoes in the proper sizes—as its major wartime contribution. The increased sophistication in attention paid to conditions of the foot was evidenced in the pioneering work of an Army surgeon, Col. Edward L. Munson, MC, who published a handbook on foot care and who is remembered by the Munson last, a genuine improvement in shoe design that was a blessing to soldiers who spent so much time on their feet. "The footwear of the soldier," said Munson, "is the very last article of his apparel upon which to practice economy." Chiropodists, the forerunners of podiatrists, were employed by the Medical Department as civilians under the supervision of orthopedic surgeons to handle foot ailments in the training camps. The department also employed enlisted chiropodists. The surgeon general solicited the assistance of the National Association of Podiatrists in identifying chiropodists as they were drafted so that they could be transferred to duty with the Medical Department.[95]

About 9 percent of soldiers during World War I had a refractive error which required them to wear eyeglasses.[96] However, the Medical Department's ability to give soldiers proper eye examinations was a hit-or-miss proposition. Few physicians other than ophthalmologists could perform an accurate refraction, and there was no provision for commissioning optometrists. Optometrists could enlist in the Hospital Corps, and an occasional few could practice their specialty. An example was Edward J. Perkins, O.D., the first optometrist to have official authority to practice in the Army. Perkins enlisted in the 30th Infantry in 1914 after studies at the California College of Optics. In 1915 his unit moved to Plattsburg Barracks, New York, where the post surgeon allowed him to practice optometry at the base hospital. Perkins' efforts were appreciated by line commanders who saw improved marksmanship scores by their soldiers. Another pioneer was Otto R. Englemann, O.D., who served as an enlisted optometrist at the eye, ear, nose, and throat clinic of the base hospital at Camp Grant, Illinois. The clinic chief, a Medical Corps major who knew his limits in refraction, would use prearranged signals to recall himself from the examining room when he had to examine general officers. That was so that Englemann could enter and actually perform the procedure.[97]

The need for proper eyewear led to the development of a program in 1917 to furnish spectacles to officers and recruits for a price 10 percent over the government's cost for the frame and lenses. The following year the Army authorized the free issue of spectacles to enlisted personnel. Officers, nurses, and civilian employees were authorized to purchase eyeglasses through the post exchange. The Army purchased frames for 45 cents, cases for 15 cents, and lenses for 95 cents up to four dollars. The surgeon general authorized hospital commanders to designate enlisted "oculists" to order and fit spectacles.

The need for a spectacle fabrication capability in the Army resulted in the formation of optical manufacturing units. Optometrists and optical technicians could enlist as privates and seek assignment to those units.[98] The department organized a base optical unit consisting of eight auxiliary manufacturing sections. Commanded by Capt. F. H. Edmonds, SnC, in civilian life the head of an optical firm and the unit's only officer, it deployed to France in April 1918. There the auxiliary units were stationed with base hospitals, where they also made dark lenses for gas casualties undergoing atropine or belladonna therapy and experimented with aluminum frames.[99]

Summary

The formation of the Sanitary Corps was a major event in the history of the Medical Service Corps. Indeed, today's MSC is almost a mirror image of its precursor. When the United States entered the war, the Medical Department needed a wide array of specialties in order to fight a European conflict, but it could commission only graduates of medical, dental, or veterinary schools. Medical Corps officers filled a range of administrative positions in the medical force structure and provided what coverage they could for the scientific specialties. However, that practice removed physicians from clinical duties and used them in roles for which they were unprepared. Furthermore, in many cases the department simply did not have access to the specialties it needed.

The diversification of medical specialties in turn reflected the enormous improvement in scientific medicine. The practical benefits of medical progress to the Army were immense. Sanitary Corps officers can be credited with helping the Medical Department give American generals freedom to concentrate on enemy threats and not epidemic threats. The department had learned lessons from its previous conflicts, and there was no need for a sanitary commission to prod it into action in World War I. For the first time, the ratio of battle deaths to deaths from disease was 1:1 overall, and much more than that in the theater of operations. General Gorgas boasted that the Medical Department had prevented a half million cases of disease and saved ten thousand lives in the first six months of mobilization alone.[100]

New management technology enabled the department to commission officers in the varied skills it needed for an increasingly sophisticated industrial organization. The administrative specialty officers of the Sanitary Corps and the U.S. Army Ambulance Service gave the Medical Department access to the businesslike skills necessary to support the nation's huge new army. Those officers brought a depth of skill, talent, and dedication to the Medical Department that presaged the future Medical Service Corps administrative specialty officers in a remarkable way.

The ability to commission officers in a wide variety of administrative and scientific specialties resulted in their substitution for other commissioned Medical Department officers, i.e., physicians. While this process was beneficial for the department's mission and generally recognized as such, it did produce some underlying tension, as the debate over the adjutant position and the introduction of psychology reflected. That internal tension would surface again in the future.

The question still to be answered in 1918 was what would happen after the war. Both the Sanitary Corps and the U.S. Army Ambulance Service were wartime entities formed for the national emergency. Would there be an opportunity for full and rewarding careers for administrative and scientific specialty officers in a peacetime Army Medical Department? Or would the Medical Department return to its old ways until reawakened by a new emergency?

Notes

[1]1. Gorgas: Phalen, *Chiefs of the Medical Department*, pp. 88–93. Quoted words: U.S. Congress, House, *Hearings before the Committee on Military Affairs*, 6 Jan–11 Feb 16, p. 694, hereafter cited as House, *Hearings*, 1916.

[2]2. Testimony: House, *Hearings*, 1916, pp. 694–95. Gorgas testified "almost daily." Gorgas and Hendrick, *William Crawford Gorgas*, p. 305.

[3]3. Quoted words: Lynch, *The Surgeon General's Office*, p. 152. Lt. Jerome Jeffrey, Sanitary Corps (SnC), an x-ray equipment expert, said he never understood the origin of the name, since he never knew of any of those officers in World War I who had anything to do with sanitation. Jeffrey to THU, 14 May 58, MSC-USACMH.

[4] Quoted words: WDGO 80, 30 Jun 17, PL.

[5] Numbers: See also William A. Hardenbergh and James A. Tobey, "The Sanitary Corps of the Army; Its Scope and Functions," *Military Surgeon* 65 (July 1929): 46–52.

[6] Ireland's assessment: Ireland, transmittal ltr in Lynch, *The Surgeon General's Office*, p. 6.

[7] Contributions: E. Alexander Powell, *The Army Behind the Army* (New York: Charles Scribner's Sons, 1919), pp. 437–38. New specialties: *SG Report*, 1918, pp. 245–46, 251, 273. Movie makers: The Adjutant General (TAG) to TSG, 16 May 18, sub: Personnel for the Sanitary Corps, Medical Department, MSC-USACMH.

[8] Numbers: *SG Report*, 1918, p. 393; Table J, Sanitary Corps, Dec 17, MSC-USACMH; *SG Report*, 1919, 2: 1117; Lynch, *The Surgeon General's Office*, p. 152; Col. William A. Hardenbergh et al., draft chapter, sub: The Sanitary Corps, undated, folder 83, box 6/18, MSC-USACMH. Positions: Memo, SGO no. 333.054–1, 8 Dec 17, MSC-USACMH. Projected strength: TSG to TAG, 12 Nov 18, MSC-USACMH.

[9] Signature: Lt Col William D. Wrightson, SnC, to Col C. L. Furbush, 10 Jun 18, MSC-USACMH.

[10] Change: SGO Office Orders no. 55, 11 Jun 18, MSC-USACMH. An organizational change in June 1918 transferred personnel functions performed by Wrightson to the chief of the Personnel Division. However, Gorgas directed that Wrightson continue as head of the Sanitary Corps to resolve issues related to corps policy and organization. Wrightson to Furbush, 20 Jun 14, MSC-USACMH.

[11]11. Wrightson: Biographical sketch, THU, OTSG; 1st Lt R.W. Bamberg, MSC, citing Memo, TSG for Wrightson, in draft rpt, sub: History of the Medical Service Corps, 20 Sep 54, THU, OTSG, folder 260, box 16/18, all in MSC-USACMH; Lynch, *The Surgeon General's Office*, p. 4; Gorgas and Hendrick, *William Crawford Gorgas*, pp. 297–301. Wrightson was released from active duty in January 1919.

[12] TSG wishes: TSG to TAG, 11 Aug 17; Memo, Henry N. Fuller, SGO, sub: Notes Related to the Medical Administrative Corps, 4 May 37, MSC-USACMH.

[13] Authority: WDGO 113, 22 Aug 17, PL; Wrightson to Heads of Divisions, SGO, 8 Jun 18, MSC-USACMH.

[14] Reassignment: Lt Col S.P. Upshur, Commander (Cdr), U.S. General Hospital #3, Colonia, N.J., to TSG, 7 Jun 18, sub: Sanitary Corps Personnel at Hospitals, MSC-USACMH. Gorgas complaints: Gorgas to TAG, sub: Commissions in the Sanitary Corps, 14 Aug 17, MSC-USACMH.

[15] Shortages: Regimental history, 42d Division (Div), sub: Iodine and Gasoline: A History of the 117th Sanitation Team, Lt. Col. Wilbur S. Conklin, MC, commander, 1919, copy in Library of Congress. The 117th's performance was noted by Brig. Gen. Douglas MacArthur, Div Chief of Staff (COS).

[16] Substitution: Memo, Col Winfred A. Smith for Col Miller, SGO, 8 Aug 18, folder 109, box 8/18, MSC-USACMH.

[17] Quartermaster Corps: Lynch, *Field Operations*, p. 172. Upshur: Lt Col A.P. Upshur, MC, to TSG, 7 Jun 18, sub: Sanitary Corps Personnel at Hospitals, MSC-USACMH.

[18] Course: Lynch, *Field Operations*, p. 172. Physicians who completed the course reported to the Fort Riley hospital for on-the-job training. There they received a special report on their aptitude for administration and, if acceptable, were assigned to a hospital as an adjutant.

[19] Increase: TAG to TSG, 16 May 18, sub: Personnel for the Sanitary Corps, Medical

Department, MSC-USACMH.

[20] Shortages: Ibid., pp. 18–20; *SG Report*, 1919, 2: 1290–91. AEF, 1919: Joseph H. Ford, *Administration, American Expeditionary Forces*, vol. 2 of *The Medical Department of the United States Army in the World War* (Washington, D.C.: War Department, 1927), pp. 100–101, hereafter cited as Ford, *Administration, AEF*.

[21] Dickson: Biographical sketch, THU, OTSG, MSC-USACMH; Hume, *The Medical Book of Merit*, p. 26.

[22] Mail: Ford, *Administration, AEF*, p. 85. The same problem arose in 1990 in Operation DESERT SHIELD.

[23] Minderbender: Joseph Heller, *Catch 22* (New York: Dell, 1963), pp. 270–71.

[24] Quoted words: Alfred E. Cornebise, *Typhus and Doughboys; The American Polish Typhus Relief Expedition, 1919–1921* (Newark: University of Delaware Press, 1982), pp. 27–28, 33. Herbert Hoover headed the effort as the director general of relief and rehabilitation for the Supreme Economic Council of the Allies.

[25] Quoted words: House, *Hearings*, 1916, p. 580.

[26] Quoted words: *SG Report*, 1919, 2: 1505. Also see Ltr, Brig Gen John S. Winn, IG, Services of Supply (SOS), to IG, AEF, sub: Conditions in SOS, 26 Jul 16, RG 120, Entry 588, Box 122, NARA-NA. The chief of the Surgeon General's Finance and Supply Division said it was "absolutely necessary that the supplies for the care of the sick and wounded be on hand at all times wherever required." Col Carl R. Darnall to Col Miller, 8 Aug 18, sub: Officers of the Sanitary Corps Required by the Finance and Supply Division, MSC-USACMH; also see *SG Report*, 1919, 2: 1501.

[27] Expansion: *SG Report*, 1919, 2: 227; *SG Report*, 1918, pp. 20, 320; Lynch, *The Surgeon General's Office*, p. 218.

[28] Quoted words: *SG Report*, 1919, 2: 1505.

[29] Number: *SG Report*, 1918, p. 20.

[30] Problems: Ibid., p. 320. Functions: Edwin P. Wolfe, *Finance and Supply*, vol. 3 of *The Medical Department of the United States Army in the World War* (Washington, D.C.: Government Printing Office, 1928), p. 414, hereafter cited as Wolfe, *Finance and Supply*.

[31] Supply depots: *SG Report*, 1918, pp. 320–21. Training: Lynch, *The Surgeon General's Office*, p. 234. Russia and England: TAG to TSG, 16 May 18, sub: Personnel for the Sanitary Corps, Medical Department, MSC-USACMH; Lynch, *The Surgeon General's Office*, p. 234.

[32] Procurement: *SG Report*, 1918, pp. 320–24. Standardization: Lynch, *The Surgeon General's Office*, p. 221.

[33] Burkard: A native of Germany, Burkard enlisted in 1898 and advanced to the rank of master hospital sergeant. As a Hospital Corps private he was decorated for bravery in action against Chippewa Indians at Leech Lake in northern Minnesota on 5 October 1898. Burkard was "the hero of the day," who dragged fellow soldiers to safety "without paying any attention to the bullets which were sprinkling him with sand and cutting the grass all around him. As soon as this was done he would return to the firing line and fire as coolly as he dressed wounds." Biographical sketch, THU, OTSG, undated, MSC-USACMH; Elbridge Colby, "Our Last Indian War," *Infantry Journal* 43 (March–April 1936): 109; Quoted words from Richard K. Kolb, "Last Stand at Leech Lake," *Army* 37 (June 1987): 74.

[34] Mobile units: Jeffrey to THU, 14 May 58, MSC-USACMH. One of the Renault trucks was located in 1937 in a private collection near Morristown, N.J. G. Burling Jarrett, "Notes," *Military Affairs* 1 (Fall 1937): 133–34.

[35] Celebration: Jeffrey to THU, 14 May 58, MSC-USACMH.

[36] Resources management: *SG Report*, 1918, pp. 270–72; Wolfe, *Finance and Supply*, pp. 767, 817–18.

[37] Hospitals: Duncan Neuhauser, *Coming of Age: A Fifty-Year History of the American College of Hospital Administrators and the Profession It Serves* (Chicago: Pluribus Press, 1983), pp. 38–39.

[38] Medical schools: House, *Hearings*, 1916, p. 636; U.S. Department of Labor, Bulletin no. 863, *Postwar Outlook for Physicians* (Washington, D.C.: U.S. Bureau of Labor Statistics, 12 February 1946), p. 3; Kenneth M. Ludmerer, *Learning To Heal: The Development of American Medical Education* (New York: Basic Books, 1985), pp. 72–74, 87–88, 166–90; Abraham Flexner, *Medical Education in the United States and Canada: A Report to the Carnegie Foundation for the Advancement

of Teaching (1910; reprint, New York: Arno Press and the New York Times, 1972); Paul Starr, *The Social Transformation of American Medicine* (New York: Basic Books, 1982), pp. 119–20. See Ludmerer for development of medical schools; 1885 is his date.

[39] American College of Surgeons (ACS): Shryock, *The Development of Modern Medicine*, p. 348; American College of Surgeons, *Manual of Hospital Standardization* (Chicago: American College of Surgeons, 1937), p. 5; Neuhauser, *Coming of Age*, p. 39; George W. Stephenson, "The College's Role in Hospital Standardization," *Bulletin of the American College of Surgeons* (February 1981): 21; Loyal Davis, *Fellowship of Surgeons* (Springfield, Ill.: Charles C. Thomas, 1960), pp. 221–22.

[40] Administration: Neuhauser, *Coming of Age*, pp. 41–65, 105.

[41] Quoted words: Charles E. Rosenberg, *The Care of Strangers* (New York: Basic Books, 1987), p. 279.

[42] Army staff: Lynch, *The Surgeon General's Office*, p. 1053. Hospital planning: Memo, Winford Smith for Col Miller, SGO, 24 Oct 18, MSC-USACMH.

[43] Registrar: Albert G. Love, Eugene L. Hamilton, and Ida L. Hellman, *Tabulating Equipment and Army Medical Statistics* (Washington, D.C.: Office of the Surgeon General, Department of the Army, 1958), pp. 70–75, hereafter cited as Love, *Tabulating Equipment.*

[44] Draftee exams: Albert G. Love and Charles B. Davenport, *Defects Found in Drafted Men* (Washington, D.C.: Senate Committee on Military Affairs, 1919), pp. 27, 259; this is an abbreviated version of Love and Davenport, *Defects Found in Drafted Men* (Washington, D.C.: War Department, 1920). Equipment: Use of mechanical equipment dated from 1880 when Maj. John Shaw Billings, head of the Surgeon General's Medical Library and consultant to the Census Office, persuaded a statistician, Herman Hollerith, Ph.D., to develop machines for tabulating census data. Hollerith incorporated his firm in 1896 as the Tabulating Machine Company located in Georgetown, Washington, D.C. Through various mergers this evolved into IBM. Love, *Tabulating Equipment*, pp. 36–51; Mark Walston, "Fast Calculating in Georgetown," *Washingtonian* 22 (September 1987): 19.

[45] Gorgas: He "had always been more interested in disease prevention than in office administration." Phalen, *Chiefs of the Medical Department*, p. 92.

[46] Quoted words: Hans Zinsser, *Rats, Lice and History* (Boston: Little, Brown and Company, 1935), p. 298. Typhus vector: Shryock, *The Development of Modern Medicine*, p. 290. Epidemic: Zinsser, *Rats, Lice and History*, pp. 296–98; Richard P. Strong, "Typhus Fever with Particular Reference to the Serbian Epidemic," in *Typhus Fever with Particular Reference to the Serbian Epidemic,* Part I (Cambridge: Harvard University Press, 1920), pp. 7–10; William Hunter, "The Serbian Epidemics of Typhus and Relapsing Fever in 1915," in *Proceedings of the Royal Society of Medicine, Section of Epidemiology and State Medicine* 13 (December 1919): 41, 75.

[47] Advances: Unfortunately, that capability did not include success with the respiratory infections, principally pneumonia secondary to the measles and influenza that were common in training camps and on troop transports. For example, an influenza outbreak on a ship in 1918 killed 60 of 1,400 soldiers during a six-day crossing of the Atlantic. Rpt, Maj Edward E. Brinton, IG, to Base Area 3, SOS, sub: Observations Concerning Embarkation and Transport of Troops During Epidemic of Influenza, 19 Oct 18, RG 159, Entry 26, Box 301, File 333.7, NARA-NA. They were also helped by German preventive medicine practices that stopped epidemics in the east from traveling to the west.

[48] Numbers: Stanhope Bayne-Jones, *The Evolution of Preventive Medicine in the United States Army, 1707–1939* (Washington, D.C.: Office of the Surgeon General, 1968), p. 151, hereafter cited as Bayne-Jones, *Preventive Medicine*; Armed Forces Information Service, *Almanac: Defense 83* (Arlington, Va.: Government Printing Office, 1983), p. 46. Pershing reported 81,141 deaths in the AEF, of which 24,786 were from disease. Pershing, *Final Report*, p. 77. Quoted words: Elbert E. Persons, "The Organization, Management, Duties, Training, etc., of the Sanitary Service with a Newly Raised Regiment," in Sanitary Field Service School for Medical Officers, *Sanitary Field Service* (Fort Leavenworth, Kans.: Field Service School for Medical Officers, 1912), pp. 6–7.

[49] Gorgas: James S. Simmons, "The Division of Preventive Medicine, Office of the Surgeon General," *Medical Bulletin* (July 1941): 63; Weston P. Chamberlain and Frank W. Weed, *Sanitation*, vol. 6 of *The Medical Department of the United States Army in the World War* (Washington, D.C.: Government Printing Office, 1926), pp. 65–68, hereafter cited as

Chamberlain and Weed, *Sanitation*; Gorgas and Hendrick, *William Crawford Gorgas*, p. 312. Inspectors general (IG) inspected hospitals as a matter of routine. The Army Inspector General, Maj. Gen. John L. Chamberlin, inspected American Expeditionary Forces (AEF) hospitals in France, where he found at least one hospital "positively dirty." Rpt, Lt Col Charles H. Patterson, sub: Diary of Events Connected with the Visit of the Inspector General of the Army to France, July 9, 1918, to September 18, 1918, RG 159, Entry 26B, Box 8, File 333, AEF IG, NARA-NA. The hospital referred to was Clermont Base Hospital No. 30, organized at the University of California. Quoted words: Chamberlain and Weed, *Sanitation*, p. 303. Venereal disease (VD): As an example, organizations with a VD rate of 2 percent or higher were restricted and their commanders received an unfavorable comment in their officers' record books, the forerunner of officer efficiency reports. Chamberlain and Weed, *Sanitation*, p. 951.

[50] Sanitary engineers: *SG Report*, 1918, pp. 224, 265. Competition: In one group of 2,000 applicants for enlisted and commissioned status only 250 were selected. Lynch, *The Surgeon General's Office*, p. 266. Course: TSG to TAG, 12 Jun 18, sub: Personnel, Sanitary Corps—Sanitary Engineering Division, MSC-USACMH. The course for sanitary engineers was initially conducted in the School of Applied Hygiene and Sanitation. A School of Sanitary Engineering was formed in March 1918. It became autonomous in May 1918. Payoff: Simmons, "The Division of Preventive Medicine," p. 62.

[51] Tinsman: *Medical Bulletin* (July 1932): 23; *SG Report*, 1919, 2: 1436; Biographical summary, THU, OTSG, undated, MSC-USACMH.

[52] Equipment: Frederick Palmer, *Newton D. Baker; America at War*, 2 vols. (New York: Dodd, Mead, 1931), 1: 313. "The manufacturer of an incinerator might assure us that it would work; but, alas, in practice it often did not work any better than some of the boasted sewage-disposal systems did." Design problems: *SG Report*, 1918, p. 268.

[53] Quoted words: TSG to TAG, 12 Jun 18, MSC-USACMH.

[54] Plants: *SG Report*, 1919, 2: 1334; Rpt, Behrman, sub: Experience of Colonel A.S. Behrman in the Sanitary Corps, World War I, undated (1959), folder 81, box 6/18, MSC-USACMH.

[55] Responsibilities: WD Cir 67, 15 Nov 18, PL; William B. Hermes, "Malaria Drainage Operations at the Port of Embarkation, New Port News, Virginia," *Military Surgeon* 47 (July 1920): 21–23. Number in May 1918: TSG to TAG, 12 Jun 68, MSC-USACMH. The surgeon general argued that the number authorized was inadequate.

[56] Pershing's request: TSG to TAG, 3 Dec 17, MSC-USACMH. Hisock: Summary of 201 file in Joseph Israeloff, draft chapter, sub: Gearing for Global Conflict, undated (1968), MSC History Project, box 1/18, MSC-USACMH. The unit was the 30th Division.

[57] Quoted words: *SG Report*, 1919, 2: 1578.

[58] Entomology: Perez Simmons, "A House Fly Plague in the American Expeditionary Forces," *Journal of Economic Entomology* 16 (August 1923): 359–61, 363; quoted words, ibid., p. 361. Dysentery attacked 188 of 207 soldiers. What Simmons referred to as the "Spanish Flu" was actually the first wave of the 1918 influenza pandemic, which killed about thirty million people worldwide. It was the worst infectious disease outbreak of the twentieth century. See K. David Patterson and Gerald F. Pyle, "The Geography and Mortality of the 1918 Influenza Pandemic," *Bulletin of the History of Medicine* 65 (Spring 1991): 4–7, 21.

[59] X-ray: Chief, Div of Roentgenology, OTSG, to TSG, 8 Oct 18, MSC-USACMH; Lynch, *The Surgeon General's Office*, pp. 468–69. Jeffrey: Jeffrey to THU, 14 May 58, MSC-USACMH.

[60] Schearer: Jeffrey to THU, 14 May 58, MSC-USACMH. Bedside x-ray: Wolfe, *Finance and Supply*, pp. 582–83.

[61] Laboratory officer duties: *SG Report*, 1918, p. 328; *SG Report*, 1919, 2: 1324–35; Lynch, *The Surgeon General's Office*, pp. 290–91; Col Frederick F. Russell, MC, SGO, inclosure (Incl) to TSG to TAG, 12 Nov 18, MSC-USACMH. Hookworm: Charles A. Kofoid, "Intestinal Parasites," in Joseph F. Silers, ed., *Communicable and Other Diseases*, vol. 9 of *The Medical Department of the United States Army in the World War* (Washington, D.C.: Government Printing Office, 1918), p. 532–33, 541; Kofoid, "Rapid Method for Detection of Ova of Intestinal Parasites in Human Stools," *Journal of the American Medical Association* 71 (1918): 1557.

[62] Training: *SG Report*, 1918, p. 328.

[63] Quoted words: Rpt, THU, OTSG, sub: Advisory Editorial Board for MSC History, 13 Nov 58,

pp. R–I, 21–22, MSC-USACMH. Training: *SG Report*, 1918, p. 439. Rockefeller program: Donald Van Slyke to Thomas Jeffries, 29 Jul 65, MSC-USACMH. Yale and Fort Leavenworth: William N. Bispham, *Training*, vol. 7 of *The Medical Department of the United States Army in the World War* (Washington, D.C.: War Department, 1927), p. 460, hereafter cited as Bispham, *Training*.

[64] Mobile laboratories: Lynch, *Field Operations*, pp. 213–17; Gorgas, *Inspection of AEF Medical Services*, p. 39.

[65] Statistics: U.S. Congress, Senate, "Vocational Rehabilitation of Disabled Soldiers and Sailors," 65th Cong., 2d sess., 30 Jan 1918, S. Doc. 166, p. 11. Congressional direction: U.S. Congress, Senate, "A Bill to Provide for Vocational Rehabilitation and Return to Civil Employment of Disabled Persons Discharged from the Military or Naval Forces of the United States," 65th Cong., 2d sess., 20 May 1918, S. 4557. The Vocational Rehabilitation Act, also known as the Smith-Sears Act, was signed into law 27 June 1918. Division established: Lynch, *The Surgeon General's Office*, pp. 474–75, 479. Veterans benefits: Pershing, *Final Report*, pp. 835–36, and *Encyclopedia Britannica* (1912), s.v. "Veterans Administration." Veterans Administration: Eli Ginzberg, "Federal Hospitalization," *Modern Hospital* 72 (April 1949): 63. Responsibility: TSG to Chief of Staff, Army (CSA), 25 Jun 18, and 1st Indorsement (Ind), AGO to TSG, 31 Jul 18, sub: Reconstruction, Physical, MSC-USACMH. Sanitary Corps numbers: *SG Report*, 1918, p. 403; 1st Ind, AGO to TSG, 31 Jul 18, MSC-USACMH.

[66] Baldwin: See Bird T. Baldwin, *Physical Growth and School Progress, A Study in Experimental Education*, U.S. Bureau of Education Bulletin no. 10 (Washington, D.C.: Government Printing Office, 1914); Baldwin, *Occupational Therapy Applied to Restoration of Movement* (Washington, D.C.: Walter Reed General Hospital, 1919), pp. 5–7, 64.

[67] Establishment: *SG Report*, 1918, p. 377; John R. Murlin to McConnell, 26 Oct 43, MSC-USACMH; Lt Col Robert Ryer, MSC, draft chapter, sub: Nutrition, in draft MSC History, undated (1961), folder 256, box 16/18, MSC-USACMH; Murlin and Caspar W. Miller, "Preliminary Results of Nutritional Surveys in U.S. Army Camps," *American Journal of Public Health* 9 (June 1919): 407. After the war Murlin would serve as chairman of the National Research Council's Committee on Food and Nutrition, as editor of the *Journal of Nutrition*, and, in 1930, as a member of the White House Conference on Child Health and Protection.

[68] Quoted words: Ryer, draft chapter, p. 26.

[69] Improvements: Paul E. Howe, "The Effect of Recent Developments in Nutrition on the Rationing of the Army," *Connecticut State Medical Journal* 6 (March 1942): 157.

[70] Prescott's course: Ruckman, *Technology's War Record*, pp. 28–29. Duties: Memo, Chief, Food and Nutrition Div, for Pers Div, SGO, 22 Oct 18, MSC-USACMH.

[71] Bug Juice: *Stars and Stripes* (27 September 1918): 6.

[72] Organizing: Robert M. Yerkes, "Psychology in Relation to the War," in NAS, *Memoirs of the National Academy of Sciences*, vol. 25 (Washington, D.C.: Government Printing Office, March 1918), p. 85; Yerkes, "Report of the Psychology Committee of the National Research Council," *Psychology Review* 26 (March 1919): 87; Maj Yerkes to TSG, sub: Estimated Number of Psychologists Appointed in the Sanitary Corps for Military Service, 25 Oct 17, MSC-USACMH. Yerkes held an organizing meeting 6 April 1917 at Harvard. Yerkes, *Psychological Examining in the United States Army*, vol. 15 of *Memoirs of the National Academy of Sciences* (Washington, D.C.: Government Printing Office, 1921), p. 7. Tests: Yerkes, "Psychology in Relation to the War," pp. 94–105; TSG to TAG, 7 Dec 17, MSC-USACMH; Lynch, *The Surgeon General's Office*, pp. 397–98; *SG Report*, 1918, p. 373; Louis M. Termon, "The Use of Intelligence Tests in the Army," *Psychological Bulletin* 15 (June 1918), pp. 177–87. Staff: *SG Report*, 1918, p. 372, and Edwin G. Boring to Lt Col Joseph Israeloff, 3 Mar 67, MSC-USACMH. Pioneers: Philip I. Sperling, "A New Direction for Military Psychology: Political Psychology," *American Psychologist* 23 (February 1968): 97–98. Stanford test: Morton A. Seidenfield, "Clinical Psychology," in Albert J. Glass and Robert J. Bernucci, eds., *Neuropsychiatry in World War II*, vol. 1 of *The Medical Department of the United States Army in World War II* (Washington, D.C.: Office of the Surgeon General of the Army, 1966), p. 568.

[73] Low scores: Yerkes, *Psychological Examining in the United States Army*, pp. 518–19. The branches in "order of excellence" were Engineers, Artillery, Infantry, Quartermaster, Medical, Dental, and Veterinary, based on tests of 5,563 officers at four training camps. Special report: Col Henry A. Shaw, MC, to TSG, sub: Psychological Tests, Camp Lee, Virginia, 16 Nov 17, and Shaw to TSG,

sub: Psychological Ratings of Medical Officers, Camp Lee, Virginia, 19 Nov 17, both in ibid., pp. 18–19, 22–23. "I believe that the time has come when we must insist on a higher standard of professional ability and must exercise greater care in the selection of candidates."

[74] Intelligence testing: *Medical Bulletin* (January 1935): 40–42; *SG Report*, 1919, 2: 1074; and Lynch, *The Surgeon General's Office*, pp. 400–401. Army impetus: Kevin McKean, "Intelligence: New Ways to Discover the Wisdom of Man," *Discover* (October 1985): 25–41.

[75] School: Lynch, *The Surgeon General's Office*, p. 398; Yerkes, "Report of the Psychology Committee," p. 88.

[76] Tests: *Medical Bulletin* (January 1935): pp. 40–42; *SG Report*, 1919, 2: 1074. Numbers: *SG Report*, 1918, pp. 373–74; *SG Report*, 1919, 2: 1075; Yerkes to Wrightson, sub: Estimated Personnel for Psychological Service, 6 Apr 18, MSC-USACMH; Yerkes to Div of Commissioned Personnel, OTSG, 24 Oct 18, MSC-USACMH; Lynch, *The Surgeon General's Office*, p. 399.

[77] Aviation: U.S. War Department (WD), Division of Military Aeronautics, *Air Service Medical* (Washington, D.C.: Government Printing Office, 1919), pp. 24–25, 382–85 (interleaved photos), hereafter cited as WD, *Air Service Medical*; David M. Lam, "From Balloon to Black Hawk: The Origins," pt. 1, *U.S. Army Aviation Digest* 27 (June 1981): 44–45. In July 1918 all airfields were required to convert one airplane to an ambulance. SnC officers: Gapen to Col Miller, Pers Div, OTSG, 30 Oct 18, MSC-USACMH. Aviation medicine: WD, *Air Service Medical*, pp. 99–100; Lynch, *The Surgeon General's Office*, p. 486, 488–89; Ayers, *The War with Germany*, p. 85; Yerkes, "Report of the Psychology Committee," p. 97.

[78] Quoted words: WD, *Air Service Medical*, p. 22.

[79] Research: Knight Dunlap, "Psychological Research in Aviation," *Science* 49 (24 January 1919): 94; Edward C. Schneider, "Physiologic Observations and Methods," pt. 1 of "Medical Studies in Aviation," *Journal of the American Medical Association* 71 (26 October 1918): 1388, and Dunlap, "Psychological Observations and Methods," pt. 2 of ibid.: 1392–93.

[80] Board request: Seibert to Air Service Div, OTSG, 17 Jun 18; TSG to TAG, 4 Jun 18 and Ind, AGO, 1 Jul 18; TSG to Col G. H. Crabtree, 6 Jul 18; TSG to TAG, 12 Nov 18, all in MSC-USACMH. Quoted words: TSG (Lt Col W. D. Wrightson, SnC) to TAG, sub: Sanitary Corps Personnel for Air Service Division, 4 Jun 18.

[81] Laboratory: The unit, consisting of thirty-three officers and fifteen enlisted, arrived at Issoudon, France, 2 September 1918. William H. Wilmer, *Aviation Medicine in the A.E.F.* (Washington, D.C.: Government Printing Office, 1920), pp. 16–17, hereafter cited as Wilmer, *Aviation Medicine*.

[82] Physiology: Edward C. Schneider, "Physiology," in Wilmer, *Aviation Medicine*, pp. 59–112. Also see WD, *Air Service Medical*, pp. 137–227.

[83] Psychology: Floyd C. Dockeray, "Psychology," in *Aviation Medicine*, pp. 113–32.

[84] Ideas and issues: Yerkes to Div of Commissioned Personnel, 24 Oct 18, MSC-USACMH.

[85] Poison gas: Ayers, *The War with Germany*, pp. 78, 84. Gas defense: Amos A. Fries and Clarence J. West, *Chemical Warfare* (New York: McGraw-Hill, 1921), pp. 34–35, 77, 103; Lynch, *The Surgeon General's Office*, pp. 504–07. Dunlap: Yerkes, "Report of the Psychology Committee," p. 97.

[86] Quoted words: Fries and West, *Chemical Warfare*, p. 77. Transfer: WDGO 62, 26 Jun 18, PL, and 1st Ind, AGO to TSG, sub: Chemical Warfare Service (CWS), 13 Jul 18, MSC-USACMH. Maj. Gen. William L. Sibert was appointed the first director of the CWS on 11 May 1918.

[87] Delousing: H.L. Gilchrist, "Delousing the American Army in France," *Military Surgeon* 47 (August 1920): 131, 146.

[88] Venereal disease: Raymond B. Fosdick, *Chronicle of a Generation* (New York: Harper and Brothers, 1958), pp. 144–45. Public Health Service: Fitzhaugh Mullan, *Plagues and Politics: The Story of the United States Public Health Service* (New York: Basic Books, 1989), pp. 73–74.

[89] Quoted words: Edward Frank Allen, "Keeping Our Men Fit Physically and Morally," in vol. 7 (October–November 1918) of *The New York Times Current History, The European War* (New York: New York Times, 1918), p. 127.

[90] Rates: Chamberlain and Weed, *Sanitation*, p. 983.

[91] AEF VD control: TSG to TAG, 12 Nov 18, MSC-USACMH; and Chamberlain and Weed, *Sanitation*, pp. 973–79.

[92] Photography: Robert S. Henry, *The Armed Forces Institute of Pathology, Its First Century*

1862–1962 (Washington, D.C.: Office of the Surgeon General, Department of the Army, 1964), pp. 171–74, hereafter cited as Henry, *AFIP*; *Stars and Stripes* (9 May 1919): 3. The unit operated out of the Elysee Palace in Paris.

[93] Henry, *AFIP*, p. 174.

[94] Pharmacy: Edward Kremers and George Urdang, *History of Pharmacy*, 3d ed., revised by Glenn Sonnedecker (Philadelphia: J.B. Lippincott, 1963), p. 302; Caswell Mayo, "Why the Pharmaceutical Corps Should Be Established," *American Druggist* 66 (April 1918): 25–27, hereafter cited as Mayo, "Pharmaceutical Corps." Quoted words: Mayo, "Pharmaceutical Corps," p. 26.

[95] Quoted words: *SG Report*, 1918, p. 361. Chiropody: Division of Orthopedic Surgery, OTSG, "Foot Care in Military Service," *Marine Corps Gazette* 3 (March 1918): 3; Lynch, *The Surgeon General's Office*, pp. 432–34; *SG Report*, 1918, pp. 361–62. Munson last: Edward L. Munson, *The Soldier's Foot and the Military Shoe: A Handbook for Officers and Noncommissioned Officers of the Line* (Menasha, Wisc.: George B. Banta Publishing Co., 1917), pp. 55–65, quoted words, p. 39. Munson served as president of the Army Shoe Board, which pioneered innovations in shoe design and foot care based on a study of 2,000 soldiers conducted over four years. Enlisted chiropodists: Frank W. Weed and Loy McAfee, *Surgery*, vol. 11 of *The Medical Department of the United States Army in the World War* (Washington, D.C.: Government Printing Office, 1927), p. 593. "Those secured by transfer early in the war soon demonstrated their usefulness to such an extent that the desirability of having all qualified chiropodists who might be accepted in the draft made available for this work became evident."

[96] Optometry: SGO Cir Ltr, 27 Nov 17, in Lynch, *The Surgeon General's Office*, p. 1143; TSG to TAG, sub: Spectacles for Military Personnel, 11 Jul and 9 Sep 18; WDGO 35, 15 Apr 18, all in RG 112, Accession No. 69A–127, Box 10/32, NARA, Washington National Records Center, Suitland, Md., hereafter cited as NARA-WNRC.

[97] No optometrists: "No provision is made in the Medical Department for Optometrists" (SGO to W.F. Hellberg, O.D., Marshalltown, Iowa, 10 Nov 17, folder 58, box 5/18, MSC-USACMH). First optometrist: Edward J. Perkins, O.D., Portland, Ore., to Capt Albert L. Paul, MSC, 3 Jan 60, folder 55, box 5/18, MSC-USACMH. Englemann: Otto R. Englemann, O.D., Chicago, Ill., to Capt Paul, 27 Jan 60, folder 55, box 5/18, MSC-USACMH.

[98] No commissions: The Surgeon General's Office received hundreds of inquiries from optometrists. Their only option was to enlist as medical soldiers and hope to have their professional expertise capitalized upon by a hospital commanding officer. Lt C.T. Cunningham, SnC, to Editor, *Optical Journal*, New York, 18 Dec 17, folder 51, box 5/18, MSC-USACMH.

[99] Optical units: Lt Col Francis Fitts, MC, SGO, to Mr. Samuel A. Bocolter, Philadelphia, 26 Sep 39, folder 51, box 5/18, MSC-USACMH; *Stars and Stripes* (23 August 1918): 1–2. Edmonds had been president of an optical company. The first three units were outfitted by Bausch & Lomb Optical Co. Howard Trimby, Sales Mgr, Ophthalmic Instruments, Bausch & Lomb, to Capt Albert L. Paul, MSC, OTSG, 13 Jan 60, folder 55, box 5/18, MSC-USACMH.

[100] Ratio: 51,417 deaths from disease: 50,510 battle deaths (Bayne-Jones, *Preventive Medicine*, p. 151).Claim: *SG Report*, 1918, p. 236.

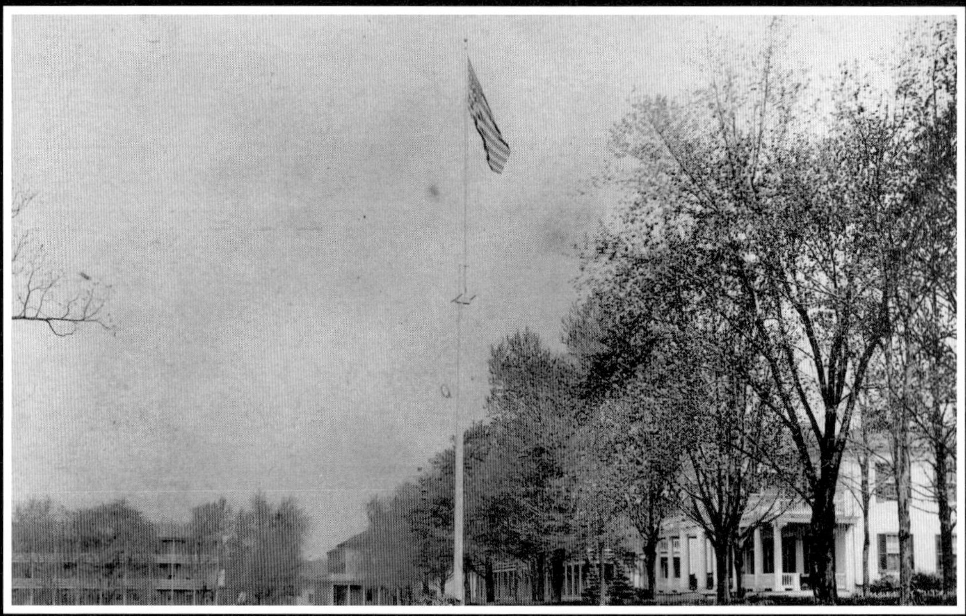

Parade ground at Carlisle Barracks, 1925

4

BETWEEN THE WORLD WARS

The Armistice that ended World War I also eclipsed the Medical Department's ability to commission officers for administrative and scientific specialties. The wartime expedients of the U.S. Army Ambulance Service (USAAS) and the Sanitary Corps began to disappear as the United States rapidly demobilized. All USAAS officers had to leave active duty, and their numbers dropped from a peak of 209 officers in November 1918 to 3 in July 1920. A few Sanitary Corps officers could be retained on active duty upon the specific request of the surgeon general. Nevertheless, the corps went from 2,919 officers to 219 in the same period, and Col. William Wrightson, SnC, who had served as its de facto chief, returned to civilian life. Medical Department reductions were part of the overall military drawdown as the Army's strength dropped from 3,685,458 in November 1918 to 131,959 in 1923. The Medical Department shrank from a peak wartime strength of 353,572 to a low point of 11,535 in 1939, and the Surgeon General's Office went from a staff numbering over 2,100 to a mere 177 in 1934.[1]

Meanwhile the economic, cultural, social, and political upheavals caused by World War I set the stage for World War II. The United States, after the flush of victory in Europe, withdrew into isolationism and stumbled into its worst economic depression.[2] The times were bad, and in 1932 the American people turned Herbert Hoover out of office. They elected Franklin Roosevelt, who ushered in the New Deal and went on to an unprecedented four terms as president. Yet, despite FDR's activism, the Great Depression refused to release its grip on the American economy until after the United States entered World War II.

Meanwhile, the Army endured a time of genteel poverty. George Marshall reverted in 1920 from his wartime rank of colonel (and a recommendation for promotion to brigadier general) to his permanent grade of major. Dwight Eisenhower and George Patton also reverted to major from colonel in 1920. (Patton would spend fourteen years as a major, Eisenhower sixteen.) In 1935 Marshall wrote that he was "fast getting too old to have any future of importance in the Army."[3]

However, the officers destined for greatness in World War II benefited from Army schools that provided a progressive series of courses unlike anything that had existed before. The branch schools taught Army management and tactics to company grade officers in advanced courses. The Command and General Staff College at Fort Leavenworth, Kansas, guided field grade officers through the complex problems of maneuvering and sustaining large formations. Officers at the Army Industrial College in Washington, D.C., explored the strategic impact of

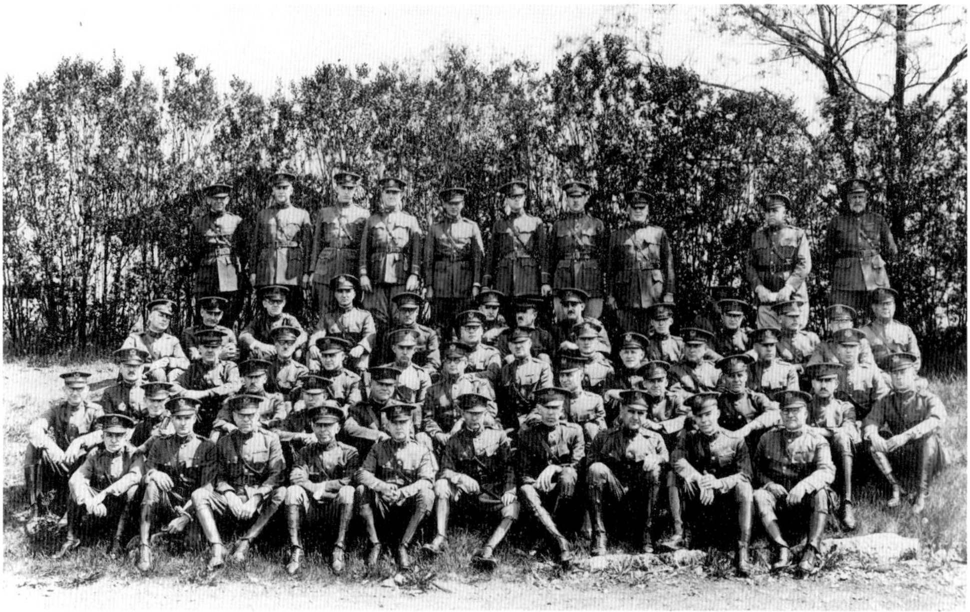

Basic course students, Medical Field Service School, 1925

logistics, and the Army's premier school, the Army War College—also in Washington—instructed senior officers in strategic planning. Eisenhower was first in his Leavenworth class. George Patton, a Leavenworth honor graduate, was first in his War College class.[4]

In 1920 the Medical Department established the Medical Field Service School at Carlisle Barracks, Pennsylvania, to teach department officers "the military side of their work."[5] The school conducted a four-month officer basic course, a two-week officer advanced course, and a six-week field officer course for National Guard and reserve officers. By the early 1930s the basic course had lengthened to a five-month program conducted eight hours a day on Monday through Friday plus classes on Saturday morning. Instruction covered tactics, military organization, military law, logistics, leadership, administration, map reading, and field medical service, the last featuring two weeks of field exercises. The officer advanced course had expanded to a two-month program. The Medical Field Service School established a fine reputation, and a report of an inspector from the Army Inspector General's Office declared that "someone besides the Medical Department ought to know how good it is."[6]

The Army experimented with new technology during the interwar period, and the Medical Department was affected by those developments. As the department had accommodated motorized vehicles, it now took some tentative steps at adapting its doctrine to the airplane. It took delivery of two airplane ambulances in 1926, stationing one plane at Kelly Field, San Antonio, Texas, and the other in the Canal Zone, Republic of Panama. The marines tested a Pitcairn XOP–1 autogyro in the evacuation of casualties in Nicaragua, and the Medical Department

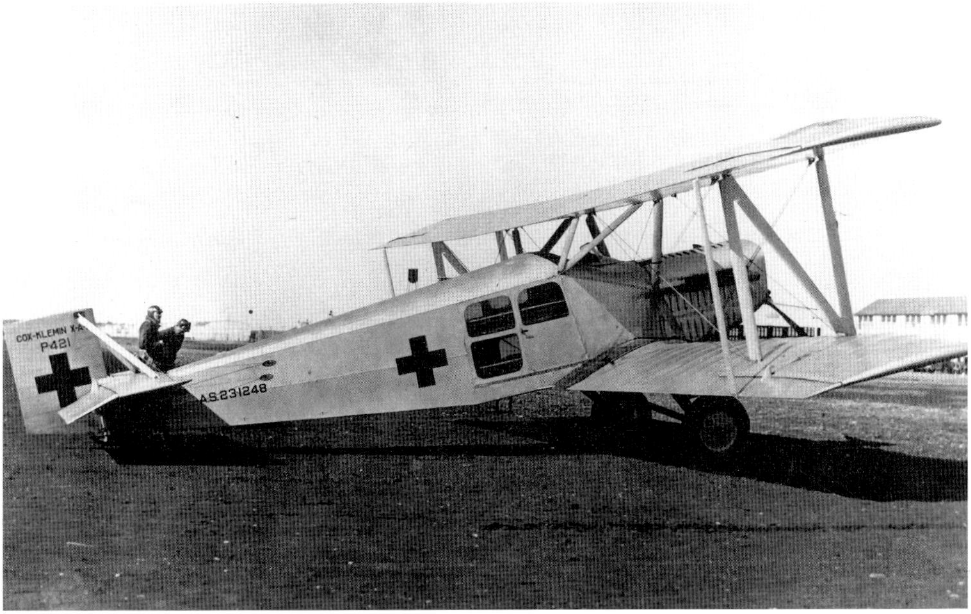

Cox-Klemin airplane ambulance at Kelly Field, Texas, 1926

tested this forerunner of the helicopter at the Medical Field Service School in 1936. Both tests showed that it was underpowered for use as a forward evacuation vehicle. Overall, there was little progress in the development of air ambulance technology and doctrine. Although many predicted that aviation would revolutionize field medical support, there remained considerable inertia as well as skepticism about its safety, medical efficacy, and military usefulness.[7]

Formation of the Medical Administrative Corps

The Medical Department's experience in World War I had demonstrated the importance of medical administrative and scientific specialty officers as members of the military medical team. Losing that capability after the war, the department searched for a solution. The establishment of a Sanitary Section of the Quartermaster Reserve was a partial remedy, and by 1920 413 Sanitary Corps officers had accepted appointments and transferred to the Quartermaster Corps. Col. Michael Blew, SnC, a sanitary engineer, was one of the officers who resigned his Sanitary Corps commission after the war and received a reserve commission in the Quartermaster Corps Sanitary Section.[8]

However, opportunity for commissioning in the reserves did nothing to alleviate the Medical Department's staffing problems for the Regular Army and provided only a tenuous source of officers. The absence of Regular Army officers in the specialties that had been provided by the USAAS and the Sanitary Corps again compelled the department to place physicians—as well as some dentists and veterinarians—in administrative positions as medical supply officers, adjutants,

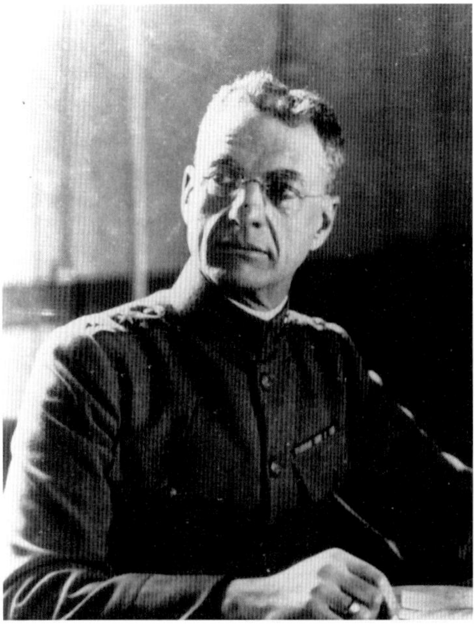

General Ireland

registrars, and commanders of field units and in charge of ambulances and transportation. The department estimated that about 20 percent of its uniformed physicians were engaged in nonclinical duties during this period. Maj. Gen. George E. Armstrong, who would serve as surgeon general during the Korean War era, said that when he entered active duty in the 1920s Army pay for physicians was equivalent to the incomes of their civilian peers, but the administrative jobs given to them made Army medicine unattractive. "We didn't go seven or eight years to medical school to become administrators; we wanted to take care of sick people."[9]

Brig. Gen. Harold W. Glattly, MC, later chief of personnel in the Surgeon General's Office, recalled the interwar period as a time of promotion "by senility" in the Medical Department.[10] The department was held in high esteem by neither the civilian medical establishment nor the Army, and it experienced difficulty in recruiting qualified applicants. In 1927 only thirty-five physicians took the entrance examination for the Medical Corps, and only sixteen of those qualified. Not until the Great Depression did the number of applicants in a single year exceed 100.[11]

Such problems prompted Maj. Gen. Merritte W. Ireland, General Gorgas' successor as surgeon general from 1918 to 1931, to recommend formation of a Regular Army "Medical Service Corps." Ireland, in testimony on 4 September 1919 before the Senate Subcommittee on Military Affairs, proposed a corps of officers in grades from lieutenant to major who would perform the administrative specialties the department needed. It would provide commissioning opportunities for enlisted soldiers who had a minimum of five years' service, including at least three years as a noncommissioned officer.[12]

General Ireland was willing to give up authorizations for Medical Corps officers in order to establish a Medical Service Corps because he wanted to forestall any revival of the Civil War practice of detailing line officers for duty with the Medical Department. "The line officer you want for that kind of work is not at all willing to accept it. He wants to be with his organization in time of war."[13] He argued that a Medical Service Corps would not only resolve that problem but would serve as an encouragement to enlisted members of the Hospital Corps, who would then have an opportunity to earn a commission in the Medical Department. It would also improve the utilization of pharmacists, since the new corps could include a limited number of pharamacists commissioned for duties in medical supply.

TABLE 2—STRENGTH OF THE SANITARY RESERVE CORPS, 1921–1941

Date (as of 30 June)	COL	LTC	MAJ	CPT	1LT	2LT	Total
1921	1	5	30	71	74	64	245
1926	4	41	101	144	110	97	497
1931	3	27	101	108	108	118	465
1936	2	17	72	71	67	166	395
1941	2	22	51	99	283	2	45

Source: *Annual Reports of The Surgeon General*, 1921–1941

TABLE 3—STRENGTH OF THE MEDICAL ADMINISTRATIVE OFFICERS' RESERVE CORPS, 1921–1941

Date (as of 30 June)	CPT	1LT	2LT	Total
1921	134	147	185	466
1926	304	431	760	1,495
1931	406	489	1,183	2,078
1936	261	416	889	1,566
1941	236	386	426	1,048

Source: *Annual Reports of The Surgeon General*, 1921–1941.

Congress acted upon Ireland's proposal in the Army Reorganization Act of 4 June 1920. The new law, codifying a U.S. defense policy of a small regular force backed up by a large, trained reserve, defined three components: a Regular Army composed of officers and enlisted personnel on continuous active duty; a National Guard; and an Organized Reserve. It established a Regular Army Medical Administrative Corps (MAC) as a permanent part of the Medical Department. The reserves included a Medical Administrative Officers' Reserve Corps and a Sanitary Officers' Reserve Corps. Congress used the title Medical *Administrative* Corps rather than General Ireland's proposed Medical *Service* Corps in order to distinguish the new corps as an organization designated for administrative specialty officers, in contrast to the Sanitary Corps, which was set aside for scientific specialty officers. There was no restriction on grades in the Sanitary Corps, but officers appointed in the Medical Administrative Corps were limited to the grade of captain.

The law set an initial authorization for 140 Medical Administrative Corps officers in grades from second lieutenant to captain and provided for the appointment of enlisted soldiers with two or more years of active service. Examinations for appointment included tests in basic educational skills as well as written, oral, and practical tests in administrative regulations, office organization and administration, mess management, property management, military law, and drill and ceremonies. There was a good response to the opportunity for a commission in the Medical Department, and thirty-nine officers were appointed by the end of September 1920. Their principal duty assignments were adjutant, personnel adjutant, mess officer, supply officer, and office executive. By December 141 officers were on active duty, one more than the 140 authorized. All charter members of the Medical Administrative Corps were given a 1 July 1920 date of rank (*see Appendix B*).[14]

Officers with wartime service in the scientific specialties were generally appointed in the Sanitary Officer's Reserve Corps. Colonel Wrightson received such an appointment, as did 245 other World War I Sanitary Corps officers. Officers who had served in administrative specialties during the war were appointed in the Medical Administrative Corps Reserve. Some noncommissioned officers who were unable to obtain appointments in the Regular Army MAC were appointed in the MAC Reserve, which also provided for direct appointments from civilian life. By 1928 there were 1,887 officers in the MAC Reserve and 499 officers in the Sanitary Corps Reserve. A few officers were appointed in the National Guard. In 1937 the National Guard had 1 Sanitary Corps and 136 Medical Administrative Corps officers.[15]

The new corps had a rocky road to travel. The initial authorization of 140 officers—a figure based on a ratio of 1:2,000 enlisted soldiers in the active Army—was reduced in subsequent congressional action, dropping to 72 in June 1922. At that point, sixty-six MAC officers were surplus, a state of affairs not improved by the Pay Readjustment Act of 10 June 1922, which limited their income by preventing them from counting enlisted service for pay and allowances. General Ireland called that "unjust and discriminatory,"[16] and the pay restrictions were lifted in 1928. The cap on promotions remained, even though Ireland sought legislation to establish promotion opportunity for MAC officers through the grade of colonel.[17]

Lack of a permanent corps for both administrative and scientific specialty officers soon produced problems to plague the department. In 1920 General Ireland began lobbying for establishment of a medical auxiliary corps that would merge the wartime MAC and Sanitary Corps into a permanent part of the Medical Department.[18] Ireland continued his efforts throughout his long tenure as surgeon general. In April 1929 Congressman Jonathan M. Wainwright introduced legislation to replace the Medical Administrative Corps with a medical auxiliary corps of 120 officers and the enlisted personnel of the department's Hospital Corps.[19] Wainwright's proposal did not pass.

There was a trickle of appointments in the Medical Administrative Corps in the 1930s as vacancies occurred. For example, examinations conducted in the spring of 1934 resulted in nine appointments; examinations were held that fall for another ten. A disappointment for veteran officers came in 1935. Legislation was enacted that provided a special retirement option to encourage officers in the World War I "hump" to retire, speeding up promotions for those who remained on active duty. Officers who met certain criteria were eligible to retire in the grade of major with a special pay multiplier. The problem was that all but six MAC officers in that category exceeded the maximum number of years of service (thirty) allowed by the law. If they retired, they would receive less retired pay than those officers who retired with less than twenty-nine years of service. The surgeon general, believing that this discrimination was not the intent of Congress, requested remedial legislation, but no action was taken.[20]

That was the background for the most dramatic of the setbacks for the Medical Administrative Corps, which came when Congress in 1936 reduced the corps to sixteen officers, a number that held until the eve of World War II. Officers already on active duty were "grandfathered," but the law restricted future appointments in the Regular Army Medical Administrative Corps to graduates of four-year schools of pharmacy.[21]

General Ireland, called "one of the greatest champions the Medical Administrative Corps ever had,"[22] had been succeeded by Maj. Gen. Robert U. Patterson (1931–1935), who was followed by Maj. Gen. Charles R. Reynolds (1935–1939). General Reynolds, disenchanted with the corps, supported the cutback. He said that recent appointees had been "inadequate substitutes" for physicians due to their lack of technical qualifications and limited military experience. Reynolds said the department had found it necessary to extensively train the new generation of MAC officers so that they could perform adequately. In short, he believed that a Medical Administrative Corps of sixteen pharmacists was plenty for the active Army. He also believed it would satisfy the desires of pharmacists, who for fifteen years had been clamoring for commissioned status. Finally, he believed it would end appointments of enlisted personnel as MAC officers, a practice he viewed with disfavor.[23]

Reynolds was reacting to an unevenness of quality in the MAC. Many of the officers who had originally been appointed in the corps had extensive military service, some dating from the Spanish-American War. As those older officers retired in the 1920s and 1930s, the replacement stream of new officers was drawn from a pool of personnel with much less experience, but who met the minimum requirement of two or more years of enlisted service. Some were commissioned as the result of efforts by senior Medical Corps patrons doing favors for their enlisted "dog robbers." Others, "commissioned corporals," were discredited by graft, pilferage, indebtedness, marital problems, or immorality. A few problem officers cast a bad light on the corps and blinded some of the department's leaders—General Reynolds for one—to the benefit of a corps of administrative specialty officers.

Indeed, given the limits of opportunity, the Medical Department was fortunate to attract and retain superior Medical Administrative Corps officers. Col. Frederick H. Gibbs, MSC, who served during this period, pointed out that while the majority were able, some were not up to the challenges of service as an officer, a problem at least partly a creation of the department's, since it had control over the selections for appointments in the corps. Colonel Gibbs believed that MAC officers of the interwar period had to be viewed within the context of their times. They had limited opportunities for development, and the officers generally progressed to the extent of their own initiative for improvement, but without the benefit of personnel management planning by the department. Not surprisingly, MAC officer professional development was uneven.[24]

What General Reynolds said publicly he argued for more forcefully in private, to the extent of calling for the abolition of the Medical Administrative Corps. He said that in its time the MAC had been a worthwhile organization that had provided commissions for senior NCOs who had held wartime commissions in the Sanitary Corps. But that time had passed. Those old-timers were on the way out and their replacements did not have the education, experience, or potential to be officers. It would be best, he argued, to discontinue the corps. Only external pressure to create a separate pharmacy corps kept him from succeeding completely.[25]

Proposals for a Pharmacy Corps

There were proposals to establish additional Medical Department commissioned corps. One of the more unusual was an undertaking in 1935 by Congressman Frank Dorsey to establish an embalmers corps. Commissioning in that corps would have required a diploma from a recognized embalming school, three years' experience, and a qualifying examination. Successful candidates would be appointed as embalmers and assistant embalmers in the grade of first and second lieutenant, respectively, and would have an opportunity for promotion through the grade of major. The Medical Department opposed the proposal, citing insufficient workload. For example, in 1933 there were 574 Army deaths at 126 different locations, a figure that did not support the proposed solution.[26] The proposal failed to gain War Department or congressional support.

The most significant proposal was a move to create a separate pharmacy corps, or at least to recognize pharmacists as commissioned officers. The initiative took on a life of its own during the 1920s and 1930s and embroiled three surgeons general. It exemplified the evolutionary process of twentieth-century American medicine in which emerging health care specialties were striving for recognition. When the pharmacy profession encountered institutional discrimination in the Medical Department, it turned to avenues outside the Army for help. Those avenues were open through a political influence unlike other specialties. Pharmacists, respected and trusted professionals, provided a gathering place for townspeople and neighbors to exchange news and gossip in thousands of corner drug stores all over the country. Not infrequently citizens also turned to them for assessments of the quality of local physicians. Smart politicians stayed tuned in to the pharmacists in their area, some of whom ran for office themselves.

In 1918 Caswell A. Mayo, editor of the *American Druggist*, had recommended the formation of a pharmacy corps along the lines of the French Army and the armies of other major powers, which commissioned pharmacists for a variety of administrative and scientific duties. The French pharmacy corps, headed by a brigadier general, offered opportunities for its officers at all levels of the French military from the War Ministry on down in staff work, the management of manufacturing and warehouse operations, and scientific duties in clinical, toxicology, research, and quality control laboratories. The pharmacy corps of Germany, Japan, and Spain were headed by colonels; those of Italy, Belgium, Holland, and Austria by lieutenant colonels; and majors headed the corps of Switzerland, Norway, Sweden, and Australia. Caswell had cited the department's success in the war with advisory committees composed of medical supply and equipment executives. Some were pharmacists, and their expertise had greatly assisted the mobilization. He found it inconceivable that there was no means to commission such talented leaders in the Medical Department. "We ask you to let pharmacists take the place of the physician doing non-medical work."[27]

Protestations by organized pharmacy at the end of the war had been overshadowed by the formation of the Medical Administrative Corps, but the issue remained alive as time passed, and pharmacists were still unable to obtain commissions. The American Pharmaceutical Association (APA) took up the issue and passed a resolution in 1928 supporting legislation to create a pharmacy corps. In October of that year, A. L. I. Winne, the APA chairman, wrote General Ireland asking for a meeting to discuss their proposal. His letter set off correspondence that would continue in a contentious spirit for over a decade. Even the details for setting an initial meeting became fractious.[28]

Ireland responded that he did not support creation of a pharmacy corps, just as he did not support establishing separate corps for psychology, nutrition, or other specialties. The surgeon general reminded Dr. Winne of a gentleman's agreement between Lt. Col. Carl R. Darnall, MC, his representative, and Dr. E. Fullerton Cook of the APA at the time the Medical Administrative Corps was formed. The Medical Department had agreed to provide commissioning opportunity for graduate pharmacists in the Regular Army MAC, which would be further supplemented in wartime by appointments in the Sanitary Corps Reserve. For its part, the APA had agreed to cease lobbying for a pharmacy corps. "Now with this perfectly frank statement on my part, I see no reason to put your committee to the trouble of visiting Washington for an interview." Of course, Ireland's office "was always open for visits by any gentleman who wants to see me." He added that he would be in his office during the period suggested by Winne.[29]

Winne was insulted by the surgeon general's putting off his committee. In the ensuing exchange of letters, Ireland denied that he had refused, but Winne insisted he had.[30] He was certain that no "self-respecting committee would intrude themselves upon your presence on the strength of your statement that your office is open, and they may come in if they want to."[31] There is no record that such a meeting occurred that year, and the controversy continued to simmer. General Ireland's continuing effort to get a medical auxiliary corps for all administrative and scientific specialties—including commissioned pharmacists—did not satisfy those who continued to seek a separate corps for pharmacists.[32]

The dispute went public in 1928 when Murray Breese, editor of the *American Druggist*, bitterly complained that restricting pharmacists to enlisted status ranked them no higher than cooks. For two decades pharmacists had been "shuttlecock to the Medical Corps' battledore," and the recognition accorded them in the Revolution and the Civil War had been lost. Patriotic labors of pharmacists had been met with "sweet words to the face and kicks from the rear." Breese feared that General Ireland's medical auxiliary corps would result in a token number of commissions for pharmacists so that the department could argue that it had adequately provided for the specialty. He urged his readers to fight for their own corps, and he called on every pharmacist to join the fray.[33]

In January 1930 Senator Royal Copeland countered the proposal for a medical auxiliary corps with legislation for a pharmacy corps. This prompted Ireland to write a lengthy letter to the American Pharmaceutical Association expressing his support of the Wainwright Bill and his opposition to Copeland's. In private he was convinced that his proposal for a medical auxiliary corps would deflect the APA lobbying for a separate corps.[34] In fact, it did please the moderate wing of the APA, as reflected when E. Fullerton Cook, Ph.D., head of a special committee of the APA, wrote Ireland to express his hope that the surgeon general would have the full support of the pharmacy profession for the Wainwright Bill. Ireland, encouraged by this, told Congressman Wainwright that he opposed the establishment of a pharmacy corps but was attempting to reach agreement with American Pharmaceutical Association representatives.[35]

Neither legislative proposal passed, but the issue of commissioning pharmacists did not die. In 1932 the surgeon general, General Patterson, wrote the APA that there were thirty graduate or registered pharmacists on active duty as enlisted pharmacists in Medical Department facilities. His office had canvassed Army hospital commanders and determined that there was a requirement for ten more, but no requirement for commissioned officers. Consequently he had closed the door on any support for commissioning, a position he reiterated in 1934. However, the APA persisted, and in 1935 its president wrote Patterson that there continued to be considerable support for a separate pharmacy corps. Patterson would not hear it. He did not support efforts that would create an "unwieldy and illogical organization."[36]

The legislative drumbeat continued. General Patterson supported a proposal to establish a medical auxiliary corps that was introduced by Congressman Jed Johnson in 1935, but he opposed another that would increase the Medical Administrative Corps by forty spaces for commissioned pharmacists. He again called for the establishment of a medical auxiliary corps. Another House legislative proposal called for appointment of pharmacists in the Medical Corps.[37]

In May 1935, his final month as surgeon general, Patterson wrote of his exasperation with the whole business. He complained that a great deal of the agitation by organized pharmacy was "based upon the desires of certain men in the enlisted ranks of the Army who were trying to force themselves into a better status in the Medical Department without having the necessary educational qualifications." Patterson declared that in many hospitals "there wouldn't be one full hour's work a day" for a pharmacist. The truth was that he believed there was a requirement for no more than fifteen or seventeen pharmacists in the entire Medical Department.[38]

General Reynolds became entangled in this issue shortly after succeeding Patterson as surgeon general. Reynolds supported his predecessor's proposal for a medical auxiliary corps and opposed the formation of a pharmacy corps. However, he soon learned that organized pharmacy had not abandoned hope for a separate corps. In January 1936 Dr. H. Evert Kendig, head of an APA committee formed to promote a pharmacy corps, wrote to Reynolds asking for his help in commissioning pharmacists. Kending said he was under considerable pressure to support a separate corps and was being rapidly forced into a nonnegotiable position by members of his profession.[39]

General Reynolds, changing the department's tune, came out in favor of commissioning pharmacists, pointing to recent increases in the Army's enlisted strength, which had created new patient care workload requirements for the Medical Department. A study conducted by the Surgeon General's Office identified requirements for twenty-one commissioned pharmacists. Seven were at general hospitals, eight at station hospitals, one at a general dispensary in Washington, D.C., four in depots, and one in the Surgeon General's Office. Commissioning pharmacists in the MAC would be an obvious solution, but the problem was that the two-year enlisted service requirement precluded commissioning officers from outside the enlisted ranks.[40]

In March 1936 Senator Norm Sheppard of the Senate Committee on Military Affairs sent Reynolds a copy of a bill he had introduced to restrict Medical Administrative Corps appointments to pharmacists. The surgeon general was not in a receptive mood since he was now pushing for abolition of the Medical Administrative Corps. His previous spirit of accommodation had vanished, and he opposed commissioning pharmacists. He believed the Army's pharmacy requirements were adequately met by the nearly forty graduate pharmacists who were serving as enlisted technicians under the direct control of physicians. Wartime needs would be handled by appointing pharmacists in the Officer Reserve Corps. In short, pharmacists were just one of a number of groups—osteopaths, chiropractors, chiropodists, and embalmers were others—"definitely not essential to the medical service of the Army."[41]

That was not the end of it, for General Reynolds would soon reverse himself again when he saw a way to, in effect, eliminate the Medical Administrative Corps by restricting it to pharmacists. Testifying in hearings on Sheppard's bill on 26 May 1936, Reynolds supported the appointment of sixteen pharmacists in the Medical Administrative Corps. He stated that these officers could serve in a variety of positions useful to the Medical Department, including procurement of medical materiel and training enlisted pharmacy technicians.[42]

The effort to commission pharmacists at last succeeded when, on 24 June 1936, Congress required the Army to appoint graduates of recognized four-year pharmacy programs as officers in the Medical Administrative Corps. The Medical Department conducted examinations and commissioned two of eighty-five applicants: 2d Lt. Glenn K. Smith, MAC, and 2d Lt. Howard B. Nelson, MAC. By 1939 there were eleven graduate pharmacists in the MAC, and examinations were conducted that November to fill five vacancies. General Reynolds' move to eliminate the Medical Administrative Corps turned another corner on 3 April 1939, when Congress limited the Regular Army Medical Administrative Corps to sixteen pharmacists, thereby restricting future appointments to pharmacists. There were just sixty-eight Regular Army MAC officers on active duty when the United States entered World War II.[43]

In the end, resolution of the issue was a compromise. Pharmacists had gained the opportunity to serve as commissioned officers in the Medical Department. The department had acquiesced to that ambition but had prevented the establishment of yet another separate corps by restricting new appointments in the Regular Army MAC to pharmacists. Unfortunately, the department had achieved a Pyrrhic victory, because it had lost from the Regular Army the range of administrative specialties the Sanitary Corps had provided it in World War I. Those officers were vital for wartime readiness, and the loss of that capability would hamper the department's performance in the early years of World War II. It was a loss that could have been devastating if the nation had not enjoyed the luxury of a long period to mobilize.

Administrative Specialty Officers

Medical Administrative Corps officers were scattered throughout the Army, but their small numbers did not preclude their use in emergency situations. A relief expedition sent to Japan after an earthquake in 1923 included two MAC officers who assisted in establishing a 1,000-bed base hospital and a field hospital in Tokyo. Some MAC officers filled administrative positions in the Medical Division of the Air Corps, the forerunner of the U.S. Air Force Medical Service and a component of the Medical Department that operated semiautonomously.[44]

A large post would have only two or three MAC officers. In 1925 2d Lt. Robert L. Black, MAC, who as a colonel would become the second chief of the Medical Service Corps, enlisted, and in 1928 he successfully competed for one of four Medical Administrative Corps vacancies. Commissioned that December, he reported to Fitzsimons General Hospital, Denver, Colorado, where he joined the hospital's adjutant and the officers club manager as one of three MAC officers on the post, each of whom assumed a number of additional responsibilities. Black was assigned as the medical supply officer, but one of his extra duties was management of a pig farm, which the hospital maintained to handle the disposal of edible garbage. When Black moved the following year to the hospital at Schofield Barracks, Hawaii, he was the sole Medical Administrative Corps officer. There he served as medical supply officer, adjutant, mess officer, registrar, troop commander, recreation officer, and summary courts-martial officer.[45]

Duty conditions were not necessarily unpleasant. After Hawaii, Black reported to Fort Benning, Georgia, where he was one of two MACs. There, as in Hawaii, the duty day ended at 1300, a situation that made it possible for the Black family to take up golf and horseback riding. Yet, however pleasant the working conditions might have been, they did not fully compensate for the shortcomings of military service in the interwar period. Black was promoted to first lieutenant in 1931, but a cut in military spending meant that promotions would result in no increase in pay, and he continued on the salary of a second lieutenant. Injury was added to insult when Congress imposed a 15 percent pay cut.[46]

A few officers attended the basic officers course at the Medical Field Service School, Carlisle Barracks, Pennsylvania. There 1st Lt. Glenn K. Smith was the only Medical Administrative Corps officer among fifty-eight graduates in the audience when Army Chief of Staff Maj. Gen. Malin Craig addressed the class in June 1938. Attendance at the advanced course was practically unknown for MAC officers, and none attended the Army Command and General Staff College at Leavenworth or the Army War College. Two attended the Army Industrial College during the interwar period.[47]

Reserve officers were supposed to receive two weeks of training each year, but that was not always the case.[48] Despite the fact that reserve training was erratic, some Medical Department reservists were able to attend two-week summer camps throughout the country; 223 Medical Administrative Corps and 51 Sanitary Corps reserve officers attended those camps in 1931, a representative year. Other reserve MAC and Sanitary Corps officers served as instructors with Medical Department Reserve Officer Training Corps (ROTC) summer camps for medical, dental, and veterinary students at Carlisle Barracks, Pennsylvania; Fort Snelling, Minnesota; Fort Lewis, Washington; Fort Sam Houston, Texas; and Fort Oglethorpe, Georgia.[49]

The Medical Department benefited from the service of MAC officers who stuck it out during the interwar period. One was Lt. Col. Thomas M. England, MAC, an officer whose services received special recognition when England General Hospital, a 3,650-bed hospital in Atlantic City, New Jersey, was named after him during World War II. England had enlisted in the Army in 1899 and served in the occupation of Cuba. While there, he volunteered for Walter Reed's yellow fever experiments, whose protocol required him to sleep twenty nights in a bed formerly occupied by a yellow fever patient, in the clothing worn by a victim of the disease, and with his head lying "on a towel stained with the blood of a case of yellow-fever." In 1931 England was awarded the Yellow Fever Medal for this act of courage, a congressional award consisting of a gold medal, annual listing in the Army's Roll of Honor, and payment of $250 per month for life.

England was a master hospital sergeant when commissioned in the Sanitary Corps in 1918. He had served as a medical supply officer in the United States and France during World War I and in Washington, D.C., after the war. He was in the original group of officers appointed in the Medical Administrative Corps. England retired in October 1940 upon reaching the statutory age limit of sixty-four. He was recalled to active duty a week later, promoted to major when the Medical Administrative Corps grade limitation of captain was lifted, and later promoted to lieutenant colonel. He died on active duty in 1943 while serving as the Executive Officer and Chief, Medical Branch Office, Headquarters, Fifth Service Command, Fort Hayes, Ohio. He was sixty-seven years old and in his forty-fifth year of active federal service at the time of his death.[50]

Another early Medical Administrative Corps officer was Capt. Robert A. Dickson, the Sanitary Corps officer awarded the Distinguished Service Medal for his service in France in World War I. Appointed as a captain in the Medical Administrative Corps at age forty-five, he performed in a variety of assignments

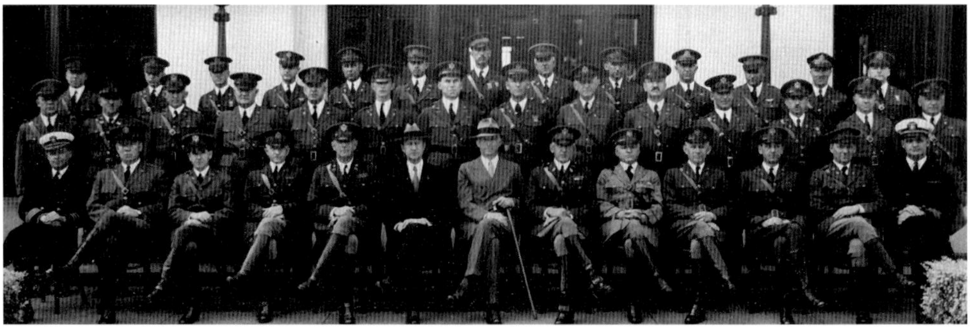

Army Industrial College Class of 1929–30. Captain England is fourth from left and Captain Dickson is sixth from right in the second row.

in the 1920s and 1930s, including adjutant, enlisted detachment commander, and post exchange officer. He retired as a captain in 1934. Dickson and England were the only MAC officers to attend the Army Industrial College during this period. Capt. Oscar Burkard, the Sanitary Corps holder of the Medal of Honor, was also one of the first Medical Administrative Corps officers. Burkard served at various posts in the 1920s and retired as a captain in 1930.[51]

Some MAC officers would later be leaders in the Medical Service Corps and retire as MSC colonels. One was Joseph Carmack, who enlisted in 1924. In 1930 he was commissioned as one of three successful candidates out of 300 applicants. Another was Harry Nelson, who enlisted in 1932 and later applied for an MAC commission. He passed the appointment examination in Omaha, Nebraska, in October 1934, but a shortage of vacancies delayed his appointment until August 1935. In December 1935 he reported to the basic officers course at Carlisle Barracks, which was followed by assignment to the 11th Medical Regiment, Schofield Barracks, Hawaii. There he served with the ambulance company, as commander of the headquarters and service company, and later as hospital medical supply officer. In 1935 he was assigned to Fort Jay, New York, where he was promoted to first lieutenant after five years in grade as second lieutenant, a wait that was normal for that period. At Fort Jay he was the only Medical Administrative Corps officer assigned to the hospital. He was promoted to captain in 1940 but, due to congressional funding limits for the military, continued at the salary of his previous grade.[52]

Col. Louis "Bill" Williams, MSC, enlisted in 1923 and was commissioned in the Medical Administrative Corps in 1931. "General MacArthur was on one end of the promotion list and I was on the other." He concentrated in medical logistics, a specialty that particularly appealed to him because, unlike people, supplies did not talk back. Officers were identified only by their branch, for this was before the Army established military occupational specialties (MOSs) for officers, and Williams handled the various duties common for MAC officers. "You did not tell the old man that was not your MOS, you just did the job," he later recalled. Army life appealed to him. "I came out of a tobacco patch in Tennessee, so every day in the Army was like Sunday on the farm."[53]

Medical Logistics

Medical logistics began to expand greatly as American medicine underwent a technological revolution. The Army supply table listed 74 drugs and 18 surgical instruments in 1918; by 1927 the table listed 4,300 items in these categories. Medical Administrative Corps officers handled the overseas responsibilities for medical logistics. One was Capt. W. Harvey Kernan, MAC, who from 1925 to 1928 served as the medical supply officer in Panama where he was instrumental in organizing the medical supply depot on the Atlantic side of the Panama Canal Zone. The depot was named in his honor in 1967. In 1935 MAC Capts. John D. Foley, Richard E. Humes, and Edward D. Sykes were in charge of medical supply operations in Panama, Hawaii, and the Philippines, respectively.[54]

The minuscule size of the Medical Administrative Corps limited the use of MAC officers, and it again fell to physicians in the active Army to assume duties as medical supply officers. In 1934 the medical supply officers of the New York, Eighth Corps Area, San Francisco, and Chicago quartermaster depots and the commander of the St. Louis Medical Depot were all physicians. Colonel Black was assigned in 1937 to Fort Sam Houston, San Antonio, Texas, as the medical supply officer, replacing a Medical Corps officer who believed that "no lay person could ever successfully hold such a position."[55] At least some efforts were made during the interwar years to plan for mobilization. In 1924 sixty-two medical supply industry executives were commissioned in the Sanitary Corps Reserve for that purpose.

That the Medical Department retained its medical supply function at all was in itself an accomplishment. Maj. Gen. George W. Goethals, who had directed the completion of the Panama Canal—and had been General Gorgas' nemesis—was recalled to active duty in World War I as the Army's director of purchase, storage, and traffic.[56] At the end of the war Goethals succeeded in transferring the medical supply functions of the surgeon general to his office where it remained for about two years, shifting back only after Goethals retired. The surgeon general reported that the experiment was a failure, having "demonstrated that a single supply system is too complicated for general use in providing supply for the Army."[57]

Goethals saw it differently. Called to testify in the congressional hearings for the 1920 Army Reorganization Act, he argued for creation of a department of supply for the Army that would handle all Army standard supply and transportation functions, including medical items. He once again clashed with the surgeon general. He recalled his experience during the war:

> They stated I could not buy medicines. Well, the doctors can not buy medicines, either. They get chemists in to do their purchasing, and I could get chemists in to do the purchasing, and those chemists could buy other chemical goods that are required by the other bureaus. . . . [Army physicians] could then look after the sick. That is their proper function.[58]

Goethal's proposal was not adopted, and the Medical Department retained its medical logistics responsibilities.

Training was principally a matter of detailing junior officers to medical supply depots for on-the-job experience. Some Medical Administrative Corps, Medical Corps, and Veterinary Corps officers attended a two-year Medical

Supply Training School established in 1922 at the New York General Depot, which had the largest medical section of all the depots. The school also offered an advanced medical supply training program designed to prepare Army physicians for the highest positions in medical supply. This program consisted of a series of rotations beginning with twenty-one months at the New York Depot, followed by twelve months' experience in the Surgeon General's Office and the ten-month course of the Army Industrial College. Colonel Black applied for the advanced program, but the Surgeon General's Office "quite definitely closed the door for other than Medical Corps pupils."[59]

There were attempts to increase the training of reserve medical logisticians as war threatened in Europe. The most advanced program was at the New York Depot, where in the late 1930s the department could rely upon about 125 reserve medical supply officers in the New York City area. Many of the reserve officers worked in areas allied to their Medical Department specialties as hospital purchasing agents, drug company executives, chemists, and plant managers. The department's training program consisted of lectures, demonstrations, and exhibits. Fifty-four officers attended the 1938 session.[60]

The military buildup in the years just before the United States entered World War II created additional requirements for medical logistics officers. Accordingly, the Medical Department requested authority in 1940 to commission lieutenants in the Sanitary Corps Reserve to serve as purchasing agents, and it regularly brought the shortage of medical supply officers to the attention of the assistant secretary of war. Those shortages and others caused the War Department to bring additional reserve and National Guard MAC and Sanitary Corps officers on active duty in the year prior to America's entrance into the war. There were twelve MAC and Sanitary Corps Reserve officers on active duty in June 1940. A year later there were 1,233.[61]

There was a lighter side to the medical supply business. In Hawaii, Colonel Black managed the medical war reserve stock of supplies and equipment, mostly World War I surplus. This included 55-gallon drums of alcohol, which the depot repackaged into 5-gallon containers for issue to medical units. The drums had originally been filled in a cold climate, and when opened in Hawaii would erupt in a fountain of spray. Black devised a way to capture the surplus, which when mixed in charcoal barrels made a satisfactory gin. He never lacked for associates willing to help in his "surplus disposal activities."[62]

A medical supply officer for Schofield Barracks, 1st Lt. Joseph E. McKnight, MAC, demonstrated innovation of a different sort when asked to repair a hopelessly overloaded air compressor for the dental clinic. McKnight rounded up an old Kelvinator compressor, a one-half-horsepower electric motor from a dishwasher, an automatic switch, and a forty-gallon tank. He talked the post electrician into assembling that collection of parts into a suitable replacement compressor, which ended complaints about compressed air.[63]

Hospital Administration

Health care had become a billion-dollar business in the United States. American hospitals were on their way to being important institutions, although the Great Depression whittled their number from 6,852 in 1928 to 6,166 in 1938.[64] Their buildings became more imposing structures as Elisha Otis' successful development of the elevator enabled vertical rather than pavilion-style construction. Pressure from external influences, such as the American College of Surgeons (ACS), pushed hospitals into management improvements. The ACS conducted more than forty thousand surveys of American hospitals from 1918 to 1936. It approved 76 percent of the 3,564 hospitals it surveyed in 1939—over 93 percent of the large hospitals passed—a great improvement since its first surveys in 1918.[65] The number of American medical schools dropped to ninety-six in 1915 and to seventy-six in 1930 as the institutional revolution of American medical schools from 1885 to 1925 was completed, and medical schools assumed the corporate form they would retain for the rest of the century. That development had given rise to the modern teaching hospital, another pressure for professional hospital administration.[66]

Army hospitals also became considerable enterprises demanding professional management. The Medical Department operated seven general hospitals and eight smaller station hospitals in the United States and the Philippines, the largest of which in 1936 were two 1,200-bed hospitals, the Walter Reed General Hospital in Washington, D.C., and the Fitzsimons General Hospital in Denver, Colorado. In 1925 all government hospitals submitted to the survey program of the ACS, and all passed.[67] Yet, while the civilian practice of hospital administration was maturing into a clearly defined profession, change occurred slowly in the Army. A shortage of military physicians in the expanding prewar Army became acute during the winter of 1940–41, and some MAC officers replaced physicians in administrative specialty positions to help alleviate the staffing problems. But substitution of that sort did not materially progress during the interwar years. It would take World War II to spur the growth of professionalism in Army hospital administration.[68]

While evolving, hospital administration did not yet possess the attractiveness as a profession that it would later have. It was still "generally viewed as an inferior calling, offering a berth rather than an opportunity."[69] Educational levels reflected that perception: of 2,196 administrators responding to a survey in 1935, 12 percent had no education beyond high school. While 67 percent of the men had university degrees, that figure was misleading because two-thirds of all administrators were women, and only 8 percent of the women had college degrees. Furthermore, half of all male respondents were physicians whose training was not related to management.[70]

The American College of Hospital Administrators (ACHA) was an important factor in the development of the profession both in civilian life and in the Army. Formed in 1933 to enhance the professional growth and development of its members, it both influenced and was influenced by Medical Administrative Corps and, later, Medical Service Corps officers. University training in hospital administration began, and in 1934 Michael M. Davis at the University of Chicago started the first successful graduate program. However, the Medical Department offered its officers no programs to improve their skills in hospital administration during the interwar period.[71]

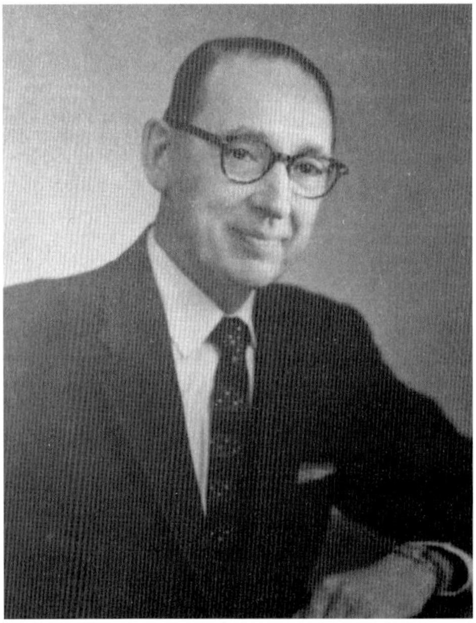

Professor Gibbs

Frederick H. Gibbs was a pioneer in hospital administration whose career exemplified the noncommissioned officers who developed expertise in various administrative specialties and went on to obtain appointments in the Medical Administrative Corps. Gibbs enlisted in 1925 and his Medical Department assignments led to commissioning in 1941 and to various hospital administration assignments, including duty during World War II as the 4th Service Command hospital inspector. Following the war Gibbs served as chief of the Surgeon General's Management Improvement Branch and as the second director of the Army-Baylor Program in Hospital Administration. In 1956 Colonel Gibbs became director of the Interagency Institute for Federal Health Care Executives. He founded the graduate program in Health Services Administration of the George Washington University after his retirement from the Army.[72]

Scientific Specialty Officers

The absence of a Sanitary Corps in the Regular Army prevented the flowering of the scientific specialties provided by that corps in World War I. A small number of Sanitary Corps officers maintained an Army affiliation during the interwar years through the reserve or National Guard. The importance of that corps as a Medical Department wartime asset was recognized in the Medical Department's *Handbook for the Medical Soldier*:

> It is composed of officers qualified as sanitary engineers, hospital architects, public health licentiates who are not graduates in medicine, experts on food and nutrition, psychologists, chemists, laboratory and x-ray experts, and business and technical men engaged in the production of supplies and appliances used by the Medical Department.[73]

Annual training of Sanitary Corps Reserve officers began with four officers attending summer training in 1923 and 1924. A two-week course for Medical Department officers began in 1925 at the Medical Field Service School, Carlisle Barracks, that was attended by twenty-five Sanitary Corps and twenty-six Medical Administrative Corps Reserve officers the first year. During the 1927 session Lt. Col. William A. Hardenbergh, SnC, recognized a need for training physicians and Sanitary Corps officers in the distinctive requirements of military preventive medicine; he led the other sixteen Sanitary Corps officers attending summer camp in developing a military sanitation course that was conducted each summer from 1928 to 1940 for both Medical Corps and Sanitary Corps officers. The course included instruction in epidemiology, sanitary engineering, and preventive medicine administration. The reserve officers also used the time at summer camp to develop wartime preventive medicine doctrine and plans for the utilization of scientific specialty officers, principally sanitary engineers. That effort included plans drawn up in 1935 by Lt. Col. Paul E. Howell, SnC, and Maj. Rudolph J. Anderson, SnC, for the use of nutrition officers. The efforts of these officers during the interwar years helped to offset the absence of their expertise on active duty and ensured that the Army had a nucleus of preventive medicine specialists and doctrine to draw from when the United States entered World War II. A small reserve corps devoted to preventive medicine purposes provided the department and the nation with a capability that had not existed in previous interwar periods.[74]

Sanitary Engineering

Sanitary engineers were prominent in the Medical Department's planning efforts. Led by Colonel Hardenbergh, a prominent sanitary engineer who published standard texts on water purification and sewage treatment during this period, they maintained their currency with military medicine and with each other through correspondence courses, meetings of local reserve groups, and annual training. Hardenbergh, Lt. Col. Michael Blew, SnC, and others directed the two-week training sessions at Carlisle.[75]

The wartime doctrine, as they developed it under Hardenbergh's leadership in 1934, called for sanitary engineers to gather preventive medicine data and to supervise sanitation efforts within each corps area during the mobilization period. They envisioned that sanitation for a field army would be the responsibility of Sanitary Corps public health specialists assigned to the army surgeon who would have a sanitary battalion to execute the preventive medicine efforts throughout the field army area of operations. Hardenbergh and other planners believed that the structure they proposed would both improve the Army's sanitation efforts and provide increased opportunity for field grade promotions for Sanitary Corps officers.[76]

Their planning, which was based on the concept of a small reserve Sanitary Corps without any Regular Army counterpart, gave pause to some outside observers. The editor of the *American Journal of Public Health* argued that only 100 of the 400 Sanitary Corps Reserve officers were "qualified sanitarians." That number would be insufficient for the public health capability to support the Army's planning for the mobilization of over 1.5 million soldiers in four months. Their plans were not the precise blueprint; a sanitary battalion would not come to pass, for example. Yet the effort had catalyzed organizations representing the interests of sanitary engineers into a posture of careful oversight that would intensify after World War II.[77]

Perhaps most important, the department had an enthusiastic nucleus of officers who were devoted to the objectives of preventive medicine. Their training ended each summer with a meeting of the Loyal Order of the Boar, a fraternal group

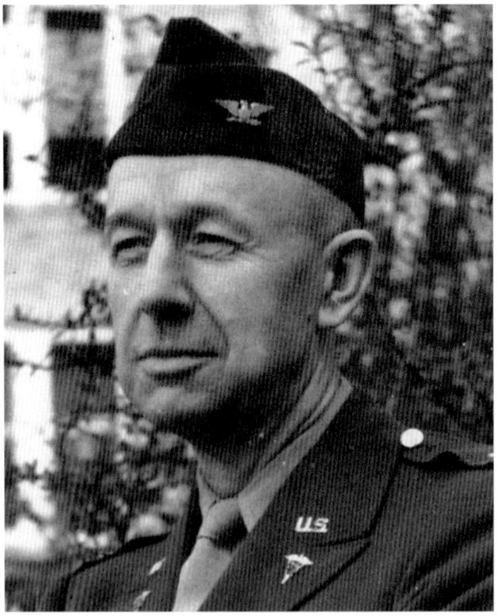

Colonel Hardenbergh
(Photo taken in 1941.)

formed at Carlisle in 1928. Membership was by invitation for a select group of Sanitary Corps and Medical Corps officers who were "interested primarily in sanitation and the promotion of good fellowship between officers of the Regular and Reserve components of the Army." Its mottos were *Fratres Suilis* and "In Union There Is Strength." Its logo was two hogs pointing in opposite directions with their tails entwined. Meetings followed an agenda of "banquet, Boar business, and the initiation of the shoats into the Order." Officers included a president, vice president, secretary-treasurer, and "The Boar." The Loyal Order of the Boar continued to generate a fraternal spirit among officers affiliated with the preventive medicine mission during the interwar period as well as after World War II.[78]

Chiropody and Optometry

No state regulated chiropody prior to 1895, and barbers, masseurs, shoemakers, and shoe clerks cut corns as a sideline along with itinerant corn-cutters. By the early 1930s chiropody had come to include the treatment of a variety of foot conditions such as bunions, abnormal nails, and defective arches. It was becoming established as a distinct health care specialty, partly "because chiropodists are able to supply service at a price which physicians cannot and will not meet."[79] H.R. 3738, introduced in 1941, proposed establishment of an Army chiropody corps of the same number of officers as the Dental Corps. Candidates would have to be graduates of established colleges of chiropody and pass a Medical Department examination in the specialty. This legislation, as in the case of the embalmers corps, failed to gain congressional support and died.[80]

By 1932 there were 20,000 optometrists practicing in the United States, and the profession was exhibiting a widening scope of practice based on a broader range of diagnostic procedures. Their bread-and-butter procedure of refraction was becoming viewed as a technical application for which the ophthalmologist was overtrained. When a physician performed that procedure "his general medical knowledge lies idle and constitutes an unused overhead for which patients must pay." However, the absence of military optometrists required Army physicians to perform the examinations.[81]

The program of free issue of spectacles to enlisted personnel begun in 1918 was extended to officers in 1920 and then dropped in 1922. While Army physicians could prescribe spectacles, the government would not as a rule supply them free of charge. The Medical Department got back in the business—although not for soldiers—in the 1930s when it was tasked with providing medical support to the Civilian Conservation Corps (CCC), one of FDR's New Deal programs. The Army charged the CCC enrollees an average of $2.60 for a pair of eyeglasses. This was during a time when spectacle prices generally ranged between $5 and $10, although some larger drug chains would sell them for as low as $3.35.[82]

Summary

The Army needed commissioned officers in a variety of administrative and scientific specialties to form the team necessary for a modern military medical support system. As a result, the Medical Department struggled to retain in peacetime the capabilities that had been created during war, and Surgeon Generals Ireland and Patterson fought to establish a full-time corps, which they called the Medical Auxiliary Corps. But their dream was not to become reality during the interwar period. The formation of the Medical Administrative Corps in the Regular Army and reserve components and the retention of the Sanitary Corps in the reserve components was as far as Congress was prepared to go.

The need for officers in administrative specialties was met only marginally, and the department again resorted to using clinicians—principally physicians and dentists—to fill administrative positions. The need to return such specialists to clinical practice (and to enable them to retain their professional skills), the increasing sophistication of health care institutions, and the advances in administrative specialties were building a demand not met by the Medical Department's structure. The professionalization of hospital administration in the civilian sector—as exemplified in the formation of the American College of Hospital Administrators—represented advances in the civilian health care industry not matched by the Army. The move to provide additional reserve component officers qualified in medical supply was an encouraging development, but not enough for a department charged with preparing an industrial capability to support a world power.

The growth of scientific medicine was producing emerging specialties that sought professional recognition by the Army. Chiropody knocked on the door with a proposal for a separate corps, and the Army's tentative steps in establishing an optical program for soldiers was a glimpse at the future of optometry. Sanitary engineers established a position of prominence, to the credit of Col. William Hardenbergh and his fellow reserve officers. Their work in developing a sanitary engineering doctrine for wartime preventive medicine exhibited the progressive thinking necessary for a modern army.

Pharmacy's lobbying for a place in the commissioned officer ranks was one of the larger stories, both as an example of an emerging scientific specialty and as a demonstration of the effect of external influences upon the Medical Department. The pharmacy struggle entangled three surgeons general in a protracted debate with representatives of a politically influential specialty's professional guilds and trade press. It resulted in the addition of a needed commissioned specialty, but only at the cost of losing others.

Opportunities for career advancement remained small. The Army offered Regular Army careers for a small number of officers commissioned in administrative and scientific specialties, the latter restricted to pharmacy. For those few officers, their opportunity in the Army beyond commissioning was circumscribed by limited chances for training, positions, promotions, and sometimes pay. Those constraints made it difficult to build professionalism in the Medical Administrative Corps. Another small group had an opportunity for Army affiliation on a part-time basis through the reserve and National Guard, but the active and reserve components together did not provide the numbers or expertise for the department to assume global responsibilities.

Nevertheless, a small group of Medical Administrative Corps officers kept the flame alive in the Regular Army during the interwar period. They formed a slender thread of continuity between the world wars. Years later, Col. Othmar Goriup, the first chief of the Medical Service Corps, saluted the officers who stuck it out, "little, old, gray-haired people who were still captains." He hoped that young officers just entering active duty would be told about "the real black days" when opportunity was so limited. "If it hadn't been for these people, God knows we probably wouldn't have . . . the Corps that we have today."[83]

Notes

[1] Demobilization: See Marvin A. Kreidberg and Merton G. Henry, *History of Military Mobilization in the United States Army, 1775–1945* (Washington, D.C.: Government Printing Office, 1955), pp. 374, 379. Numbers: *SG Report*, 1919, 2: 1112; *SG Report*, 1920, p. 284; Lynch, *The Surgeon General's Office*, p. 138. Reductions: John H. McMinn and Max Levin, *Personnel in World War II*, vol. 14 of *Medical Department, United States Army in World War II*, ed. John B. Coates, Jr. (Washington, D.C.: Office of the Surgeon General, Department of the Army, 1963), pp. 23, 113; *Medical Bulletin* (April 1938): 1. SGO cut: *Medical Bulletin* (October 1934): 4. USAAS and SnC: *SG Report*, 1919, 2: 1118. Wrightson: Biographical summary, U.S. Army Center of Military History, in MSC-USACMH.

[2] Great Depression: John J. Ward, who would eventually retire as an MSC colonel, entered college in 1929, the year of the stock market crash. He worked in a steel mill for 17¢ an hour in order to pay $5 a week for room and board. *Stack Arms*, newsletter of the Willow Grove Chapter of the Retired Officers Association, Incl to Ltr, Col John J. Ward, USA, Ret., to Col Walter F. Johnson III, MSC, 18 Mar 85, in MSC history files, DASG-MS.

[3] Interwar period: Biographical information based on lectures and typed summaries by D. Clayton James, Ph.D., Morrison Professor of History, U.S. Army Command and General Staff College, Fort Leavenworth, Kans., 2 Apr–2 Jun 81, author's notes. See also Thomas W. Collier, "The Army and the Great Depression," *Parameters* 18 (September 1988): 105; Peter Lyon, *Eisenhower: Portrait of the Hero* (Boston: Little, Brown, and Company, 1974), p. 53. Quoted words: Forrest C. Pogue, *George C. Marshall: Education of a General, 1880–1939*, vol. 1 of 3 (New York: Viking, 1963), p. 297. Marshall was a lieutenant for fourteen years after his graduation from Virginia Military Institute in 1901.

[4] Schools: See also Weigley, *History of the United States Army*, pp. 477–78. They also wrote. In 1920 Eisenhower and Patton published articles in the *Infantry Journal* promoting the tank, an action that got Eisenhower in hot water with the chief of infantry. See George S. Patton, "Tanks in Future Wars," *Infantry Journal* 13 (May 1920): 958–62; Dwight D. Eisenhower, "A Tank Discussion," *Infantry Journal* 13 (November 1920): 453–58; Eisenhower, *At Ease: Stories I Tell to Friends* (New York: Doubleday, 1967), p. 173.

[5] Quoted words: *SG Report*, 1922, p. 242.

[6] Medical Field Service School (MFSS): *SG Report*, 1922, pp. 243–44; Interv, Col Henry J. Nelson, MSC, Ret., with Col Harral A. Bigham, MSC, Denver, Colo., 2 Jan 85, DASG-MS. Quoted words: Maj C. H. Rice, Inspector General Department (IGD), War Department Inspector General (WDIG), in Rpt, sub: Inspection and Survey of Carlisle Barracks, Pennsylvania, June 3–7, 1929, 22 Jun 29, RG 159, E11, Box 185, NARA-WNRC.

[7] Air ambulances: *SG Report*, 1926, p. 304, and 1930, p. 395; *Medical Bulletin* 26 (September 1931): 122–31; Richard Tierney and Fred Montgomery, *The Army Aviation Story* (Northport, Ala.: Colonial Press, 1963), p. 204; David M. Lam, "From Balloon to Black Hawk: The Origins," pp. 46–48. The Panama plane flew five missions evacuating seven patients before it was destroyed in a crash. Each mission averaged five hours, a savings of twenty-four hours. The Kelly Field plane received national attention when it evacuated casualties from a tornado in Rocksprings, Texas, in 1927; in 1930 it evacuated thirty-four patients.

[8] Colonel Blew: THU, OTSG, Minutes of the First Meeting of the Advisory Editorial Board for the History of the U.S. Army Medical Service Corps, held at Forest Glen, Maryland, 13 November 1958, MSC-USACMH, cited hereafter as 1958 MSC History Project. Appointments: *SG Report*, 1920, p. 293. SnC Reserve: Speech, Lt Col Joseph J. Gilbert, SnC, at Sanitary Corps, U.S. Army, Conference of Sanitary Corps Officers, Headquarters (HQ), 2d Service Command, 24 Nov 44, MSC-USACMH.

[9] 20 percent: *Medical Bulletin* (February 1922): 45. Quoted words: Interv, Maj Gen George E. Armstrong, MC, Ret., with Col Joseph Israeloff, MSC, THU, OTSG, 12 Mar 76, interv files, USACMH.

[10] Quoted words: Interv, Brig Gen Harold W. Glattly, MC, Ret., with Samuel Milner, CMH, 22 Oct 63, USACMH.

[11] Problems: James A. Tobey, *The Medical Department of the Army*, Institute for Government Research Monograph no. 45 (Baltimore: Johns Hopkins, 1927), pp. 68, 84–92, hereafter cited as Tobey, *The Medical Department*; Maj Gen Norman T. Kirk to Brig Gen Elliot G. Cutler, Harvard University Medical School, sub: The Procurement of Medical Officers for the Post War Army, 1 Jul 46, MSC-USACMH. "They were looked down upon by the line, and had little to do with civilian medicine, who didn't think much of them either" (Interv, Col Frederick H. Gibbs, MSC, Ret., with Samuel Milner, CMH, 18 Mar 64, USACMH).

[12] MSC proposal: U.S. Congress, Senate, Hearings on S. 2715, *A Bill To Increase the Efficiency of the United States Army, and for Other Purposes*, 66th Cong., 1st sess., 1919, p. 612. In fact a "Medical Service Corps" already existed. The Council of National Defense, in an action on 31 January 1918 that was approved by President Wilson on 12 August, formed a "Volunteer Medical Service Corps" for the purpose of enrolling all physicians who were not eligible for reasons such as age, physical disability, etc., for service in the Medical Reserve Corps of the Army or Navy. This was a creature of the moment when there was patriotic fervor to "go over there," and the catalyst for the group ended with the armistice. Franklin Martin, "Volunteer Medical Service Corps," *New York Medical Journal* 108 (1918): 291–93.

[13] Quoted words: Ibid.

[14] MAC formation: 41 Stat. 767, 4 June 1920; Memo, Capt E. R. Taylor, Judge Advocate General Corps (JAGC), for Col Kintz, sub: Brief Summary of Medical Administrative Corps Legislation, 12 Feb 46, MSC-USACMH; Fact Sheet, OTSG, sub: Army Medical Service Corps, 1957, DASG-MS. Appointments: *SG Report*, 1921, p. 109. Positions: Charles V. Lewis, "Medical Administrative Corps," *Military Surgeon* 80 (April 1937): 304–05.

[15] Reserves: *SG Report*, 1921, pp. 117–18; *Medical Bulletin* (1 January 1931); War Department, *Annual Report of the Chief of the National Guard Bureau*, 1937; Crossland and Currie, *Twice the Citizen*, p. 37.

[16] Quoted words: *SG Report*, 1926, p. 222.

[17] Reductions: 42 Stat. 721, 30 June 1922. Ceiling on pay: 42 Stat. 625, 10 June 1922. MAC positions: SGO Cir Ltr 2, 10 Jan 23, MSC-USACMH. TSG proposal: Memo, Brig Gen F. R. Koefer, Asst Surg Gen, for Col David L. Stone, General Staff (GS), Office of the Chief of Staff, Army (OCSA), sub: Letter of Captain C. R. Dabbs re Discrimination Against M.A.C., 6 Apr 27, MSC-USACMH. Pay restriction lifted: 45 Stat. 788, 28 May 1928.

[18] 1924 efforts: Maj Gen Merritte W. Ireland, TSG, to A. L. I. Winne, Chairman (Chm), American Pharmaceutical Association (APA), 9 Nov 28, MSC-USACMH.

[19] Wainwright bill: U.S. Congress, House, H.R. 1248, 71st Cong., 1st sess., 18 April 1929.

[20] 1934 accessions: *Medical Bulletin* (October 1934): 17–18. Promotion "hump": 49 Stat. 505, 31 Jul 35; *Medical Bulletin* (October 1935): 70; Memo, Henry N. Fuller, sub: Notes Relative to the Medical Administrative Corps, 4 May 37, MSC-USACMH.

[21] MAC reduced: 49 Stat. 36, 24 June 1936.

[22] Quoted words: Speech, Maj Gen James P. Cooney, Dep Surg Gen, sub: Some Notes on the Historical Development of the Medical Service Corps, at monthly MSC meeting, Forest Glen annex, Walter Reed General Hospital, 25 Oct 56, box 2/18, MSC-USACMH. "Ireland did everything possible to dissolve the inequities under which the Corps labored at the time."

[23] Reynold's views: Charles R. Reynolds, "Legislation Affecting the Medical Department," *Medical Bulletin* (July 1936): 7, 9.

[24] Problems: Interv, Col Louis F. Williams, MSC, Ret., with Lt Col Richard V. N. Ginn, MSC, Clearwater, Fla., 15 Nov 84, DASG-MS; Interv, Col Frederick H. Gibbs, with Milner, CMH, 24 Oct 63, MSC-USACMH. Colonel Williams served on the court-martial of one of the MAC officers convicted of wrongdoing during this period.

[25] Reynold's views: Memo, Reynolds, sub: Commissioning of Pharmacists in the Army, 4 Apr 36, MSC-USACMH.

[26] Embalmers corps: U.S. Congress, House, H.R. 8282, *A Bill Amending the Act of June 3, 1916, entitled "The National Defense Act,"* 74th Cong., 1st sess., 31 May 1935; *Medical Bulletin* (July 1935): 14.

[27] Pharmacy Corps: Caswell A. Mayo, "Why the Pharmaceutical Corps Should Be Established," *American Druggist* 66 (April 1918): 25–27.

[28] Winne letter: A. L. I. Winne, Chm, APA, to Maj Gen Merritte W. Ireland, TSG, 15 Oct 28, MSC-USACMH.

[29] Ireland: Ireland to Winne, 10 Oct 28, MSC-USACMH.

[30] Exchange of letters: Winne to Ireland, 22 Oct 28; Ireland to Winne, 24 Oct 28, both MSC-USACMH.

[31] Quoted words: Winne to Ireland, 25 Oct 85, MSC-USACMH.

[32] Controversy continues: Winne to Ireland, 1 Nov 28; Ireland to Winne, 9 Nov 28, both MSC-USACMH.

[33] Quoted words: Murray Breese, "Will Pharmacy Again Be a Joke in the Next War," *American Druggist* (October 1928): 18–19, 70, 72.

[34] Copeland bill: U.S. Congress, Senate, S. 3211, *A Bill To Amend the National Defense Act by Providing for a Pharmacy Corps in the Medical Department*, 71st Cong., 2d sess., 6 January 1930. 21-page letter: Ireland to Special Conference of the APA Committee, 15 Nov 30; Lt Col G. L. McKinney, MC, Planning and Training Div, SGO, to Lt Col A. D. Tuttle, MC, Spec Asst to TSG, 1 Dec 30, MSC-USACMH.

[35] APA delighted: E. Fullerton Cook, P.D., Philadelphia College of Pharmacy and Science, to Ireland, 24 Nov 30, MSC-USACMH. Opposition: Ireland to Rep Jonathan M. Wainwright, 3 Dec 30, MSC-USACMH.

[36] Pharmacy survey: Memo, Col S. J. Morris, MC, Spec Asst to TSG, for TSG, 10 May 32. No need for change: Maj Gen Robert U. Patterson, TSG, to E. F. Kelly, Secretary (Secy), APA, 20 Jun 32. TSG position not changed: Lt Col Robert C. McDonald, MC, Executive Officer (XO), SGO, to E. F. Kelly, 11 Apr 34. APA president under pressure: Robert P. Fischelis, Pres, APA, to Patterson, 7 Mar 35. Quoted words: Patterson to Fischelis, 11 Mar 35, all in MSC-USACMH.

[37] Medical Auxiliary Corps: U.S. Congress, House, H.R. 5594, 74th Cong., 1st sess., 12 February 1935; *Medical Bulletin* (April 1935): 24. Johnson bill: Rep Jed Johnson to Patterson, 8 Apr 35; Patterson to Johnson, 15 Apr 35, MSC-USACMH; U.S. Congress, House, H.R. 7485, 74th Cong., 1st sess., 12 April 1935; *Medical Bulletin* (July 1935): 14–15. Pharmacists in the MC: U.S. Congress, House, H.R. 7455, 74th Cong., 1st sess., 11 April 1935.

[38] Exasperation: Patterson to Fischelis, 2 May 35. Medical Auxiliary Corps: Patterson to ACS, G–1, sub: Pharmacy Bill (HR 7485), 6 May 35, both in MSC-USACMH.

[39] Reynold's opposition: Maj Gen Charles R. Reynolds, TSG, to Johnson, 12 Jul 35, MSC-USACMH. APA: H. Evert Kending, Chm, Committee on Pharmacy Corps in the U.S. Army, to Reynolds, 16 Jan 36, MSC-USACMH.

[40] Response: Reynolds to Kending, 22 Jan 36, MSC-USACMH. Requirements: Memo, Maj J. A. Rogers, MC, for TSG, 25 Jan 36, MSC-USACMH.

[41] Sheppard bill: U.S. Congress, Senate, S. 4390, 74th Cong., 2d sess., 30 March 1936; and Sen Norm Sheppard to Reynolds, 31 Mar 36, MSC-USACMH. Quoted words: Memo, Reynolds, 4 Apr 36, MSC-USACMH.

[42] Reynold's testimony: U.S. Congress, House, Military Affairs Committee, Hearings, 26 May 1926.

[43] Commissions: 49 Stat. 1907, 24 June 1936. Examinations: *Medical Bulletin* (April 1937): 30; *SG Report*, 1939, p. 171. Candidates were required to be male U.S. citizens, between the ages of twenty-one and thirty-two, possessing a BS in pharmacy from an acceptable four-year college. The examination process included a physical examination, an assessment of the candidate's adaptability for military service, and a written test in the practice of pharmacy, pharmaceutical chemistry, pharmacognosy, pharmacology, bacteriology, and hygiene and sanitation. *Medical Bulletin* (October 1938): 113–14. 16 officers: 53 Stat. 555, 3 April 1939. 68 officers: McMinn and Levin, *Personnel in World War II*, p. 113.

[44] Japan: *SG Report*, 1924, p. 300. Aviation: See *SG Report*, 1930, p. 394.

[45] Lieutenant Black: Transcript, Lt Col Richard V. N. Ginn, MSC, Asst to Chief, MSC, sub: Panel Discussion with Former Chiefs of the Medical Service Corps, Washington, D.C., 6 May 83, DASG-MS; Interv, Col Robert L. Black, USA, Ret., with Lt Col Michael C. Baker, MSC, Palm Springs, Calif., 7 Mar 84, Project 84–16, Senior Officers Oral History Program, U.S. Army Military History Institute (USAMHI) and the U.S. Army War College, Carlisle Barracks, Pa., USAMHI, hereafter cited as Black, Baker Interv. Schofield: Black to Ginn, 24 Dec 84, DASG-MS.

[46] Fort Benning: MSC Panel, 6 May 83; Isadore S. Falk, *Organized Medical Service at Fort Benning* (Chicago: University of Chicago, 1937), p. 3. Pay cut: Black, Baker Interv.

[47] Training: Memo, Col Charles R. Reynolds, MC, CDT, MFSS, sub: The Medical Field Service School, 9 Nov 29, in Stimson Library, Academy of Health Sciences, Fort Sam Houston, Tex.; *SG Report*, 1931, p. 346. Also see Black, Baker Interv. In other examples: no MACs attended any course in 1926; six attended the basic course in 1935 and one attended in 1940, but no other courses either year. *SG Report*, 1926, p. 328; 1927, p. 332; 1935, p. 143; 1940, p. 180. In 1929 a report of the Army inspector general singled out Capt. Samuel W. Pennington, MAC, for special praise for his food service operation at Carlisle. Rpt, WD IG, sub: Inspection and Survey of Carlisle Barracks, Pennsylvania, Made June 3–7, 1929, by Maj. C. H. Rice, IGD, 22 Jun 29, RG 159, E11, Box 185, NARA-NA. The first advanced course was conducted 11 February to 15 December 1926 for five MC officers. The course was divided into three sections: mobilization, industrial procurement, and medical planning. *SG Report*, 1927, p. 332. Lieutenant Smith: *Medical Bulletin* (July 1938): 96.

[48] Reserves: Crossland and Currie, *Twice the Citizen*, p. 40.

[49] Reserve training: *SG Report*, 1931, p. 344.

[50] Colonel England: "Captain Thomas M. England," *Military Surgeon* 87 (October 1940): 384–85; Biographical summary, THU, OTSG, undated, MSC-USACMH; WDGO 57, 21 Sep 43, PL; Clarence M. Smith, *The Medical Department: Hospitalization and Evacuation, Zone of the Interior*, in the series United States Army in World War II (Washington, D.C.: Office of the Chief of Military History, Department of the Army, 1956), p. 306, hereafter cited as Smith, *Hospitalization and Evacuation*. Used as an amputation center, its closure in 1946 became a cause celebre as amputees staged protests in Atlantic City. MS, Tracy S. Voorhees, "A Lawyer Among the Doctors," USACMH, p. 218.

[51] Dickson and Burkard: Biographical data cards, THU, OTSG, USACMH.

[52] Carmack: Interv, Col Joseph Carmack, MSC, Ret., with Israeloff, 25 Jan 67, USACMH. Nelson: Nelson, Bigham Interv, DASG-MS.

[53] Williams: Williams to Col R. L. Parker, MSC, 13 Jun 60; Williams to Ginn, 7 Nov 84; Williams, Ginn Interv, DASG-MS.

[54] Increase: M. A. Reasoner, "The Development of the Medical Supply Service," *Military Surgeon* 63 (July 1928): 2. Overseas: *Medical Bulletin* (October 1935): 18–19. Kernan: "Medical Supply Renamed After Pioneer Corpsman," *Southern Command News*, 10 November 1967; "Medical Officer's Widow Unveils Memorial Plaque," *Southern Command News*, 12 November 1967, DASG-MS. His son, Col. William F. Kernan, USARSO Dep Cdr, assisted Mrs. Kernan in the ceremony. Appointments in reserves: *SG Report*, 1924, p. 227.

[55] Shortage: *Medical Bulletin* (15 October 1922): 177. Black: Black to Col R. L. Parker, MSC, 17 May 60, MSC-USACMH.

[56] Feud: See Gorgas and Hendrick, *William Crawford Gorgas*, pp. 222–33; McCullough, *The Path Between the Seas*, pp. 572–73; Harrison, *Mosquitoes, Malaria and Man*, p. 166; Joseph Baldwin Bishop and Farnham Bishop, *Goethals, Genius of the Panama Canal* (New York: Harper and Brothers, 1930), pp. 171–75.

[57] Transfer: Wolfe, *Finance and Supply*, pp. 75–81; WD Cir 102, 24 Oct 18, PL. Quoted words: Wolfe, *Finance and Supply*, p. 81.

[58] Clash: Bishop and Bishop, *Goethals, Genius of the Panama Canal*, p. 378. Quoted words: U.S. Congress, Senate, Hearings on S. 2715, 66th Cong., 1st sess., 29 September 1919, pp. 1031–32.

[59] Supply training: Wolfe, *Finance and Supply*, p. 663. MC emphasis: *Medical Bulletin* (April 1938): 34. General depot program: *Medical Bulletin* (October 1922): 179; Robert J. Parks, *Medical Training in World War II* (Washington, D.C.: Office of the Surgeon General, Department of the Army, 1974), in the series Medical Department in World War II, p. 48. Black: Black to Parker, 17 May 60, MSC-USACMH.

[60] Reserve supply training: *Medical Bulletin* (July 1938): 99–100.

[61] SnC Reserve: OTSG, Supply Service Notes, Sep–Dec 44, MSC-USACMH. Asst Secy: Lt Col Charles F. Shook, MC, Finance and Supply Div, SGO, to Maj Paul I. Robinson, MC, sub: Assistant Secretary of War's Weekly Report, 10 Sep 40, MSC-USACMH. Increase: McMinn and Levin, *Personnel in World War II*, p. 113.

[62] Quoted words: Black, Baker Interv.

[63] McKnight: *Medical Bulletin* (January 1936): 77–78.

[64] Hospitals: Neuhauser, *Coming of Age*, pp. 41–42; Siegfried Giedeon, *Space, Time and Architecture* (Cambridge: Harvard, 1956), pp. 206–09.

[65] ACS: American College of Surgeons, *Manual of Hospital Standardization* (Chicago: ACS, 1937), p. 7. The ACS classified hospitals of 100 beds or more as large hospitals.

[66] Medical schools: U.S. Department of Labor, *Postwar Outlook for Physicians*, Bulletin 863 (Washington, D.C.: U.S. Bureau of Labor Statistics, 12 February 1946), p. 3. Teaching hospitals: Ludmerer, *Learning To Heal*, pp. 219–33, 257. The dates are Ludmerer's.

[67] Army hospitals: Memo, Maj John A. Rogers, MC, for TSG, 25 Jan 36, MSC-USACMH; Tobey, *The Medical Department*, p. 103.

[68] Substitution: Smith, *Hospitalization and Evacuation*, pp. 30–31.

[69] Quoted words: Neuhauser, *Coming of Age*, p. 57.

[70] 1935 survey: Ibid., p. 58.

[71] ACHA: American College of Hospital Administrators, *ACHA News* 15 (January 1957); Neuhauser, *Coming of Age*, p. 15. Reports: James A. Tobey, "The Mission of the Sanitary Corps (Sanitation Section) in War Time," *Military Surgeon* 76 (April 1935): 73. First program: Michael M. Davis, *Hospital Administration: A Career* (New York: Rockefeller Foundation, 1927), pp. 58–88; Neuhauser, *Coming of Age*, pp. 92–93.

[72] Gibbs: Interv, Col Frederick H. Gibbs, MSC, Ret., with Ginn, St. Petersburg, Fla., 15 Nov 84, DASG-MS.

[73] Quoted words: Arnold D. Tuttle, *Handbook for the Medical Soldier* (New York: William Wood, 1927), p. 39.

[74] Training: Cols William A. Hardenbergh, Michael J. Blew, and Raymond J. Karpen, draft chapter, sub: The Sanitary Corps, undated, folder 83, box 6/18; Rpt, Lt Col Paul E. Howe, SnC, and Maj Rudolph J. Anderson, SnC, sub: Proposal for the Use of Officers of the Sanitary Corps Trained in Food and Nutrition, MFSS, 1935, folder 109, box 8/18, both in MSC-USACMH. The 1925 course also included 252 Medical Corps (MC), 24 Dental Corps (DC), and 7 Veterinary Corps (VC) officers. The Military Sanitation Course was not held in 1933 because the Reserve Army instructors were on Civilian Conservation Corps duty.

[75] Sanitary engineers: Speech, Lt Col Joseph J. Gilbert, MSC, sub: The Sanitary Corps—U.S. Army, presented at the meeting of the Association of Military Surgeons, Sanitary Engineering panel, 2 Nov 44; Col Stanley J. Weidenkopf, draft chapter, sub: Sanitary Engineering, in THU, MSC history project, 1965, pp. 14–15, all in MSC-USACMH. Hardenbergh: William A. Hardenbergh (Lt. Col., SnCR), *Sewerage and Sewage Treatment* (Scranton, Pa.: International Textbook Company, 1936); Hardenbergh, *Operation of Sewage-Treatment Plants* (Scranton: International Textbook Company, 1939); Hardenbergh, *Purification of Water* (Scranton: International Textbook Company, 1938).

[76] Sanitation plan: Tobey, "The Mission of the Sanitary Corps," pp. 180–81.

[77] 1938 editorial: Cited in *Military Surgeon* 83 (November 1938): 459–60.

[78] The Boar: Maj Gen Paul H. Streit, MC, to Lt Col Elwood Camp, MSC, 8 Jul 50; Col Raymond J. Karpen, MSC, Ret., to Lt Col Joseph Israeloff, MSC, sub: Observations on the Formative Period of the Medical Service Corps, 14 Apr 76, both in DASG-MS.

[79] Chiropody: Louis S. Reed, *Midwives, Chiropodists and Optometrists: Their Place in Medical Care*, pamphlet no. 15 (Washington, D.C.: Committee on the Costs of Medical Care, March 1932), pp. 6–8.

[80] Chiropody corps: U.S. Congress, House, H.R. 3738, *A Bill To Establish a Chiropody (Podiatry) Corps in the Medical Corps of the United States Army*, 77th Cong., 1st sess., 3 March 1941.

[81] Optometry: Reed, *Midwives, Chiropodists and Optometrists*, pp. 3–9.

[82] Optical program: TSG Cir Ltr 99, 25 Aug 20, RG 112, Accession 69A–127, Box 10/32; TSG Cir Ltr 20, 4 Apr 22, RG 112, 69A–127, Box 10/32; Memos, Jones for the Executive Officer, SGO, 1 Aug 34 and 12 Aug 37, RG 112, 44A–0041, Box 1/1; TAG to CG, 1st Army Corps Area, 5 Jun 41, and TSG to TAG, 5 Jun 41, RG 112, 69A–127, Box 10/32, all in NARA-WNRC; WDGO 14, 31 Mar 22, PL. Prices: Advertising, *Optometric Weekly*, 23 November 1933 and 15 February 1934, and Ltr to the editor, J. H. Lepper, 14 December 1933, p. 1208; Editorials, *Journal of the American Optometric Association*, November 1931, p. 30, and November 1939, pp. 14, 15.

[83] Quoted words: THU, 1958 MSC History, p. R–2 (1–2).

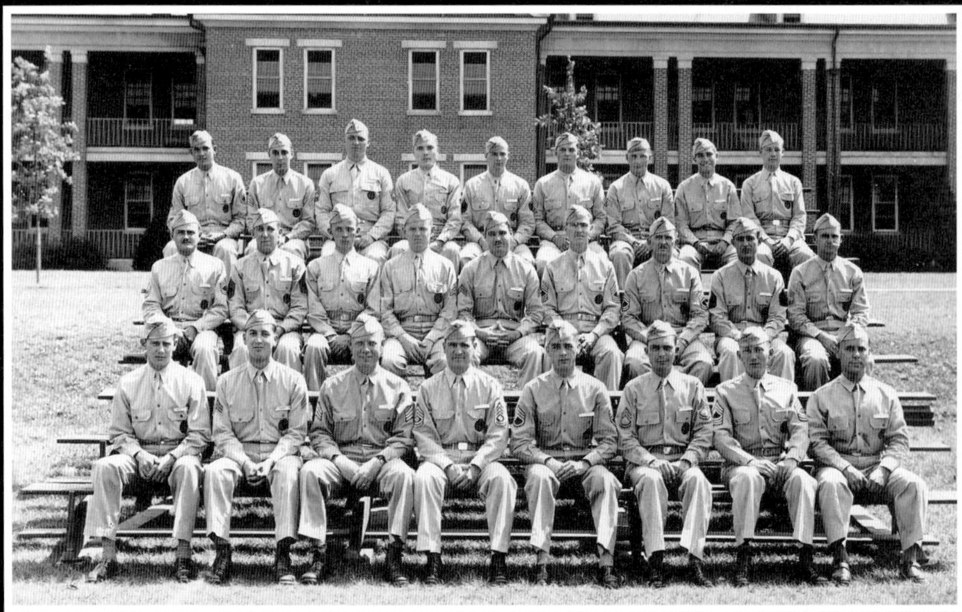

Officer Candidate School class at Carlisle Barracks, September 1941

5

World War II: The Administrative Specialties

It was in World War II that the Medical Administrative Corps (MAC) became essential to the medical support of American military operations.[1] The war was the largest task the Medical Department had ever been called upon to undertake, and in meeting its new responsibilities the MAC, "long the Cinderella of the Medical Department," grew from 1,343 active duty officers in December 1941 to a peak of 19,867 in August 1945.[2] Demand was so great for administrative officers that officer candidate schools (OCS) set up to commission MACs grew to be the third largest OCS program in the Army. Forty-five MAC officers were lost as battle deaths, and another forty-five died from nonbattle causes.[3]

On 7 December 1941, the Japanese attack on Pearl Harbor thrust the American people into a conflict that had been raging since September 1939, when Hitler invaded Poland. By the time the war ended the United States had buried 291,557 soldiers, sailors, marines, and airmen and had moved to center stage as the world's leader.[4] The war was an epic of destruction that placed enormous demands on military medicine, and the Army Medical Department expanded to over eight hundred thousand military and civilian personnel to meet the challenge.[5] Estimates of the total number of people killed in the war range up to sixty million worldwide but will never be accurately determined. Military deaths totaled nearly seventeen million for all belligerents, but for the first time more civilians than military died in war. Attacks on civilian population centers required the department to be prepared for the care of refugees and others displaced and injured by the war. The Nazis also declared a racial war against all races deemed inferior, and genocide was undertaken on an unprecedented scale. In the "final solution" the Nazis exterminated five to six million Jews and up to a half million Gypsies. An additional nine to ten million Slavs were killed by execution or starvation.[6]

Mobilization by the United States of over sixteen million citizens for military service gave the Medical Department a large support mission. More than eleven million men and women served in the Army, which mushroomed from fewer than 265,000 personnel in 1940 to a peak of nearly 8.3 million in 1945, deployed in eleven theaters of operations. Seventy percent of the Army was in support units, including a wide variety of medical organizations.[7] The Medical Department became a massive industrial organization, which required the latest in management skills. The prewar department had operated fewer than 79,000

CHART 2—WORLD WAR II ECHELONS OF MEDICAL SUPPORT

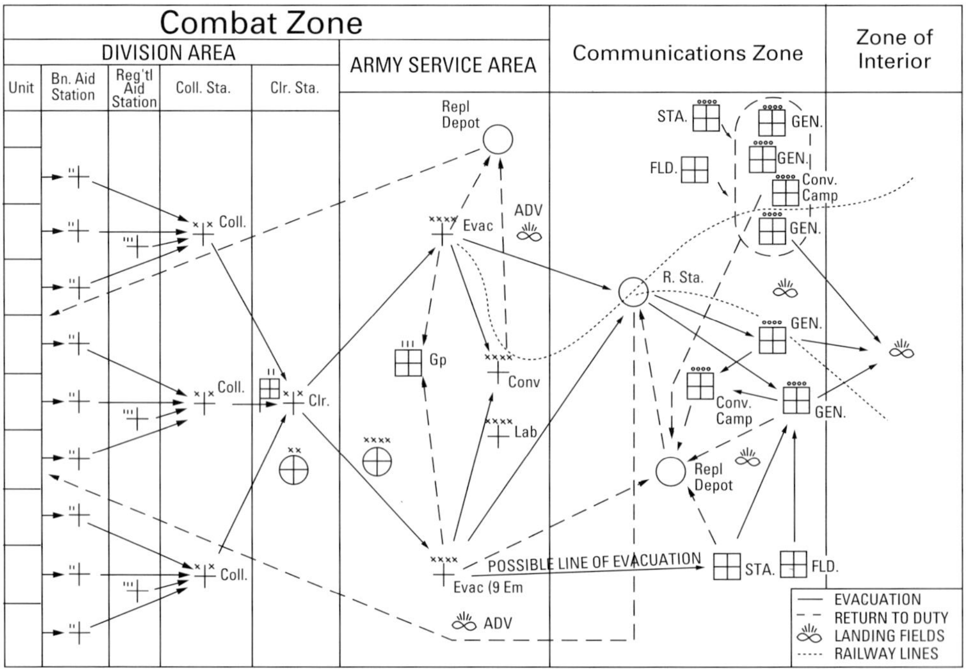

Source: *Military Medical Manual*, 6th edition, revised October 1944 (Harrisburg, Pa.: Military Service Publishing Company, 1945), p. 546.

hospital beds, but by the end of the war it maintained nearly 750,000, of which 425,000 were overseas.[8]

Medical doctrine continued to be based on a chain of treatment and evacuation under complete medical control. As in World War I, the chain stretched from the company aidman to the general hospital in the United States and included both field and fixed units in an integrated system (*Chart 2*). Sorting of the wounded by severity of injury occurred constantly at every level, and medical units evacuated casualties back to their location from areas to their front. The three echelons of medical support in World War I were, with boundary adjustments, renamed the combat zone, communications zone, and zone of the interior. The combat zone was further divided into three echelons of medical service. The first echelon was provided by the regimental medical detachment's company aidmen and aid stations. The second was provided by the clearing company and three collecting companies of the division medical battalion. The third echelon was provided by the evacuation hospitals of the field army. The first three echelons plus the communications zone (numbered station and general hospitals) and zone of the interior (named general hospitals in the United States, Brooke General Hospital at Fort Sam Houston, San Antonio, Texas, being an example) added up to five echelons of medical service.[9]

Medical Administrative Corps Expansion

Supporting a global war expanded the number of duty assignments for Medical Administrative Corps officers from fourteen to fifty-two and moved them into positions previously filled by Medical, Dental, or Veterinary Corps officers.[10] The Medical Department had begun to open up positions for MACs on the eve of World War II, but the highest hospital job to which they could aspire was adjutant (*see Appendix C*). The department initially attempted to expand its pool of administrative specialty officers by training more physicians as administrators but, as in World War I, that program was short lived.[11]

The movement of MAC officers into positions formerly the domain of Army physicians resulted basically from the inability of the Medical Department to manage its great expansion competently. This was not entirely the department's fault. In early 1942 Chief of Staff General George C. Marshall interposed a layer between himself and the surgeon general—and other key figures—through the "Marshall reorganization." By creating super commands—air, ground, and service forces—he hoped to maintain his executive control of the Army while freeing himself to concentrate on national strategy.[12] Marshall selected Lt. Gen. Brehon B. Somervell, described as "dynamite in a Tiffany box," to command the service forces. Somervell became a powerful force and his "catchall command," the Services of Supply (later renamed the Army Service Forces), controlled the Army's support establishment, including the Medical Department. The surgeon general, Maj. Gen. James C. Magee, was subordinated to a headquarters that reported to the Army Staff, losing the direct access to the chief of staff his predecessors had enjoyed. Marshall was already unhappy with the surgeon general, and Somervell agreed that change was necessary. Magee soon found out his new boss was not going to wait for the department to move at its own pace.[13]

Somervell appointed a panel to investigate charges of mismanagement; the Committee To Study the Medical Department began its deliberations on 25 September. Called the Wadhams Committee for its chairman, Col. Sanford H. Wadhams, MC, USA, Ret., it reviewed the entire scope of the department's operations. Its investigation brought into sharp relief the necessity to modernize, and it opened the way for greatly expanded use of the MAC.[14] The Wadhams Committee met daily for two months, and its report, while not as corrosive as anticipated, took the Medical Department sharply to task. Irrespective of that outcome, the chief of staff's loss of confidence in the surgeon general was permanent. Marshall said he was "determinedly opposed" to Magee's retention beyond his first term, and he replaced Magee with Maj. Gen. Norman T. Kirk in 1943, even though the war was far from over.[15]

A major finding of the committee was that the surgeon general had lost control over medical logistics. This the Wadhams Committee blamed on a lack of executive talent caused in part by placing physicians in nonclinical duties while failing to use officers commissioned and trained for medical administrative specialties.[16] Physician misutilization was a principal issue. The committee recommended the use of trained hospital administrators, the substitution of Medical Corps officers with MAC officers in administrative roles, and the immediate expansion of the MAC. For example, the committee learned that there were thirty-four physicians working in the Surgeon General's Office alone. Governor Paul V. McNutt, chairman of the War Manpower Commission and a member of the committee, was appalled. "The complaint of doctors not doing medical work is one we hear most frequently. My desk has been flooded with such complaints."[17] The conclusion was unequivocal. "The Committee recommends that the practice of assigning medical officers, even temporarily, to any type of work that could be performed by non-professional personnel be discontinued promptly."[18] The surgeon general attempted to reject that recommendation—along with many others—but was ordered by Somervell to comply.[19] The resulting Army policy directed that physician shortages would be resolved by utilizing MAC officers "wherever practicable."[20]

Closely related to actions of the Wadhams Committee was political pressure from community leaders across the country who were angered when local physicians were drafted but not used to practice medicine. Those political stirrings found a powerful voice in the Procurement and Assignment Service, a federal coordinating agency formed in October 1941 at the urging of the American Medical Association. The AMA desired to control the department's procurement of physicians in order "to prevent medical personnel from being put into positions where their special qualifications were not utilized."[21] Efforts by the surgeon general to turn off that pressure were to no avail.[22]

Other pressures also forced the department to fill administrative positions with MACs and to use physicians, dentists, and veterinarians in positions requiring their special training. The sheer number of clinicians needed for patient care was one. The department estimated that there were 176,000 physicians in the United States in 1942. The military had initially planned to tap about one-third for the Army and Navy, but the political fallout forced a reappraisal. The Army lowered its requirement to 45,000, a figure that closely approximated the number actually placed on active duty during the war, but even the higher estimate could be accommodated only through greatly expanded substitution of administrative officers for clinicians.[23]

Common sense and the desires of physicians were other pressures. "The younger AUS doctors were very angry at being used as company commanders, mess officers and sanitation officers and were insistent that what they wanted was to practice their profession."[24] Brig. Gen. Raymond W. Bliss, MC, a physician who served as the surgeon general's chief of operations, thought this was such an important point that he kept in his notebook file an extract of an interview with a Medical Corps major who had served for three and a half years as a regimental surgeon in the Pacific. The Army physician was angered by the deterioration of his clinical skills. "Fully half of the medical officers in the field are wasted and few have the opportunity to do more than glorified first aid work."[25]

The Wadhams Committee findings were later echoed in the report of the Kenner Board, an internal Medical Department panel established in 1943 by General Kirk, Magee's successor as surgeon general. It was headed by Brig. Gen. Albert W. Kenner, MC, who had been surgeon of the Western Task Force during the North African invasion. General Kirk asked the board to develop plans for the more efficient use of all medical personnel, but his principal emphasis was upon the utilization of physicians. Although the department had predicted a shortage of nearly fifty-five hundred Medical Corps officers, the Kenner Board found that there were still nearly four hundred physicians serving as executive officers, detachment commanders, registrars, mess officers, supply officers, adjutants, and hospital inspectors. The board recommended assigning MAC officers to those duties. It also identified additional positions in medical logistics, Air Forces organizations, the surgeon general's staff, field medical units, and Army schools. Altogether the Kenner Board identified 5,289 Medical Corps officers who could be replaced with MAC officers.[26]

Demands to fill positions with MAC officers encountered resistance. Lt. Gen. Leonard Heaton, surgeon general from 1959 to 1969, later observed that it had been "repugnant to many officers steeped in the traditions of the prewar Medical Department . . . some urging was necessary."[27] Some of the resistance was from physicians unsuited for clinical duties either through incompetence, failure to remain current, or both. For others more competent, their careers as they advanced in rank were by necessity a succession of administrative jobs. The rank and experience of the small number of Regular Army physicians made their wartime service in staff and command positions inevitable, and the problem of Army physicians remaining current with American medicine continued.[28]

The effort to admit nonphysicians to some positions was strongly resisted, especially the posts of hospital executive officer, registrar, and inspector. The conclusions of various official Army assessments after the war were not complimentary on that score. The Army Service Forces concluded that, although the ASF kept the pressure on the surgeon general to economize in the use of physicians and other medical specialties, their efficient and full-time use was never fully achieved.[29] The Army's account of its stateside hospitals faulted the department's recalcitrance. "Problems of hospital commanders would have been fewer and the possibility of adverse effects upon professional care less if changes eventually made had been initiated early in the war by the Medical Department itself."[30]

But wholesale substitutions did occur, to the benefit of the Army and the Medical Department. Maj. Gen. John F. Bohlender, MC, commander of Fitzsimons General Hospital, said MAC officers "rapidly proved their worth."[31] The postwar report of the European Theater of Operations applauded the expanded use of MAC officers. "Good Medical Administrative Corps officers have performed their duties in a manner far superior to anything that had been anticipated."[32]

Substitution yielded expanded opportunity for MAC officers to serve in a diversity of duties that exceeded those of World War I. They served as hospital administrators, statisticians, physical training directors, medical equipment maintenance officers, historians, morale officers, litter officers, training officers, and public relations officers, to name a few.[33] Improvement in position opportunity was accompanied by improvement in promotion opportunity in 1942, when the War Department, acting upon a Wadhams Committee recommendation, provided for advancement of MAC officers beyond the grade of captain. In previous years young officer candidates had accurately sized up the situation: "If we go into the infantry we can wear four stars, but if we go into the Medical Administrative Corps, we wear two bars. That is as high as we can get."[34] But now there was opportunity for promotion to any rank, including the potential for general officer.

Officer Candidate Schools

Substitution was initially constrained by the limited availability of Medical Administrative Corps replacements, and some shortages persisted.[35] The department was compelled to rapidly expand the MAC to meet the demand, so it established an MAC officer candidate school (OCS) in July 1941 at Carlisle Barracks, Pennsylvania, that a War Department inspector later called the best OCS in the Army. Increasing use of MAC officers and the activation of new medical units produced a demand that outstripped Carlisle's capacity. Consequently, in May 1942 the department opened a second OCS at Camp Barkeley, a post located eleven miles southwest of Abilene, Texas.[36] Between them, Carlisle and Barkeley commissioned 17,094 officers in the third largest of the eighteen Army OCS programs. Another 200 were commissioned through special OCS programs in England, New Caledonia, Hawaii, and Australia—the last near Brisbane, which, its director lamented, was "on the deserted side as far as the Yanks go."[37]

Throughout the war the vicissitudes of class sizes and the closing and reopening of the schools were creatures of imperfect projections of MAC requirements. That imprecision arose from changes in force requirements as well as in policy. Rapidly expanding opportunities for MAC officers produced burgeoning OCS classes by the fall of 1942. However, projected requirements had overstated the positions actually available, and the department began placing graduates into replacement pools pending reassignment.

As a result of the changing requirements, Carlisle suspended operations at the end of February 1943 and reopened in May 1944. Barkeley had no classes in February, March, and April 1944. In July 1943 the Army predicted a surplus of over twenty-eight hundred Medical Administrative Corps officers by the end of the year, and nearly fifteen hundred officers were in replacement pools that fall. At that point the Army decided to replace the second physician in maneuver battalions—the assistant battalion surgeon—with an MAC officer. In addition, increasing casualty loads created staffing problems at the stateside hospitals. Those changes created a resurgence of demand, which required the schools to resume full operation until the United States accepted the surrender of Japan.

Carlisle and Barkeley shared a common curriculum divided into six basic subjects: tactics, administration, logistics, training, sanitation, and chemical warfare. Tactics consisted of map reading, Army and Medical Department organization, military operations, employment of medical units, and a field training exercise. Administration included general and company-level administration and military law. Logistics embraced vehicle maintenance, troop movements, and logistics in the field. The training portion prepared candidates to be instructors and, in addition, encompassed drill and ceremonies, first aid, and inspections. Sanitation included preventive medicine and field sanitation. Chemical warfare classes trained candidates for duties as medical unit gas officers.

Lessons learned in the war influenced curriculum changes. For example, the department's medical logistics problems caused modification of the supply portions, and reports of deficiencies in land navigation led to increased emphasis on map reading. Academic progress was measured with tests and quizzes. A passing grade of 75 was required in all subjects, and failure in two or more subjects required review of the candidate by a board of officers.

The candidates' day began at 0545 with first call and ended at 1700 with retreat, followed by two hours of supervised study from 1800–2000. Classes were scheduled based on eight fifty-minute periods with ten-minute breaks. Classroom instruction was interspersed with outdoor problems and demonstrations, drill, and road marches. Physical activity included daily calisthenics, obstacle courses, and interplatoon sports. Free time for social activities normally occurred on Saturday afternoon.

Basic prerequisites for MAC OCS were the same as for any Army OCS. Applicants were required to have scores greater than 100 on the Army General Classification Test and a minimum of three months' enlisted service, although that could be waived for education, experience, or prior service. In any case, the applicant was required to have completed basic training.[38] The background of Peter A. Luppen, a member of the second class, was typical of the early candidates. As a soldier in the 7th Division, Luppen had learned "how to wash a horse's rear end, front end and underneath" before he went to OCS.[39]

Each Army branch identified additional prerequisites it desired, and MAC OCS applicants were also expected to meet at least one of the following additional requirements: (a.) successful completion of one year of college; (b.) practical experience in management, for example as head of a business department, an athletic coach, or a noncommissioned officer; (c.) one year of experience in a business specialty, for example as an accountant, records supervisor, or sales manager; or, (d.) practical experience in hospital management, medical records management, medical supply, mess management in large institutions, or pharmacy.[40]

The Carlisle and Barkeley schools graduated 17,094 of 24,929 candidates for an overall pass rate of 68.6 percent. Carlisle's pass rate of 79 percent was significantly better than Barkeley's 65.3 percent. In fact, of seventeen Barkeley classes from January 1943 through June 1944, thirteen had more candidates failing than passing, and the "unlucky" Class Number 13 had only a 43.5 percent pass rate. Barkeley set up a special four-week Command School in 1943 in an attempt to salvage some of the candidates who appeared promising. Selected candidates were withdrawn from the regular OCS course in groups of eight to nine students to undergo extensive training in drill and command, calisthenics, public speaking, and practice teaching. Sixty-seven of the eighty-four candidates placed in this program successfully completed OCS.

The Barkeley attrition rate became so high that the Army Service Forces headquarters asked for an explanation. The school faulted poor selection methods, which sent students to OCS who had no chance of success, had inadequate prior military training, and were held to the exacting standards of their platoon leaders. The poor living conditions at Barkeley added to the rigors of the training environment. Some students decided it was all a mistake and took advantage of the privilege of voluntary withdrawals.

CHART 3—ORGANIZATION OF THE MEDICAL ADMINISTRATIVE CORPS OFFICER CANDIDATE SCHOOL, CARLISLE BARRACKS, PENNSYLVANIA, 1942

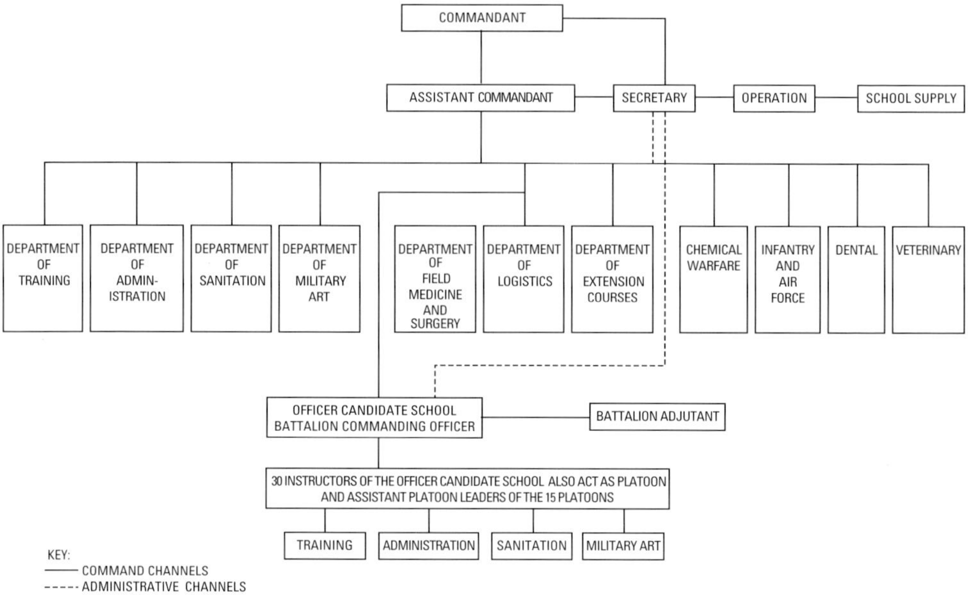

Source: Robert J. Parks, *Medical Training in World War II*, in the series Medical Department of the United States in World War II (Washington, D.C.: Office of the Surgeon General, Department of the Army, 1974), p. 103.

The surgeon general's director of training saw it differently and argued that the difference in attrition between the two schools was due to a difference in philosophy. The idea at Carlisle was "to help as many through as possible," but at Barkeley the approach was to "see how many candidates can be kept from becoming officers." OCS candidates witnessed many of their classmates fail.[41] One who watched was Joseph P. Peters, later a nationally prominent health care administration consultant. Peter's barracks was half empty by the time he graduated from Barkeley.[42]

Most candidates who failed did so for leadership deficiencies. Peters said that most of those who washed out at Barkeley lacked "command presence." Candidates had to learn to bark out orders, and a good set of lungs helped.[43] Carlisle counted 311 of the 441 failures in its first thirteen classes as leadership deficiencies.[44] Barkeley had 5,348 failures in its first thirty-one classes. Of those, 2,942 were voluntary resignations, an option not available at Carlisle. The next highest category encompassed the 1,149 candidates dropped for leadership deficiencies, followed by 614 separated for academic problems. College graduates had the lowest attrition rates.

An Officer Candidate Preparatory School was established at Barkeley in April 1942 to help reduce the failure rate. The four-week course was designed by 1st Lt. Edward Marks, MAC, assisted by 1st Lt. Robert L. Parker, MAC, and

Marks served as its first commandant. It had a cadre of five MAC officers and six enlisted personnel, and classes ranged from 150 to 400 students. Similar schools were established at all medical replacement training centers. Not surprisingly, OCS candidates who had completed that course did better than those who had not.[45]

Carlisle Barracks

The Medical Field Service School at Carlisle Barracks expanded its staff of 108 by another 40 officers, 87 enlisted personnel, and 4 civilian typists to operate the OCS. The instructors were mainly Medical Corps officers at first, but that changed as instructors and key staff officers were replaced with OCS graduates. Capt. Louis F. Williams, MAC, was the school secretary for the first class, and four other MAC officers were on the staff. Students were organized into a battalion, and platoon leaders and assistant platoon leaders also served as instructors. The commandant of the Medical Field Service School acted as the OCS commandant, with day-to-day operations vested in the assistant commandant (*Chart 3*). The Carlisle OCS was able to take advantage of the established facilities at Carlisle Barracks, and its candidates enjoyed better billets, classrooms, and recreation facilities than their peers in the more Spartan surroundings at Barkeley. The OCS used thirty-one buildings, a number that included seventeen barracks, three 300-seat auditoriums, and five 250-seat classrooms.[46]

The inaugural class of 100 officer candidates began on 1 July 1941, and enrollment increased to 250 students by the third class. With the fourth class the school shifted to staggered rather than consecutive scheduling and began enrolling a new class of 250 candidates every thirty days for a capacity of 750 candidates at any given time. The course initially totaled 561 hours of instruction conducted over twelve weeks. It increased to 576 hours by 1942, and by July 1943 was a seventeen-week program of 808 hours.[47]

Carlisle operated without interruption until 27 February 1943, when declining requirements for MAC officers caused its suspension. It reopened on 25 May 1944 and enrolled a class of 250 students in each of the ensuing twelve months. The thirteenth class, of only thirty-four candidates, continued after the war had ended, and when that class graduated on 17 October 1945, Carlisle OCS ceased operation permanently. It had commissioned 4,688 officers during its existence, and its graduates played important roles in the Army and in the Medical Department. One, John E. Haggerty, was promoted to brigadier general and appointed chief of the Medical Service Corps in 1973. Another, Leo Benade, later transferred to the Adjutant General's Corps and retired as a lieutenant general.[48]

There was also some opportunity for black Americans. Army OCS in World War II was integrated, and the Medical Administrative Corps OCS graduated 387 black officers. By September 1945 there were 213 black MAC officers as well as 8 black Sanitary Corps officers serving in a variety of staff and command positions in black field medical units and fixed facilities stateside and overseas. One was the 93d Infantry Division at Fort Huachuca, Arizona. Others were the 268th, 335th, and 383d Station Hospitals in Burma and the Philippines. Stateside assignments included the hospitals at Tuskegee, Alabama, and Fort Huachuca,

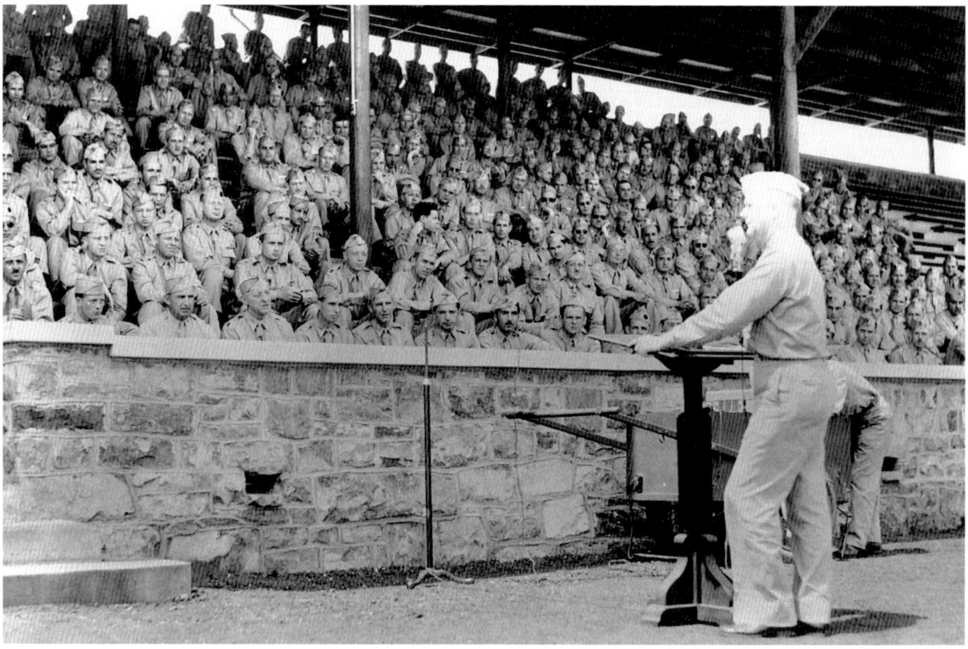

Capt. Louis F. Williams lectures at the Medical Field Service School, Carlisle Barracks, June 1941.

Arizona, but black officers had difficulty finding suitable housing and they were not assigned unless segregated quarters were available. The limited opportunities in the Medical Department resulted in a few officers' being sent for training at the Infantry School, Fort Benning, Georgia. Sixteen black MAC officers were detailed to the infantry by mid-1945.[49]

The Army formed sanitary companies specifically for staffing by black soldiers and officers. The companies initially had a nonspecific mission and were assigned to hospitals when requested by hospital commanders; the first two were established at Fort Bragg, North Carolina, and at Camp Livingston, Louisiana, where the hospitals had all-black wards. Col. William A. Hardenbergh, SnC, chief of the Surgeon General's Sanitary Engineering Division, recommended the company's use in insect and mosquito control, and the Army formed 87 medical sanitary companies of 3 officers and 112 enlisted soldiers. The company was organized in two platoons to drain swampy land or lowlands, perform sanitary surveys, and provide insect and rodent control.[50]

The presence of black candidates in the first classes was a milestone. When Col. Elliotte J. Williams, MSC, entered Carlisle in March 1942, he was 1 of only 6 black candidates in a class of 300; the class just before his had only 1 black candidate. Four of his black classmates were eliminated by the end of the first month, and he began to suspect that discrimination was at work because two of the four were college graduates and the other two had more enlisted experience than he did. However, Williams and his remaining black classmate were assured

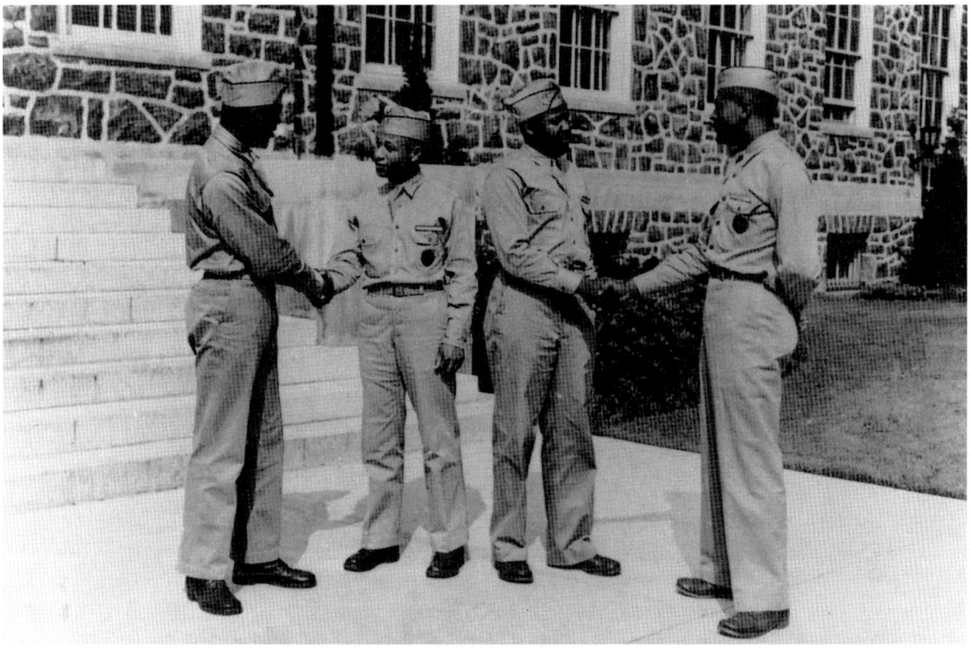

2d Lt. Elliotte J. Williams (second from left) *greets incoming OCS students, May 1942.*

that race was not a factor in the fate of the others. They had simply been unable to meet the standards expected of an Army officer. "Thus advised, we relaxed, worked together on our study assignments, and enjoyed the meager spare time that was available."[51]

Williams described the program that provided so many with the gold bars of a second lieutenant:

> We made friends of fellow candidates and attacked with new vigor our program in military sanitation, field medicine and surgery, administration, training management, logistics, and military art. We learned how to build and maintain a compost heap for the cavalry, the principles of battlefield triage of the wounded, execution of motor marches, and the development and conduct of training programs. We learned how to conduct a sanitary inspection, manage a mess hall or motor pool, the principles of medical supply, and personnel administration. We were to be the generalists in medical administration, prepared to assume any medical administrative duty in a hospital or field unit.[52]

Williams and his friend graduated in May 1942 and were posted to the 93d Infantry Division, where Williams was assigned as executive officer for the division surgeon. There he found the post facilities were completely segregated, including the tables in the officers' mess. Later he requested transfer to the Army hospital at Tuskegee, Alabama, where he served as the enlisted detachment commander. Lieutenant Williams and his wife and baby daughter encountered the humiliations that awaited a black family traveling in the South when they moved

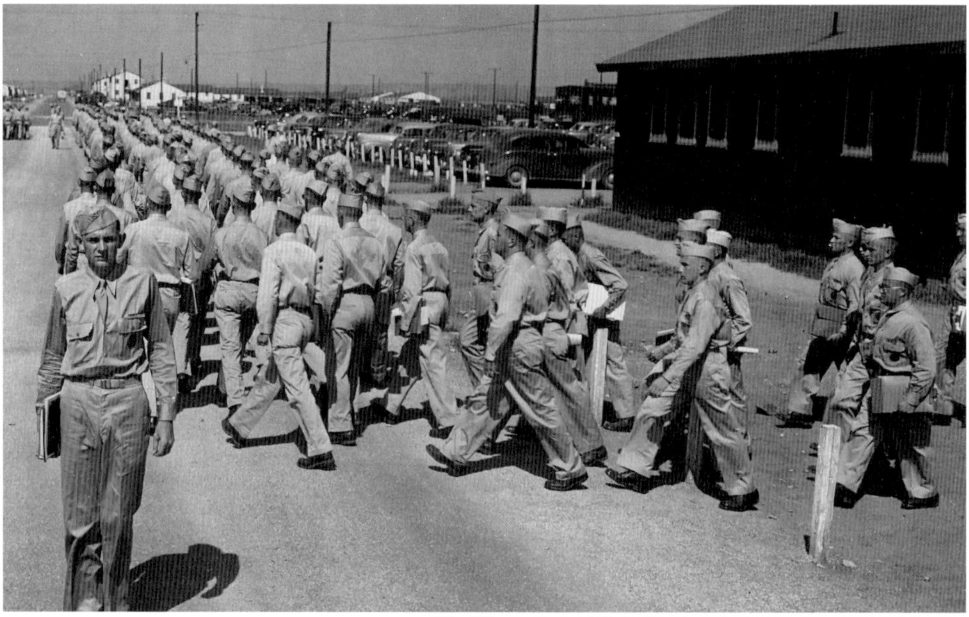

OCS candidates march to class at Camp Barkeley, Texas.

to their new assignment. They negotiated restroom privileges at service stations and prayed that their car would not break down on the road.

Camp Barkeley

> Take off those stripes, wipe off that grin
> Cut off that hair, shave off that chin
> Polish those shoes, shine that brass
> Get on the stick and show some class.
> Now double time with all your power,
> Then stand in line for half an hour.[53]

The first Camp Barkeley OCS class of 253 candidates began on 11 May 1942. The cadre consisted of twelve MAC officers transferred from the Carlisle staff who arrived in Texas just four days ahead of the students. Another fourteen officers arrived from Carlisle two weeks after the school opened, and later additions to the cadre came from Barkeley graduating classes. Initially department heads trained new instructors. Later, the school established a fourteen-hour faculty development course that included graded practice presentations. Barkeley adopted the staggered scheduling used by Carlisle and enrolled an additional class of 250 students each month until a capacity of 750 candidates at one time was reached. The capacity increased in June 1942 to 1,000 students, and by the end of September 1942 Barkeley was enrolling a new class of 500 students every two weeks.[54]

In July 1943, as the student census reached 2,969, the school had a staff of 564, with 173 officers, 376 enlisted, and 15 civilians (*Chart 4*). Barkeley reached

Chart 4—Organization of the Medical Administrative Corps Officer Candidate School, Camp Barkeley, Texas, 1942–43

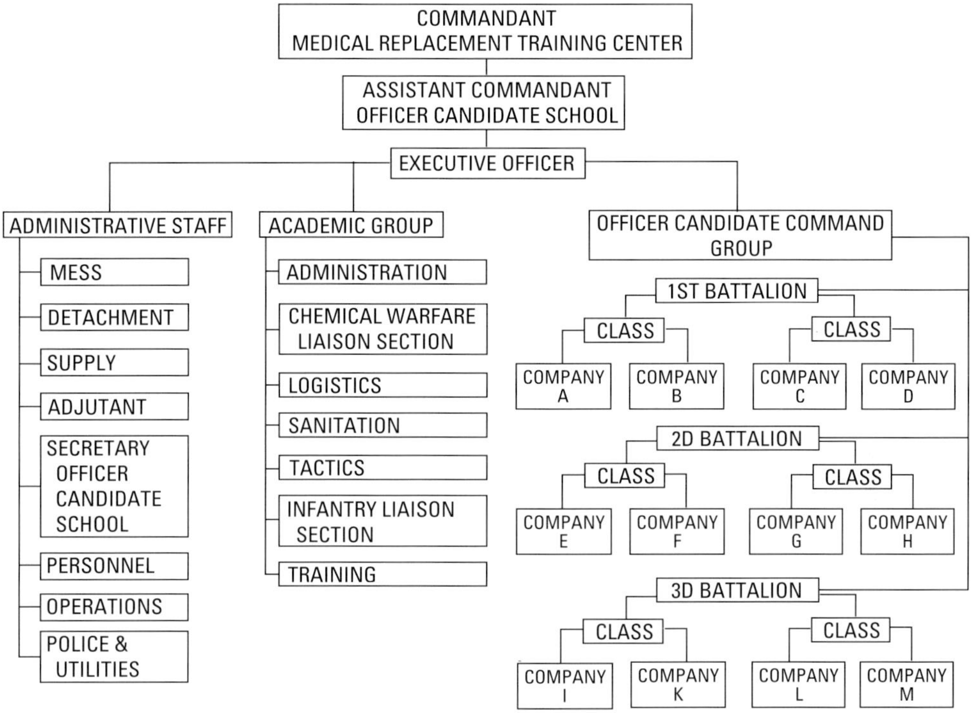

Source: Robert J. Parks, *Medical Training in World War II*, in series *Medical Department of the United States in World War II* (Washington, D.C.: Office of the Surgeon General, Department of the Army, 1974), p. 104.

its peak of 3,011 candidates in attendance in July 1943. Class size then dropped monthly until January 1944 when the class numbered 106 candidates, the smallest. Barkeley enrolled no more classes after that until May 1944 when it again enrolled 250 students. In June 1944, as Carlisle reopened, Barkeley expanded to classes of 500 students. Barkeley graduated its fortieth and final class on 15 March 1945, having commissioned 12,406 officers since May 1942. The highest course average in the school's history, 90.22, was posted by 2d Lt. Thomas P. Glassmayer, MAC, Class 40.[55]

The OCS occupied stark, treeless terrain in an area formerly belonging to the 120th Medical Regiment of the 45th Division. It used ninety-three buildings, temporary structures of the wood construction typical of Army camps. Those included 58 fifteen-man "hutments," 12 five-man hutments, and 9 mess halls in areas nicknamed Kings Row, the Black Outs, and Tortilla Flats (also called Pneumonia Flats). Hutments were tarpaper-covered wood-frame structures with no amenities and "were cold as tombs" in winter.[56] Training followed the typical OCS regimen of copious harassment, drill, and ceremonies. Sometimes the ceremonies went poorly; when a British Royal Army Medical Corps colonel visited in

July 1942, a canopy erected to shield the colonel from the Texas sun fell down, nearly smothering him.[57]

Morale was reported as exceptionally high. Entertainment included facilities for all seasonal sports, and dances were held with the cooperation of the YMCA, the USO, and nearby colleges. The highlight was a class graduation dance held in the school's gymnasium the night before graduation.[58] However, high attrition rates colored some candidates' perceptions. There were rumors of a snitch in the barracks and a belief that "the walls had ears." While there is no evidence that a system of informers existed, the suspicion that it did reflected the stressful environment. A peer review system that required each candidate to rate fellow candidates on personal characteristics added to the pressure.[59]

By April 1945, 158 black candidates had completed Barkeley OCS, with a completion success rate the same as white candidates. Life was not easy for those pioneering officers. Abilene, Texas, was rigidly segregated, and most recreational facilities were denied to blacks. The effect upon their morale was such that the surgeon general requested special authority to transfer black candidates to Carlisle. That did not occur, however, because the Carlisle facilities were overcrowded.[60]

Training exhibits at Barkeley included two elaborate outdoor displays. One was a sanitation exhibit with sections demonstrating disposal of human, kitchen, and animal wastes; sanitation of field messes; delousing; and mosquito control. The other was a miniature battlefield measuring 60 by 349 feet that illustrated the three zones of medical support, with models of the medical installations in each zone. The portion for the communications zone and the zone of the interior was 212 feet long and incorporated an artificial pond, representing the oceans that separated them.

One of the field exercises was a four-hour class on evacuation techniques in which candidates alternated duties as collecting company commander, clearing company commander, litter bearer platoon leader, and ambulance platoon leader. Candidates were graded on their knowledge of emergency medical treatment and their ability to evacuate simulated casualties. A six-day bivouac included a series of training exercises in a field setting.

Elliot Richardson completed the Barkeley OCS in 1943. He later held some of the highest positions in the United States government, including secretary of defense. Richardson began his military career after surmounting several difficulties. His repeated efforts to volunteer had been defeated by poor eyesight; he was drafted in December 1942, and although he had memorized the eye chart, his glasses gave him away. He was classified as a noncombatant and ordered to enlisted medical training at Camp Pickett, Virginia. There he completed OCS prep school, then went to Barkeley. "I've been a candidate for elective office," he later recalled, "and I've been elected to various things, but I think my proudest moment in any election was being elected platoon leader of my OCS platoon." He thought Barkeley was "a *very* tough school."[61]

Another distinguished alumnus was Col. Vernon McKenzie, MSC, who retired in 1984 as the principal deputy assistant secretary of defense for health affairs, a position he held with some intermissions for nearly ten years during the period following his retirement from the Army in 1967. McKenzie was drafted in

1941 and after basic training was stationed in Brisbane, Australia. There he applied for OCS. "I went to a miserable place called Camp Barkeley, Texas, and decided shortly thereafter that I could withstand any form of psychological warfare that the Army could wish to apply to me for three months."[62] His company commander was Capt. John Haggerty, MAC, later brigadier general and chief of the Medical Service Corps. Col. Knute Tofte-Nielsen, MSC, had a different experience. Tofte-Nielsen came to Barkeley after service as an enlisted medic with the 76th Division at Camp McCoy, Wisconsin. He found Barkeley "very pleasant, basically," an experience in which his enlisted background helped immeasurably.[63]

OCS candidates stood regular inspections. During one, the inspecting officer asked a candidate to turn over his brass belt buckle. It turned out to be very dirty. "That's brass, too, isn't it?" challenged the inspector. Without hesitation the candidate lifted one foot and pointed to the bottom of his shoe. "That's leather, too, but I don't polish it." The candidate was hauled before a cadre board, which decided he should be retained in the program. The Army needed an officer who could think on his feet.[64]

Administrative Specialty Officers

By the end of the war administrative specialty officers routinely filled all hospital administrative positions except those of commander and executive officer.[65] By 1944 the number of Medical Corps officers in a 1,000-bed general hospital in the zone of the interior decreased from thirty-seven to thirty-two while the number of MAC officers increased from seven to ten. The same was true in the Army Air Forces, where most administrative positions in dispensaries and station hospitals were filled by MAC officers who also served with the early air evacuation units.[66]

As medical registrars, MACs contributed advances in medical records management at a time when progressive measures of any sort were welcome in a system faced with enormous demands. The addressograph, a "seemingly small" advance, eliminated the need to type orders and rosters. This was no minor assistance for a facility such as Stark General Hospital, Charleston, South Carolina, which admitted over 44,000 patients in the first nine months of 1945. MAC officers were responsible for all levels of the system. Capt. Stephen Tucker, MAC, served as chief of the Medical Records Division for the European Theater of Operations (ETO). In Washington, Maj. Harold F. Dorn, MAC, received the Legion of Merit for his service as chief of the Surgeon General's Medical Statistics Section. Major Dorn, a Sanitary Corps officer in World War I and later a Public Health Service statistician, revamped the department's methods for statistical compilations.[67]

Some officers served in personnel management duties. One was Capt. Burt Langhenry, MAC, a personnel officer in the Surgeon General's Office who handled the assignment of MAC officers worldwide. In Europe, Lt. Col. James T. Richards, MAC, was assigned to the Surgeon's Division of the European Theater of Operations as chief of readjustment and redeployment. "If you asked me 'what was the biggest job you ever did, or the most responsible job,' I'd have to say that was it," he later declared. Richards' section had the responsibility of computing adjusted service rating scores for 70,000 Medical Department officers and 254,000

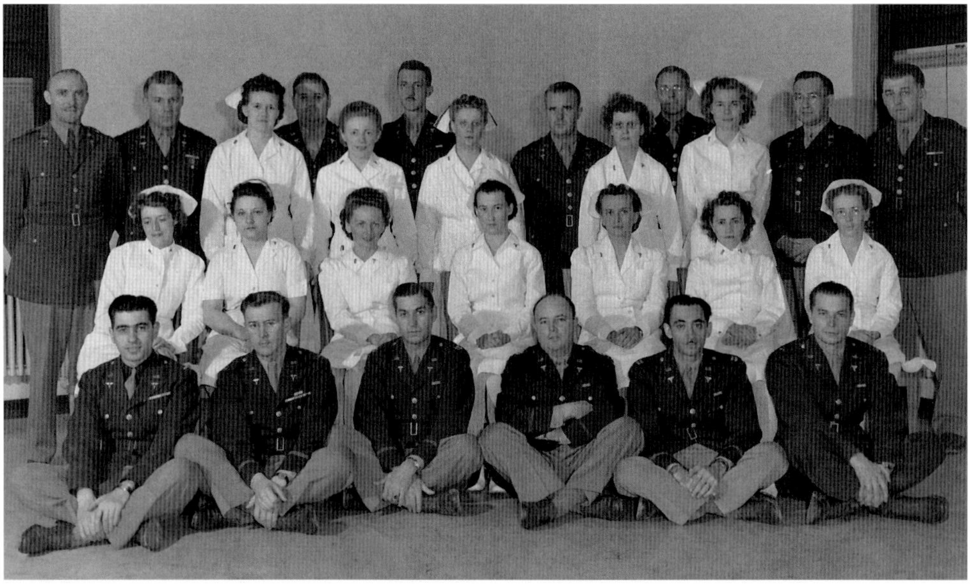

Staff of the Station Hospital at Fort Pepperrell, Newfoundland, September 1943

enlisted personnel in order to determine who would return to the United States. A card-sort mechanism failed, and his staff had to resort to the use of index cards. He communicated movement orders directly to the units by telephone, irritating some commanders in the process.[68]

Other MAC officers served as regulating officers in the theaters of operations and the zone of the interior. They were "medical traffic cops" who controlled patient movement by matching a patient's disease or injury with the availability of beds in the hospitals. Stateside they were stationed at embarkation ports and the Surgeon General's Medical Regulating Office where they controlled movement of patients to the military hospitals nearest their homes that were equipped to handle their problems. The processing of large numbers of patients was a matter of keen interest to congressmen and was performed almost exclusively as an MAC function. The success of the system was called "one of the great achievements" of the war.[69]

The financial management field also opened. Maj. Nepthune Fogelberg, SnC, who had received a Master of Business Administration from Harvard in 1929, was commissioned as a Sanitary Corps officer in 1942. He established a nine-state regional fiscal office in Chicago and in 1943 moved to the Office of the Surgeon General where in 1945 he became chief of the Fiscal Division. Fogelberg stayed on in the same capacity as a civilian employee following his release from active duty and was one of the key officials in the Office of the Surgeon General for years afterward.[70]

The use of trained hospital administrators accelerated during the war. General Armstrong described most Army hospital administrators before the war as physicians who were "out of the mainstream" of medicine,[71] a situation that did not meet wartime needs. The department thus established a program in 1942 to commission civilian hospital administrators. Appointment grade was related to a civilian's rank in the American College of Hospital Administrators. A college nominee rated appointment as a second lieutenant, a member as first lieutenant, and a fellow as captain. The program had produced 250 MAC officers by the summer of 1943, when it ended.[72]

Effective utilization of MAC hospital administrators depended upon opening up the key positions. The job of hospital commander remained closed to MACs, but wartime needs gradually forced the executive officer (XO) position open. That was an important change, because the XOs were in effect the hospitals' chief operating officers. One of those early nonphysician XOs was Maj. Raymond H. Tolbertt, MAC, appointed in August 1943 as the XO of Borden General Hospital, Chickasha, Oklahoma. Tolbertt, who had risen from private to staff sergeant in Regular Army service from 1931 to 1940, was respected by the enlisted soldiers as an officer who had come up through the ranks.[73] In 1944 the War Department mandated the use of MACs as the XOs of all stateside hospitals. The surgeon general vigorously protested, and the following month the War Department partly reversed itself. It allowed continued use of physicians as XOs of the general hospitals, especially stateside, but it permitted the use of carefully selected MAC officers as executive officers of station hospitals.[74]

There were more openings at the lower levels of the hospital organization. Newly commissioned physicians were not familiar with Army procedures, and some MAC officers proved invaluable as administrative assistants for the medical, surgical, and physical medicine departments of the larger hospitals. Their duties included property and supply management, reports, and, in some cases, preparation of medical histories on new patients.[75]

Movement into administrative positions in fixed facilities was mirrored by the assignment of over fifteen thousand MAC officers to field medical units and headquarters staffs. Assignments ranged from instructors of enlisted recruits to staff officers for the surgeon general, and MACs were key figures in management of the evacuation and treatment chain at all points from the battlefield to the stateside hospitals. MAC officers, like their forbears in the Civil War, were recognized for heroism under fire, and 1st Lt. Lester Dannenburg, of the U.S. Army Forces in the Far East, was awarded the Distinguished Service Cross in 1945. Some served as historians of the epic military medical events of World War II. One, Capt. James H. Stone, MAC, edited a compellingly candid account of medical support by men and women of the medical team who labored at the end of the line in the China-Burma-India Theater. Over fifty years later, *Crisis Fleeting* remains an essential source for those charged with medical plans and operations for Asian countries or the tropics.[76]

Enlisted medical soldiers were almost exclusively trained by MAC and Sanitary Corps officers during World War II. MAC officers performed principal command and staff duties of the seven medical replacement training centers where the Medical Department enlisted recruits received their basic training, which for the first time included weapons training. The average training center had 350 MAC officers assigned. MAC officers were also assigned as instructors

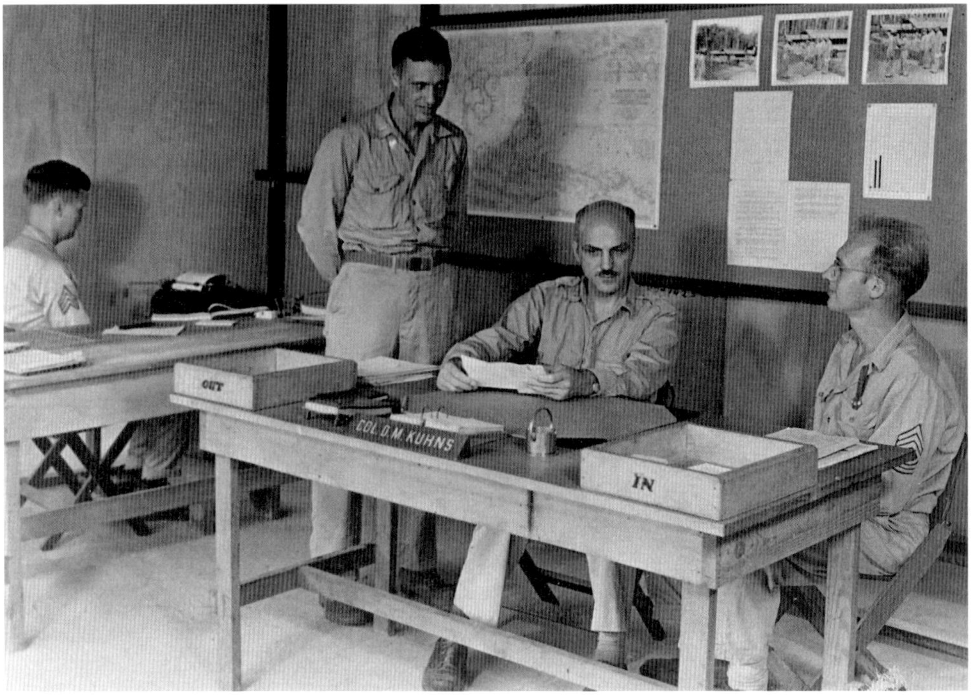

Medical administration staff discuss plans at the headquarters, 19th Medical Service Detachment, in Hollandia, New Guinea, March 1945.

and key staff officers for the nine Medical Department enlisted technician schools where soldiers received their advanced training. Thus the school at Fitzsimons General Hospital, Denver, Colorado, had forty MAC and four Sanitary Corps officers.[77]

MAC officers led litter bearer and ambulance platoons and served in the administrative positions of medical collecting companies, clearing companies, and ambulance companies. Third Army ambulance platoon leaders kept their ambulances "as close to the front lines as possible" as they moved through France and Belgium into Germany.[78] Basil V. Everin, MAC, a first lieutenant, was an ambulance platoon leader in the 585th Ambulance Company. Everin was evacuated back to the States after he was shot in the mouth in action near Mayen, Germany, in March 1945. His platoon sergeant remembered him as an officer "whose example of bravery and leadership based upon integrity and fairness was a source of constant encouragement to us all."[79]

In India, 1st Lt. William R. Odahl, MAC, was executive officer of Company B, 151st Medical Battalion, headquartered in Ledo. Odahl's duty as pay officer made him the company's link with the small medical teams at aid stations dispersed throughout the inhospitable terrain in which engineer units were laboriously building the Ledo Road. A legendary rapid walker, 1st Lt. Kenneth D. Harris, MAC, of the 896th Clearing Company (Seagrave's Hospital), was the "walking link" between his company's detachments in Burma and India. Patients delivered to evacuation and field hospitals were moved in the field ambulances of separate medical detachments and companies commanded by Medical Administrative Corps officers, who also staffed the medical battalions and groups that served as the parent units. Capt. John Lada, MAC, the S–3 (operations officer) of the 33d Medical Ambulance Battalion located at Weymouth, England, handled the operational planning for his battalion's support of the Normandy invasion. The 33d moved casualties from the landing ships to the general hospitals in England. It evacuated 823 casualties during one 24-hour period.[80]

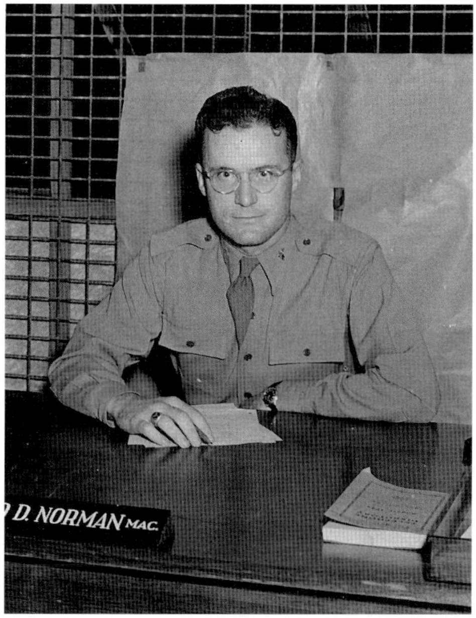

Lt. David D. Norman, historian and public relations officer, Brisbane, Australia, August 1944

Elliot Richardson, who had attended Barkeley, was commissioned as a second lieutenant, MAC, and served as a litter bearer platoon leader in the 4th Infantry Division from its D-day landing on Utah Beach through V-E Day. His platoon was part of a medical collecting company that supported the 12th Infantry Regiment, a unit authorized about three thousand soldiers that sustained nine thousand casualties in its eleven months of combat operations. The casualty rate translated into a 500 percent turnover of personnel in some rifle companies.[81]

Richardson quickly learned that there was no role for litter bearers to the rear of battalion aid stations because field ambulances handled evacuation from that level of the evacuation chain. Therefore, he employed his squads as relief teams for the litter bearers of the maneuver battalions. He used his jeep as a field ambulance, and his record was eighteen casualties carried in and upon the vehicle at one time. Richardson experienced the exhilaration of danger, but at the same time he learned the satisfaction of service for its own sake during experiences that remained vivid the rest of his life. Twice wounded and twice recommended for the Distinguished Service Cross, he was intensely proud of his contribution as a MAC officer. "I will never do anything that I feel better about," he told an interviewer.[82]

MAC officers served in a variety of positions in the general, evacuation, convalescent, station, and field hospitals.[83] MAC registrars handled responsibilities that required some of the most able officers assigned to a hospital. Capt. Charles D. Witenbower, MAC, registrar of the 21st General Hospital, which served in Italy and France, attributed his section's success to hard-working and conscientious soldiers.[84] MAC officers supervised hospital mess operations assisted by the hospital dietitian. MAC officers were responsible for medical and general supply functions, and MAC adjutants handled the administrative procedures expected of Army units. Philip U. Farley, MAC, a second lieutenant, had the dual responsibilities of adjutant and hospital inspector for the 48th Evacuation Hospital at Hellsgate, a 750-bed semimobile unit on the Ledo Road in India.[85]

In the Philippines, Capt. Jack F. Lemire, MAC, was adjutant of General Hospital Number 1. The hospital was captured by the Japanese in the fall of Bataan and relocated to Camp O'Donnell in northern Luzon, a prisoner-of-war (POW) camp just north of Clark Air Force Base at the terminus of the Bataan death march. There, Lemire's hospital supported a population that at its peak numbered over 45,000 in a prison camp designed for 9,000. The Filipino and American POWs faced starvation, disease, and ill-treatment in the "Andersonville of the Pacific." Lemire was later moved to the large American POW camp at Cabanatuan, east of Camp O'Donnell, where Capts. Henry Siegrist and Rex Axton, MAC, were members of the prison hospital staff. Lemire, accused of being a spy, was placed in the camp brig where he was kept on a starvation diet and beaten regularly. Lemire later died aboard an unmarked Japanese "hell ship" transporting POWs to Japan under bestial conditions.[86]

Some officers were assigned as enlisted and patient detachment commanders. They served as ward administrators and transportation and utilities officers in the larger hospitals, and as company commanders and training officers for hospital rehabilitation units established to ensure that convalescing soldiers returned to full duty. For example, the 5th General Hospital at Toul, France, was collocated with a replacement depot through which convalescent troops passed on their return to the front. The hospital represented the last chance for those soldiers to escape combat, and it became inundated with "surly, hostile and defiant" patients.[87] Establishment of a rehabilitation unit led by MAC officers turned around a bad situation.

MAC officers were the "Jacks of all trades" in the field hospitals of the communications zone. When the hospital broke into three separate hospital units (platoons), an MAC officer assumed administrative responsibilities for each 100-bed component. Dorothy S. Davis, a second lieutenant in the Army Nurse Corps (ANC), served with the 57th Field Hospital south of Strasbourg, France, in the winter of 1945, where it received casualties from the Battle of the Bulge. Capt. William V. Davis, MAC, whom she later married, was the adjutant. Dorothy Davis said the MAC officers were greatly respected. They ran the ambulance support and "were right up in front with the infantry officers."[88]

One of the MAC hospital executive officers was Maj. Gilbert A. Bishop of the 59th Evacuation Hospital. Bishop had been the hospital's adjutant as it deployed in North Africa in support of Operation TORCH. There, the executive officer, a physician, was killed, and Bishop was promoted to major and placed in the slot, continuing in that position in North Africa, Italy, France, and Germany.[89] Another MAC executive officer was Capt. William D. Schaefer, who entered politics after the war and was elected governor of Maryland in 1986 after fifteen years as mayor of Baltimore. Schaefer said that his tour as a hospital executive officer in England taught him the principles of management. "I learned then that if you want to get things done you can do it two ways, ordering people around or asking them to work."[90]

Medical units above division level were organized into medical groups whose principal staff (other than the commander and executive officer) were MAC officers. Maj. Thomas S. Prideaux, a Carlisle OCS graduate, was S–3 of the 1st Medical Group, which supported Ninth Army from the crossing of the Roer River to the fall of Germany. Prideaux provided the operational planning and execution for eight months of combat support, relocating the group headquarters nine times (including five times in one two-week period). At one point the group was responsible for the hospitalization of nearly forty thousand civilians and German and Allied POWs in areas occupied by the advancing American units. Maj. Bernard Aabel, MAC, served as the S–2 (Intelligence) and liaison officer of the 68th Medical Group, which had 2,500 personnel in four medical battalions and five field hospitals supporting First Army. From June 1944 to May 1945 the group's ambulances traveled over 2.6 million miles transporting 207,060 patients. It put eight million miles on its vehicles during the European campaign.[91]

MAC assignments within the evacuation chain included hospital trains. Other patients moved by sea, and beginning in 1943 some MACs served on twenty-eight hospital ships, whose crews included one Sanitary Corps and three to five MAC officers, depending on the ship's size. Some MACs served as beachmasters during amphibious operations. They coordinated evacuation of casualties to the hospital ships and received medical materiel ashore and won praise for keeping the blood distribution system running at night on the beachheads.[92]

MACs contributed to the development of the Air Force Medical Service and its establishment of intertheater, long-range air evacuation using large aircraft. MAC officers in the Army Air Forces served as administrative assistants and executive officers for base and section surgeons and in administrative positions in medical air evacuation squadrons which were formed to provide the medical and nursing staffs for air evacuation flights. An example is 1st Lt. Clement J. Quarantiello, MAC, who served as the adjutant, supply officer, and personnel officer for a medical air evacuation squadron assigned to the Fifth Air Force in New Guinea. His unit provided medical staffing for C–47s which evacuated patients from six locations in New Guinea to Doboduru and Port Moresby in Papua. The evacuation squadrons were organized into six flights, each headed by a Medical Corps flight surgeon. A Twelfth Air Force report recommended replacing the physicians with MACs, since their principal function was to maintain liaison between the airfields and the hospitals, a task that did not require a physician.[93]

MACs also contributed to the development of forward air evacuation of casualties with small Army aircraft. In 1945 1st Lt. Ernest C. Townsend, MAC, was instrumental in setting up an air evacuation system in Luzon for the Sixth Army surgeon during the Philippines campaign, adopting techniques developed in the China-Burma-India Theater where a squadron of light aircraft had evacuated 700 wounded in northern Burma during a one-month period in 1944. An air commando group provided squadrons of Stinson L–5s, Cub-like planes that could carry one patient either sitting up or on a litter. Up to thirty planes oper-

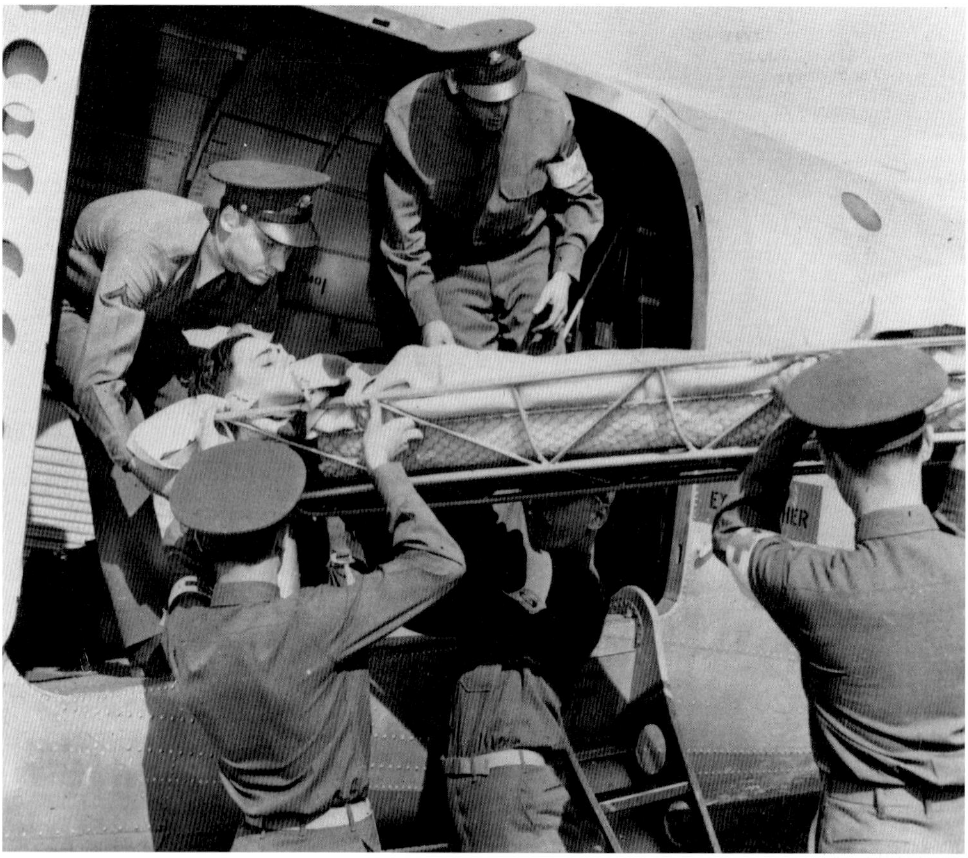

Douglas transport plane adapted for use as an air ambulance; below, *Piper Cub modified for use as an air ambulance. Raised fuselage shows position of litter with patient.*

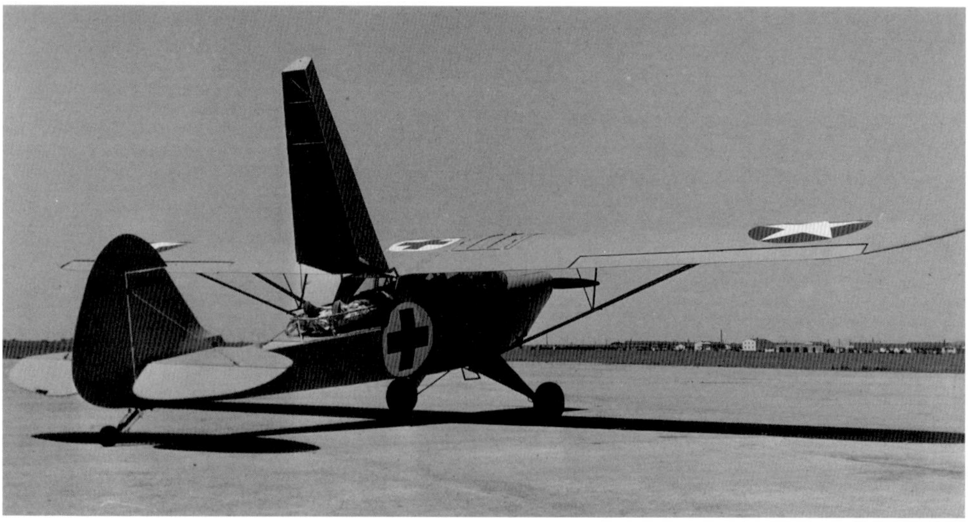

ating daily in a one-month period evacuated over three thousand patients from a network of forty landing strips, while also delivering medical supplies to the forward positions.[94]

Other developments included using Piper Cub L–4s and –5s in the European Theater, the Pacific, and Burma for the movement of medical supplies and blood plasma. The use of air ambulances in forward evacuation was fairly common in some areas, even though there was no widespread development of doctrine and organization to make it a systematic practice. Further development of the helicopter was needed to make it fully possible. The two-seat Sikorsky R–4 helicopter was used in northern Burma in 1943 for patient evacuation, but a proposal that year to organize helicopter air ambulance units foundered on the question of whether patients should be carried internally or externally.[95]

Battalion Surgeon's Assistant

The decision in November 1943 to substitute a MAC officer for the assistant battalion surgeon was controversial. The idea of the battalion surgeon's assistant (BSA) had surfaced as a recommendation of the Kenner Board, a dramatic departure from previous practice that was necessitated by a shortage of physicians. The use of Army Nurse Corps officers was not contemplated since there was no provision for commissioning male nurses in that corps and the Army did not permit the employment of female nurses that far forward. The BSAs worked out well,[96] and their success presaged the establishment of the warrant officer physician assistants in the post-Vietnam era.

The primary role of BSAs was to ensure the rapid evacuation of wounded soldiers and the quick return to duty of those with minor wounds or illness. BSAs took over the administrative responsibilities of the battalion surgeon, including operation of the field ambulances as well as some clinical duties. On occasion the clinical duties—principally routine treatment of minor illnesses—would predominate. This was especially true for BSAs assigned as surgeons aboard the smaller troop transports, where they conducted sick call. In combat their medical treatment duties centered on emergency treatment: arresting hemorrhage, fixing fractures, preventing shock by the infusion of blood expanders, administering pain-killing drugs, and preparing casualties for further evacuation. In some cases the BSA was the only officer in an aid station during battle. While MAC officers were not primarily intended to perform medical treatment, they were expected to be able to render emergency medical care and were trained accordingly in field medicine and surgery.[97]

Not all physicians were happy with this development. Maj. Gen. Morrison C. Stayer, MC, chief surgeon of the North African Theater of Operations, was sufficiently distressed to write Surgeon General Kirk that it could be a "real source of danger" if BSAs were tempted to provide clinical care beyond their capability.[98] Kirk responded that he found it difficult to get agreement by medical officers on any issue, and this one was no different. The primary purpose for the BSA was not patient care. "He is put in there to do the administrative work of the detachment, command the litter bearers, and *assist* the battalion surgeon as he does in hospitals. We have no trouble with MAC officers trying to do surgery or write diagnoses on patients in hospitals. Why should we with assistant battalion surgeons?"[99]

Some BSAs were medical sergeants who received battlefield commissions in the MAC. An example in the ETO was S. Sgt. Samuel G. Calhoon, the noncommissioned officer of a battalion medical section in the 398th Infantry Regiment of the 100th Division. When Calhoon received his new rank his soldiers applauded this recognition of "his wonderful work on the battlefield."[100] Most BSAs were MAC officers who completed the BSA course, a six-week school begun in January 1944 as an affiliate of the Barkeley OCS. It graduated its first class of 250 students in March, and in all trained 1,974 officers in seven classes ending in January 1945, two months before Barkeley closed. About half of the instruction was in field medicine and surgery, with the balance in tactical employment of battalion aid stations, administration, and field sanitation. When planning for the invasion of Japan created a requirement for another 500 BSAs, the course had to be reinstituted at Carlisle Barracks; it reopened there on 7 July 1945 and had graduated another 102 officers by the time Japan surrendered.[101] Lt. Richardson was delighted when the 4th Infantry Division received its first BSAs as it fought through France, because that gave him counterparts in each battalion to assist in rotating the litter bearer teams and in getting the jeeps as far forward as possible, a task he had been doing alone up to that point.[102]

Capt. Klaus H. Huebner, MC, a battalion surgeon in the 88th Infantry Division in Italy, welcomed the arrival of an MAC lieutenant as "an innovation" who relieved him of administrative duties.[103] In the South Pacific, Sgt. Czar Hertzell received a battlefield commission as an MAC second lieutenant in the 6th Infantry Division and was twice decorated for valor. His battalion surgeon, faced with "overwhelming" paperwork and unit administration, said Lieutenant Hertzell was a "big help and timesaver" as the BSA, especially with his coordination of evacuation and medical supply during combat.[104]

Col. Jimmie Kanaya, MSC, a BSA in World War II, believed the use of MAC officers in this role was a sensible improvement in the utilization of Army physicians. Kanaya was the medical detachment sergeant for a regimental combat team attached to the 34th Infantry Division in Italy. He received a battlefield commission and was appointed the BSA in September 1944 when the assistant battalion surgeon was wounded and evacuated. Kanaya received the Silver Star for his actions in Italy and was redeployed with his regiment to southeastern France where it was attached to the 36th Infantry Division. He was captured in the Vosges mountains and remained a prisoner of war until his liberation in April 1945. Initially held by the Germans in Schubin, Poland, Kanaya, along with another MAC officer, 1st Lt. Les Brown, was force-marched 360 miles to Nuernberg, Germany, in the winter of 1945. Kanaya, the only non-Caucasian of 1,400 POWs, kept a prohibited diary in which he described liberation by a task force from Patton's Third Army. Kanaya worked in the POW dispensary and at one point escaped execution by a ruse. "Attempt was made by the Germans to move out all American officers during this period. Feigned illness in the dispensary bed with actual temperature (fever) so the Germans let me stay."[105]

World War II: The Administrative Specialties

Medical Logistics

The Medical Department's World War II history characterized its logistical performance as marked by "numerous shortcomings, tragedies, handicaps and errors."[106] The lack of an adequate capability at the beginning of the war was hard to overcome, a matter of "too little and not early enough."[107] That the department recovered was to the credit of MAC officers serving in medical logistics duties, a number that reached about five thousand by the end of 1943. Administrative specialty officers held key positions at all levels of the medical logistics system.

These officers commanded virtually all the overseas depots and filled the positions in the Army Air Forces, which created its own medical logistics system in 1942. They served as medical supply officers of hospitals of every size, enabling those units to meet the demands of combat support. An example was the 23d General Hospital, which used 90 miles of gauze, 12,000 pounds of plaster of paris, 3,600 cans of ether, and over 2,000 liters of normal saline in 1944. Inevitably, some of the officers encountered resistance to their assumption of duties formerly performed by physicians. Capt. Claude C. Britell, MAC, commander of the 30th Medical Depot, took his unit to Fort Lewis for predeployment training. The post surgeon adamantly believed that only physicians should command medical units, and only the intercession of higher headquarters prevented him from relieving Britell of his command.[108]

The importance of officers competent in medical logistics was again underscored. General Kirk spoke to a meeting of medical logisticians shortly after his appointment as surgeon general, and he recalled for the group just how frustrating the early logistical failures had been. In some areas there had been no suction equipment for surgery and the medics would have to hook up a hose to a truck's windshield wiper vacuum line. Scissors would not cut and the fluoroscopic glass in every x-ray machine had broken during shipping. There were no intestinal sutures, no washing machines to do the hospital laundry, sterilizers without gauges, and "warehouses full of junk left from the last war."[109]

Assessments after the war cited a number of reasons for the early failures,[110] but the vital ingredient in turning the situation around was Medical Administrative Corps officers. Col. Louis F. Williams, MSC, one of the officers who contributed to the effort, recalled that: "No one was trained for anything, and we made all the mistakes that are possible to make. How we got through, I don't know, except probably we were able to produce so much."[111] New techniques were introduced, such as the wooden pallet, which in combination with the forklift truck reduced manual operations to a minimum. But most important, MAC officers succeeded in meeting unbending demands. "The old phrase 'ain't got any' was 'out.'"[112]

Initially, the procurement of medical materiel was the sole domain of Sanitary Corps officers who were recruited in the interwar program of commissioning officers from industry. MAC officers concentrated on warehousing, storage, and issue of medical items. But the distinction between MAC and Sanitary Corps officers in procurement duties disappeared when it became evident that the department could not meet all its requirements with the Sanitary Corps program.[113] One officer who specialized in procurement was Maj. C. W. Torbet, SnC, deputy director of the Surgeon General's Procurement Division. He reported in June 1943 that the classified drug "penicillum" was being procured for experimental use by the Army. With the exception of the atomic bomb project, the penicillin program had the highest priority of any military item during the war. The Army's requirement went from slightly more than half of the monthly U.S. production of 50,000 vials in June to 1.5 million vials in December 1943. Other procurement actions ranged from an order for 364,125 gross of prophylactics (this required the intervention of the Office of the Rubber Director) to contracts for 1,000 glass eyes per month.[114]

Medical administrative specialty officers operated at all levels of a vastly expanding medical logistics operation. The growth of the Surgeon General's Supply Service reflected this movement. In September 1939, as the Finance and Supply Division, it numbered 4 officers and 27 civilians. By June 1943 it totaled 73 officers and 522 civilians. Fifty-three officers were MAC and Sanitary Corps officers; only 7 were physicians. By then the Medical Department had 800 officers and 15,000 civilians handling its stateside medical logistics operations.[115]

Changes in the depot system reflected the assumption of responsibilities by MACs. In February 1942 Capt. Eugene G. Cooper, MAC, was assigned to the Richmond General Depot as the first MAC officer to activate the medical section of a general depot. The St. Louis Medical Depot had 4 Medical Corps and 25 MAC or Sanitary Corps officers in March 1942. Three years later it had 2 MC and 87 MAC officers.[116]

Medical administrative specialty officers also ran the medical portion of the United States Lend-Lease program, which began in 1941 as a small section in the Surgeon General's Office headed by Capt. Burwell B. Smythe, MAC. Renamed the International Division (dubbed the "International Gift Society") and headed by Lt. Col. Francis C. Little, MAC, it directed the shipment of $150 million of medical materiel during the war, 23 percent of which went to the Soviet Union, the largest single recipient.[117]

MACs provided medical supply support around the world. Capt. Orion V. Kempf, MAC, commander of the medical supply depot in the Philippines, was captured by the Japanese in the fall of the Philippines. He died on 9 January 1945 aboard the unmarked Japanese vessel *Enoura Maru*, which was transporting POWs to Japan and was attacked by Allied aircraft in Takao Harbor, Formosa.[118] In the China-Burma-India Theater, Lts. George J. DeBroeck and Philip U. Farley, MAC, served as medical supply officers supporting the 10th (Chinese) Engineer Regiment and several American units in building the Ledo Road from Burma to China, a road "that was pushed across the hills by a band of gallant and hardy giants."[119]

Medical logistics training was conducted by the depots. In 1942 the St. Louis Medical Depot organized a two-week orientation course for officers commissioned from industry. In March 1943, expanded to one month, it was incorporated into the Army Service Forces Depot Course, which 412 Medical Department officers completed by June 1944. The other two phases were a month at the Quartermaster School, Fort Lee, Virginia, and a one-month practical experience

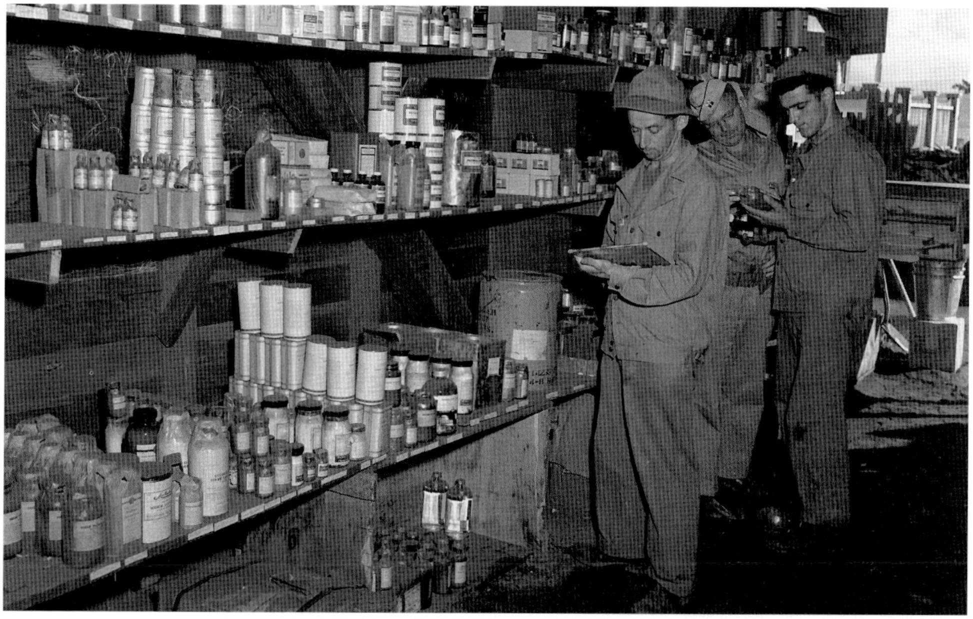

U.S. Army Medical Supply Depot in New Caledonia, 1942

at the medical supply section of a general depot. In addition, the St. Louis Medical Depot trained ninety-eight officers as medical equipment maintenance officers, and a smaller number completed an optical repair course. OCS graduates were a primary source of students.[120]

Actions to resolve medical logistics difficulties also led to the first general officer among the precursors of the Medical Service Corps. The promotion of Col. Edward Reynolds, MAC, to brigadier general in 1945 boosted the morale of MAC officers. "That Reynolds, an MAC, could become a brigadier general, tickled the vanity of the MACs and enhanced their image very substantially."[121]

Reynolds' promotion had a lot to do with the actions of Col. Tracy S. Voorhees, an attorney who, with other talented civilian leaders, joined the staff of the Surgeon General's Office. Commissioned as a colonel in the Judge Advocate General Department, Voorhees organized a legal division for the surgeon general and later served as director of the Control Division (a Somervell development). In 1945 he was appointed assistant secretary of war and after the war became under secretary of war.[122]

In November 1942 Voorhees, alarmed by the Wadhams Committee hearings, convinced the surgeon general to appoint a businessman with a national reputation as chief of supply in order to improve the department's logistics and defuse the attacks. Even though the surgeon general was a physician and not a businessman, Voorhees warned that "he was operating what was in effect a national chain store enterprise," and he needed expert help.[123]

Magee reluctantly took Voorhees' advice and appointed Edward Reynolds, the president of Columbia Gas and Electric Corporation, New York, as his spe-

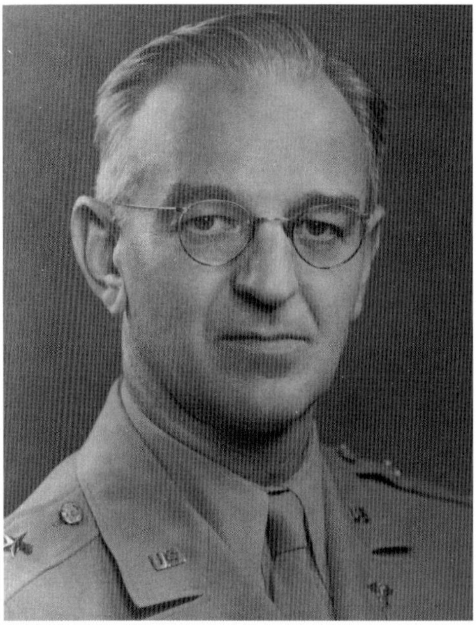

General Reynolds

cial assistant. A Harvard graduate, Reynolds had seen action in 1916 as a first lieutenant in the Mexican Punitive Expedition, joined Columbia Gas and Electric in 1922, and became the company's president in 1936.[124] Reynolds' role was initially not well defined, at least publicly, but Voorhees' plan was to transfer all medical supply authority to Reynolds. Voorhees believed that Reynolds' appointment helped soften the report of the Wadhams Committee. "The Committee's findings concerning the surgeon general were not particularly flattering," he noted, "but were much milder than they otherwise might have been."[125]

Reynolds' position solidified in June 1943 when General Kirk, the new surgeon general, appointed Reynolds as the acting chief of the Supply Service and in August as the chief. Reynolds was commissioned an MAC colonel in April 1944.[126] In the spring of 1945 General Kirk asked Colonel Voorhees for assistance in promoting Reynolds to brigadier general, something that Kirk had promised. Voorhees interceded with his friend Judge Robert P. Patterson, the under secretary of war. "I saw the 'Judge' the next day," Voorhees said. Reynolds was promoted on 17 June 1945, "but I don't think he ever knew how it came about."[127]

MACs were members of three troubleshooting teams led by Colonel Voorhees in 1944 to correct major medical logistics problems overseas. The most dramatic occurred from January to April 1944, when a team composed of Voorhees; Lt. Col. Leonard H. Beers, MAC; Herman C. Hangen (on loan to the Medical Department from the J.C. Penney Company); and Lt. Col. Byron C. T. Fenton, MC, visited the ETO headquarters in England.[128] There they found that medical support deficiencies were about to derail the Normandy invasion. Maj. Gen. Paul R. Hawley, the ETO chief surgeon, called it "a horrible mess. It was really terrible."[129]

American forces required an additional 44,000 beds to support the invasion, yet by mid-February only 7,000 were available. The problems were endless. For one thing, all the First Army's mobile hospital sets had been opened for inspection, thereby destroying the integrity of their original amphibious packing. For another, the Americans had difficulties accommodating to the supply systems of its allies. Examples were many: U.S. oxygen tanks were green, the color that the British used for carbon dioxide—a problem that would cause several deaths early in the invasion. There were infinite differences in detail between the systems: Americans issued aspirins in 500-tablet bottles, for example, while the British issued 50,000 tablets in a stove pipe that had each end plugged.[130]

Voorhees' team reported that an immediate reorganization was required.[131] The team moved quickly. Col. Silas B. Hays, MC, was put in charge of the medical supply service and Colonels Beers and Fenton remained in England on Hays' staff. Capt. William B. Walker, MAC, arrived in late February to supervise the repacking of the fifteen First Army hospitals.[132] Medical support was ready in time for the invasion, which began on 6 June, although medical logisticians would face great demands as the invasion proceeded. After the war the General Board of the European Theater of Operations concluded that the medical logistics system "would not have been able to support operation 'Overlord' had not certain changes been effected as a result of the Voorhees Committee investigation."[133]

The summer of 1944, Voorhees, Hangen, and Louis F. Williams (then a Pharmacy Corps [PhC] lieutenant colonel) investigated medical supply problems in the China-Burma-India (CBI) Theater.[134] There they found that the Surgeon, Services of Supply (the chief administrative officer for the CBI medical support) had ignored complaints of medical supply problems.[135] There were shortages throughout the theater because until the assignment of a competent medical supply officer, Maj. Claud D. La Fors, PhC, the theater had not requisitioned any supplies. His predecessor, a personal choice of the SOS surgeon, had been a dental officer. "Our suspicion was that the dentist must have pulled teeth in the morning and become so tired in the afternoon he could not even order what he could get merely for the asking."[136] The commander of the largest activity, the medical depot in Calcutta, had been the "$125-a-month proprietor of an ice cream parlor" prior to the war and was quite incompetent.[137] They removed him on the spot.

A final Voorhees mission traveled to Hawaii, New Guinea, the Philippines, Saipan, and the South Pacific in the fall of 1944. Voorhees, accompanied by Colonel Williams; Maj. Gordon S. Kjolsrud, MAC; and Charles W. Harris, deputy chief of the Supply Service, found enough medical supplies in the South Pacific Base Command for the current war and the next one as well. Requisitions submitted since August by units in Guadalcanal had not been filled by November because the forms were not properly filled out.[138] Medical supply in MacArthur's Southwest Pacific Area was an "utterly red-tape organization." Subordinate depots were not permitted to requisition directly from outside the theater unless the item was not present within the theater. This caused insurmountable difficulties for an area of operations that spanned more than twenty-five hundred miles and lacked dependable transportation. "If the theater was short of an item, a lot would be on requisition, all of which might go to the Philippines and none to New Guinea or vice versa." Corrective actions ranged from modifying stockage levels and requisitioning practices to immediate personnel changes.[139]

Summary

The principal story of medical administrative specialty officers in World War II was the breadth and depth of their movement into positions throughout the Medical Department as it woke from the somnolence of the interwar years. The revolution was propelled by pressure from a number of sources working in tandem: national and departmental politics, civilian associations and guilds, the burgeoning demands of wartime patient care, the influence of modernization within the American health care industry, the need for trained executives, and the desires of physicians to practice medicine rather than occupy their time with nonclinical duties.

The department resisted those pressures, but the time was long overdue for modernization. Administrative specialty officers and their scientific specialty colleagues enabled the department to accomplish its enormously complex task. Opportunity for commissioning, training, and meaningful positions flourished. Promotion opportunity also opened during the war and was distinguished by the first selection of a general officer among this group of Medical Department officers.

During World War I the Army had learned all the lessons it needed on the necessity for a complete medical team. Yet the Medical Department's failure to select, train, and nurture a sufficient number of administrative specialty officers during the interwar years continued to plague the department throughout World War II. A premier example was medical logistics. The trained and experienced senior medical logisticians the Army needed did not exist because no one had "grown" them in the necessary numbers before the war. Even with enormous efforts to turn around the medical logistics system, the absence of adequate planning and execution at the theater level seriously impaired the medical supply support in the China-Burma-India Theater and nearly derailed the invasion of Europe.

Medical administrative specialty officers were needed in great numbers to handle medical logistics worldwide, as well as the full range of management functions that were essential for a global industrial capability. The Army rapidly selected, trained, and pressed into service thousands of officers in the attempt to overcome the problems of medical support that had not been planned for before the war. Through their performance and contributions they were reshaping the Medical Department into a new kind of organization.

Notes

[1] MAC: Most administrative specialty officers were commissioned in the MAC, although a handful served in the Sanitary Corps and the Pharmacy Corps, the latter a wartime creation.

[2] Quoted words: Albert E. Cowdrey, *The Medics' War*, volume in the series U.S. Army in the Korean War (Washington, D.C.: U.S. Army Center of Military History, 1987), p. 53.

[3] MAC numbers: McMinn and Levin, *Personnel in World War II*, pp. 15, 113, 376, 436; Disposition form (DF), Samuel Kier to Maj Israeloff, THU, OTSG, sub: Comparative Statistical Data, 17 Dec 65, MSC-USACMH; Bernard P. C. Aabel, "The Medical Administrative Corps," *Medical Bulletin* (June 1947): 518, hereafter cited as Aabel, "The MAC." The 1,343 MAC officers in June 1941 consisted of 68 Regular Army, 933 Reserve, 266 National Guard, and 76 Army of the United States officers, the last a wartime temporary component. In October 1944 over half of the corps was overseas. In all, 20,213 officers served in the MAC during World War II. Other August 1945 figures were Army Nurse Corps (ANC): 55,950; MC: 46,980; DC: 14,170; VC: 2,070; and enlisted: 493,209.

[4] U.S. casualties: Pamphlet, Armed Forces Information Service, *Defense 83 Almanac* (Arlington, Va.: Department of Defense, September 1983), p. 46, hereafter cited as *Defense 83*.

[5] Peak strength: McMinn and Levin, *Personnel in World War II*, pp. 12, 15, 247–66, 499. The Medical Department by the fall of 1944 was three times the size of the entire Regular Army in 1937. Kent Roberts Greenfield, *The Historian and the Army* (New Brunswick, N.J.: Rutgers University, 1954), p. 73, citing comparisons by Donald O. Wagner, Ph.D., TSG's chief historian. In August 1945 the strength of the MAC was 19,867, the SnC was 2,490, and the PC was 68. These are TSG numbers; TAG numbers were slightly different.

[6] Casualties: *Encyclopedia Americana*, 57th edition, s.v. "World War II," section by John R. Elting on "Costs, Casualties, and Other Data." The estimate of the killed during the war is from Henry J. Gwiazda II, "World War II and Nazi Racism," *Prologue* (quarterly of the National Archives) 25 (Spring 1993): 65. The figures remain very imprecise. For example, estimates of the number killed in the Soviet Union and China remain very fluid. Racial war: Gwiazda, "World War II and Nazi Racism," pp. 65, 67; Rudolph J. Rummell, *Democide: Nazi Genocide and Mass Murder* (New Brunswick, N.J.: Transaction Publishers, 1992). The "final solution" of the Nazis was a deliberately planned and implemented genocide of the Jews. It was one aspect of a Nazi ideology that sought to preserve Aryan blood over all others. Rummell in a detailed examination of this complex and horrifying subject concludes that the Nazis probably murdered over 16.3 million (and possibly as many as 24 million) people because of race, religion, ethnicity, or sexual preference. Ibid., p. 100.

[7] Armed Forces: *Defense 83*, p. 46. Theaters: John B. Coates, "The US Army Medical Department in World War II," *Journal of the American Medical Association* 165 (September 21, 1957): 244. The major theaters and the numbers of soldiers in each were: European Theater of Operations (ETO), 3,000,000; Southwest Pacific Theater, 340,000; Pacific Ocean Areas, 450,000; and Mediterranean Theater of Operations, 500,000. Army buildup: Greenfield, *The Historian and the Army*, pp. 70, 86. Logistical burdens of fighting a global war caused Army Chief of Staff General George C. Marshall to suspend creation of new divisions in the summer of 1943 so as to concentrate on building up the support base. The Army finished the war with 89 divisions rather than the 215 originally envisioned.

[8] Prewar capacity: *SG Report*, 1941, p. 253. There were 78,734 beds on 30 June 1941, of which 41,051 were occupied, reflecting the buildup.Wartime capacity: Army Service Forces, *Statistical Review: World War II*, pp. 243, 245, 248, copy in JML; Eli Ginzberg, "Federal Hospitalization: II—Current Trends," *Modern Hospital* 72 (April 1949): 73. Zone of the Interior hospitals: Eli Ginzberg, "Army Hospitalization, Retrospect and Prospect," *Medical Bulletin* (January 1948): 38–44, hereafter cited as Ginzberg, "Army Hospitalization." That there was sufficient stateside capacity to receive those patients was a tribute to TSG's strenuous efforts before the Normandy invasion to preserve hospital beds in the face of enormous pressure from the War Department Staff to reduce hospital capacity. Ibid., p. 44.

[9] Doctrine: Medical Field Service School, *Service of a Field Force*, pamphlet no. 6 (Carlisle Barracks, Pa.: U.S. Army Medical Field Service School, 1932), p. 47; *Military Medical Manual*, 6th ed., rev. October 1944 (Harrisburg, Pa.: Military Service Publishing Company, 1945), pp.

545–47; Monograph, Donald E. Hall, *From the Roer to the Elbe with the 1st Medical Group: Medical Support of the Deliberate River Crossing* (Fort Leavenworth, Kans.: Combat Studies Institute, U.S. Army Command and General Staff College, 1992), pp. 6–15. Lessons: Some lessons learned are in Rpt, ETO, U.S. Army, sub: Reports of the General Board, United States Forces, European Theater, established by GO 128, HQ, ETO, USA, 17 Jun 45, USACMH, hereafter cited as ETO, General Board. Medical doctrine is covered in report number 90. Experience in Europe taught that cellular units were impracticable and that a large and immediately available bed capacity was essential for combat support. See also Memo, Ginzberg for Director, History Division (Dir, Hist Div), OTSG, 5 Sep 45, MSC-USACMH; Ginzberg, "Army Hospitalization," pp. 38, 42. Ginzberg was a noted economist (still publishing in 1991) who was a key figure in SGO during the war.

[10] MAC positions: Samuel M. Goodman, Training (Tng) Doctrine Branch (Br), Tng Div, OTSG, sub: A Report on the History of the Medical Administrative Corps Officer Candidate Schools, 1 Nov 44, with Supplement, 1 Jul 44–30 Jun 45, pp. 14, 56, MSC-USACMH, hereafter cited as Goodman, OCS Report.

[11] MAC positions: Col Joseph Israeloff, MSC, draft chapter, sub: Medical Officer Substitutions, THU, OTSG, 1965 MSC History Project (Israeloff revision, winter 76), pp. 13, 66, MSC-USACMH, hereafter cited as Israeloff, Medical Officer Substitutions.

[12] Reorganization: Maj. Gen. Henry H. Arnold assumed command of the Army Air Forces. Lt. Gen. Lesley J. McNair headed the Army Ground Forces, a command which formed the U.S. training base and put together the divisions that were furnished to theater commanders. This account is based on several sources: Blanche B. Armfield, *Organization and Administration in World War II*, volume in the series Medical Department of the United States Army in World War II (Washington D.C.: Office of the Surgeon General, Department of the Army, 1962), pp. 145–85; Smith, *Hospitalization and Evacuation*, pp. 54–61; James E. Hewes, Jr., *From Root to McNamara: Army Organization and Administration, 1900–1963* (Washington, D.C.: U.S. Army Center of Military History, 1975), pp. 57–103; John D. Millet, *The Organization and Role of the Army Service Forces*, volume in the series United States Army in World War II (Washington, D.C.: U.S. Army Center of Military History, 1954), pp. 36–38. Access regained: See Ms, Tracy S. Voorhees, A Lawyer Among Army Doctors, pp. 79–80, USACMH.

[13] Quoted words: Charles Murphy, "Somervell of the S.O.S.," *Life* (8 March 1943): 43. TSG: Millet, *The Organization and Role of the Army Service Forces*, p. 93.

[14] Wadhams Committee: Account drawn from Millet, *The Organization and Role of the Army Service Forces*, pp. 145–200; Smith, *Hospitalization and Evacuation*, p. 61; Rpt, War Department, sub: Committee To Study the Medical Department, Col. Sanford H. Wadhams, MC, USA, Ret., Chm, 9 volumes of testimony, 1942, copy in MSC-USACMH, hereafter cited as Wadhams Committee.

[15] Marshall and Magee: Interv, Eli Ginzberg with Samuel Milner, 10 Sep 63; Interv, Maj Gen Raymond W. Bliss, MC (TSG), Ret., with Milner, 14–15 Jun 63, both in interv files, USACMH; Armfield, *Organization and Administration in World War II*, p. 185, quoted words, p. 200.

[16] Logistics: One witness described seventeen medical procurement employees working up to twelve hours a day in a room adequate for six people. "They work until they get the jitters." Wadhams Committee, testimony by Col Albert J. Browning, Dir, Purchasing Div, SOS (formerly President [Pres], United Wall Paper Factories), 7 Oct 42. TSG received the report in late February 1943, after Secretary of War Henry L. Stimson approved it.

[17] The total staff numbered 337. Quoted words: Paul V. McNutt (Chm of the Board, United Artists; previously Governor of Indiana, 1933–37), testimony 3 Oct 42, Wadhams Committee, MSC-USACMH. For a perspective on this from within the Medical Department see Gibbs, Milner interv, 24 Jun 64.

[18] Wadhams Committee, Recommendation 95.

[19] ASF supervision: Brig Gen James B. Wharton, Dir Mil Pers, HQ SOS, to TSG, sub: Availability of Physicians, 22 May 42, Wadhams Committee, MSC-USACMH. TSG was directed to remove physicians from "administrative or executive positions which do not require professionally trained medical personnel."

[20] WD policy: Smith, *Hospitalization and Evacuation*, p. 133, citing TAG to CGs of AGF, AAF, and all CAs (Corps Areas), sub: Relief of MC Officers from Duties Which Do Not Require

Professional Medical Training, 13 Jul 42; WD Cir 99, 9 Mar 44, sub: Conservation of Medical Officers, PL.

[21] AMA: It was also an effort by organized medicine to control the allocation of medical resources.

[22] Physician draft: McMinn and Levin, *Personnel in World War II*, pp. 73–74, 134, 175, 185–88, including quoted words, p. 73.

[23] Physician requirement: McMinn and Levin, *Personnel in World War II*, pp. 67, 73–74; Israeloff, Medical Officer Substitutions, pp. 21, 31–32; Gerald H. Teasley, "Personnel Problems of the Medical Department," *Southern Medical Journal* 36 (March 1943): 211. MC: The Medical Corps strength peaked at 46,970 in January 1945. McMinn and Levin, *Personnel in World War II*, p. 12.

[24] Quoted words: Gibbs, Milner Interv, 24 Oct 63.

[25] Report: Operations Service (Ops Svc), OTSG, General Bliss Notebook, Rpt, sub: Utilization of Medical Personnel in the Field, 31 Oct 44, folder 176, box 11/18, MSC-USACMH.

[26] Kenner Board: SGO, Medical Department Personnel Board, Brig Gen Albert W. Kenner, MC, Chm, Rpt to Chief, Ops Svc, SGO, sub: Study of Medical Department Personnel, 28 October 1943, Board established by SGO Office Orders no. 715, 16 Sep 43, MSC-USACMH, hereafter cited as Kenner Board; also see Israeloff, Medical Officer Substitution, pp. 50–65.

[27] Heaton on substitution: Leonard D. Heaton, foreword to McMinn and Levin, *Personnel in World War II*, p. xi.

[28] Incompetence: "Our hospital administrators were generally medical officers who were not too successful in their practices." Interv, Maj Gen George E. Armstrong, MC (TSG), Ret., Dir, New York University Medical Center, with Samuel Milner, 13 Jul 67, USACMH. See also Gibbs, Milner Interv, 18 Mar 64. Regular Army (RA) MC: All but six RA MCs served in staff or administrative positions during the war. THU, OTSG, Mtg of the Advisory Editorial Board for the Medical Service Corps History, 13 Nov 58, p. PR 3–5, 1, MSC-USACMH, hereafter cited as THU, AEB for MSC History.

[29] Pressure on TSG: Millet, *The Organization and Role of the Army Service Forces*, p. 95–96.

[30] Resistance: Smith, *Hospitalization and Evacuation*, pp. 259–60. SGO announced a test of substitution in June 1942 and asked fourteen hospitals to respond with their findings. Guidance from SGO in August 1942 said that the executive officer and registrar positions in large hospitals must be physicians. Col John A. Rogers, MC, XO, SGO, to hospital cdrs, 29 Jun 42; Lt Col J. R. Hudnall, MC, SGO, to Lt Col Arthur J. Redland, 5th Service Command, 10 Aug 42, both folder 44, box 4/18, MSC-USACMH.

[31] Command: Maj Gen John F. Bohlender to Col Gene Quinn, MSC, 19 Jun 59, MSC-USACMH.

[32] ETO: ETO, General Board, Rpt 89, USACMH.

[33] MAC positions: Goodman, OCS Rpt, p. 56.

[34] Quoted words: 5 Sep 42, Wadhams Committee.

[35] Shortages: Smith, *Hospitalization and Evacuation*, pp. 133–34; Army Service Forces (ASF), *Statistical Review, World War II* (1945), p. 73; Memo, Albert H. Schwichtenberg for Col Higgins, G–4, drafted by Eli Ginzberg, Special Asst to Dir, Hosp Div, OTSG, sub: Station and Regional Hospital Bed Requirements, 31 Oct 44; THU, AEB for MSC History, 13 Nov 58, all in MSC-USACMH. ASF was reporting a shortage of 512 MACs as late as the fall of 1944.

[36] MAC Officer Candidate Schools (OCS): Unless otherwise noted, this discussion is based on Goodman, OCS Rpt; Rpt, MAC OCS, sub: Annual Rpt, 30 Jun 42, Medical Replacement Training Center, Camp Barkeley, Tex., folder 145, box 9/18, MSC-USACMH; Parks, *Medical Training in World War II*, pp. 97–123; and Col Joseph Israeloff, MSC, draft chapter, sub: Officer Candidate Schools for Medical Administrative Corps Officers, THU, 1965 MSC History Project (Israeloff revision, winter 1976), MSC-USACMH. Demand: The Medical Department projected that it could supply only 1,600 of the 2,450 officers required by January 1943, causing the start of a second OCS.

[37] Australia: Lt Col A. B. Miller, MC, to Capt John W. Harvey, OTSG, HQ, SOS, 20 Mar 45, folder 185, box 12/18, MSC-USACMH.

[38] OCS prerequisites: WD Army Regulation (AR) 625–5, "Officer Candidates," 26 Nov 42, PL.

[39] Quoted words: Rpt, Capt Peter A. Luppen, MAC, sub: Autobiography, 1945, folder 142, box 17/18, MSC-USACMH.

[40] MAC requirements: WD AR 625–5, "Officer Candidates," 26 Nov 42, PL.

[41] Quoted words: Goodman, OCS Rpt, p. 12.

[42] Barracks: Notes of telephone interv, Joseph P. Peters, Consultant in Strategic Planning and Health Care Services, Philadelphia, with Lt. Col. Richard V. N. Ginn, MSC, 24 Apr 85, DASG-MS.

[43] Peters: Ibid.

[44] Failures: Goodman, OCS Rpt, p. 31.

[45] Prep school: Bernard Aabel, "History and Mission of the Medical Administrative Corps," *Armored Cavalry Journal* 56 (May–June 1947): 50, hereafter cited as Aabel, "History of the MAC."

[46] MAC officers: Other MACs on the staff were Capts. Elmer W. Lindquist and Early E. Morton and 1st Lts. Vincent B. McFadden and Don D. Sherrill. Better conditions: Interv, Cols Otto H. Sandman, Jr., MSC, and Frank L. Lawford, MSC, with Lt Col Joseph Israeloff, MSC, THU, OTSG, 6 Oct 67, USACMH.

[47] Best OCS: Statement of Lt Col Mott, WD inspector, as reported in Col Paul R. Hawley, MC, Asst Commandant (Cmdt) MFSS, Carlisle Barracks, Pa., to Maj Frank B. Wakeman, MC, OTSG, 8 Sep 41, folder 185, box 12/18, MSC-USACMH.

[48] Benade: Interv, Lt Gen Leo F. Benade, USA, Ret., with Ginn, Alexandria, Va., 25 Jan 84, DASG-MS. Benade transferred as an MSC colonel.

[49]Black graduates: Carlisle OCS graduated 127, and Barkeley graduated 260. Parks, *Medical Training in World War II*, pp. 97–123. Segregation: See Col Elliotte J. Williams, MSC, Ret., to Ginn, 25 Nov 85, DASG-MS. This essay on the experiences of a young black officer during this period is a moving, valuable insight. Infantry: Memo, Maj H. M. Rexrode, MAC, for Ch, Pers Svc, 29 May 45, sub: Semi-Annual History of MAC & SnC for Period 1 Jan–31 May 1945, in file Research Notes WWII, box 2/18, MSC-USACMH.

[50] Black company: WD T/O 8–117, Sanitary Company, 1 Nov 40, USAMHI; McMinn and Levin, *Personnel in World War II*, pp. 320–21, 411–12; Smith, *Hospitalization and Evacuation*, pp. 223–24; Israeloff, draft chapter, sub: Winning the War, THU, 1965 MSC History Project, pp. 93–101, DASG-MS, hereafter cited as Israeloff, Winning the War; WD T/O 8–117, Medical Sanitary Company, 13 May 44, *Military Medical Manual* (4th ed., 1945), pp. 645, 817.

[51] Integration: Col Elliotte J. Williams, MSC, Ret., to Ginn, 15 May 85 and 25 Nov 85, DASG-MS.

[52] Quoted words: Williams to Ginn, 15 May 85. Blacks: McMinn and Levin, *Personnel in World War II*, p. 321.

[53] Verse: Rpt, 1st Lt Edwin H. Potts, MAC, sub: History of the Medical Administrative Corps Officer Candidate School, Camp Barkeley, Tex., 15 Mar 45, folder 185, box 12/18, MSC-USACMH, hereafter cited as Potts, History of the MAC OCS.

[54] Enrollment in September 1942: "One Thousand Administrative Officers a Month at Camp Barkeley," *Journal of the American Medical Association* 121 (1943): 437. The article claimed that MACs were "releasing doctors of medicine for medical and surgical work."

[55] Barkeley history: Potts, History of the MAC OCS.

[56] Quoted words: Interv, Lt Col Woodus Carter, MSC, with Israeloff, 13 Oct 67, USACMH.

[57] Canopy fall: Unpublished paper, Owen J. Brady, "A Memorial: The Hotel de Gink Association, MAC-OCS, Abilene, Texas, 1942–1945," prepared for 8th reunion in Laguna, Calif., Oct 75, MSC-USACMH.

[58] Entertainment: Extract from MFSS, Annual Rpt 1942 and 1943, in file Research Notes WWII, box 2/18, MSC-USACMH.

[59] Conditions: Also see Carter, Israeloff Interv. Quoted words: Telephone Interv, Peters with Ginn. Peer review: Notes of discussion, Col William B. O'Neill, MSC, Ret., with Ginn, Falls Church, Va., 20 Nov 85, DASG-MS; Maj Gen George E. Armstrong, Jr., Ret., and Lt Col John A. Ey, Jr., MSC, Ret., draft chapter, sub: Medical Administrative Corps Officer Candidate School, 1961, in 1958 MSC History Project, folder 243, box 15/18, MSC-USACMH.

[60] Blacks: Extract, Barkeley MAC OCS Annual Rpt, FY 1942–43, annex to pt. 2, Statistical Information, in file Research Notes WWII, box 2/18, MSC-USACMH; Israeloff, Winning the War, p. 101.

[61] Quoted words: Interv, Elliot L. Richardson with Ginn, Washington, D.C., 29 Jan 86, DASG-MS. He was also attorney general; secretary of commerce; secretary of health, education, and wel-

fare; and ambassador to the Court of St. James. He is remembered for his resignation as attorney general during the Watergate scandal rather than follow President Nixon's order to fire Special Prosecutor Archibald Cox.

[62] Quoted words: Interv, Col Vernon McKenzie, USA, Ret., Principal Deputy Assistant Secretary of Defense, Office of the Assistant Secretary of Defense for Health Affairs (OASD-HA), with Ginn, Washington, D.C., 17 May 84, DASG-MS.

[63] Quoted words: Interv, Col Knute A. Tofte-Nielsen, MSC, USA, Ret., Chief, Doctrine and International Activities Br, OTSG, with Ginn, Washington D.C., 23 Oct 84, DASG-MS.

[64] Anecdote: Notes of Telephone Interv, Donald J. Pletsch, Ph.D., with Ginn, 9 Jan 86, DASG-MS.

[65] Duties: An occasional MAC was assigned to scientific specialty duties. Capt. Markus Ring, MAC, was assigned as the designing officer, Fort McPherson, Georgia, Dental Laboratory. See Ring, "Laboratory Procedures in Restoring Mastication, Vertical Dimension and Esthetics," *Journal of the American Dental Association* 33 (October 1946): 1346–49; M. L. Mills and Ring, "Deflashing Techniques," *Medical Bulletin* (November 1945): 599–601.

[66] Hospitals: Smith, *Hospitalization and Evacuation*, pp. 132, 251, 280; Mae Mills Link and Hubert A. Coleman, *Medical Support of the Army Air Forces in World War II* (Washington, D.C.: Office of the Surgeon General, Department of the Air Force, 1955), pp. 371–73; Israeloff, Winning the War, p. 80. The Army Air Forces School of Air Evacuation at Bowman Field, Kentucky, opened a special training program for MAC officers in June 1943.

[67] Registrar: ETO, General Board, no. 89; George W. Mallory, "Utilization of Medical Administrative Officers in Hospitals," *Military Surgeon* 101 (October 1947): 319, hereafter cited as Mallory, "Utilization of Medical Administrative Officers"; Israeloff, Winning the War, p. 80. Tucker: Israeloff, Winning the War, p. 80. Dorn: Biographical summary, THU, OTSG, USACMH; Albert G. Love, Eugene L. Hamilton, and Ida L. Helman, *Tabulating Equipment and Army Medical Statistics* (Washington, D.C.: Office of the Surgeon General, Department of the Army, 1958), pp. 111, 183. Addressograph: Smith, *Hospitalization and Evacuation*, p. 345.

[68] Langhenry: Lt Col Franklin P. Boeckman, MSC, HQ, USA Log Mgmt Ctr, Fort Lee, Va., to Col Gene Quinn, MSC, THU, OTSG, 10 Jun 59, MSC-USACMH. Langhenry stayed in the D.C. area after the war as a vice president of Acacia Mutual Insurance Company. Quoted words: Ltr, Col James T. Richards, MSC, Ret., to Ginn, sub: Here's My Story, 28 Feb 86, DASG-MS. Richards' calls angered some ETO senior medical officers who believed he "really rode roughshod." See comments (to Maj Gen Paul R. Hawley, ETO surgeon) by Col John B. Coates, Jr., MC, and Brig Gen James B. Mason, MC, in Rpt, THU, sub: Meeting of the Advisory Editorial Board for the History of the Medical Service in the European Theater in World War II, 9–10 Oct 62, USACMH, hereafter cited as THU, Medical Service in the European Theater.

[69] Regulating: James R. Francis, "Medical Administrative Corps Officers in the Chain of Evacuation," *Military Surgeon* 100 (May 1947): 417, hereafter cited as Francis, "MAC Officers"; Aabel, "History of the MAC." Quoted words: Ginzberg, "Army Hospitalization," p. 44. Also see Interv, Maj Gen Albert H. Schwichtenberg, USAF, with Milner, THU, 4 Oct 1967, USACMH.

[70] Fogelberg: Office of the Surgeon General, Current Trends Conference, 1966, USACMH; Biographical data card, THU, OTSG, USACMH.

[71] Quoted words: Armstrong, Milner Interv; also see Notes of Telephone Interv, Gibbs with Milner, 29 Jun 69, USACMH.

[72] Commissions: Memo, Lt Gen Brehon Somervell, HQ, SOS, for Chief of Staff of the Army (CSA), sub: Increase in Procurement Objective, 10 Jun 42, MSC-USACMH; DF, Lt Col Durwood G. Hall, MC, to Ch, Pers Svc, SGO, to Dir, Mil Pers Div, ASF, 29 Jul 43, and Address, Hall to Officer Procurement Service District Officers, Palmer House, Chicago, 17 Jun 43, both in folder 64, box 5/18, MSC-USACMH. Grade: Telephone Interv, Peters with Ginn.

[73] Maj. Tolbert: "Major Raymond F. Tolbert," Borden General Hospital newspaper, n.d. (1943), and Mrs. Josephine J. Tolbert to Ginn, 30 Oct 93, both in DASG-MS.

[74] XO: WD Cir 99, 9 Mar 44; Cir 122, 28 Mar 44; Cir 152, 17 Apr 44, all in PL; Smith, *Hospitalization and Evacuation,* p. 280.

[75] MAC positions: Mallory, "Utilization of Medical Administrative Officers," pp. 318–19; Robert S. Anderson, ed., *Army Medical Specialist Corps* (Washington, D.C., Office of the Surgeon General, Department of the Army, 1968), p. 136.

[76] Field unit positions: Francis, "MAC Officers," pp. 415–17; Aabel, "The MAC," pp. 517–18; Israeloff, Winning the War, pp. 80–92. See also Interv, Lt Gen Hal B. Jennings, MC, USA, Ret., with Col Kenneth K. Yamanouchi, MSC, USAMHI Senior Officer Oral History Program, 8 Jan 1983, in USAMHI, Carlisle Barracks, Pa. Jennings, a retired surgeon general, described his experience with the continued use of MC and DC officers early in the war. For examples see WD T/O 8–15P, 1 Oct 39, Medical Battalion (a new unit that replaced the medical regiment in division medical service, which initially had no MAC officers but was changed in revisions of 1 April 1942 and 1 March 1943); T/O 8–504, 1 Nov 40, Medical General Lab, which authorized sixteen SnC officers; T/O 688–W, Hospital Center (no MAC officers in 1 April 1942 version, but five MACs in that of 23 April 1944); T/O 8–22, 20 May 43, HHD, Medical Group (every staff section headed by MACs); T/O 8–75, Med Bn, Armored Division (MAC major as XO); T/O 8–661, Medical Supply Depot, Army or COMMZ, 2 Apr 43 (officer staff almost entirely MAC and SnC); T/O 8–317, 5 Dec 44, Ambulance Company (Separate), (MAC commander), all in USAMHI. Numbers: Francis, "MAC Officers," p. 417. Dannenburg: GO 131, U.S. Army Forces in the Far East, 15 Jan 45, cited in Joe Kralich, Ranchos, N.Mex., to Ginn, 4 Jan 93, DASG-MS. Historian: James H. Stone, ed., *Crisis Fleeting* (Washington, D.C.: Office of the Surgeon General, Department of the Army, 1969). Lt. Gen. Leonard Heaton, TSG, called Stone's account "unique and distinctive" (p. vii).

[77] Training: Israeloff, Winning the War, pp. 88–92. The seven Medical Replacement Training Centers were at Camps Lee and Pickett, Virginia; Camp Grant, Illinois; Camp Barkeley, Texas; Camp Joseph T. Robinson, Arkansas; Fort Lewis, Washington; and Camp Crowder, Missouri. The nine Medical Department Enlisted Technician Schools were at the Army Medical Center, Washington, D.C.; William Beaumont General Hospital, El Paso, Texas; Billings General Hospital, Fort Benjamin Harrison, Indianapolis, Indiana; Brooke General Hospital, Fort Sam Houston, San Antonio, Texas; Fitzsimons General Hospital, Denver, Colorado; Lawson General Hospital, Atlanta, Georgia; and O'Reilly General Hospital, Springfield, Missouri. Weapons training: Mobilization Training Program (MTP) 21–3, 1 May 44, and MTP 8–5, 1 Jun 44, established requirements for training in the bayonet, carbine, grenade, and rifle for the defense of medical personnel and patients. See Col Edward A. Zimmerman, MC, draft chapter, sub: Training Programs of Medical Replacement Training Centers, training Ms, n.d., THU, OTSG, folder 251, box 16/18, MSC-USACMH.

[78] Quoted words: Arthur W. Wolde, *Ambulance #11* (New York: Vantage Press, 1982), p. 52. See this account for an enlisted ambulance driver's perspective.

[79] Quoted words: Jack C. Coleman, *The Second* (Santa Anna, Calif.: privately published, 1985), p. 9.

[80] Odahl: Stone, *Crisis Fleeting*, pp. 2, 26–27. Harris: Ibid., pp. 25, 28, 64. Seagrave's Hospital: Named for Lt. Col. Gordon S. Seagrave, MC. Seagrave, who is highly praised by Stone, had come to Burma in 1922 as a medical missionary. When war broke out, he provided medical support to the Burmese and set up a series of small hospitals in support of the Chinese Sixth Army. See Gordon S. Seagrave, *Burma Surgeon* (New York: W. W. Norton, 1943), pp. 162–73. General Stilwell commissioned him as a Medical Corps officer in 1942, and his hospital was later absorbed into the American forces. Lada: Col John Lada, MSC, Ret., to Col Tim Jackman, Asst to Ch, MSC, 6 Dec 89, DASG-MS. With the exception of the commander and executive officers, the key staff and three company commanders were MAC officers. The battalion was expanded with the addition of four ambulance companies and three sanitary companies.

[81] Richardson: Richardson, Ginn Interv; David S. Broder, "Richardson: Diverse Career," *Washington Post*, 29 November 1972.

[82] Quoted words: Richardson, Ginn Interv. See also Richardson, "A Cause Worth Dying For," *Washington Post*, 16 February 1986.

[83] Hospital duties: Francis, "MAC Officers," p. 415.

[84] Need for quality: ETO, General Board, no. 89. 21st GH: 21st General Hospital (GH) historical rpt, 1944, folder 152, box 10/18, MSC-USACMH.

[85] Farley: Stone, *Crisis Fleeting*, pp. 5, 110, 131.

[86] Philippines: Julien M. Goodman, *M.D.P.O.W.* (New York: Exposition Press, 1972), pp. 3, 43, 61, 67; Alfred A. Weinstein, *Barbed Wire Surgeon* (New York: MacMillan Co., 1948), pp. 50–51, 243, 275; John E. Olson, *O'Donnell, Andersonville of the Pacific* (Lake Quivira, Kans.: self-published,

1985), p. 78. The Japanese confiscated medical supplies and issued only small amounts to the prison hospitals. Olson, *O'Donnell*, pp. 114–19.

[87] Rehabilitation: 5th GH historical rpt, 1945, folder 149, box 9/18, MSC-USACMH.

[88] Davis: Interv, Dorothy S. Davis, R.N., HQ, American Red Cross, with Ginn, Washington, D.C., 8 Nov 84, DASG-MS. Captain Davis was later Colonel Davis, MSC. Field hospital: WD T/O 8–510, 28 Sep 43, *Military Medical Manual*, 6th ed., 1945, pp. 644, 830. The title was misleading because the hospital was not designed for employment in the combat zone. The portable surgical hospital (T/O 8–572S), developed in the Pacific, was (ibid., pp. 643–44).

[89] XO: Interv, Lt Col Gilbert A. Bishop, MSC, with Israeloff, 29 Dec 66, USACMH.

[90] Schaefer: Gov William D. Schaefer to Ginn, 8 Apr 87, DASG-MS. Quoted words: Gwen Ifill, "A Complex Big-City Mayor Who Defies the Conventional," *Washington Post*, 2 June 1986.

[91] Prideaux: Hall, *From the Roer to the Elbe with the 1st Medical Group*, p. 21. Aabel: U.S. Congress, House, Committee on Armed Services, Hearings on H.R. 1982, *To Establish a Permanent Medical Service Corps in the Medical Department of the Regular Army*, beginning 20 February 1947, testimony 12 March 1947, 80th Cong., 1st sess.; Francis P. Kintz and John Edgar, "Medical Groups of First U.S. Army in European Campaign, I: Beach Head, Break Through and Pursuit," *Military Surgeon* 106 (January 1950): 39, and "II: Siegfried Line, Ardennes, Rhine River and German Collapse" (February 1950): 142, 144.

[92] Hospital ships: WD T/O 8–537T, Hospital Ship Complement, 7 Dec 43, USAMHI; Howard A. Donald, "The Hospital Ship Program," *Medical Bulletin* (February 1944): 37, 41. Of the twenty-eight, twenty-five were transports converted and used by the Army as hospital ships and three were ships built expressly for that purpose. Blood: THU, Medical Service in the European Theater.

[93] New Guinea: "Air Evacuation of Patients in New Guinea," *Medical Bulletin* (August 1945): 185–90. Evacuation squadrons: Rpt, Robert F. Futrell, USAF Historical Division, Air University, Maxwell Air Force Base, Montgomery, Ala., USAF Historical Studies no. 23, sub: Development of Aeromedical Evacuation in the USAF, 1909–1960, May 1960, DASG-MS.

[94] Air ambulance: M. J. Musser, Jr., and Emmett C. Townsend, "Use of Small Airplanes for Medical Evacuation on Luzon," *Medical Bulletin* (August 1945): 191–97; Richard Tierney and Fred Montgomery, *The Army Aviation Story* (Northport, Ala.: Colonial Press, 1963), pp. 77, 141, 161, 204–06; David M. Lam, "From Balloon to Black Hawk: World War II," part 2 of 4-part series, *U.S. Army Aviation Digest* 27 (July 1981): 44–47.

[95] Burma: Tierney and Montgomery, *The Army Aviation Story*, pp. 205–06.

[96] BSAs: Smith, *Hospitalization and Evacuation*, p. 148; Francis, "MAC Officers," p. 415; Aabel, "History of the MAC," p. 51; Kenner Board, 1944; WD Cir 99, 9 Mar 44; WD Cir 327, 8 Aug 44, PL.The ETO General Board said the BSAs did "an especially fine job." ETO, General Board, no. 88, p. 6.

[97] Duties: Israeloff, Medical Officer Substitutions; Carter, Israeloff Interv, 13 Oct 67. Carter, a graduate of the second Barkeley class, was a BSA in the 4th Armored Division.Transports: Aabel, "History of the MAC," p. 50. The use of MAC officers as troop transport surgeons was limited to trips not exceeding 3,000 troop transport days (e.g., 300 troops for ten days).

[98] Stayer: Maj Gen Morrison C. Stayer, Surg, North African Theater of Operations, U.S. Army (later, Mediterranean Theater of Operations), to Maj Gen Norman T. Kirk, TSG, 3 Sep 44, MSC-USACMH.

[99] Quoted words: Kirk to Stayer, 11 Sep 44, MSC-USACMH; Extract from Pers Div, Office of Chief Surg, ETO, Annual Rpt, 1944, in file Research Notes WWII, box 3/18, MSC-USACMH.

[100] Quoted words: Keith Winston, *V–Mail; Letters of a World War II Combat Medic* (Chapel Hill, N.C.: Algonquin Books, 1985), p. 254.

[101] BSA school: Parks, *Medical Training*, pp. 123–24; Goodman, OCS Rpt, pp. 15–16; Potts, History of the MAC.

[102] 4th Infantry Division: Richardson, Ginn Interv.

[103] Quoted words: Klaus H. Huebner, *Long Walk Through War: A Combat Doctor's Diary* (College Station: Texas A&M Press, 1987), p. 118.

[104] Hertzell: George Sharpe, *Brothers Beyond Blood* (Austin, Tex.: Diamond Books, 1989), pp. 159–60, 196. For a private's view of an MAC lieutenant in a medical platoon of the 87th Division in the ETO see Lester Atwell, *Private* (New York: Simon and Schuster, 1958). Unfortunately,

Atwell's lieutenant folded under the pressure of the fighting through France and Belgium. "From the beginning he had neglected, or avoided, much of his actual work—that of locating the companies in an attack, establishing collecting points. . . . His face had grown small and haggard, and his eyes were rheumy with dark circles beneath them." Ibid., pp. 213–14.

[105] Kanaya: Col Jimmie Kanaya, MSC, Ret., Gig Harbor, Wash., to Ginn, 23 Aug 83 and 12 Oct 84, including copy of diaries at Oflag 64, Schubin, Poland, and Oflag XIII–D, Nuernberg, Germany, DASG-MS. On 26 October 1984, Kanaya and about three hundred of his fellow unit members were honored in France at the fortieth anniversary of the liberation of Bruguieres.

[106] Quoted words: Charles M. Wiltse, ed., *Medical Supply in World War II*, volume in the series Medical Department of the United States Army in World War II (Washington, D.C.: Office of the Surgeon General, Department of the Army, 1968), p. 562.

[107] Quoted words: Col Robert L. Black, MSC, Ret., to Col R. L. Parker, MSC, 20 Jun 60, box 19/18, MSC-USACMH.

[108] Logistics: Israeloff, Winning the War, pp. 70–71, 77; Rpt, Capt Charles G. Langham, Jr., MAC, sub: Activities of Medical Administrative Corps, Sanitary Corps and Pharmacy Corps Officers in the European Theater of Operations, THU, OTSG, 1965, folder 142, box 17/18, MSC-USACMH. 23d GH: 23d General Hospital, Historical Rpt, 1944, folder 154, box 10/18, MSC-USACMH. The 23d operated in Italy and France. ETO chief: Col. Robert A. Black, PhC, replaced Col. Silas B. Hays, MC, as ETO chief of medical supply on 1 October 1945. Britell: Col Claude C. Britell, MSC, account in Lt Col Andrew Colyer, MSC, draft chapter, sub: Medical Field Service, 1961, in 1958 MSC History Project, folder 243, box 15/18, MSC-USACMH.

[109] Kirk: Speech, Maj Gen Norman T. Kirk, MC, sub: Address to the Storage Operations Field Clinic, Denver, Colo., 24 Sep 43, MSC-USACMH.

[110] Logistics lessons: Col Silas B. Hays, MC, Lt Col Louis F. Williams, PhC, and Maj Robert L. Parker, MAC, to Dir, Planning Div, ASF, sub: Supplementary Material to be Included in ASF Manual M409, 18 Feb 46, DASG-MS; Wiltse, *Medical Supply in World War II*, pp. 29, 559–62.

[111] Quoted words: Williams, Ginn Interv, 15 Nov 84.

[112] Pallets: Rpt, Capt Richard E. Yates, MAC, sub: The Procurement and Distribution of Medical Supplies in the Zone of the Interior During World War II, OTSG, 31 May 46, folder 269, box 17/18, MSC-USACMH, hereafter cited as Yates, Medical Supplies, 1946. Quoted words: Alan Pappas, "Responsibilities of the Medical Supply Officer," *Medical Bulletin of the North Africa Theater of Operations* 2 (October 1944): 90, USACMH.

[113] Vacancies: Ltr, Shook to Robinson, 9 Dec 40, MSC-USACMH. Procurement: Memo, 1st Lt George A. A. Muller, SnC, Office Manager (Mgr), Procurement Div, for Col M. E. Griffin, Dir, Procurement Div, OTSG, Supply Service Notes, March–December 1943, MSC-USACMH.

[114] "Penicillum": Memo, Maj C. W. Torbet, SnC, Dep Dir, Procurement Div, for Maj Kibler in Supply Service, OTSG, sub: Supply Service Notes for the Surgeon General's Notebook, March–December 1943, DASG-MS, hereafter cited as OTSG, Supply Service Notes, plus date; Yates, Medical Supplies, 1946; Memos, Edward Reynolds, Actg Chief, Supply Service, for Under Secretary of War, 4 Nov 43, 2 Dec 43, DASG-MS; Each vial contained 100,000 units. In Italy the 23d General Hospital received its first two vials on 6 January 1944. 23d GH, Historical Rpt 1944, folder 154, box 10/18, MSC-USACMH. Secrecy: Early reports on penicillin were classified. After the war the U.S. Strategic Bombing Survey found that German scientists were surprised that the Allies had been able to keep from the scientific literature several details essential for production. Cortez F. Enloe, Jr., "Medical Supplies: Development, Production and Distribution," in U.S. Strategic Bombing Survey, *Effect of Bombing on Health and Medical Care in Germany* (Washington, D.C.: War Department, 1945), p. 338.

[115] Supply personnel: Memo, Col Reuel E. Hewitt, MC, for Col Albert G. Love, Historical Div, OTSG, 12 Jul 43, MSC-USACMH; and Wiltse, *Medical Supply in World War II*, pp. 9, 23, 559.

[116] Depot staff: St. Louis Medical Depot unit rosters, 1942–45, folder 115, box 8/18, MSC-USACMH. Duties: Col Joseph C. Thompson, MSC, XO, 34th GH, to Col R. L. Parker, 3 Apr 61, MSC-USACMH; Gibbs, Milner Interv, 24 Jun 64; Interv, Maj Gen Silas B. Hays, MC, USA, Ret., with Milner, 25 Oct 63, USACMH. Cooper: Thompson to Parker, 3 Apr 61, MSC-USACMH. MAC and SnC: Memo, Col Charles F. Shook, MC, for Col Paden, 10 Sep 42, MSC-USACMH. SnC officers: Memo, Shook for Maj Robinson, sub: Assistant Secretary of War's Weekly Report, 10

Sep 40, DASG-MS; OTSG, Memo, sub: Qualification for Appointment as First Lieutenant, Sanitary Corps, signed Lt Col John A. Rogers, MC, XO, 7 Jan 42, MSC-USACMH.

[117] Lend-Lease: Maj R. E. Wilson, MAC, Historical Rpt, Apr 46, and other documents in SGO Lend-Lease Historical Files, folders 22, 23, 24, box 4/18, MSC-USACMH.

[118] Kempf: Biographical data card, based on report of death, THU, OTSG, 27 May 47, USACMH. For a description of the conditions aboard ship and the attack see extracts from the war crimes trials in Paul Ashton, *Bataan Diary* (published privately, 1984), pp. 292–332.

[119] Quoted words: Rpt, Maj Walter S. Jones, MC, liaison officer, 10th (Chinese) Engineer Regiment, sub: Chinese Liaison Detail (May to December 1943), 1 Aug 45, folder 273, box 17/18, MSC-USACMH. DeBroeck and Farley were assigned to the 69th Medical Supply Platoon.

[120] Supply training: Parks, *Medical Training in World War II*, pp. 48–49; Wiltse, *Medical Supply in World War II*, pp. 6–7, 23, 43–44. Maintenance: Rpt, OTSG, sub: History of Maintenance of Medical Department Equipment, n.d., in Medical Supply Files, MSC-USACMH.

[121] Quoted words: Gibbs, Milner Interv, 1 Nov 63.

[122] Voorhees: Voorhees, "A Lawyer Among Army Doctors," p. 201.

[123] Quoted words: Ibid., p. 18.

[124] Magee's action: Armfield, *Organization and Administration in World War II*, pp. 161–62. Reynolds: Lt. Gen. Leonard D. Heaton, TSG, Statement before the Committee on Armed Services, House of Representatives, 20 July 1966, DASG-MS; Biographical data card, USACMH.

[125] Quoted words: Voorhees, "A Lawyer Among Army Doctors," p. 20.

[126] Reynolds' appointment: Reynolds replaced Col. Francis C. Tyng, MC. Wiltse, *Medical Supply in World War II*, p. 19; see also Memos for the Undersecretary of War, 1 Jun 43 from Tyng, Chief, Supply Service, and 8 Jun 43 from Edward Reynolds, Actg Chief, Supply Service, MSC-USACMH.

[127] Reynolds' promotion: Voorhees, "A Lawyer Among Army Doctors," pp. 86–87. He was not, as McMinn and Levin called him, "Chief, Medical Administrative Corps." McMinn and Levin, *Personnel in World War II*, p. 78. Reynolds left active duty 8 January 1946 and became administrative vice president of Harvard University.

[128] Normandy invasion: Voorhees, "A Lawyer Among Army Doctors," pp. 101–10; Wiltse, *Medical Supply in World War II*, pp. 280–83; THU, Medical Service in the European Theater.

[129] Quoted words: Interv, Maj Gen Paul R. Hawley, MC, Ret., with Col John B. Coates, Jr., MC, Charles M. Wiltse, Ph.D., and Hubert E. Potter, THU, OTSG, 16 and 18 Jun 62, USACMH.

[130] Glitches: Williams, Ginn Interv; THU, Medical Service in the European Theater.

[131] Quoted words: Voorhees, "A Lawyer Among Army Doctors," p. 101.

[132] Repacking: Walker repacked ten 400-bed and one 750-bed evacuation hospitals plus four field hospitals. THU, OTSG, draft chapter, sub: Medical Preparations for the Invasion of the Continent, n.d., in draft history, sub: Medical Support for the European Theater of Operations, 15 January–6 June 1944, folder 267, box 17/18, MSC-USACMH.

[133] Quoted words: ETO, General Board, no. 93.

[134] CBI: Voorhees, JAGD, Dir, Control Div, SGO, sub: Visit to China-Burma-India Theater to Survey Medical Supply, 11 Sep 44, DASG-MS; Voorhees, "A Lawyer Among Army Doctors," pp. 116–21; Wiltse, *Medical Supply in World War II*, pp. 522–24.

[135] CBI: Stone, *Crisis Fleeting*, p. 176. Stone was highly critical of the SOS surgeon, Col. John M. Tamraz, MC.

[136] Quoted words: Voorhees, "A Lawyer Among Army Doctors," pp. 119–20; Williams, Ginn Interv, 15 Nov 84.

[137] Quoted words: Voorhees, "A Lawyer Among Army Doctors," p. 121.

[138] Pacific: Rpt, Voorhees, sub: Story of Pacific Trip, October thru December 1944, n.d., DASG-MS; Voorhees, "A Lawyer Among Army Doctors," pp. 152–200; Wiltse, *Medical Supply in World War II*, pp. 478–80.

[139] Quoted words: Voorhees, Story of Pacific Trip.

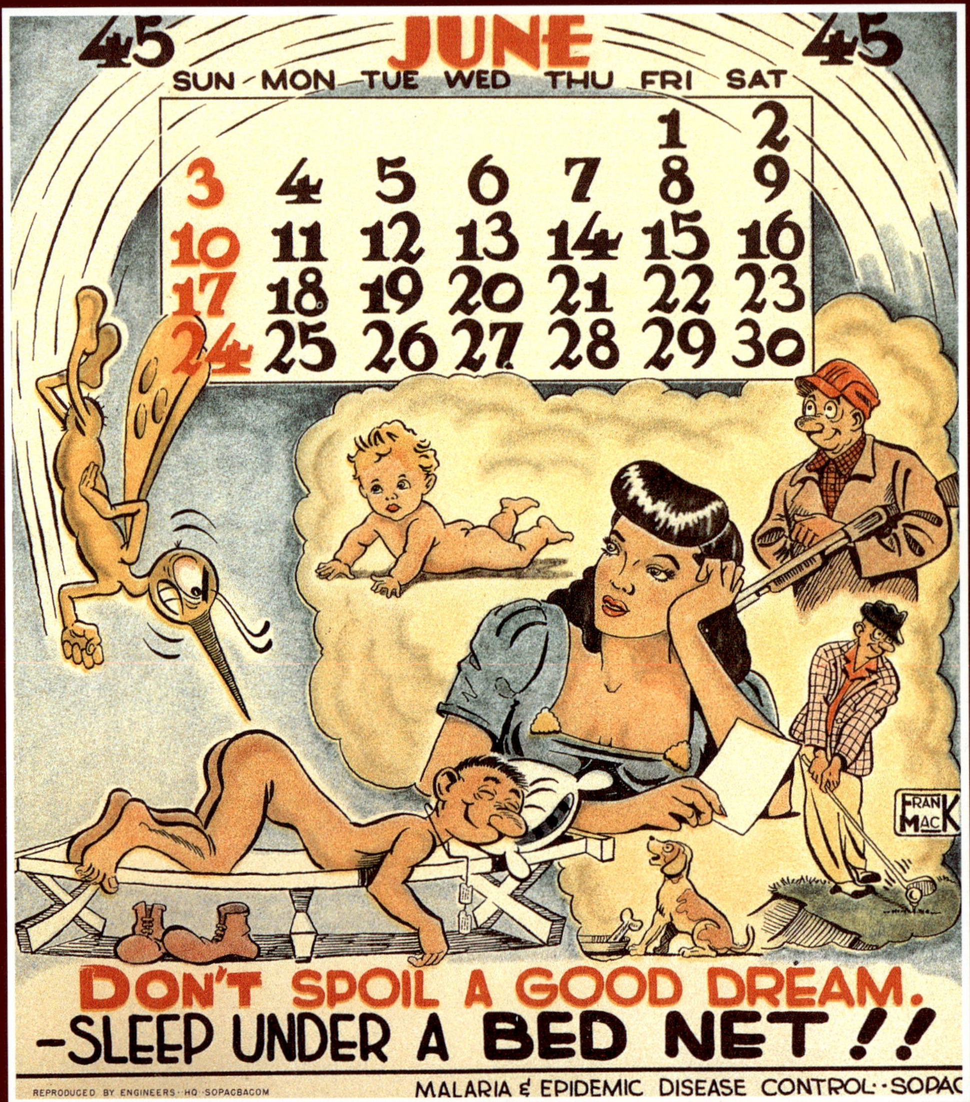

June 1945 calendar promoting malaria and epidemic disease control

6

World War II
The Scientific Specialties

The nearly twenty-six hundred scientific specialty officers who served in the Medical Department during World War II played essential roles in the Army's wartime preventive medicine and treatment activities. Their use demonstrated several major trends: the modernization of the military medical team, the beginning of a standing medical research and development program, the increasing role of preventive medicine, and the growing influence of professional guilds.

Early mobilization efforts had increased the number of Sanitary Corps officers on active duty from 8 in June 1940 to 227 when Japan attacked Pearl Harbor. The need for those officers was so acute that by July 1943 the Army listed seven groups—sanitary engineer, bacteriologist, biochemist, serologist, parasitologist, nutritionist, and medical photographer—in the category of "scarce" specialties. That made civilians with the proper skills eligible for direct commissioning as Sanitary Corps first lieutenants without the requirement for completing OCS.[1] Appointment required a baccalaureate degree and four years' experience. Recruitment took a variety of forms, including articles in professional journals and solicitation of universities, industrial organizations, and professional societies. The effort worked, and by December 1943 there were 2,365 Sanitary Corps officers on active duty. The corps peaked in April 1945 with 2,560 officers. A new entity, the Pharmacy Corps, was established in 1943 as a Regular Army component. By April 1945 it reached its top strength of seventy officers, about a third of whom were pharmacists.[2]

Brig. Gen. James S. Simmons, MC, the surgeon general's World War II preventive medicine chief, said that the importance of having scientific specialty officers was one of the three major lessons of the war and that the Sanitary Corps had made possible the Medical Department's success in preventive medicine. The increased sophistication of medical technology, the demands of meeting medical support requirements worldwide, and the health care requirements of occupied areas greatly expanded the use of these officers. They did not necessarily substitute for medical officers, since they often represented specialties not otherwise present in the department. For example, medical training did not prepare physicians for duties as sanitary engineers, entomologists, or nutritionists.[3]

War Department policy restricted appointments to applicants over the age of thirty because the government wished to preserve officer candidate school as the preferred route for commissioning draft-age applicants. The Surgeon General's Office desired relief from the minimum age requirement because it limited the pool the Medical Department could draw from in the scientific specialties. That made it difficult to comply with the War Department's policy that directed the maximum substitution of nonmedical for Medical Corps officers in positions not requiring medical training. The Medical Department wanted the latitude to appoint younger, draft-age applicants who possessed the necessary educational background and to compensate for their lack of experience with additional Army training. The War Department accepted the Surgeon General's Office's argument, and the rules were modified in 1943 to allow the commissioning of scientific specialty applicants with two years' experience as second lieutenants.[4]

A Modernized Medical Team

Officers who were experts in emerging technologies enabled an expansion and modernization of the Medical Department team that would otherwise have been impossible. The influence of psychologists, sanitary engineers, entomologists, nutritionists, laboratory officers, social workers, chiropodists, and optometrists illustrated that progress, and the accounts of those specialties reveal different facets of the modernization. Intertwined in those accounts is the desire of each group for professional recognition, especially for the last three, who did not achieve commissioned officer status during the war. Overall, there was an effort to mold the disparate specialties into a unified team operating within the fundamental evacuation and treatment doctrine. The totality of the team that evolved was greater than the sum of its parts.[5]

Psychology

Demand for psychologists accelerated in World War II as a spiraling psychiatric workload overwhelmed psychiatrists and dictated the acceptance of clinical psychologists into the mental health team for diagnostic testing and therapy—a change from the use of psychologists strictly for personnel management where their testing expertise was utilized in screening recruits and in assessing applicants for various specialties and schools. Part of the workload was caused by psychiatric casualties from combat exhaustion (a condition referred to as "shell shock" and war neurosis in World War I), which inundated the medical treatment capacity in some areas. Psychiatric admissions far exceeded all other nonsurgical admissions in some Army divisions.[6]

Initially, all psychologists were commissioned in the Adjutant General's Department where their testing expertise was employed in the classification of recruits. As such they had no prospect of clinical duties, but the Medical Department soon found that they were needed in the hospital setting as members of the emerging mental health team. In 1942 Lt. Col. Patrick S. Madigan, MC, chief of the Surgeon General's Neuropsychiatric Division, arranged for commissioning six clinical psychologists as Sanitary Corps first lieutenants and assigning them to general hospitals in the Zone of the Interior, where they were well received. Commissioning in the Sanitary Corps halted when the surgeon general agreed that all psychologists would be commissioned in the Adjutant General's Department and the adjutant general agreed to assign clinical psychologists to all hospitals of 1,000 or more beds. That arrangement held during most of the war.[7]

Consequently, Army psychologists in World War II performed both personnel management and clinical functions, with the Adjutant General Corps absorbing the former and the Medical Department the latter. The adjutant general appointed Lt. Col. Morton A. Seidenfeld, AG, as the chief clinical psychologist to coordinate their joint use. This required frequent coordination between the Adjutant General's and Surgeon General's Offices.

The opening of clinical opportunities integrated clinical psychologists into the mental health team in the largest program of its kind anywhere. It was strongly supported by successive chiefs of the Surgeon General's Neuropsychiatric Division, and especially by Brig. Gen. William C. Menninger, MC, of Menninger Clinic fame. In 1945 Menninger succeeded in transferring total responsibility for clinical psychology to the Medical Department, and 340 psychologists were transferred to the Medical Administrative Corps. In addition, five women were commissioned in 1945 as clinical psychologists in the Adjutant General for duty with the Medical Department, one of the earlier programs of opportunity for women in the military.[8]

Clinical psychologists were usually assigned to general and convalescent hospitals, rehabilitation centers, and disciplinary barracks. They administered tests previously unavailable in Army hospitals, such as Weschler-Bellevue and Babcock-Levy. They performed other diagnostic studies, maintained liaison with Red Cross social workers for social histories of patients, and assisted psychiatrists in certain electroencephalographic studies. The Medical Department found that the use of uniformed, rather than civilian, psychologists enhanced their effectiveness because they were "compelled to live in day-to-day contact with military folk and military problems."[9] In this way they worked on problems that were directly related to the needs of the military.

A survey of fifty clinical psychologists revealed that their principal activity was the administration and interpretation of a battery of tests selected especially for each patient. Psychiatrists used the results of that testing in a way analogous to the use of x-ray pictures by surgeons. The testing, used as it was for clinical diagnosis and treatment, went beyond that performed by psychologists to serve personnel classification needs in the Adjutant General Department. For example, IQ (intelligence quotient) tests conducted by Sanitary Corps officers were supplemented by personality tests such as the Army Weschler and Weschler-Bellevue and used for differential diagnosis. Sanitary Corps psychologists reported that individual therapy performed under the direct supervision of a psychiatrist was their second most common function. Their third principal area of responsibility was the administration and supervision of the clinical psychology staff.[10]

Some psychologists participated in the Aviation Psychology Program, an effort more closely related to the functions of the Adjutant General's Office than to those of the Surgeon General's Office. It carried on the work begun in World War I of selecting and classifying candidates for aircrew training. Sanitary Corps psychologists developed the Army Air Forces Qualifying Examination, which was used to screen one million applicants. Over six hundred thousand aviators took another test, the Aircrew Classification Battery, which was used to predict success in pilot, bombardier, and navigator training.[11]

Social Work

While the use of social workers was expanded in the Army during World War II, they did not achieve commissioned status during the war. They performed in their specialty either as Red Cross civilians or as nonmedical enlisted soldiers. Although some social workers served as officers in the Army, they worked in other branches and not in their professional specialty.

Social workers focused their attention on the human side of medical care, serving as the bridge between the perplexing complexity of hospitals and the reality of patient lives which if not attended to could interfere with or negate the efforts of health care providers. "It is the area of social functioning, coping, and adapting that social workers address as they relate to the needs of the whole patient."[12] In 1905 Richard C. Cabot, M.D., head of outpatient services for Boston's Massachusetts General Hospital, established a medical social service that set a trend in American medicine. Cabot portrayed the situation he was attempting to rectify in everyday terms. "Without any sense of the humor of the situation, we say (in substance) to many patients: 'take a vacation,' or 'get a job,' 'get a set of teeth' or 'get a truss.' There is none in sight and no means of getting any. What do we do? We pass cheerfully to the next patient."[13] Social work services for Army hospitals were first provided by American Red Cross social workers in a program begun in late 1918 and continued during the interwar years at seventeen Army and Navy hospitals. The Red Cross and enlisted social workers during World War II supported mental health units, convalescent and rehabilitation centers, disciplinary barracks, and general hospitals in the United States. At the end of the war there were 711 social workers stateside and 25 overseas.[14]

The importance of social work was increasingly apparent during the war. This was especially the case as General Menninger developed the mental hygiene consultative service, an interdisciplinary mental health team of psychiatrists, psychologists, and social workers, the first of which opened at Fort Monmouth, New Jersey, on 4 March 1942. Menninger lobbied for establishment of a social work branch as part of the Neuropsychiatric Division, and he saw that come to fruition in July 1945, when Lt. Col. David E. O'Keefe, AG, became the first chief.[15]

Sanitary Engineers

Sanitary engineers again played an important part in the Medical Department's preventive medicine effort, their numbers increasing from sixty-five in 1941 to nearly one thousand by the end of the war. They were assigned to headquarters staffs, to research and development roles, as post medical inspectors, and to positions controlling the environmental factors of water, sewage, and garbage. One hundred officers commanded malaria control units stateside and overseas.[16]

Col. William A. Hardenbergh, SnC, who had remained active in the Sanitary Corps Reserve during the interwar period, served as chief of the Sanitary Engineering Division. His assistant was Capt. Joseph J. Gilbert, SnC, who also served as chief of the Waste Disposal Branch. Capt. James B. Baty, SnC, was chief

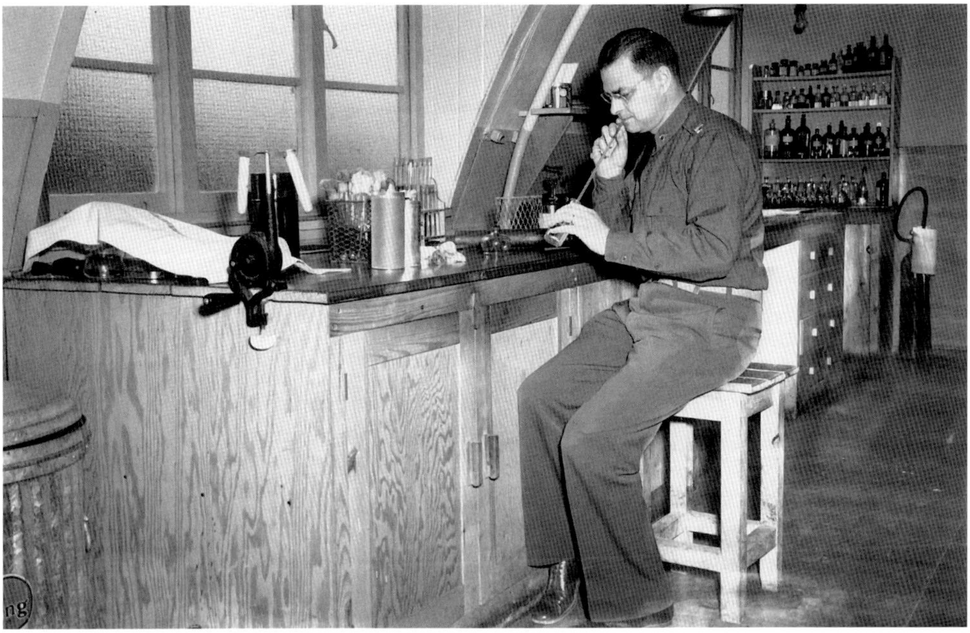

Sanitary Corps officer at a base hospital in Iceland tests water specimens from camps nearby.

of the Water Supply Branch, and Capt. David F. Smallhorst, SnC, headed the Insect and Rodent Control Branch. While he was credited by some accounts as serving as chief of the Sanitary Corps, as Colonel Wrightson had in World War I, Hardenbergh's attention was principally directed toward sanitary engineers and entomologists. Other scientific specialties were handled elsewhere in the Surgeon General's Office. All the same, his decisions influenced the direction of the corps. One of his first actions was to release about half of the reserve officers "because they had no training in what we considered to be recognized by our program. This may seem unimportant now, but it was one of the essential steps toward getting the Sanitary Corps truly professional, and so recognized." Brig. Gen. Stanhope Bayne-Jones, MC, deputy chief of the Surgeon General's Preventive Medicine Service, credited Colonel Hardenbergh and other Sanitary Corps officers with important contributions to typhus control.[17]

Another senior sanitary engineer was Col. Michael J. Blew, SnC. Blew had been a Sanitary Corps lieutenant with the 82d Division during World War I, had served in the Sanitary Corps Reserve during the interwar years, and was part of a group that performed its annual training at Carlisle each summer. An engineer with the City of Philadelphia, Blew reentered active duty in 1941. He found the greatest change over the years had occurred in the development of a sense of teamwork among physicians and scientific specialists. Army physicians in World War I had not understood the capabilities of Sanitary Corps officers.[18]

Sanitary needs varied greatly from one theater of war to another. Waste disposal posed difficult problems for sanitary engineers in England who supported the troop buildup prior to the Normandy invasion. Terrain and population density prevented use of routine disposal methods. American units employed "honey bucket" latrines, but emptying the buckets was a most unpleasant chore and "not a task undertaken voluntarily by American soldiers." Later, on the Continent, they found that the French, like the British, had no sewage system in the provinces, but instead used cesspits whose contents were pumped into trucks for disposal. The GIs ranked the French system above the British, at least from an aesthetic point of view.[19]

Sanitary engineers were important figures in carrying out the department's public health responsibilities in occupied areas. In the Philippines, Maj. Lloyd K. Clark, SnC, worked closely with Corps of Engineers units and local civilian officials to reestablish the Manila public water supply. He entered northern Manila on 9 February 1945 with advance elements of Sixth Army engineer units and found the city without water in its distribution system. Restoration of water supplies required repair of the damage from combat action and sabotage by the retreating Japanese forces. It was a difficult undertaking, sometimes done in the face of enemy action.[20]

Capts. Lawrence S. Farrell, SnC, and Paul J. Houser, SnC, served as sanitary engineers on the Strategic Bombing Survey of Germany in 1944, a study commissioned by President Roosevelt. Farrell and Houser found that bombing hampered the essential services of water supply and sewage and garbage disposal but did not materially alter public health conditions. Certainly the damage was impressive. Water mains and sewer pipes twenty feet below the surface were ripped open by bombing attacks. Air raids on Munich in July and August 1944 caused severe damage to that city's water distribution system, severing all five main lines feeding the city and breaking the lines themselves in about 850 places. In some cities subjected to fire raids—for example, Stuttgart in 1944—raw sewage was pumped on the fires because of water shortages. Yet the destruction did not cause an increase in communicable disease to the extent anticipated by the team. Farrell and Houser credited that paradoxical result to an excellent public health system, but they also believed that Germany could not have maintained essential services for long if the war had continued.[21]

Captain Houser also coauthored the environmental sanitation section in the report of the Strategic Bombing Survey of Japan, a study ordered in 1945 by President Harry S. Truman. As in Germany, the study found disruption of basic services without the degree of increase in communicable disease anticipated by the team, but the similar result could not be explained with the same reasons as in the case of Germany. Two factors worked in favor of Japan. Unlike the demolition bombing of Germany, Japan was principally fire-bombed, which may have temporarily sterilized the bombed areas. Second, the common practice of using night soil as a valued fertilizer, while contributing to enteric diseases, rendered waste water in Japan less polluted than in Europe. On the other hand, the authors did not find evidence of an individual understanding of personal hygiene in Japan nor attempts by the government to instruct the population in its principles. Those factors complicate understanding of their finding of an absence of a serious epidemic disease problem.[22]

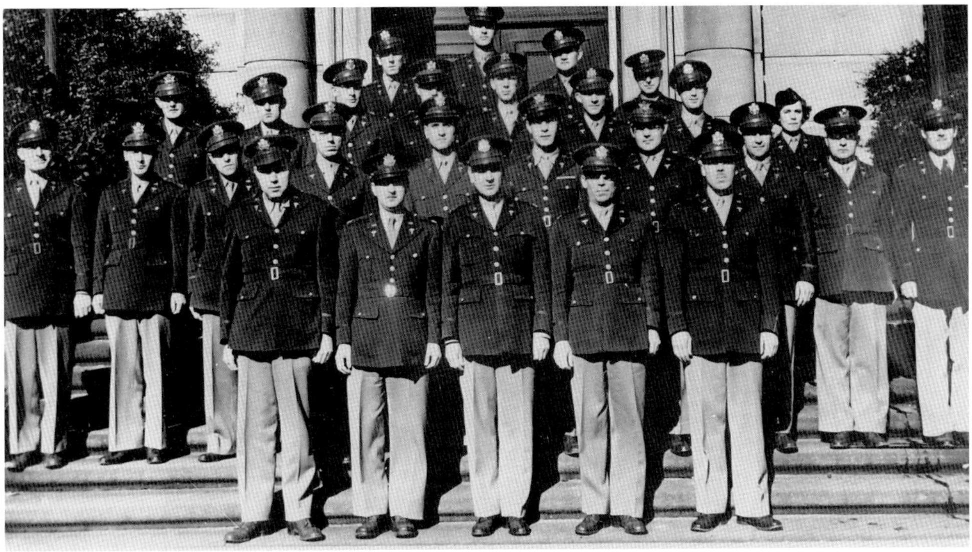

Army Industrial Hygiene Laboratory personnel, Johns Hopkins School of Public Health, 1944

Some sanitary engineers contributed to the use of industrial hygiene, especially in the design of military equipment, in order to enhance the ability of soldiers to operate in hostile environments.[23] Lt. Col. Theodore F. Hatch, SnC, a sanitary engineer, was assigned to the Armored Force Medical Research Laboratory at Fort Knox, Kentucky, from 1942 to 1945. There, he participated in tests of the M4 tank that revealed that when the tank was "buttoned up" there was no air exchange for the crew. The project manager disapproved a recommendation to install ventilation fans because "the tank already had too many gadgets." Hatch broke this impasse by arranging for two general officers to take part in test-firing ten 75-mm. shells; one general acted as the gunner, the other was the loader, and Hatch was the tank commander. "When the ammonia reached about 400 ppm after firing four rounds, the generals were weeping copiously and ready to quit." The fans were installed.[24]

Entomology

One of the few insects to play a leading role in literature was Archy the cockroach in Don Marquis' delightful tale of life among the unwashed, *Archy and Mehitabel.* When Archy declared war on mankind, he declared he would "fling a billion times a billion risen insects in an army at the throats of all you humans."[25] The first line in the Army's defense against Archy's hordes was the Sanitary Corps entomologist. There were 239 entomologists serving as Sanitary Corps officers in February 1945, up from 13 in the Sanitary Corps Reserve at the end of 1940. They were essential members of the preventive medicine team that fought diseases transmitted by insect vectors, often with notable success, such as in the Far East where the reduction in the malaria attack rate was termed an "achievement of historic importance." One of the entomologists was John N. Belkin, Ph.D.,

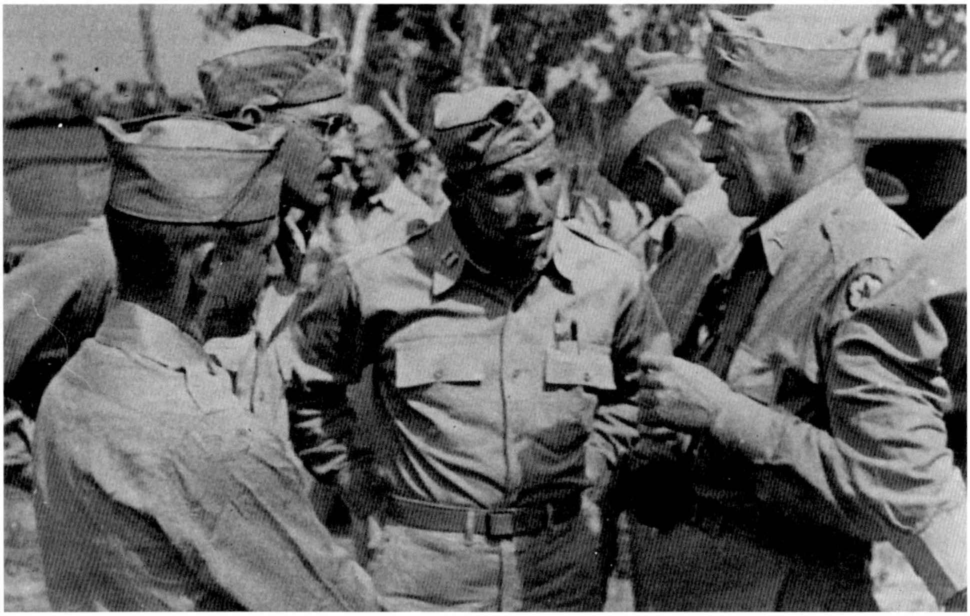

*Captain Pletsch (*center*) in New Caledonia, 1945*

who as a Sanitary Corps captain commanded a malaria survey unit in Guadalcanal and the Philippines. Belkin became a prominent figure in mosquito taxonomy after the war, and he named a number of new species after soldiers who had served in his unit.[26]

Donald J. Pletsch, Ph.D., a professor of entomology at Montana State College, was commissioned in 1942 as a first lieutenant in the Sanitary Corps. In 1944 he took command of the 218th Malaria Survey Detachment, which was initially employed in malaria control efforts in Texas, Louisiana, and Florida. In January 1945 the 218th moved to the Philippines where it was attached to the 81st Infantry Division for mopping-up actions in Leyte and New Caledonia. When Japan fell, the detachment drew winter clothing and went from the Philippines by landing ship, tank (LST), to Hokkaido, Japan. Landing in snow, they undertook operations to control an outbreak of louse-borne typhus among Chinese and Korean laborers who had been used by the Japanese as coal miners. The Americans formed a close association with the Zoology Department of the Hokkaido Imperial University, and their colleagues hosted a Thanksgiving dinner to honor the American medical soldiers. The Japanese went to great lengths to make the dinner a special event, a task made quite difficult by food rationing.[27]

Entomologists were indispensable in combating arthropod-borne disease, especially typhus and relapsing fever (lice), plague (fleas), and yellow fever and malaria (mosquitoes). DDT (dichloro-diphenyl-trichloroethane) was a spectacular addition to their armamentarium, although it was only one factor of many. It became available for mosquito control in the summer of 1944, but by that point the malaria rates had already decreased as the result of actions by malaria control and survey units. DDT in powder form was highly valued for delousing operations in the battle with typhus, especially in refugee populations.[28] Entomologists in the Southwest Pacific Area established a rodent-control training program in the Philippines as part of the typhus control program there. In yet another function, they served in the U.S. occupation of Germany. Maj. John W. Bailey, SnC, a staff officer of the U.S. Military Government for Germany, surveyed the insect collections in forty-eight museums in eleven countries. He found that there had been universal effort to preserve the collections, and thirty-six collections were unharmed. Six had been totally destroyed. He arranged for the return of valuable entomological collections that had been removed from Holland to Germany.[29]

Nutrition

Col. Paul E. Howe, SnC, headed the Food and Nutrition Subdivision of the Surgeon General's Office. Howe was a charter member of the American Institute of Nutrition and a leading biochemist and nutritionist who had been instrumental in popularizing iodization of table salt and enrichment of flour in the United States. He had served as a nutrition officer during World War I and remained in the Sanitary Corps Reserve during the interwar period. He was on the staff of Princeton University when recalled to active duty for World War II.[30]

Nutrition officers advised commanders on the adequacy of food supply for soldiers. Howe directed a series of 455 food consumption surveys at fifty camps and posts that demonstrated that soldiers at Army training camps had a nutritionally adequate diet—one that averaged 3,700 calories per day, plus another 350 to 400 calories at the post canteens. At the peak, there were 185 Sanitary Corps nutrition officers. They were closely monitored by the Surgeon General's Office to ensure they were not sidetracked into duties outside their specialty.[31]

The need for expertise in the medical aspects of food and nutrition as they affected soldier performance (as opposed to the Quartermaster General's concern with food technology and supply) led to the formation of the Army Medical Nutrition Laboratory at the Army Medical School, Washington, D.C., in 1942. Sanitary Corps officers were part of that effort from the beginning, and in 1944, when the school moved to Chicago, Illinois, it was commanded by Maj. George H. Berryman, SnC.[32]

Sanitary Corps nutrition officers were a necessary asset in civil affairs operations. In the occupation of Germany, the Army estimated in 1945 that 60 percent of the German population was existing on a diet that could result in disease or malnutrition. In May a team of nutrition officers was assigned to the Belsen Concentration Camp near Hanover, Germany, to evaluate the nutritional status of the survivors and to assist in relief efforts. They found 60,000 men, women, and children in extremely serious condition, so poor that even after two weeks of effort by the team inmates were still dying at the rate of 300 per day from starvation or tuberculosis, pneumonia, and other infectious diseases. Other teams visited American-guarded prisoner of war camps. Surveys of fifteen camps in May 1945 established that the caloric intake of the German prisoners was only slightly below that of American soldiers in the field. Later surveys showed much malnutrition.[33]

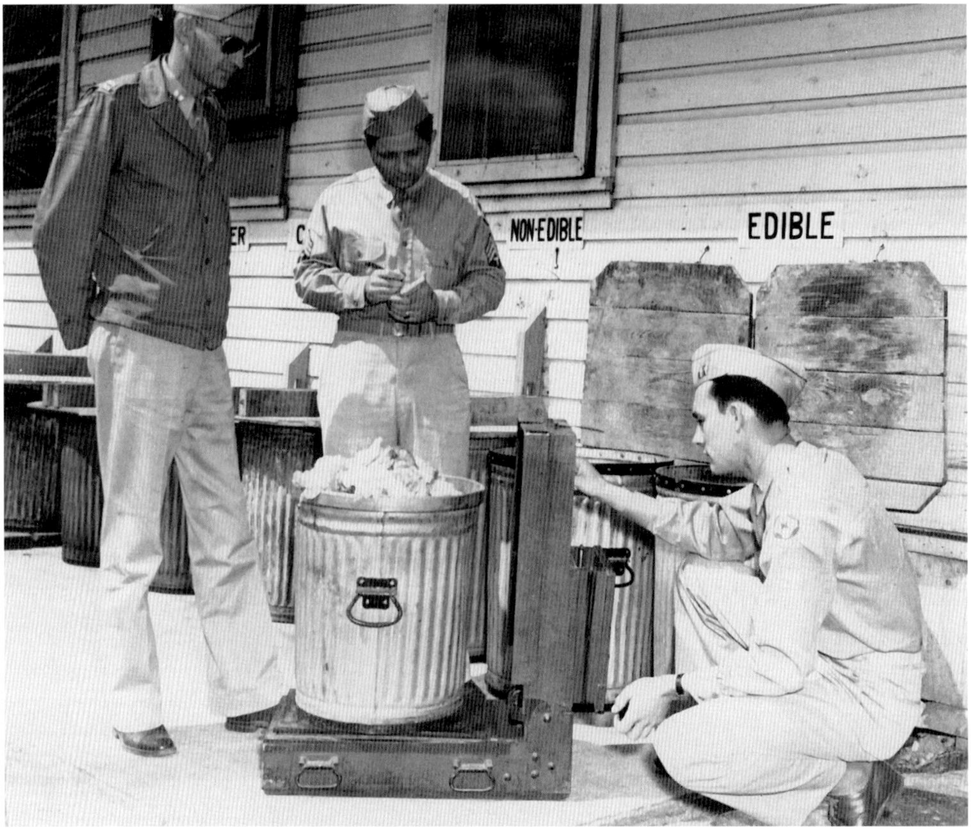

*Nutrition officer (*right*) weighs plate waste during a mess survey at Camp Shelby, Mississippi, 1942.*

While on an inspection trip, Colonel Howe observed swelling in the necks of soldiers engaged in arctic and desert training, a sign of goiters caused by iodine deficiency. Howe was able to persuade the Quartermaster Corps to enforce the use of iodized salt. He also found that the American soldiers' ingenuity had conquered a thoroughly despised antiscorbutic artificial lemonade.[34] Howe reported to the National Research Council that the GIs had twenty-one uses for the lemonade powder, ranging from tooth cleansing to scouring field ovens.

Laboratory Officers

By August 1944 there were 1,030 Sanitary Corps laboratory officers, a number consisting of 895 bacteriologists and biochemists, 101 parasitologists, 24 serologists, 9 medical photographers, and 1 neuroanatomist. Maj. Arthur Stull, SnC, served as the wartime chief of the Laboratories Division of the Surgeon General's Office and, as such, as the spokesman for the specialty. Stull had been the first Sanitary Corps officer assigned to that office. Newly commissioned officers were usually former noncommissioned officers who possessed baccalaureate

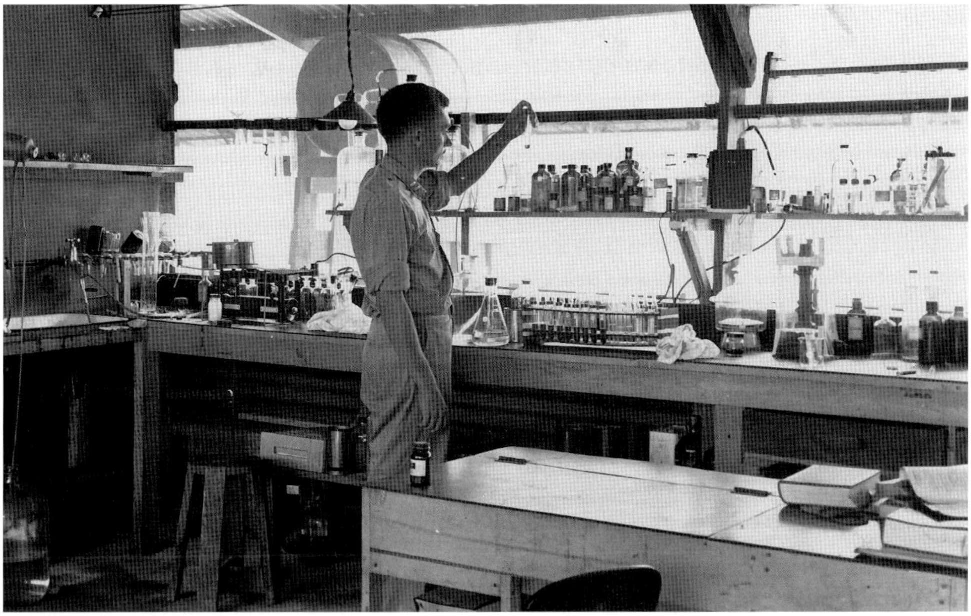

Sanitary Corps officer in the chemical section of the 9th General Hospital laboratory, Biak Island, New Guinea, 1944

and sometimes master's or doctoral degrees coupled with one to two years' experience in laboratory procedures. Nearly 50 percent of the laboratory officers had advanced degrees, and 29 percent had doctorates. Although their functions proliferated, they were not permitted to serve as chiefs of laboratories. The department continued to restrict those assignments to physicians "because of the broad field of training required." Maj. Roy D. Maxwell, SnC, broke new ground in 1945 as the first scientific specialty officer to attend the Command and General Staff College at Fort Leavenworth, Kansas.[35]

Experience in World War II demonstrated that such specialist officers were essential for the operation of a good hospital laboratory—one of the significant advances that came out of the war. The department needed as many laboratory officers as it could obtain, but by the end of 1944 found that the manpower pool had dried up. In June 1944 the Surgeon General's Office estimated that 250 officers were needed but only 100 men were qualified.[36]

The department considered commissioning women, since some enlisted members of the Women's Army Corps were qualified by training and experience as biochemists, serologists, parasitologists, and bacteriologists. The Judge Advocate General ruled that no women could be commissioned in the Sanitary Corps, but that they could be enlisted or commissioned in the WAC and detailed for duty with the Sanitary Corps. Therefore, qualified applicants were commissioned in the Women's Army Corps upon completion of WAC basic training and were assigned to the Medical Department after a one-month course for laboratory officers. They were detailed to the Sanitary Corps and wore the insignia of their new corps after

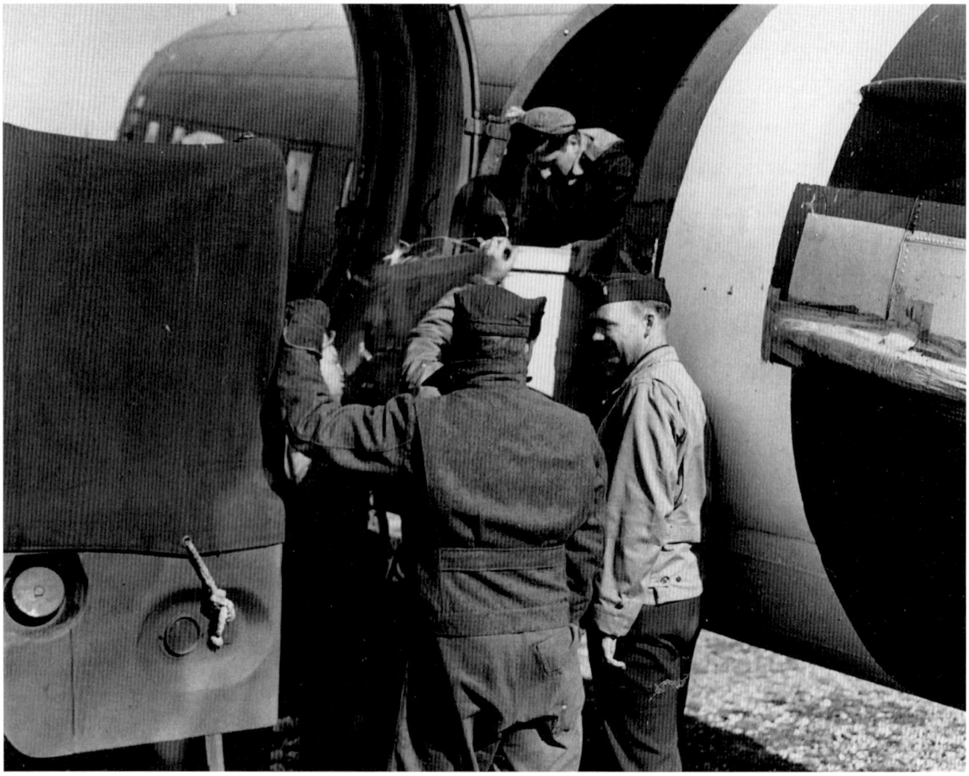

*Lieutenant Pryor (*right*) oversees the loading of medical supplies onto a C–47 at Greenham Common, England, June 1944.*

a six-month probationary period. Col. Oveta Culp Hobby, director of the Women's Army Corps, agreed to the arrangement because those officers, by being detailed to the Medical Department, would not reduce her quota of officer candidates. The first group of twenty-four WAC enlisted soldiers was commissioned in the fall of 1944, detailed to the Sanitary Corps, and attended a special orientation course at Billings General Hospital, Fort Benjamin Harrison, Indiana. By March 1945 thirty-one women were serving as Sanitary Corps officers.[37]

Some laboratory officers had participated in the Sanitary Corps Reserve during the interwar period. One was Maj. Reuben L. Kahn, SnC, who published *Serology in Syphilis Control* in 1942, a book based on lectures he had delivered at the Army and Navy Medical Schools in Washington. Kahn, a professor of bacteriology and serology at the University of Michigan Medical School, had developed the Kahn test, a Wassermann-type serological test for syphilis, in 1934.[38]

Sanitary Corps laboratory officers were members of blood collecting and distribution detachments that collected over thirteen million pints of blood during the war. One of those officers, Capt. Ralph H. Maurer, SnC, a laboratory officer at the 300th General Hospital in Italy, demonstrated that blood could be safely stored up to seven days and that the incidence of reaction from stored blood was not greater than fresh blood if it was handled by a competent blood bank team. Maurer's team prepared 7,150 transfusions of stored blood in one year without a fatality. Medical Administrative Corps officers joined their Sanitary Corps colleagues in transporting blood. In 1944, 2d Lt. Robert E. Pryor, MAC, as head of the medical section of the Army depot at Greenham Common, England, arranged for the use of an air transport squadron to move blood and medical supplies forward and to evacuate casualties to the rear. In a three-month period the squadron moved 30,000 pints of blood.[39]

Chiropody

The Medical Department's wartime experience also demonstrated a requirement for chiropody. Basic training in World War II was a seventeen-week course, over twice as long as that of World War I, and marching was intentionally performed over difficult terrain. The orthopedic consultant for the Zone of the Interior believed that the long treks contributed to a higher incidence of foot disability, and the demand for foot care was very high in some units. Seventy percent of the orthopedic clinic visits in the Fourth Service Command, a training organization that covered the southeastern United States, were for foot problems. The regional hospital at Camp Swift, Texas, reported that 30 percent of its orthopedic clinic visits in 1944 were for foot problems. A study of the 29th Infantry Division in Europe, most of whose troops had been in the Army for about two years, revealed that 12 percent of the division went on sick call for foot pain and disability during a two-week training period in the fall of 1942. Navy experience was similar. One report revealed that 17.6 percent of all dispensary visits were for foot problems. Another indicated that women had a much higher rate of minor foot pathology; this was the cause of over 52 percent of dispensary visits by Navy female sailors in another study.[40]

There was no provision for commissioning chiropodists, but the Medical Department hired civilian practitioners with a Doctor of Surgical Chiropody (D.S.C.) from programs approved by the National Association of Chiropodists. In other cases, chiropodists who had been drafted were assigned to the Medical Department as enlisted soldiers and used in their specialty. The civilian and enlisted chiropodists performed within a tightly defined range of functions under the supervision of orthopedic surgeons. Their practice was limited to diagnosis and treatment of minor foot ailments, minor surgery, and prescribing correct footgear. Surgery was limited to the removal of corns, calluses, and plantar warts. Yet that limited scope of practice enabled them to assume a large workload.[41]

Optometry

Optometrists were not commissioned either, but the Medical Department allowed the use of enlisted optometrists to perform refractions. There was movement toward more comprehensive eye care for soldiers with the restoration of a spectacle issue program. That was prompted by the surgeon of the IV Corps Area at Fort McClellan, Alabama, who recommended that the Army provide soldiers free replacement spectacles. While claims of broken glasses while performing official duties were not always totally convincing, it was certainly clear that training ceased once a soldier was unable to see.[42]

The surgeon general took the proposal forward to the War Department, which agreed in 1941 to provide spectacles to active duty soldiers. The surgeon general's staff attempted to determine an estimated requirement but, unable to obtain "the barest hint" of actual usage records for World War I, estimated that 10 percent of military personnel would have defective vision, a number they "pulled out of the air." They also assumed that one-half of those soldiers would enter active duty owning their own glasses. Based on those assumptions, the Surgeon General's Office projected a requirement for 200,000 pairs of spectacles in 1942.[43]

Unfortunately, they had not allowed for replacements of lost or broken spectacles. Neither had they anticipated that most of those who came in the Army with their own spectacles had glasses that could not withstand the rigors of military life. Indeed, the department discovered that 18 to 20 percent—not 10 percent—of soldiers required corrective lenses. The Medical Department issued well over two million pairs of spectacles in 1943, ten times the original estimate, and the initial lack of an optical program was described as "shortsightedness."[44]

In addition to support for soldiers, the Army found a need for optometric support for civilian populations in the areas it occupied. For example, local optical services ceased to function in Germany when that country capitulated. A small forerunner of the Marshall Plan was the Army's establishment of a bifocal manufacturing capability in Bavaria using ex-POW optometrists.[45]

There was a requirement for fabrication and distribution of spectacles both in the Zone of the Interior and within the theaters of operation. The necessity for that was underscored by the ophthalmology consultant for the European Theater of Operations, who believed it would have been necessary to evacuate 10,000 soldiers out of the theater monthly if there had been no fabrication capability during the invasion of Europe. Capt. Alfred T. Wells, SnC, was awarded the Legion of Merit for designing and developing a mobile, self-sustained optical unit, and a prototype built by the Medical Field Service School at Carlisle Barracks, Pennsylvania, was approved by the Surgeon General's Optical Advisory Board in November 1943. The field optical unit stocked semifinished lenses in the sizes, shape, and smoothness that would meet most of the demand and reduce the requirements for grinding and surfacing. Its mobility enabled the Medical Department to place optical support near the front lines.[46]

The mobile optical repair unit was mounted on a 2 1/2-ton truck and was staffed by one Sanitary Corps officer and six enlisted soldiers. It had the capability of repairing or replacing 100 pairs of spectacles a day. A smaller, portable version consisted of two chests that could be carried in a jeep and was operated by two enlisted soldiers who could handle up to twenty jobs per day. The officers and enlisted technicians completed a six-week course at the St. Louis Medical Depot. Officers were selected from candidates with an optical shop background; some were optometrists.[47]

The effort to place optical support as close as possible to the combat soldiers paid off. "Line officers noted with pleasure, but with little astonishment, that the

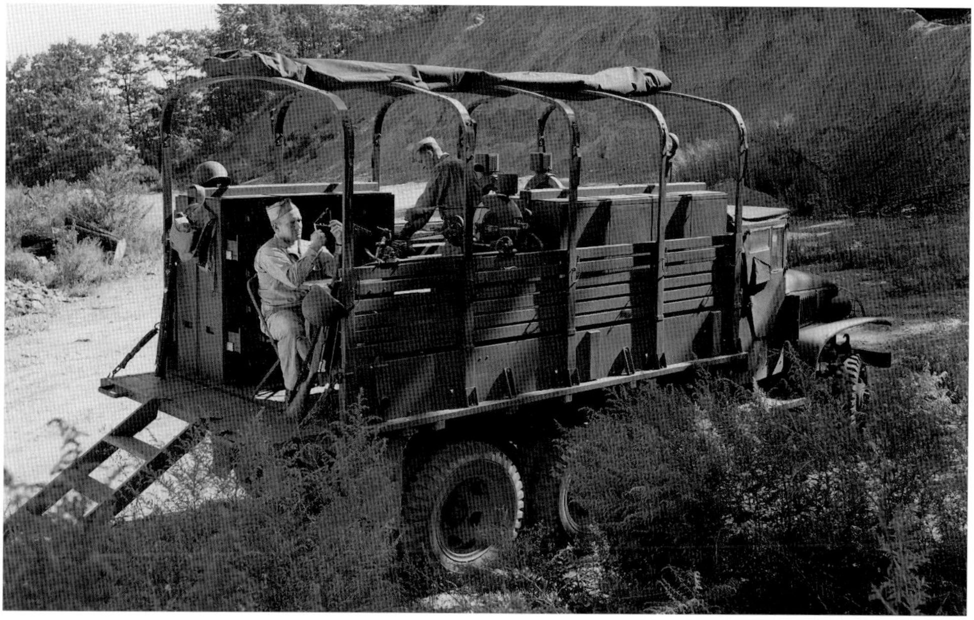

Mobile optical repair unit

need for spectacle repairs diminished when the repair units began to operate near the front."[48] One hundred and fifty optical units produced one-half million pairs of glasses in fiscal year 1945. The units repaired or replaced about 160,000 pairs of spectacles in the first six months following the Normandy invasion.[49]

There were no opportunities for commissions as an optometrist, but for some, whether enlisted or officer, the duty was satisfying. Cpl. Herbert Gordon, O.D., for example, was stationed at a Miami Beach hotel in Florida and assigned to an Army Air Forces clinic on Lincoln Road that screened and treated aviation cadets. Cpl. Ernest F. Ames, O.D., was assigned to the optical laboratory at Norcross, England, where he and his compatriots had a sideline of designing cigarette lighters from cartridges, coins, and, in one case, a glass eye—all inscribed with the American flag and the slogan "Cheers."[50]

A Medical Research and Development Team

Scientific specialty officers found a natural home in Army medical research and development, a program that became much more sophisticated and broadly based during World War II. As the Medical Department improved its medical technology, it also improved its organizational ability to take advantage of those technological advances. The Research and Development Section was added to the Surgeon General's Office in 1940, and the Board for the Investigation and Control of Influenza and Other Epidemic Diseases in the Army, later called the Army Epidemiological Board, was formed in 1941.[51] Consisting of seven civilian members directing ten commissions of M.D. and Ph.D. specialists in biochemistry, infectious disease, preventive medicine, bacteriology, and immunology, the board provided the Surgeon General's Office with access to some of the best expertise available in the control of epidemic diseases. Furthermore, the externally based group of civilian advisers provided direction and focus for Army medical research and development and was influential in building permanency into the program after the war.[52]

The scientific talent of Sanitary Corps officers was also available to the Medical Department for a variety of medical intelligence activities, such as collecting health and medical data on a geographical basis and assessing enemy medical capabilities. In 1944 Sanitary Corps officers headed three medical teams that collected captured medical equipment and materiel in the Pacific and Europe. One item they analyzed was a high-quality folding microscope developed by the Japanese. In Europe, a sanitary engineer, Lt. Col. John H. Watkins, SnC, served on the U.S. Strategic Bombing Survey. Watkins coauthored two chapters of the medical portion of the report, a study remarkable for the fact that it documented the absence of any epidemics in Germany resulting from the Allied bombing.

Other officers contributed research that helped the United States develop alternate sources of medical equipment for those shut off by the war. For example, Germany had been the principal supplier of surgical instruments, and it was quite important for the United States to develop its own manufacturing capability. It was so important that Maj. Joseph A. Calamari, SnC, received the Legion of Merit for identifying the cause of corrosion in surgical instruments made from stainless steel and plated carbon steel and devising a method of prevention.[53]

Sanitary Corps laboratory officers contributed to the demonstration of the effectiveness of sulfadiazine prophylaxis in lowering the meningococcus carrier rate among new recruits and to the development of new biochemical methods for the determination of antimalarial drugs in body fluids. They were members of research teams that worked on typhoid, typhus, dysentery, and cholera vaccines and, in tandem with sanitary engineers, developed chemical warfare detection kits for testing food and water supplies. They participated in studies on atypical pneumonia, typhus, and respiratory infections.[54]

At the Army Medical School, Washington, D.C., 1st Lts. Kenneth Wertman, SnC, and Reginald L. Reagan, SnC, under the leadership of Col. Henry Plotz, MC, operated the Division of Virus and Rickettsial Diseases, the first military or civilian laboratory to provide a single diagnostic source for those infections. They established the division in January 1941, when Wertman and Bergman were still enlisted technicians, and in 1942 Plotz and Wertman confirmed the etiologic agent of Brill's disease. Soldiers benefited from the research efforts of such scientific specialty officers as 2d Lt. I. Gordon Fels, SnC, of the 67th General Hospital in France, who developed a new test for the rapid identification of gas gangrene, an important development for wound management. In Alaska, 2d Lt. Charles D. Graber, SnC, a bacteriologist, alerted the Army to a deadly flaw in the woolen clothing issued to soldiers when he discovered that gas gangrene bacilli had been introduced into the wool during manufacturing. Soldiers wearing uniforms made from that material who were wounded during a Japanese attack on Attu Island had their wounds contaminated with the lethal infection.[55]

In 1943 Capt. Ludwig R. Kuhn, SnC, a bacteriologist, demonstrated that sulfadiazine could prevent the spread of cerebrospinal meningitis in Army camps. In Italy, an outbreak of atypical pneumonia in early 1945 was identified by another bacteriologist, 1st Lt. Robert Rustigian, SnC, as Q fever. Rustigian, who contracted the disease in the course of his laboratory work, developed findings that led to scientific recognition of the worldwide distribution of Q fever, believed until then to be isolated in certain areas of Australia.[56]

Typhus commanded the attention of a number of Sanitary Corps officers. Lts. Byron Bennett and E. John Bell, SnC, and Capt. Trygve O. Berge, SnC, were among fourteen Sanitary Corps and seven Medical Administrative Corps officers detailed to the U.S. Typhus Commission, which, with its Army and Navy membership, was one of the earliest joint service agencies. The Sanitary Corps officers contributed to worldwide field studies of louse-borne typhus, particularly in North Africa and Italy, and they were important figures in the mastery of this disease. Twelve officers were awarded the Typhus Commission Medal. Brig. Gen. Stanhope Bayne-Jones, MC, the commission's director, singled out Maj. George Zinneman, MAC, for handling its European support requirements "under incredibly difficult conditions." Col. Ira V. Hisock, SnC, received the Legion of Merit for his typhus control work in Italy, where his efforts ensured that not a single case of typhus occurred among the thousands of troops who passed through the Naples area.[57]

Maj. Emory C. Cushing, SnC, an entomologist recruited from the U.S. Department of Agriculture (USDA), was the Army's liaison for research conducted by the USDA at its Bureau of Entomology and Plant Quarantine laboratory in Orlando, Florida. An important product of that effort was the development of the "aerosol bomb" for dispensing insecticides. After the war this invention spawned a multibillion-dollar aerosol industry for everything from hair spray to paint.[58] The Orlando research effort was also responsible for the military use of DDT, one of the major technological advances of the war. DDT is a synthetic compound first used as an insecticide in Switzerland, and it was tested in the Orlando laboratory beginning in November 1942. Sanitary Corps entomologists who participated in field studies of DDT were astounded with the potency of their new weapon, one so militarily significant that it was initially classified secret.[59]

Much of the research that involved Sanitary Corps officers was centered in the Army Medical School, which had been the focus of medical research and development during the interwar period. The school had a tradition of research and teaching in an atmosphere of teamwork among diverse scientific specialties. George W. Hunter III, SnC, was commissioned as a captain in the Sanitary Corps in 1942 and joined the faculty of the Tropical and Military Medicine Course, which expanded from 23 to 200 students. The course prepared medical officers to combat the diseases to which soldiers were exposed in the Army's worldwide operations.[60]

Hunter suggested using the outline of the course as the basis for a textbook. It was published by the National Research Council in 1945 as the *Manual of Tropical Medicine* and became the standard reference in its field. Hunter's name was not listed first among the principal authors because the company believed that a physi-

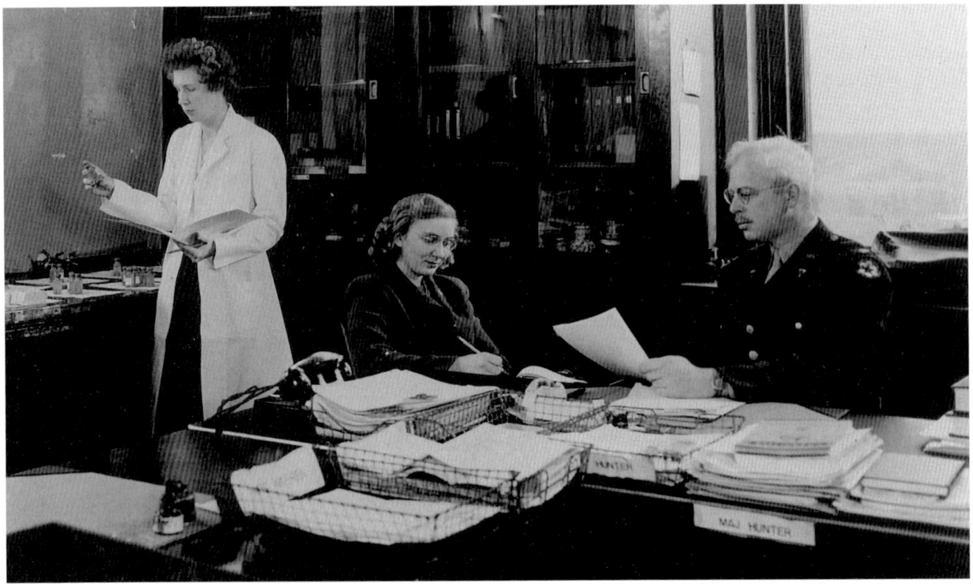

*Major Hunter (*right*) in his office at the Army Medical Department Research and Graduate School, Army Medical Center, Washington, D.C., June 1949*

cian's name would improve sales, but it was retitled *Hunter's Tropical Medicine* in later editions. With the printing of the sixth edition in 1984, Hunter, then a professor in the School of Medicine, University of California, San Diego, was recognized as "the glue that has held this book together from the very first edition."[61]

The medical research effort also included the efforts of psychologists, both in the clinical and testing aspects of the specialty. Some psychologists were employed in the design of military equipment. Others contributed to the refinement of aviator screening and classification tests. But the future of psychological research in the Army was uncertain. Maj. Anthony C. Tucker, PhC, the chief of the Air Surgeon's Psychology Research Division, cautioned that it would be difficult to retain a sufficient number of commissioned psychologists in the Army. He believed the military did not fully appreciate their value, and his reservations presaged a postwar debate. Robert M. Yerkes, Ph.D., who as a Sanitary Corps officer had headed the Surgeon General's Psychology Division in World War I, convened two meetings at the National Research Council in 1944 to review plans for the postwar utilization of military psychologists. The conference report recommended formation of a research and development corps for all scientists, including clinical psychologists. That did not occur, but at least the issue of providing a sustaining base for psychological research had surfaced.[62]

Malaria

Sanitary Corps officers were significant figures in the battle against malaria, the most militarily significant of the arthropod-borne diseases, especially in the

Pacific, Far East, and Mediterranean. Malaria had the capability of stopping an army in its tracks, and it accounted for nearly half a million hospital admissions and over three hundred deaths during the war. The early campaigns in the Solomons and New Guinea encountered rates so high that operations in some areas of the Pacific and Asia were dependent upon bringing malaria under control. When the 32d Infantry Division withdrew from New Guinea in March 1943, 67 percent of the division exhibited clinical signs of malaria. The 32d had evacuated 4,500 soldiers with malaria in five months of combat operations; most of those soldiers were lost to their units for months. The Sicilian campaign of the Seventh Army from 9 July to 10 September 1943 produced 21,482 hospital admissions for malaria as compared to 17,535 for battle casualties. In Burma, the 5307th Composite Unit (Provisional)—Merrill's Marauders—was conquered by illness, especially malaria, which in November 1943 was at an annual rate of 4,300 cases per 1,000 troops. Over half of the regiment had suffered one or more attacks of malaria, but a proposal to place soldiers on convalescence following a fourth attack of malaria was rejected because of the desperate combat situation. It was a horror of medical failure that Capt. James H. Stone, MAC, starkly portrayed in his book *Crisis Fleeting*. "In the end, amoebae and plasmodia, bacteria and rickettsia, rather than Japanese soldiers, vanquished Merrill's Marauders."[63]

The war with malaria needed experts who could advise surgeons and their commanders on how to prevent the disease, train soldiers and their leaders in preventive measures, and operate the specialized units used for survey and control of the mosquito vector. Sanitary Corps officers provided their talents to all of those aspects of the team effort, as well as contributing to the development of the technology, including DDT, used in the campaign. The Medical Department had an extremely limited number of physicians who were knowledgeable in the epidemiology and control of malaria. Sanitary Corps officers with expertise in entomology, sanitary engineering, parasitology, and other fields were thus critically important in the department's campaign against malaria, and some served as malariologists, the special advisers on malaria to unit surgeons. It was also necessary to set up a special military organization to plan and execute preventive measures.

The effectiveness of Sanitary Corps officers and the Medical Department team can be measured in the Pacific and Asiatic campaigns, which were made possible by the control of malaria. The American rates peaked in 1943, but dropped as the malaria survey and control units were fielded, even though military operations continued in highly malarious areas and with greater troop concentrations. In the Southwest Pacific Theater the rate dropped from 245 per 1,000 troops per year in 1943 to 41 per 1,000 by the end of 1944. In the Pacific Ocean Areas, including the South Pacific, the rate was reduced from 208 cases per 1,000 troops per year in 1943 to 5 cases per 1,000 in 1945. Of course this reflected to a great extent the fact that combat ceased in the South Pacific Area after Bougainville.

The malaria control effort began with control of the mosquito populations near Army bases in the United States. As part of that effort, the department called nine Sanitary Corps Reserve officers to active duty in 1941 and ordered them to training camps in the South. Their number was expanded by entomologists who were commissioned in the Sanitary Corps directly from universities and government agencies to conduct entomological surveys and reports and to provide technical supervision of insect control. One, Capt. Stanley J. Carpenter, SnC, was assigned to Camp Robinson, Arkansas, and conducted surveys in 1941 at four Army bases in Arkansas and Missouri. Captain Carpenter found that mosquitos constituted a major problem at Camp Robinson, and his efforts resulted in command action to resolve the situation. Soldiers in Captain Pletsch's 218th Malaria Survey Detachment who conducted mosquito surveys in Louisiana found that offers of jeep rides and candy made children much more likely to cooperate with the blood testing program.[64]

The responsibilities for malaria control were divided between the Surgeon General's Office and the Office of the Chief of Engineers when the Corps of Engineers assumed responsibility for control activities in the Zone of the Interior in 1942. Capt. William D. Reed, SnC, headed an Insect and Rodent Control Section that was organized in the Office of the Chief of Engineers, and Sanitary Corps officers served on the War Department staffs that coordinated the overall effort worldwide. The Medical Department remained responsible for surveys, recommendations, and technical supervision of control activities, and its capability for that requirement expanded in 1943 when Maj. Franklin S. Blanton, SnC, was recruited from the Department of Agriculture as the first entomologist on the surgeon general's staff. Training efforts included a malariology course at Camp Plauche, Louisiana, as well as a four-week course in Panama at the School of Malariology, Fort Clayton, Canal Zone. The Panama school, whose staff included Sanitary Corps entomologists, graduated 200 Medical Corps and Sanitary Corps officers between February 1944 and September 1945.[65]

The Medical Department formed two specialized organizations for the war against malaria. Malaria survey units (perhaps more appropriately called *vector* survey units) consisted of two Sanitary Corps officers—an entomologist and a parasitologist—and enlisted personnel who conducted studies and analyzed conditions in malarial areas. Malaria control units had one Sanitary Corps officer, a sanitary engineer, and eleven enlisted personnel who conducted control measures of clearing and cleaning standing water, ditching, filling, oiling, and applying larvicides. The units were allocated in malarious areas on the basis of one control unit per 7,500 troops and one survey unit per 20,000 troops.[66]

They battled not only malaria, but other diseases as well. One of those was scrub typhus, of which there were 5,441 cases during the war, with 283 deaths. While statistically unimportant in terms of the total number of cases, scrub typhus was a very dangerous disease. There were some serious outbreaks, notably at Sausapor and Biak during the New Guinea fighting, which strained the medical support capability with heavy nursing requirements and the diversion of medical resources. The fear that scrub typhus engendered far outweighed its incidence, and it became a morale problem in Burma, particularly among troops who patrolled in grassy scrub.

At the end of the war 300 Sanitary Corps officers and 2,700 enlisted soldiers were assigned to 146 malaria control units and 68 malaria survey units overseas, as well as another 16 control units and 3 survey units pending deploy-

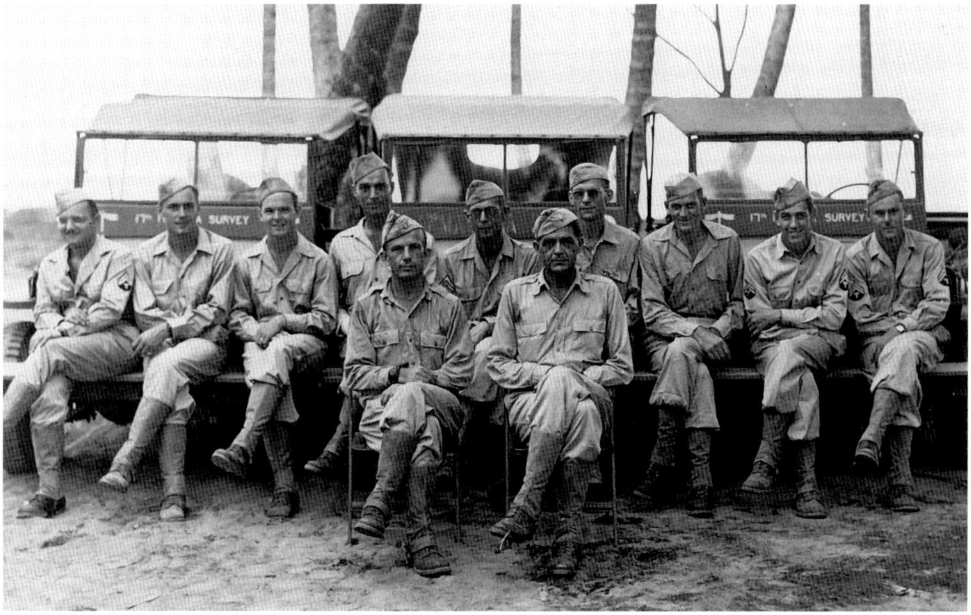

Personnel of the 17th Malaria Survey Unit, Ora Bay, New Guinea, July 1943

ment from the Zone of the Interior. The majority of the units were deployed in the extremely malarious Southwest Pacific. Mosquitos were so bad in an area occupied by the 81st Infantry Division in New Caledonia that training was repeatedly interrupted. The 218th Malaria Survey Detachment conducted mosquito control surveys to pinpoint the breeding areas. This required setting up biting studies in which a 218th soldier, acting as human bait, stripped to the waist, while another member of the unit as quickly as possible used chloroformed tubes to trap the mosquitos that collected on the first soldier's back. The record was 235 mosquitos in 15 minutes.[67]

The Sanitary Corps officers assigned to malaria units faced a variety of challenges. Capt. Samuel C. Billings, SnC, commanded the 8th Malaria Survey Unit, which deployed to China in March 1942, the only unit of its type in southwest China. He initially established his unit at an airfield near Chungking where it conducted surveys in the Kunming area. His team was furnished an old British car for transportation. "We nursed this car along for several months with no starter, much engine trouble and many broken springs." Later the team received an oversupply of insect repellent. They used it for hair tonic, spot remover, lubricant, and "almost any conceivable other use."[68]

Capt. Richard F. Peters, SnC, flew aboard a Flying Fortress to New Guinea in early 1943 to organize a malaria survey unit in an area where malaria had devastated Australian and American divisions. He instituted an area-wide program that dramatically reduced the malaria rates, and later, with Capt. Russ Fontaine, SnC, established a malaria control school for medical officers in New Guinea. Capt. Albert W. Grundmann, SnC, commander of the 15th Malaria Survey Unit, landed on Guadalcanal in June 1943. His unit's landing craft was stranded on a sandbar and refloated. It was then dive-bombed, strafed, and sunk, whereupon Grundmann and his unit made their way ashore without any equipment. Capt. Henry M. Chick, SnC, commander of the 20th Malaria Control Unit, demonstrated a secondary use for the power sprayer intended for insecticide dispersal in his attempt to control a fire at an ammunition dump in Mateur, Tunisia. Captain Chick received the Soldier's Medal for his heroism in the face of shrapnel and exploding ammunition.[69]

The standard operating procedure for amphibious operations in the Pacific was to attach one survey unit and one control unit to each assaulting division. Beachheads were aerially sprayed with insecticide during the landings in order to protect the soldiers in the amphibious assault waves. The malaria units would go ashore two to five days after the initial landings. Sanitary Corps officers participated in establishing programs for the routine spraying of malarious areas. One officer in charge of aerial spraying of bases from Hawaii to Shanghai logged over 3,400 hours of flight time in carrying out this preventive measure.[70]

External Influences

The actions of scientific specialty associations, especially pharmacy and optometry groups, reflected the ability of external guilds to influence the fortunes of their constituencies in the Army. They increased the political and War Department pressures on the Medical Department to expand the use of scientific specialty officers. This external influence was not present in the administrative specialties, which, with the exception of the American College of Hospital Administrators, did not have guilds looking out for the interests of their specialties in the military.

The field of sanitary engineering exemplifies that external influence. National leaders of sanitary engineering carefully manipulated the mechanisms that decided among competing claims for draft exemptions or for War Department recruiting objectives. They knew that the Army's requirements directly affected the needs of municipalities across the country, which depended upon sanitary engineers for the maintenance of clean water supplies and other basic public health measures. Their efforts resulted in assumption by the Procurement and Assignment Service of the same jurisdiction over sanitary engineers that it had over physicians. Abel Wolman, Ph.D., professor of sanitary engineering at the Johns Hopkins University and a nationally recognized figure, became a member of the service's board of directors and in that capacity influenced the military's utilization of practitioners of his specialty.[71]

The impact of the Army's requirements upon communities in the United States was substantial. By January 1945 about 75 percent of the 970 sanitary engineers on active duty had been recruited from state and local health departments. The Army Specialized Training Program—a program of educational assistance that had been established to supply scientific, engineering, medical, and linguistic specialists to the Army—added sanitary engineering in order to increase the numbers available for military service. Beginning in 1943, selected enlisted soldiers enrolled in sanitary engineering at five universities: Rutgers, New York University, Illinois, Michigan, and Harvard. Unlike physicians, dentists, and veterinarians, they were not commissioned upon graduation but had to complete Medical Administrative Corps OCS to become officers before being detailed to the Sanitary Corps. Of 190 graduates, 151 successfully completed OCS and were commissioned. It was the first instance of educational assistance for administrative or scientific specialty officers.[72]

Formation of the Pharmacy Corps

Pharmacy was another field where the influence of external groups was prominent. Tensions over the status of pharmacists had entangled three surgeons general during the interwar period and continued when World War II began. At the time the Medical Administrative Corps was limited to sixteen Regular Army officers, and Congress had restricted new appointments to pharmacists. But the special provision for commissioning pharmacists in the Regular Army was not matched by commissions in the Army of the United States, the wartime component of the Army, because the Medical Department continued to depend primarily on enlisted pharmacy technicians. Consequently, graduate pharmacists could enlist and attend Army Officer Candidate School, but that did not guarantee their use as pharmacy officers even if they completed Medical Administrative Corps OCS. In June 1943 there were 600 pharmacists serving as MAC officers, but none was commissioned for service as a pharmacist. In other words, nothing had really changed. This stirred up the pharmacy lobby, and cards and letters poured into the Surgeon General's Office. One writer, urging General Magee to commission pharmacists, told him to "pinch your Adam's apple and help win the war."[73]

Medical Department resistance, however, remained strong, and the surgeon general vigorously opposed the pharmacy lobby. In July 1942 Congressman Carl T. Durham, a pharmacist, introduced a bill to establish a pharmacy corps, stating that the specialty had a status comparable to medicine and dentistry. The legislation was dismissed as unnecessary by the surgeon general's spokesman, Brig. Gen. Larry B. McAfee, MC, because, as he testified, Army pharmacy was simpler than civilian practice. The department's three-month pharmacy technician course was sufficient preparation. There was little compounding. Since medications were furnished in tablet form, "any intelligent boy can read the label."[74] The surgeon general's recalcitrance angered the American Pharmaceutical Association, which claimed that the legislative proposal was nothing more than an attempt to provide soldiers with the same pharmaceutical protection as civilians.

Congressional hearings in March 1943 brought back some familiar faces. Dr. H. Evert Kendig of the American Pharmaceutical Association contradicted the surgeon general, declaring that Army pharmacy technicians were given responsibility beyond that legally permissible in civilian life even as the Army misused its professional pharmacists. He told the committee about a student at his school who was first in his class for four years, had received several prizes, but was drafted and made a dental technician. "He passes the dental ammunition, but he doesn't praise the Lord while he does it."[75]

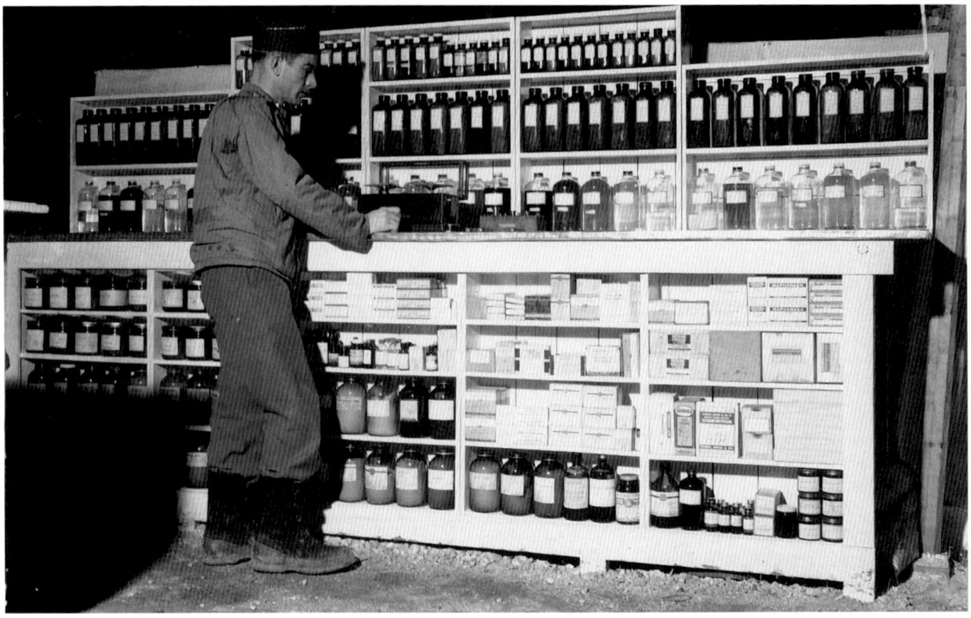

Pharmacy officer at the 8th Evacuation Hospital fills a prescription, Teano, Italy, March 1944.

Others chimed in. One was New Hampshire's governor, Robert O. Blood, M.D., who had been a medical officer with the 26th Division in World War I. Governor Blood believed the existence of a pharmacy corps would have prevented the problem he encountered of minimally trained soldiers dispensing pharmaceuticals "at great risk to our soldiers and most certainly at no economy to our Government."[76]

Congressman Durham heard the dissatisfaction of Army pharmacy officers at first hand. Capt. James T. Richards, MAC, a pharmacist assigned to the Walter Reed General Hospital, was invited to come to the American Pharmaceutical Association's Washington, D.C., office. There, Durham listened sympathetically to Richards' description of the frustrations of MAC officers with the Regular Army grade limitation of captain. (According to Richards, the Walter Reed executive officer later chastised him for "politicking" and assured him that remote assignments awaited such transgressors. That may have been, because that same month Richards was assigned to the 43d General Hospital, which was being organized at Camp Livingston, Louisiana, for deployment to Oran, Algeria.)[77]

Despite Medical Department objections, the pharmacy lobby succeeded in its fight. On 12 July 1943, President Roosevelt signed into law an act establishing the Pharmacy Corps as a component of the Regular Army. The corps was authorized seventy-two officers, with new appointments restricted to graduates of recognized schools of pharmacy. Officers who already held Regular Army commissions in the Medical Administrative Corps were moved to the Pharmacy Corps but did not count against the seventy-two authorizations for officers because so many of the

Regular Army MAC officers were not pharmacists, having been previously grandfathered by the law in 1936 that had restricted new appointments in the Regular Army MAC to pharmacists. Since the law transferred from the Medical Administrative Corps the only officers authorized for its permanent Regular Army component, this meant that the MAC was now "an empty Corps."[78]

Initially, fifty-eight Regular Army Medical Administrative Corps officers transferred to the new corps. Competition was keen for the new appointments, and of 900 applications from pharmacists in January 1944, only 12 were commissioned, having survived two days of difficult written examinations, a physical examination, and interviews.[79] By January 1945 the department had appointed eighteen pharmacists. That number, plus the forty-nine officers remaining from the Regular Army Medical Administrative Corps who had transferred, gave it a total of sixty-seven officers. The Pharmacy Corps peaked at seventy officers in April 1945.[80]

The creation of the Pharmacy Corps did not end the tension between the Medical Department and the pharmacy guild because the irony of a Pharmacy Corps that had pharmacists in the minority did not go unnoticed. By the summer of 1945 the surgeon general was again the target of complaints from across the country. Arthur H. Einbeck, chairman of the Committee on Status of Pharmacists in the Government Service, protested that the Army was dragging its heels in commissioning pharmacists, and the executive secretary of the Texas Pharmaceutical Association wrote to "deplore" General Kirk's actions. Cora Mae Briggs, the secretary of the Nebraska Pharmaceutical Association, was angered that pharmacists were being enlisted as privates to perform kitchen police and "sell beer at the officers' clubs." Briggs estimated a shortage of 500 pharmacists in Nebraska because of military conscription, and she believed the remaining pharmacists in the state were overworked. Fourteen had died the previous year, but "they didn't die of old age."[81] The protests were in vain. World War II was ending, and the celebration of victory in Europe and the Pacific would drown out their voices. That is where the matter rested when the Army went into the postwar period.

Optometry

Optometry also reflected the effect of external influences on military medicine. Although the War Department authorized the use of optometrists to perform refractions, it did not provide for their commissioning. One enlisted optometrist said that while he and his colleagues were proud to do their share in the war, he believed the Army received their service at "a bargain basement price."[82] The American Optometric Association (AOA) pressured the Army for officer status, but that did not come to pass during the war years.

An early initiative of the AOA was to establish a military occupational specialty (MOS) for optometry since none existed.[83] That achieved, their principal objective was to obtain commissioned status for optometrists who, with their graduate training in eye and visual conditions, provided a necessary health care service for which general practice physicians were trained too little but ophthalmologists were trained too much.[84] In fact, as optometry groups were quick to point out, enlisted optometrists were often compelled to straighten out the problems of patients who complained about eye examinations they had received from unqualified general medical officers. "Many came in feeling their way to the door."[85] To make things worse, enlisted optometrists would be brusquely handled by sergeants who held the opinions of privates in low regard. Further, the optical units that filled spectacle prescriptions were headed by officers, making it difficult for optometrists of low rank to demand compliance with their orders. All in all they said it was "mean trickery" that made them "underlings," and optometry journals filled with letters from disappointed optometrists.[86] One editorial, entitled "With Retinoscope and Floor Mop," fulminated that "in many cases optometrists doing refractions are privates and corporals and frequently are outranked by file clerks." If that wasn't enough, "the Army optometrist, by swinging a mop or a broom, is not enhancing his professional appearance or prestige."[87]

Not all optometrists in the Army were enlisted. About half were officers, but they were compelled to seek commissioning opportunities in branches outside the Medical Department. "As soon as they got second lieutenant's bars on they had to put the retinoscope away."[88] For example, five were commissioned in the Coast Artillery to screen antiaircraft crews for depth perception and other visual abilities and to serve as target recognition instructors.

Things took a new turn in 1942 when the AOA selected William P. MacCracken, Jr., as its Washington counsel. MacCracken, a graduate of the University of Chicago Law School, had been an Army Air Corps lieutenant during World War I, and he continued his pioneering aviation activities after the war. He was secretary of the American Bar Association from 1925 to 1936 and had served from 1926 to 1929 as the first assistant secretary of commerce for aeronautics, receiving Pilot's License No. 1. Subsequent activities as an aviation lobbyist caught him in a congressional cross fire that resulted in a ten-day jail sentence for contempt of Congress. As the AOA lobbyist he began a new career.[89]

As MacCracken described it, optometry "enjoyed only semi-respectability as a profession" in the early 1940s. It was compromised by opportunists within its own ranks and was under the firm heel of the American Medical Association. The specialty needed a systematic plan to reach its objective of professional recognition and a seasoned operator to see that through. MacCracken, it turned out, was just the person.

The AOA undertook a program to educate congressmen (and physicians) in the capabilities of optometrists, citing their wartime service as evidence, and it solicited AOA members to write their congressmen.[90] MacCracken unsuccessfully attempted to convince the deputy surgeon general that commissioning optometrists was in the department's best interest. Although the Army refused to provide this opportunity, the Navy relented and opened up its ranks. Harold Kohn, the AOA chief counsel, attributed the Navy's receptive attitude to the fact that an AOA president, Lesley R. Burdette, O.D., had played on the same college football team with the Navy's surgeon general, Rear Adm. Ross T. McIntire.[91]

Spurned by the Medical Department, MacCracken went to Congress. In 1945 Congressman Dewey Short, the ranking Republican on the House Military

Affairs Committee, introduced a bill to establish an optometry corps of sixty officers who would perform under the supervision of ophthalmologists. The bill survived two months of hearings and passed the House in the face of American Medical Association and War Department opposition (particularly that of Col. Derrick Vail, MC, the surgeon general's ophthalmology consultant and a "virulent anti-optometrist").[92] Continued opposition in the Senate made approval appear unlikely, but it passed that chamber without a dissenting vote. The legislative success was credited to MacCracken. Harold Kohn was impressed. "I don't know how it was done, but I know a miracle when I see one."[93]

The optometry corps came very close to reality, but President Truman vetoed the bill. An AOA delegation that included MacCracken and William Ezell, O.D., AOA president, met with the president to plead for reconsideration, since they believed they could again obtain congressional passage. Truman told the group that he had not changed his mind and would veto it again because the war was ending and it was time to consolidate the military and not to create new corps. However, he understood their desire for professional recognition. Consequently, before he vetoed the bill, he had received a commitment from the War Department that it would begin commissioning optometrists in the Regular Army. The AOA delegation did not leave the president's office happy, but they did leave reassured. Their optimism should have been muted. Commissioning would begin, but not until the Medical Department had stalled for another two years.[94]

Summary

The pressures that influenced the presence of scientific specialty officers on the military medical team differed in kind and scope from those that compelled the use of administrative specialty officers. The underlying imperative of releasing physicians to practice medicine was the same in both groups. In the case of the scientists, however, the process was abetted by guilds looking out for the interests of their specialty groups.

The establishment of a Pharmacy Corps was the final act in a long-running show. When it was over, no question existed that pharmacy would have a secure place in the commissioned ranks of the Medical Department. Optometry did not succeed in obtaining its own corps, and it also failed to achieve commissioning during the war. But it did succeed in getting the desires of the specialty for professional recognition placed on the national agenda, in securing a president's promise of commissioning, and in having its portfolio in the hands of a lobbyist who would keep its cause alive after the war. Sanitary engineers, through their national representation, controlled their availability for national military service during the war and their opportunities once in the military. In this way they were protected from the vagaries of conscription, something that other groups (lawyers, for example) did not achieve.

The overtones of political logrolling tend to obscure the point that the efforts of emerging specialties to secure their professional recognition was part of an evolutionary process. As in the case of the administrative specialties, there were elements of recalcitrance—resistance to commissioning of pharmacists and optometrists and to placing of laboratory officers in charge of laboratories being examples—but the process could not ultimately be halted. The scientific specialty officers made possible an expanded and modernized team that improved the diagnostic and treatment capabilities of the Medical Department. Pharmacists, optometrists, and laboratory officers were there to stay, and their success provided new opportunities for women as well as men in the scientific specialties. The Army's mental health team permanently changed its composition and improved its effectiveness with the addition of psychologists and social workers. Commissioning opportunities were available for a broader variety of specialties, and for the first time the Army provided some financial aid for university training in nonphysician specialties. Scientific and administrative specialty officers were permanently reconfiguring the department.

A component of the medical team's transformation was the emergence of a standing constituency with an external supporting base for Army medical research and development. Experience in wartime demonstrated a need for scientific specialty officers devoted to that function full time and able to respond worldwide. While the Army had sponsored medical research in the past, it had not attempted anything on the scope of what occurred in World War II. Sanitary Corps officers who contributed to medical advances opened permanent positions for themselves on the medical research team.

The United States relearned from the war the fact that global responsibilities meant the exposure of its soldiers to diseases that did not naturally occur at home. Thus, the ability to conserve the fighting strength of U.S. military forces would increasingly depend on the nation's ability to deal with the global disease threat. The program to combat malaria demonstrated the department's commitment to preventive medicine and to the application of medical research findings through the talents of scientific specialty officers: it was an extremely significant aspect of the contributions of Sanitary Corps officers. The future military medical mission would demand the full industrial model of research, development, and acquisition of new technology, coupled with the application of that technology through a modern medical system.

The Army's obligation to care for the civilian populations caught up in the aftermath of the fighting was a new dimension of warfare. American generals were beginning to comprehend B. H. Liddell Hart's admonition "to conduct war with regard to the peace you desire."[95] They needed a medical team whose scientific specialty officers not only supported soldiers in combat but could enable the United States to prosecute the peace. Those officers were indispensable in providing medical support for refugees uprooted by combat action and for people in areas liberated from the Axis Powers.

Combat units found that public health problems could overwhelm them. American forces retaking the Philippines depended upon the talents of sanitary engineers to ensure the restoration of safe drinking water, a vital necessity for civilian and soldier alike. In Europe, U.S. and Allied forces occupying a ravaged continent desperately needed the skills of the Medical Department's scientific specialty officers in meeting the enormous public health challenges. When the Third Army reached Frankfurt at the end of March 1945, it found a dying city.

"There were no telephones, no electricity, no street cars, no water mains, no gas. The sewage lines had spilled contamination into the streets, or what was left of them."[96] The Ninth Army was swamped with refugees when it reached Thuringia, Germany, in April 1945. All had suffered from malnutrition, and many had tuberculosis, typhus, or other diseases. Four and one-half million displaced persons shuffled across Europe's destitute landscape, and at one point U.S. forces were responsible for the care of hundreds of thousands of displaced persons, enemy prisoners of war, German political prisoners, and Allied prisoners of war. Lice were ubiquitous, as were delousing stations dusting civilians with DDT powder under the supervision of Sanitary Corps officers.[97]

The unanswered questions at the end of World War I were also present at the end of World War II. The military medical team had been reconfigured by the addition of administrative and scientific specialty officers, and their talents, leadership, and special expertise would be needed in the future to support a world power. Yet none of those officers had any idea of what the postwar Medical Department would offer them, either in its regular or its reserve components. Pharmacists were the only officers assured of a place in the active Army. For the rest, the future was still hazy.

Notes

[1] Shortages: DF, Lt Col Durwood G. Hall, MC, Asst to Ch Pers Svc, to Dir, Mil Pers Div, ASF, 29 Jul 43, folder 64, box 5/18, MSC-USACMH.

[2] SnC numbers: There were 226 reserve and 1 National Guard Sanitary Corps officers. McMinn and Levin, *Personnel in World War II*, pp. 15, 113. Dec 1943 SnC: This included 696 sanitary engineers, 203 entomologists, 873 laboratory specialists, 335 supply service officers, 138 nutrition officers, 44 industrial hygiene officers, and 76 officers in other duties. Rpt, Sanitary Engineering Div, Preventive Medicine (Prev Med) Svc, OTSG, sub: History of Sanitary Corps Personnel, December 1943, MSC-USACMH.

[3] Major lesson: Memo, Brig Gen James S. Simmons, Ch, Prev Med Svc, SGO, for Dir, Historical Div, 20 Sep 45, folder 173, box 11/18; Simmons to TSG, sub: Postwar Sanitary Corps, 5 Nov 45, folder 89, box 6/18, both MSC-USACMH. The other two lessons were the need for a peacetime medical research and development program and the need for dissemination of current directives, technical bulletins, manuals, and geographic assessments. Need: See Sanitary Engineering Section, History of Sanitary Corps Personnel. TSG's arguments: Memo, Thomas G. Ward, sub: Objection by the War Personnel Board to Appointment in the Sanitary Corps, Army of the United States, 17 Apr 42, MSC-USACMH.

[4] Procurement: OTSG, Cir Ltr 2, sub: Qualifications for Appointment as First Lieutenant, Sanitary Corps, 7 Jan 42, MSC-USACMH. Age: Memo, Henry L. Stimson, Sec War, sub: Appointment of Officers from Civilian Life, 12 Jan 42, MSC-USACMH. TSG opposition: Lt Col John A. Rogers, MC, XO, TSG, to ACS, G–1, sub: Increase in Sanitary Corps, 18 Feb 42; Memo, Capt Thomas G. Ward, MC, sub: Objection by the War Personnel Board to Appointment in the Sanitary Corps, Army of the United States, 17 Apr 42; TSG to CG, SOS, signed Rogers, 22 Apr 42; Col George F. Lull, MC, Asst to TSG, to CG, SOS, sub: Appointment in Sanitary Corps of the United States of Applicants Below the Age of 30, 18 Aug 1942, all in folder 36, box 4/18, MSC-USACMH. Change: OTSG, Cir Ltr 2, sub: The Sanitary Corps: Qualifications and Assignment of Its Officers, 2 Jan 43, MSC-USACMH.

[5] Team: The team also included thirty-seven acoustic officers, rehabilitation officers for the blind and deaf, and physical reconditioning officers appointed in the Medical Administrative Corps for rehabilitating disabled soldiers. SGO Annual Rpt FY 1945, file Research Notes WWII, box 2/18, MSC-USACMH.

[6] Clinical psychology: Morton A. Seidenfield, "Clinical Psychology," in Glass and Bernucci, vol. 1 of *Neuropsychiatry in World War II*, pp. 567–603, hereafter cited as Seidenfield, "Clinical Psychology"; Eli Ginzberg, "Logistics of the Neuropsychiatric Problem of the Army," *American Journal of Psychiatry* 102 (May 1946): 729–31; John G. Jenkins, "New Opportunities and New Responsibilities for the Psychologist," *Science* 103 (1946): 33–38, hereafter cited as Jenkins, "New Opportunities"; Seidenfield, "Clinical Psychology in Army Hospitals," *Psychological Bulletin* 41 (1944): 512–13; James W. Layman, "Utilization of Clinical Psychologists in the General Hospitals of the Army," *Psychological Bulletin* 40 (1943): 212–16; Max L. Hutt, "Report of Duties Performed by Clinical Psychologists," *Medical Bulletin* (February 1947): 233–35, hereafter cited as Hutt, "Clinical Psychologists"; T.G. Andrews and Mitchell Dreese, "Military Utilization of Psychologists During World War II," *American Psychologist* 3 (1948): 533–38; Notes of discussion, Charles A. Ullmann, Ed.D., Consulting Psychologist, with Ginn, Washington, D.C., Sep 83, MSC History Files, DASG-MS; WD Cirs 392, 2 Oct 44; 270, 1 Jul 44; 71, 6 Mar 45; 77, 10 Mar 45; PL. Combat exhaustion: Robert E. Hales and Franklin D. Jones, "Teaching the Principles of Combat Psychiatry to Army Psychiatry Residents," *Military Medicine* 148 (January 1983): 24; Albert J. Glass, ed., *Overseas Theaters,* vol. 2 of Glass and Bernucci, *Neuropsychiatry in World War II* (1973), p. 999; David K. Kentsmith, "Principles of Battlefield Psychiatry," *Military Medicine* 151 (February 1986): 90–92; Shabtai Noy, "Battle Intensity and the Length of Stay on the Battlefield as Determinants of the Type of Evacuation," *Military Medicine* 152 (December 1987): 605. It is estimated that there was one psychiatric admission for every two medical admissions in the First Army during the first two months following the Normandy invasion. In one division the rate was so high that the entire division would have been depleted in a year without proper treatment of the cases. Fortunately, the World War I lesson of forward treatment prevailed and reduced the losses.

[7] SnC commissions: The six SnC psychologists were 1st Lts. Michael Dunn, Robert M. Hughes, James W. Layman, William C. Murphy, Lawrence I. O'Kelly, and L. Grant Tennies (Seidenfield, "Clinical Psychology," p. 569).

[8] Transfer: WD Cir 264, 1 Sep 45; Seidenfield, "Clinical Psychology," p. 585. Women: Seidenfield, "Clinical Psychology," p. 576.

[9] Quoted words: Jenkins, "New Opportunities," p. 38.

[10] Survey: Hutt, "Clinical Psychologists," pp. 233–37.

[11] Psychology: Anthony C. Tucker, "The Role of Research Psychologists in the Military Service," *Medical Bulletin* (August 1947): 727–28.

[12] Quoted words: Bascom W. Ratliff, Elizabeth M. Timberlake, and David P. Jentsch, *Social Work in Hospitals* (Springfield, Ill.: Charles C. Thomas, 1982), p. 3.

[13] Quoted words: Thomas V. DiBacco, "Social Work's Slow Rise," *Washington Post,* 7 November 1994.

[14] Social work: Malcolm J. Farrell and Elizabeth H. Ross, "Military Psychiatric Social Work," *Bulletin of the Menninger Clinic* 8 (1944): 153–55; Daniel E. O'Keefe, "Psychiatric Social Work," in Glass and Bernucci, *Neuropsychiatry in World War II,* 1: 605–30; Israeloff, Winning the War, pp. 56–57; WD Cir 295, 13 Jul 44, PL.

[15] Menninger: O'Keefe, "Psychiatric Social Work," p. 610.

[16] Sanitary engineering: Speech, Joseph J. Gilbert, presented at the Conference of Sanitary Corps Officers, sub: Sanitary Corps, U.S. Army, 24 Nov 44, HQ, 2d Service Command, MSC-USACMH; Col Stanley J. Weidenkopf, MSC, draft chapter, sub: Sanitary Engineering, for 1958 MSC History Project, p. 66, hereafter cited as Weidenkopf, Sanitary Engineering; Sanitary Engineering Section, Medical Service Corps, OTSG, Personnel Card Files 1941–60, DASG-MS; Simmons, "The Division of Preventive Medicine," pp. 60–68; Stanley J. Weidenkopf, "Sanitary Engineers in the Army Medical Service," *Military Surgeon* 115 (July 1954): 55; Maj Raymond J. Karpen, MSC, Environmental Sanitation (Env San) Br, OTSG, to Herbert M. Bosch, Env San Div, Minnesota Dept of Health, 24 Nov 48, DASG-MS; Israeloff, Winning the War, p. 30.

[17] Duties: Ibid.; Michael J. Blew, "A Sanitary Engineer Views the Post War World," *Military Surgeon* 100 (May 1947): 410–11; THU, 1958 Board for MSC History. Hardenbergh: Stanhope Bayne-Jones, "Typhus Fever," in Ebbe C. Hoff, ed., *Communicable Diseases: Arthropodborne Diseases Other than Malaria*, vol. 7 of *Preventive Medicine in World War II,* in the series Medical Department of the United States Army in World War II (Washington, D.C.: Office of the Surgeon General, Department of the Army, 1964), pp. 185–86, 189, hereafter cited as Hoff, *Arthropodborne Diseases Other Than Malaria.* Quoted words: William A. Hardenbergh to Brig Gen Stanhope Bayne-Jones, 2 May 66, MSC-USACMH. From 1927 to 1940 Hardenbergh was vice president and general manager of *Public Works Magazine.*

[18] Blew: Sanitary Engineering Section, Medical Service Corps, OTSG, Personnel Data Cards, 1941–60, DASG-MS; Joy Day, "Oldest-Living MSC: One of First Environmentalists," *Army Medical Department Newsletter* (Fall 1971): 40, JML.

[19] Quoted words: Ralph S. Cleland, "Sanitary Engineering in the European Theater of Operations," *Military Surgeon* 101 (July 1947): 36–40; Presentation, Cleland, same sub, at the meeting of the Association of Military Surgeons of the United States, Detroit, Mich., 9–11 Oct 41, folder 110, box 7/18, MSC-USACMH. Also see Jack G. Seig, "Disposal of Liquid Wastes in the Field," *Medical Bulletin of the North Africa Theater of Operations* 2 (November 1944): 132–34, USACMH.

[20] Manila: Lloyd K. Clark, "Restoring Manila's Water System to Service," *Journal of the American Water Works Association* 38 (May 1946): 614–17.

[21] Germany: Lawrence S. Farrell and Paul J. Houser, "Environmental Sanitation," in U.S. Strategic Bombing Survey, *The Effect of Bombing on Health and Medical Care in Germany* (Washington, D.C.: Government Printing Office, 30 October 1945), pp. 238, 263. The study did not support the more extravagant claims of air power proponents.

[22] Japan: Ralph E. Tarbett and Paul J. Houser, "Environmental Sanitation," in U.S. Strategic Bombing Survey, *The Effects of Bombing on Health and Medical Services in Japan* (Washington, D.C.: Government Printing Office, 1 June 1947), pp. 119–21, and "Introduction," pp. 4–5. Brig. Gen. Crawford F. Sams was chief of the Public Health and Welfare Section of the HQ, Supreme Commander for the Allied Powers (SCAP), from 1945–1951. Sams reported that there was a high

incidence of diarrhea, probably because of the practice of using night soil. See Sams, unpublished MS, sub: Medic (an autobiography), pp. 2: 349–428, USACMH, and Cowdrey, *The Medics' War*, pp. 38–44.

[23] Industrial hygiene: Theodore F. Hatch, "The Armored Force Medical Research Laboratory in WW II," *Medical Bulletin of the U.S. Army Europe* 42 (January 1985): 22–26.

[24] Quoted words: Ibid., p. 24.

[25] Quoted words: Don Marquis, *Archy and Mehitabel* (New York: Dolphin Books, Doubleday, 1930), p. 128.

[26] Entomologists: Rpts, OTSG, sub: Entomologists on Duty with the Sanitary Corps, AUS, 4 Dec 43 and 6 Feb 45, DASG-MS. Quoted words: Henry S. Fuller, "Introduction," in Hoff, *Arthropodborne Diseases Other Than Malaria*, p. 6. 1940: Ralph W. Bunn, "Entomological Service in the Army," *Military Surgeon* 101 (July 1947): 40. Quoted words: Brig Gen Guy B. Denit, Ch Surg, Southwest Pacific Area (SWPA), Dec 44 Msg, quoted in *Medical Bulletin* (March 1945): 10. Capt. Belkin: Donald J. Pletsch, Ph.D. to Maj Joe C. Crain, MSC, Asst to Ch, MSC, 30 Jul 86, DASG-MS.

[27] 218th: Msg, HQ, Eighth U.S. Army (EUSA), to 218th Malaria Survey Unit, sub: Eichelberger, 19 Oct 45, DASG-MS; Wartime notes, Capt Donald J. Pletsch, SnC, sub: Foibles of the 218th Malaria Survey Detachment on Hokkaido, or, The Rover Boys in Japan, 24 Oct–18 Nov 45; Rpt, Capt Champion C. Coles, Jr., SnC, sub: Unit History, 218th Malaria Survey Detachment, undated [Dec 1945], hereafter cited as Coles, 218th MSD Unit History, both in DASG-MS; Notes of telephone interv, Pletsch with Ginn, 9 Jan 86, DASG-MS; "Mosquito-Fighting Detachment Holds Reunion," *Gainesville (Florida) Sun*, 22 July 1984; "WWII Medical Unit Reuniting; Generations Brought Together," *Stoddard (Missouri) County News*, 26 July 1983. Thanksgiving: Remarks, Inukai, Ph.D., Chm, Zoology Dept, Imperial University, sub: Greeting by Dr. Inukai to the Members of the 218th Malaria Survey Detachment, 25 Nov 1945, DASG-MS.

[28] DDT: James A. Baty, "Role of Auxiliary Medical Service in the Control of Tropical Diseases," *Military Surgeon* 101 (August 1947): 137; Bunn, "Entomological Service in the Army," p. 41.

[29] Rodent control: Baty, "Role of Auxiliary Medical Service in the Control of Tropical Diseases," p. 8. Occupation of Germany: John W. Bailey, "Report on the Status of the Entomological Collections in Certain European Museums, 1945," *Annals of the Entomological Society of America* 40 (1947): 203–12.

[30] Howe: Franklin C. Bing, "Paul Edward Howe (1885–1974)," *Journal of Nutrition* 115 (March 1985): 297–302; Ltr, Col David D. Schnakenberg, MSC, Dir, Nutrition Task Force, U.S. Army Research Institute of Environmental Medicine, to Ginn, sub: History of the MSC Nutrition Officer, 25 Mar 85, DASG-MS.

[31] Nutrition: OTSG, Cir Ltr 15, sub: Functions of Food and Nutrition Officers, 21 Feb 42, MSC-USACMH; Eliot F. Beach, "The Sanitary Corps Officer in Nutrition," *Military Surgeon* 101 (September 1947): 222–23. Surveys: Paul E. Howe and George H. Berryman, "Average Food Consumption in the Training Camps of the United States Army," *American Journal of Physiology* 144 (September 1954): 588–94. Also see Berryman, Cyrus E. French, and Howe, "Nutritional Evaluation of Overseas Rations," *Military Surgeon* 95 (November 1944): 391–96; Howe, "The Dietaries of Our Military Forces," *Annals of the American Academy of Political and Social Science* (January 1943): 72–79.

[32] Nutrition laboratory: Lt Col Robert Ryer, MSC, draft chapter, sub: Nutrition, 1958 MSC History Project.

[33] Occupation of Germany: Rpt, Office of the Chief Surgeon, Seventh Army, sub: Public Health in Post Hostilities Germany, undated, p. I–13; Joseph Israeloff, draft chapter, sub: Winning the War, 1965 MSC History Project, p. 45, DASG-MS, hereafter cited as Israeloff, Winning the War. POWs: SGO Annual Rpt FY 1945, file Research Notes WWII, box 2/18, MSC-USACMH. Malnutrition occurred as German soldiers were taken out of POW status and more food was allocated to Allied civilians, displaced persons, and German civilians.

[34] Lemonade: In Burma, dental officers of the 14th Evacuation Hospital found that Merrill's Marauders threw theirs away also, as they did every other preventive medicine measure. Stone, *Crisis Fleeting*, p. 303.

[35] Laboratory officers: Ibid.; Memo, Maj Arthur Stull, Ph.D., SnC, sub: Laboratory Services, Aug 1944, MSC-USACMH, hereafter cited as Stull, Laboratory Services. Stull, a Ph.D. research

chemist, was employed in the allergy department of Roosevelt Hospital, New York, prior to the war. Interv, Israeloff with Stull, 13 Jun 67, cited in Israeloff, draft chapter, sub: Gearing for Global Conflict, 1965 MSC History Project, box 1/18, MSC-USACMH, hereafter cited as Israeloff, Gearing for Global Conflict. Academic training: Laboratories Div, OTSG, extract from Annual Rpt for 1944, 23 Jan 1945, folder 183, box 12/18, MSC-USACMH; Philip R. Carlquist, "The Sanitary Corps Officer in the Laboratory," *Military Surgeon* 101 (August 1947): 131. Maxwell: Interv, Col Roy D. Maxwell, MSC, Ret., with Ginn and Col Charles R. Angel, MSC, Ret., the Pentagon, 5 Dec 83, DASG-MS.

[36] Personnel needs: Memo, Maj David A. Smith, MAC, for Dir, Officer Procurement Service, sub: Procurement of Laboratory Sanitary Corps Officers, 7 Dec 44, MSC-USACMH; Gustave J. Dammin and Elliott S.A. Robinson, "Medical Laboratories," in Ebbe Curtis Hoff, ed., *Special Fields*, vol. 9 of *Preventive Medicine in World War II*, in the series Medical Department of the United States Army in World War II (Washington, D.C.: Office of the Surgeon General, Department of the Army, 1969), p. 434.

[37] Women: Memo, Mason Ladd, Legislative (Leg) Div, for Lt Col Teasley, sub: Appointment of Female Scientists in the Sanitary Corps, Jun 44, MSC-USACMH. WAC commissions: Maj Bernard Sobol, Actg Dir, Legal Div, OTSG, to TAG, 15 Sep 43, and 1st Ind, Lt Col William T. Thurman, JAGD, Asst Ch, Mil Affairs Div, TJAG, to TSG, 30 Sep 43, folder 183, box 8/18; Col K.R. Hudnall, MC, through ASF to ACS, G–1, 1944; WD Cir 370, Section VI, sub: Sanitary Corps, 12 Sep 44, and WD Cir 462, 6 Dec 44, all in MSC-USACMH; Israeloff, Winning the War, p. 33. Also see Mattie Treadwell, *The Women's Army Corps* (Washington, D.C.: U.S. Army Center of Military History, 1954), pp. 344, 573. Special course: Rpt, History Div, OTSG, sub: The History of the Training of Medical Department Female Personnel, 1 Jul 1939 to 31 Dec 1944, undated (1945), MSC-USACMH. March 1945: Stull, Laboratory Services. At this point there were also 75 female physicians in the Medical Corps. Ch, Ops Svc, SGO, General Bliss' Notebook, vol. 1, Rpt, sub: Trend of Medical Corps Strength in Relation to Established Ceiling, 17 Jun 45, folder 176, box 11/18, MSC-USACMH.

[38] Kahn: Reuben L. Kahn, *Serology in Syphilis Control*, (Baltimore: Williams and Wilkins, 1942); also see Kahn, *Diagnosis of Syphilis by Precipitation* (Baltimore: Williams and Wilkins, 1925); Kahn, *The Kahn Test—A Practical Guide* (Baltimore: Williams and Wilkins, 1928); and Kahn, *Tissue Immunity* (Baltimore: Charles C. Thomas, 1936).

[39] Blood: Douglas B. Kendrick, *Blood Program in World War II*, in the series Medical Department of the United States Army in World War II (Washington, D.C.: Office of the Surgeon General, Department of the Army, 1964), pp. 157, 180, 465. Blood detachments: Draft MS, Donald O. Wagner, sub: The System of Field Medical Service in a Theater of Operations: Its Principles and the Types of Units Authorized, THU, OTSG, 30 Nov 59, file 258, box 16/18, MSC-USACMH. WD T/O 8–500 established two detachments, one for field army support (1 MC, 2 SnC, 26 EM) and one for corps support (1 MC, 1 SnC, 13 EM). Maurer: Ralph H. Maurer, "Blood Bank in a Fixed (General) Hospital: Analysis of 7,150 Transfusions of Stored Blood," *Medical Bulletin of the Mediterranean Theater of Operations* 3 (June 1945): 218, 223. Pryor: Kendrick, *Blood Program*, pp. 533–36.

[40] Podiatry: Cleveland Mather and Alfred R. Shands, Jr., eds., *Orthopedic Surgery in the Zone of Interior*, volume in *Surgery in World War II* in the series Medical Department of the United States Army in World War II (Washington, D.C.: Office of the Surgeon General, Department of the Army, 1970), pp. 133, 51, 227–28; Mather, ed., *Orthopedic Surgery in the European Theater of Operations*, volume in same series, 1956), pp. 23–24, 84, 187, 781–82. Navy: V.H. Witten and M. Lieder, "Minor Pathological Conditions of the Foot in Navy Personnel," *U.S. Navy Medical Bulletin* 41 (1943): 764; T.B. Marwil and Charles R. Brantingham, "Foot Problems of Women's Reserve," *Hospital Corps Quarterly* 16 (October 1943): 98–99.

[41] Use of chiropodists: Mather and Shands, *Orthopedic Surgery*, pp. 23–24, 84, 781–82.

[42] Spectacle policy: TSG to TAG, 5 Jun 41; Maj L.L. Barrow, MC, Asst to Ch, Finance and Supply (F&S) Div, SGO, to Ch, F&S Div, SGO, 22 Aug 41; TAG to CG, 1st Corps Area, Boston, sub: Repair and Replacement of Eyeglasses, 24 Sep 36. All in RG 112, Accession 69A–0127, Box 10/32, NARA-WNRC.

[43] Optical planning: Memo, Capt D.A. Peters, SnC, for Chief, Finance Br, F&S Div, OTSG, sub: Mobile Optical Unit, undated; Rpt, Capt Richard E. Yates, MAC, OTSG, sub: The

Procurement and Distribution of Medical Supplies in the Zone of the Interior During World War II, 31 May 46; Memo, Robinson for TSG, 7 Sep 42; Resume of 1943 Activities—Special Programs Branch, 24 Jan 44; Memo, Lt Col W.H. Potter, SnC, for XO, Supply Svc, OTSG, 6 Jun 44, all in RG 112, Accession 69A–0127, Box 10/32, NARA-WNRC. Actual Demand: Memo, Yates, 31 May 46; Rpt, Supply Svc, OTSG, sub: Resume of 1943 Activities, 24 Jan 44; Memo, Lt Col Paul I. Robinson, MC, Fiscal Officer, for TSG, sub: The Surgeon General's Spectacle Program, 7 Sep 42, all in RG 112, Accession 69A–0127, Box 10/32, NARA-WNRC.

[44] Expanded requirement: Rpt, Silas B. Hays, Louis F. Williams, and Robert L. Parker to Dir, Planning Div, ASF, sub: Supplementary Material To Be Included in ASF Manual M409, 18 Feb 46, DASG-MS, hereafter cited as Hays, Williams, and Parker, Supplementary Material. Quoted words: Memo, Stanley W. Ryak, Optical and Artificial Eyes Sec, Distribution Div, Supply Svc, OTSG, for Ch, Supply Svc, sub: History of the Optical Program, 28 Dec 45, RG 112, Accession 69A–0127, Box 10/32, NARA-WNRC, hereafter cited as Ryak, History of the Optical Program. Rather than costing $150,000–$200,000 a year, as originally estimated, the optical program was actually costing $8–$10 million a year by the fall of 1942.

[45] Occupation of Germany: Seventh Army, Public Health in Post Hostilities Germany, p. II–10.

[46] ETO requirement: Rpt, Lt Col James M. Greear, MC, Ophthalmology Consultant, ETO, cited in Memo, Stanley W. Ryak, Optical and Artificial Eyes Section, for Col Silas B. Hays, MC, Dep Ch, Supply Div, sub: Optical Support Program, 20 Nov 45, RG 112, Accession 69A–0127, Box 10/32, NARA-WNRC, hereafter cited as Ryak, Optical Support Program. Optical laboratory: Rpt, Special Programs Br, Supply Svc, OTSG, sub: Resume of 1943 Activities, 24 Jan 44; WD GO 76, 22 Sep 44, in file Extracts from General Orders Concerning Sanitary Corps, box 6/18, MSC-USACMH.

[47] Optical units: Hays, Williams, and Parker, Supplementary Material; Ryak, History of the Optical Program; Ryak, Optical Supply Program; Wiltsie, *Medical Supply in World War II*, pp. 82–86. Initially the Army issued one mobile and two portable units to each medical depot. This was extravagant, and in 1944 the basis of issue changed to one mobile unit per 150,000 troops, supplemented by one portable unit where troops were widely dispersed.

[48] Quoted words: Wiltsie, *Medical Supply in World War II*, p. 85.

[49] Numbers: Ibid.; Ryak, Optical Support Program.

[50] Optometrists: Robert S. Keller, O.D., to Ginn, 12 Aug 85, DASG-MS; Lt Col R.R. Patch, SnC, Chief, Liaison Br, Supply Svc, OTSG, sub: Annual Report of Liaison Branch, Purchase Division, Supply Service, FY 1944, 30 Jun 44, MSC-USACMH. Miami Beach: Herbert Gordon, O.D., to Ginn, 15 Jul 85, DASG-MS. Lighters: Ernest F. Ames, O.D., to Capt Albert L. Paul, MSC, 21 Feb 60, folder 58, box 8/18, MSC-USACMH.

[51] R&D: Blanche B. Armfield, *Organization and Administration in World War II*, volume in the series Medical Department of the U.S. Army in World War II (Washington, D.C.: Office of the Surgeon General, Department of the Army, 1963), pp. 93–96. The AEB later became the Armed Forces Epidemiological Board.

[52] Board: Stull, Laboratory Services.

[53] Commissions: James S. Simmons, "The Division of Preventive Medicine," *Medical Bulletin* (July 1941): 65. Intelligence: The officers were Maj. M.J. Plishner and Capts. Robert G. Gould and R.W. Cumley. Lt Col Raymond J. Cramer, draft chapter, sub: Intelligence, 1958 MSC History Project. Watkins: Scott V. Hitchcock and John H. Watkins, "Civilian Deaths from Air Attack," pp. 6–29; Franz K. Bauer and Watkins, "Communicable Diseases," pp. 30–82; and George A. Wulp and Watkins, "Tuberculosis," pp. 83–101, all in U.S. Strategic Bombing Survey, *Effect of Bombing on Health and Medical Care in Germany*. Calamari: WDGO 18, 15 Mar 45, cited in *Journal of the American Medical Association* 128 (19 March 1945): 210.

[54] R&D: Stull, Laboratory Services.

[55] Wertman and Reagan: Col Trygve O. Berge, MSC, draft section, sub: Virology and Immunology, 1958 MSC History Project, pp. 4–5, hereafter cited as Berge, Virology and Immunology. Fels: I. Gordon Fels, "A Rapid Cultural Method for the Presumptive Identification of Clostridium Welchi," *Medical Bulletin, Office of the Chief Surgeon, European Theater of Operations* (January 1945): 22–24, USACMH. Graber: Lt Col John R. Ransom, MSC, draft chapter, sub: Microbiology, in MSC History Project, 1961, folder 253, box 16/18, MSC-USACMH.

[56] Kuhn: Ibid. Rustigian: Berge, Virology and Immunology, pp. 9–10; Frederick C. Robbins, Robert Rustigian, Merrill J. Snyder, Joseph E. Smadel, "Q Fever in the Mediterranean Area; Report of Its Occurrence in Allied Troops. III, The Etiological Agent," *American Journal of Hygiene* 44 (1946): 62.

[57] Typhus Commission: Berge, Virology and Immunology, pp. 5, 10; Stanhope Bayne-Jones, "Typhus Fever," in Hoff, *Arthropodborne Diseases Other Than Malaria*, pp. 201–02, (quoted words, p. 240); Israeloff, Winning the War. Typhus medal: Capt. Robert Traub, Assam and Burma; Maj. Thomas H.G. Aitken, Naples; 1st Lt. Harold A. Pfreimer, ETO; Capt. Robert E. Bellamy, Naples; Maj. Charles C. Agar, ETO; Capt. Raymond C. Bushland, New Guinea; Lt. Col. Cornelius B. Philip, SW Pacific; Maj. Glen M. Kohls, New Guinea; Capt. E. John Bell, SW Pacific; Lt. Col. Emory C. Cushing, ETO; Maj. Charles M. Wheeler, Naples; Capt. Byron L. Bennett, Cairo. File, sub: Extracts from General Orders Concerning Sanitary Corps, folder 89, box 6/18, MSC-USACMH. Hisock: WDGO 28, 25 Apr 45, cited in *Journal of the American Medical Association* 128 (12 May 1945): 134; Israeloff, Gearing for Global Conflict. U.S. troops were immunized with the Cox vaccine. Hisock returned to Yale in 1945 as chairman of the Department of Public Health.

[58] Cushing: Biographical data card, THU, OTSG, USACMH. Cushing received the Typhus Commission Medal in 1945 for his service on the staff of the Chief Surgeon, European Theater of Operations. Insect control: Bunn, "Entomological Service in the Army," p. 41. Aerosols: Col Ralph W. Bunn, MSC, and Col Joseph E. Webb, Jr., MSC, draft section, sub: Entomology, 1958 MSC History Project, pp. 31, 124, hereafter cited as Bunn and Webb, Entomology; H.L. Haller, "Wartime Development of Insecticides," *Industrial and Engineering Chemistry* 39 (1947): 467–73; E.F. Knipling, "DDT Insecticides Developed for Use by the Armed Forces," *Journal of Economic Entomology* 38 (April 1945): 205, hereafter cited as Knipling, "DDT Insecticides."

[59] DDT: In the fall of 1943, the surgeon general informed the under secretary of war that the Medical Department had adopted dichloro-diphenyl-trichloroethane (DDT) to supplant pyrethrum in delousing powders and insecticides and was testing its effectiveness for mosquito control. Memo, Edward Reynolds, Actg Ch, Supply Svc, OTSG, for Under Sec of War, 4 Nov 43; Notes of discussion, Donald J. Pletsch, Ph.D., entomology consultant, with Ginn, Rosslyn, Va., 27 Feb 86, both in DASG-MS; Knipling, "DDT Insecticides," p. 205. Development: Harrison, *Mosquitos, Malaria and Man*, pp. 218–19; Knipling, "DDT Insecticides," p. 205.

[60] Army Medical School: Simmons, "The Division of Preventive Medicine," p. 61. Hunter: Rpt, Col George W. Hunter, MSC, sub: Reminiscences, 1971, DASG-MS; Notes of telephone interv, Hunter with Lt Col Richard V.N. Ginn, 1 Feb 86, DASG-MS; Lt Col Lyman P. Frick, draft section, sub: Parasitology, 1958 MSC History Project, hereafter cited as Frick, Parasitology. Hunter had resigned a reserve infantry commission in 1933 when he could not obtain an appointment in the Sanitary Corps Reserve in spite of a Ph.D. in parasitology and microbiology.

[61] Book idea: Hunter, Ginn telephone interv 1 Feb 86. *Tropical Medicine*: Thomas T. Mackie, George W. Hunter III, and C. Brooke Worth, *Manual of Tropical Medicine* (Philadelphia: W.B. Saunders, 1945). Major Hunter, SnC, and Captains Mackie and Worth, MC, were all fellow instructors in the course. Another ten Sanitary Corps officers contributed to the book: Maj. Gordon E. Davis and Capts. Luther S. West and William N. Sullivan, Jr.: entomology; Maj. Kingston S. Wilcox and Capt. Russell W.H. Gillespie: bacterial diseases; Capt. Reginald D. Manwell: malaria; 1st Lt. Joel Warren: viruses; and Capts. Curtis Saunders, A.E.A. Hudson, and William G. Jahnes, Jr.: diagnostic methods. Quoted words: G. Thomas Strickland, in introduction to *Hunter's Tropical Medicine*, 6th ed. (Philadelphia: W.B. Saunders, 1984), p. xvii.

[62] Research psychology: Hutt, "Clinical Psychologists," p. 235; Tucker, "The Role of Research Psychologists in the Military Service," p. 731; Robert M. Yerkes, "Post-War Psychological Services in the Armed Forces," *Psychological Bulletin* 42 (1945): 396–97.

[63] Malaria: Baty, "Role of Auxiliary Medical Service in the Control of Tropical Diseases," pp. 134–38; Bunn and Webb, Entomology, pp. 12, 31, 58; Ebbe C. Hoff, ed., *Communicable Diseases—Malaria*, vol. 6 of *Preventive Medicine in World War II*, in the series Medical Department of the United States Army in World War II (Washington D.C.: Office of the Surgeon General, Department of the Army, 1963), pp. 2, 6, 116, hereafter cited as Hoff, *Communicable Diseases—Malaria*; Stone, *Crisis Fleeting*, pp. 296, 304 (quoted words, p. 396).

[64] Recruitment: Bunn and Webb, Entomology, pp. 23–24, 26; Rpt, sub: Entomologists on Duty, 6 Feb 45, DASG-MS. Carpenter: Stanley J. Carpenter, "Mosquito Studies in Military Establishments in the Seventh Corps Area During 1941," *Journal of Economic Entomology* 35 (August 1942): 561. Blood smears: Coles, 218th MSD Unit History.

[65] Engineers: Bunn, "Entomological Service in the Army," p. 40. Blanton: Bunn and Webb, Entomology, p. 26. Panama: Ibid., pp. 34, 71.

[66] Vector units: Notes of Pletsch, Ginn interv, 9 Jan 86.

[67] Scrub typhus: Bunn, "Entomological Service in the Army," p. 27; Hoff, *Communicable Diseases*, p. 280; Stone, *Crisis Fleeting*, p. 123. Biting studies: Coles, 218th MSD Unit History.

[68] Billings: Rpt, Samuel C. Billings, sub: Summary Report of Military Duty as an Entomologist of the Sanitary Corps, U.S. Army—July 24, 1942 to January 30, 1946 (1954), folder 103, box 7/18, MSC-USACMH.

[69] Peters: Society for Vector Ecology, Santa Ana, Calif., *Vector Ecology Newsletter* (April 1992), DASG-MS. Peters joined the California Department of Health after the war and was head of its vector control bureau when he retired in 1978. The Society for Vector Ecology awarded him its Distinguished Service Award in 1989 and the Meritorious Service Award in 1992. Grundmann: Frick, Parasitology. Chick: GO, HQ, MTO, 15 Feb 45, in file Extracts from general orders concerning Sanitary Corps, folder 89, box 6/18, MSC-USACMH.

[70] Amphibious operations: Bunn, "Entomological Service in the Army," pp. 41–42. Bunn states the beaches were sprayed before the landings. Aerial spraying: Lloyd K. Clark, "Sanitary Corps in Forward Areas," *Military Surgeon* 101 (July 1947): 33.

[71] Personnel: McMinn and Levin, *Personnel in World War II*, pp. 201–06, 211. The change occurred in January 1943. Wolman: Wolman, active to the end, died in 1989 at the age of ninety-six. He pioneered the use of chlorine to purify water and had served as the adviser on water systems to fifty nations. *U.S. News and World Report* (6 March 1989): 16.

[72] Training program: Weidenkopf, Sanitary Engineering, p. 29; McMinn and Levin, *Personnel in World War II*, pp. 201–06.

[73] Pharmacy Corps: U.S. Congress, House, H.R. 7432, 23 July 1942; Hearings, House Military Affairs Committee, 17 November 1942 and 2 March 1943; and H.R. 997, Hearings, Senate Military Affairs Committee, 29 June 1943, MSC-USACMH; Israeloff, Winning the War, pp. 1–17; THU, Board for 1958 MSC History, pp. 5–10; "Bill Introduced to Establish Pharmacy Corps in the Army," *Journal of the American Pharmaceutical Association* 3 (November 1942): 227–28; "Army Presents Its Objections at Pharmacy Corps Bill Hearings," *Journal of the American Pharmaceutical Association* 3 (November 1942): 370–72. Quoted words: Postcard to TSG, anonymous, 25 Feb 43, folder 73, box 6/18, MSC-USACMH.

[74] Comparable status: "Bill Introduced," *Journal of the American Pharmaceutical Association* 3 (November 1942): 277. Quoted words: Hearings on H.R. 7432, p. 8.

[75] Quoted words: Hearings, H.R. 7432, 2 Mar 1943, p. 27. Kendig was chairman of the Committee on a Pharmacy Corps in the Regular Army.

[76] Quoted words: Ibid., p. 19.

[77] Quoted words: Col James T. Richards, MSC, Ret., to Ginn, 28 Feb 86, DASG-MS. The events occurred in March 1943.

[78] Pharmacy Corps: 57 Stat. 430, 12 July 1943; Memo, Capt E.R. Taylor, JAGD, Legal Div, OTSG, for Col Kintz, sub: Brief Summary of Medical Administrative Corps Legislation, 12 Feb 46; Memo, Pers Div, OTSG, sub: Problems Incident to the Utilization of Medical Service Corps Officers in Narrow Specialty Fields Upon Attaining Field Grade, 23 Dec 52; Rpt, OTSG, sub: Evolution of the Pharmacy Corps, Jan 45, all in MSC-USACMH; Samuel Milner, draft of first chapter, CMH History Project, sub: Troubled Decade: The U.S. Army Medical Service in the post World War II and Korean Eras, undated (1965), pp. 48, 67, box 1/18, MSC-USACMH. Pharmacy schools were restricted to those that required a four-year academic program for graduation.

[79] Appointments: Col Glenn K. Smith, MSC, draft chapter, sub: The Pharmacy Corps, undated (1961), in 1958 MSC History Project, folder 249, box 16/18, and Rpt, Maj Arthur H. Einbeck, MSC, Ret., sub: The History of the Pharmacy Corps, 29 Feb 56, folder 72, box 6/18, both in MSC-USACMH.

[80] Pharmacy Corps numbers: McMinn and Levin, *Personnel in World War II*, pp. 13, 15; Rpt, OTSG, sub: Evolution of the Pharmacy Corps, Jan 45, MSC-USACMH. A Pharmacy Corps song was apparently written in 1947, but was not located by the author. It is referred to in Ralph Biengang, "The History of Military Pharmacy in the United States: A Progress Report," *American Journal of Pharmaceutical Education* 11 (1947): 155.

[81] Complaint: Arthur H. Einbeck, "Army Must Be Made To Respect the Pharmacy Corps Act," *Journal of the National Association of Retail Druggists* (21 May 1945): 837. Actions Deplored: Robert G. Dillard, Executive Secretary, Texas Pharmaceutical Association, to Kirk, 20 Nov 45, folder 78, box 6/18, MSC-USACMH. Quoted words: Cora Mae Briggs, Secretary, Nebraska Pharmaceutical Association, to Sen Hugh Butler, 8 Jun 45, folder 78, box 6/18, MSC-USACMH.

[82] Quoted words: Robert S. Keller, O.D., to Ginn, 12 Aug 85, DASG-MS. Also see "Progress of an Optometrist in the Army," *Optometric Weekly* 33 (16 April 1942): 274.

[83] MOS: Otto R. Englemann, O.D., to Hon Paul McNutt, Chm, Manpower Commission, 14 Jan 43, folder 51, box 5/18, MSC-USACMH.

[84] AOA efforts: Michael Osborne and Joseph Riggs, *Mr. Mac* (Memphis, Tenn.: Southern College of Optometry, 1970), pp. 187–95.

[85] Quoted words: Ltr, John H. Smith to the editor, *Optometric Weekly* (20 December 1945): 1308.

[86] Quoted words: Carel C. Koch, "Action Now Required on Army Discrimination Against Optometrists," *American Journal of Optometry* 20 (July 1943): 252. Letters: For examples, see Daniel O. Elliott et al., "Army Recognition Through Unity," *Optical Journal and Review of Optometry* 79 (15 November 1942): 29; Daniel O. Elliott, *Optical Journal and Review of Optometry* 80 (1 February 1943): 21; Army Private, "Plaint of Optometrist in Uniform," and Just Buck Private, "The O.D. Was on K.P.," *Optical Journal and Review of Optometry* 81 (15 February 1944): 33.

[87] Quoted words: Editorial, "With Retinoscope and Floor-Mop," *Optical Journal and Review of Optometry* 80 (1 October 1943): 28–29.

[88] Quoted words: Osborne and Riggs, *Mr. Mac*, p. 194.

[89] MacCracken: Ibid., p. 216.

[90] AOA solicitation: Charles Sheard, O.D., "Report of the Council on Education and Professional Guidance," *Journal of the American Optometric Assocation* 15 (November 1943): 110. Also see Ewing Adams, O.D., President, AOA, to Otto R. Englemann, Illinois Optometric Association, 8 Feb 44, folder 51, box 5/18, MSC-USACMH. Adams encouraged Englemann to contact Governor Paul McNutt, chairman of the Wartime Manpower Commission, "using whatever influence he could to obtain proper recognition and utilization of optometry's services in the armed forces." Some optometrists in the Army noted that their prestige was rising as physicians and patients witnessed their professionalism. See Ltr, Sgt. Herbert Verner to the editor, "Prejudices Be Damned. They're Doing the Job," *Optical Journal and Review of Optometry* 81 (August 1944): 20–21.

[91] Kohn's views: Osborne and Riggs, *Mr. Mac*, pp. 194–98.

[92] Quoted words: Ibid., p. 198, quoting Harold Kohn.

[93] Proposal: Ibid., pp. 196–99; U.S. Congress, House, Rpt 7905, "Establishing an Optometry Corps in the Medical Department of the U.S. Army," 79th Cong., 1st sess., 14 July 1945. Quoted words: Osborne and Riggs, *Mr. Mac*, p. 199.

[94] Veto: Ibid., p. 197.

[95] Quoted words: B.H. Liddell Hart, *Strategy* (London: Faber and Faber, 1954), p. 366.

[96] Quoted words: Seventh Army, Public Health in Post Hostilities Germany, p. I–6.

[97] Refugees: The number was estimated at 450,000. Rpt, Army Service Forces, sub: Statistical Review: World War II, 1945, p. 68, copy in JML. Also see William M. McConahey, *Battalion Surgeon* (Rochester, Minn.: privately published, 1966), p. 159. The 90th Infantry Division occupied a sector in eastern Bavaria during May 1945, and McConahey's aid station in Maxhutte was quickly swamped with civilian health problems. Germany: Seventh Army, Public Health in Post Hostilities Germany, pp. I–6, II–18. Germany completely collapsed. Nearly 65 percent of the infants born in Berlin in 1945 died of tuberculosis or dysentery in their first year of life.

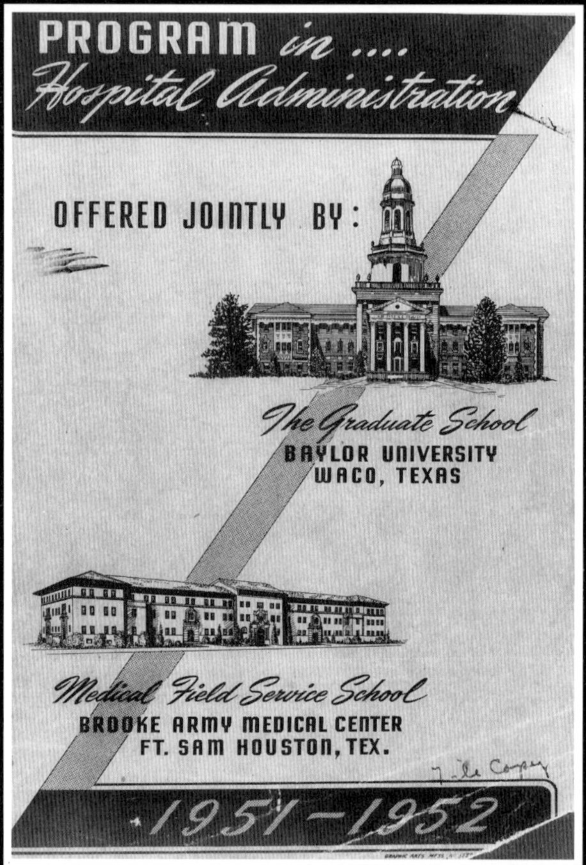

Army-Baylor Program in Hospital Administration bulletin

7

Medical Support for a World Power

The success of the medical administrative and scientific specialty officers during World War II had a profound effect on the postwar development of their role in the U.S. Army. Congressional and departmental actions consolidated them into a permanent corps, greatly increasing career opportunities for these officers and giving the Army Medical Department a much-needed permanent improvement in its mission capability. Although the Medical Department shrank during the postwar demobilization, the new corps enabled it to put together a balanced, high-quality team on a permanent basis.

The expanding global responsibilities of the United States in the evolving Cold War did not prevent it from greatly reducing the size of its armed forces. Within a year of Victory over Japan (V–J) Day, the Medical Department had dropped from a bed capacity of 750,000 to 100,000, and by June 1948 the Army and Navy combined had a capacity of only 34,000 beds. The Selective Service Act expired at the end of March 1947, and in February 1948, when the Communists seized power in Czechoslovakia, the combined strength of the Army and the Marine Corps was only 631,000. A new Selective Service Act was enacted that year, but during its two years of operation only about three hundred thousand men were drafted. In June 1950 the strength of the Army was less than six hundred thousand. As historian Russell Weigley put it, the Army had "faded to near impotence."[1]

Euphoria over winning the war was complicated by the U.S. occupation of Germany and Japan and disrupted by growing tensions with the Soviet Union. The Berlin blockade in 1948 merely underscored the deteriorating relations between the Western democracies and their former wartime ally. In response, the Truman administration in 1949 put together the North Atlantic Treaty Organization, a regional European defense alliance, but in practice the United States relied on its growing arsenal of nuclear weapons to deter Soviet expansion. Overrating the new weapon's usefulness, the nation came to rely on its nuclear supremacy as the mainstay of its defense strategy, a reliance that ultimately was at the expense of conventional forces.

But reform also became a feature of postwar military policy. The war had demonstrated the necessity for a joint service structure, and postwar pressures to economize helped to spur unification of the armed forces through the National Security Act of 1947. That law created the National Military Establishment (in 1949 renamed the Department of Defense [DOD]) with separate Departments of the Army, Navy, and Air Force. Defense medical programs were integrated through the establishment of a Medical Services Division in the Office of the Secretary of Defense in May 1949. Soon renamed the Office of Medical Services, it was the seed of central control of the military medical establishment. Although it was controversial from the beginning, in time it would offer position opportunities for MSC officers who would figure prominently in the DOD medical policy formulation process.[2]

The postwar emphasis on centralized control and efficiency severely challenged the Medical Department's planners.[3] Army medical programs now had to fit into the entire DOD medical apparatus, and issues of cost and efficiency figured prominently in planning decisions. At the same time, progress in medical technology had expanded demand for medical care from a peacetime army that was still larger than any other in U.S. history. Pressure for quality health care for both military dependents and an expanding retired military population magnified the effect. Growth in the number of eligible beneficiaries represented an increasing cost for the taxpayer and a loss of a potential source of revenue for the civilian health care industry. Nevertheless, the need to maintain a large standing army and the acceptance of the commitment to care for soldiers and their families ultimately forced the Army Medical Department to operate a substantial peacetime medical establishment.[4]

Congress' gradual acceptance of the Medical Department's expanded responsibilities, as well as the role of the nation as a world power, produced a series of policies that kept the organization of the Army's health care structure in flux. For example, Medical Administrative Corps and Sanitary Corps officers could apply for appointments in the Regular Army Pharmacy Corps, whose authorization was increased from 72 to 1,022 officers in 1946. The War Department waived the requirement for a pharmacy degree, but stipulated that applicants had to be graduates of colleges acceptable to the surgeon general and in fields that would qualify them for further training in sanitary engineering, office management, hospital administration, business administration, medical supply, parasitology, entomology, optometry, pharmacy, bacteriology, serology, clinical psychology, or social work.[5]

Over twenty-five hundred officers applied for integration into the Regular Army Pharmacy Corps. Col. Louis Williams, PC, a member of the selection board, said that the Army could pick and choose from a wide variety of candidates. He personally looked for applicants with a degree in business administration or a good background in administration—and anyone with a law degree. "So far as I know, not a single one ever let us down in a single way." Based on the board's recommendations, 728 officers were integrated into the Regular Army in 1946 and 1947. One, Capt. Jimmie Kanaya, was the first American officer of Japanese descent accepted into the Regular Army MAC. Another, Capt. William E. Gott, was the first black given a Regular Army commission in the Pharmacy Corps.[6]

Termination of the Army Specialized Training Program (ASTP) in 1946 and demobilization of the armed forces reduced the strength of the Medical Corps to a level that jeopardized the Medical Department's ability to perform its expanded health care mission. The Army found that it could persuade very few physicians to remain on active duty in a system that offered no promise of clinical excellence. The problem was so great that the under secretary of war was concerned: "Most of the civilian doctors in uniform were fed up with the Army. The situation was serious."[7]

Part of the solution to the problem resided in restoring the surgeon general's influence in management of the department's personnel so as to provide as much flexibility as possible in handling the Army's medical personnel assets. In other words it was necessary to regain the central medical direction lost during the war. In June 1947 the War Department returned career planning responsibility for all Medical Department personnel to the surgeon general and followed that up a year later with control over all assignment actions. The surgeon general now had the authority to "assign and reassign Medical Department personnel across command lines, if necessary, quickly and expeditiously as necessity dictates." It was a major policy shift.[8]

Another part of the solution was the return of physicians from administrative positions to the practice of medicine. When drafted physicians were released from military service, the Regular Army Medical Corps officers remaining on active duty had no choice but to resume clinical practice. However, all but six Regular Army physicians had been assigned to administrative positions during the war, and they had lost touch with medicine. Maj. Gen. Raymond W. Bliss, Kirk's successor as surgeon general from 1947 to 1951, believed that the prewar Medical Corps "had been isolated from the main stream of American medicine."[9] He was determined to prevent that from happening again.

The department arranged for refresher training programs at medical schools and hospitals throughout the country to infuse contemporary clinical standards into the Medical Corps and to motivate senior physicians to seek specialty training. Forty officers were placed at thirteen institutions in 1946, and MAC officers replaced those who had been serving in administrative positions. The Army's Internship and Residency Program, begun in February 1946, was an important part of the sustained effort to improve the competency of Army physicians. Simultaneously, the department stepped up the recruiting of new physicians to fill Medical Corps vacancies. Furthermore, the department vigorously pressed for dependent care and residency training as incentives to attract the best physicians to a military career.[10]

The department had also learned lessons in field medical support from its wartime experience in eleven theaters of operation. The Medical Field Service School, which moved in 1946 from Carlisle Barracks, Pennsylvania, to Fort Sam Houston, Texas, sought to incorporate those lessons into current doctrine.[11] In the process, the doctrinal dichotomy between conserving the fighting strength and clearing the battlefield was tilted in favor of the former with the idea that "treatment should be conducted as far forward as possible" in order to stem the loss of troop strength from a combat zone.[12] To put this into effect, the department estimated that the medical force available to the Army's regiments would have to be tripled.[13]

The first three echelons of medical service were thus beefed up based on the lessons of World War II. At the first echelon, the regimental level of medical service, the medical sections of the maneuver battalions became medical platoons. The regimental medical detachment became a company that fielded two collecting detachments and an evacuation detachment. This company provided the regiment with two collecting stations as well as field ambulances for evacuating patients from the battalion aid stations of the maneuver battalions.

Division medical service was the second level of the combat zone. There, the division medical battalion was changed to provide a more elaborate treatment capability. The three collecting companies of World War II were gone. The battalion now consisted of three clearing companies and an ambulance company of thirty field ambulances. The clearing companies provided a clearing station for each regiment (to back up the regimental collection stations and the battalion aid stations) as well as an ambulance platoon in support of each regimental medical company.

The third level of medical service featured an important new unit, the Mobile Army Surgical Hospital, or MASH, a field hospital added in 1948. It evolved out of the 25-bed Portable Surgical Hospital, a self-contained unit for support of divisions that had been developed for jungle fighting and amphibious operations in World War II.[14] The MASH was a mobile, sixty-bed, surgical hospital whose staff included two MSC officers, fourteen physicians, and twelve nurses. Field army medical service included other units that fleshed out the evacuation chain. Plans and operations officers could pick hospital units from the same array of hospitals used in World War II, including a 400-bed semimobile evacuation hospital established on the basis of one per division and a 750-bed evacuation hospital for each corps. Medical logistics support was to be provided throughout a theater by medical supply depots consisting of two advance platoons and a base platoon. The depot, a unit of 200 personnel, had doubled in size and its number of vehicles had increased. The fourth and fifth echelons—the communications zone and the zone of the interior—remained essentially unchanged.

There had been considerable progress during World War II in long-range air evacuation using large Air Force aircraft, but there was no comparable widespread development in forward air evacuation using light Army aircraft. Postwar progress in aviation technology advanced the capabilities of helicopters, the ideal vehicle for frontline air evacuation, and the Army tested Sikorsky H–18s for air evacuation in 1949. The tests of the helicopters, which carried two litters and an attendant, were successful, but there was no initiative to organize Army helicopter ambulance units. The stimulus for that would come later with combat action in Korea.[15]

Creation of the Medical Service Corps

There was no longer any question of the permanent need for administrative and scientific specialty officers, both to serve in positions formerly filled by physicians and to provide expertise in new technologies. The Medical Department quickly realized that it could not sustain its operations without permanent access to those specialties, but the Regular Army Pharmacy Corps was not sufficient for that purpose. As the department looked to the future, an important key to its ability to fulfill its mission would be the formation of a permanent corps for the officers on active duty in the administrative and scientific specialties, a group which numbered 3,155 at the end of 1946.[16]

In January 1946 the surgeon general, Maj. Gen. Norman T. Kirk, proposed the establishment of a medical service corps (MSC) that would consolidate the officers of the Sanitary Corps, Medical Administrative Corps, and Pharmacy Corps. General Kirk believed it was an essential step in placing the postwar department on a solid footing. The Surgeon General's Office estimated a requirement of 1,500 Regular Army MSC officers for an army of 500,000 soldiers, or 2,325 officers for an army of 750,000 soldiers, or roughly three MSC officers per 1,000 active duty soldiers.[17]

Kirk's proposal was initially opposed by leaders of organized pharmacy, who, embittered by what they viewed as cavalier treatment by the Army, wished to preserve a separate pharmacy corps. However, Kirk undertook a campaign in 1946 to sell them on his plan through a series of meetings and bargaining sessions. He was assisted by Maj. Bernard Aabel, PC, whom he had made his assistant for pharmacy affairs. Aabel was a graduate pharmacist assigned to the Surgeon General's Office as an assignment officer for members of the Medical Administrative, Sanitary, and Pharmacy Corps. He became the go-between for pharmacy issues in his new additional duty.

Aabel's lobbying paid off. In June 1946 Arthur H. Einbeck, chairman of the Committee on Status of Pharmacists in the Government Service, issued a paper that identified positions throughout the Medical Department that could be filled by pharmacists.[18] General Kirk accepted Einbeck's formulation and pledged a leading role for pharmacists in the proposed MSC. In November, Einbeck emerged from a summit meeting with the surgeon general to announce his committee's support: "The flag of pharmacy would wave just as freely and importantly" in the MSC Pharmacy Section as it would in a separate corps.[19] Harmony between the surgeon general and the leaders of organized pharmacy cleared the way for congressional action.

On 20 February 1947, the House Committee on Armed Services began hearings on H.R. 1982, a bill "to establish a permanent Medical Service Corps in the Medical Department of the Regular Army." The corps would consist of sections for pharmacy, medical administrative sciences, optometry, and other groups deemed necessary by the secretary of war. There would be a chief appointed by the secretary of war as well as assistant chiefs of the corps appointed as chiefs of the sections.

Congresswoman Margaret Chase Smith, the committee chairman, opened the hearings by observing that H.R. 1982, the Army Medical Service Corps (MSC) legislation, was quite similar to two proposals for a Navy MSC: H.R. 1361, which would establish commissioned medical administrators in the Navy's Hospital Corps, and H.R. 1603, which would establish a Navy Medical Associated Sciences Corps consisting of 205 officers. Mrs. Smith had the three bills considered as a single group since they were all dealing with the same specialties. The Army and Navy proposals differed principally in their approaches to commissioning. The Army desired a college degree as a prerequisite while the Navy wanted to keep the way open for commissioning from the ranks of enlisted personnel.[20]

The committee heard testimony from representatives of national pharmacy organizations. They agreed to support the establishment of a separate pharmacy, supply, and administration section within the Medical Service Corps if certain conditions were met, including the appointment of a pharmacist as chief of that section and a requirement that pharmacists constitute a minimum of 80 percent of its strength. The surgeon general agreed to that stipulation and further promised that he would see to it that most accessions to the section each year would be pharmacists.[21]

Representatives of other scientific specialty guilds also had their say, and then threw in with Kirk's proposed corps. Henry M. Chick, representing the National Society of Professional Engineers, feared that sanitary engineers would become a minority group and lose the advantages they had enjoyed in the Sanitary Corps. Nevertheless, he agreed to support the MSC as long as it had a separate section for sanitary engineering. William C. Ezell, O.D., former president of the American Optometric Association, reiterated the arguments for a separate optometry corps, but acquiesced in the legislative proposal for an MSC by offering an amendment requiring that the chief of the optometry section be a graduate of a recognized school or college of optometry. The MSC proposal was rolling, and Lester A. Walsh, D.P.M., representing the National Association of Chiropodists, tried to include his specialty on the bandwagon. Walsh pointed out that chiropody was recognized by the American Medical Association, and he asked that the Army follow the Navy's lead in commissioning chiropodists. The timing was not right for the inclusion of chiropody, however, and Walsh's desire was not fulfilled.[22]

Some in the Medical Department opposed consolidation. Sanitary Corps scientific specialty officers assigned to the Headquarters, Seventh Service Command, did not like the idea of being integrated with MAC officers, many of whom were OCS graduates without a college degree. The Sanitary Corps officers believed they should have an advantage over MAC officers commissioned from the ranks without an educational level comparable to theirs. As matters stood, they received no credit toward promotion for the years they spent in training. Col. William A. Hardenbergh, SnC, the senior Army sanitary engineer, was outspoken. He strenuously opposed any efforts to dismantle the Sanitary Corps, believing that it would be impossible to merge scientific and administrative specialty officers in the same group. He claimed that sanitary engineers were uniformly against formation of the MSC, and he lobbied unceasingly for preservation of the Sanitary Corps. Hardenbergh never did reconcile himself to consolidation, and he remained a vocal critic after his retirement from the Army.[23]

General Kirk, gratified by the overall support for an MSC, testified that he now envisioned an active duty requirement for 1,650 MSC officers. He told Congress that he would accept the responsibility of seeing that the best individuals would head each section of the corps. To buttress his argument for an MSC, he had two young Pharmacy Corps officers testify in support of the legislation. Maj. James B. Baty, a sanitary engineer assigned to the Surgeon General's Preventive Medicine Division, believed the new corps would be advantageous for both the Army and the members of the corps. Kirk's assistant for pharmacy, Major

Aabel, agreed. Aabel, a pharmacist in civilian life, had entered active duty from the reserves in 1941 as a Medical Administrative Corps officer, later receiving a Regular Army commission in the Pharmacy Corps. He had received a purple heart as the S–2 and liaison officer for the 68th Medical Group in the ETO. Since March 1946 he had served in the Surgeon General's Personnel Division as the assistant to the chief of the Classification and Records Branch, in which capacity he was responsible for managing Sanitary Corps, Medical Administrative Corps, and Pharmacy Corps officers. He believed that it was appropriate to consolidate the three corps in order to develop the leadership and specialization necessary for the Medical Department's execution of its mission. "I personally think it will work," he testified.[24]

Kirk's proposal became law on 4 August 1947 when Congress passed the Army-Navy Medical Services Corps Act of 1947.[25] The law established Medical Service Corps in both the Army and the Navy. It abolished the Army's Medical Administrative Corps, Sanitary Corps, and Pharmacy Corps and established the Army MSC with four sections: Pharmacy, Supply, and Administration; Medical Allied Sciences; Sanitary Engineering; and Optometry. The strength of the corps would be established by the secretary of war, but Congress set a ceiling on MSC colonels at 2 percent of the strength of the Regular Army Medical Service Corps. Unfortunately, the 2 percent figure was based on an estimate of the number of positions for Regular Army colonels which then existed among the precursor groups and was a figure considerably less than the 8 percent figure used for other branches of the Army. The 2 percent limit would bedevil the first chief of the corps.[26]

The move to establish a Regular Army Medical Service Corps for male officers paralleled the creation in 1947 of a Regular Army corps for female officers serving as physical therapists, occupational therapists, and dietitians, specialties that were at that time almost completely handled by women. It was necessary to create a separate corps because there was no provision for commissioning women in a male corps; otherwise they would have been included in the establishment of the Medical Service Corps. On 16 April President Truman signed the Army-Navy Nurses Act of 1947, which established the Women's Medical Specialist Corps (renamed the Army Medical Specialist Corps in 1955).[27]

Establishment of the Air Force led in 1949 to the formation of a third military medical department along with an Air Force Medical Service Corps. Maj. Leo Benade, MSC, along with Maj. (later Maj. Gen.) Ralph Richards, MSC, headed the Special Projects Branch of the Surgeon General's Personnel Division, which was set up to handle the transfer of Army Medical Department assets, including those of the Medical Service Corps, to the Air Force.[28]

The Formative Years of the New Corps

The formative years of the Medical Service Corps were characterized by efforts to increase the number of officers on active duty, the establishment of policies governing their employment, and planning for the variety of specialties that comprised the four sections. On 24 September 1947, a board appointed by the surgeon general selected Col. Othmar Goriup, MSC, as first chief of the corps (*see Appendix G*). Colonel Goriup was a graduate pharmacist and a fellow of the American College of Apothecaries, and General Armstrong hoped the appointment would gratify the pharmacy profession. Goriup's wartime service had been principally with the Army Air Corps, and when selected chief of the MSC he was serving in the Office of the Air Surgeon on the War Department Staff. He said that when he moved to the Surgeon General's Office it was unfamiliar territory. "I knew only about two people in the Army, and in addition to that, I knew nothing about Army operation."[29]

For the first time the Medical Department's administrative and scientific specialty officers had a permanently appointed head responsible for their organization, administration, career planning, and employment. Goriup appointed Major Benade, a most accomplished officer, as his assistant, and the two officers constituted the Office of the Chief, Medical Service Corps. The selection of the four assistant chiefs did not go as smoothly. A board selected officers for three of the four assistant chief positions in October 1947, but only one successfully made it through the nomination process—Maj. Ludwig R. Kuhn, MSC, who was sworn in as chief of the Medical Allied Sciences Section in May 1948.

The surgeon general convened a second board. Its selections were acted upon on 14 March 1949, when Brig. Gen. George E. Armstrong, the deputy surgeon general, swore in three MSC assistant chiefs. Lt. Col. Charles S. Gersoni, MSC, replaced Major Kuhn as chief of the Medical Allied Sciences Section. Maj. John V. Painter, MSC, became chief of the Pharmacy, Supply, and Administration Section, and Lt. Col. Raymond J. Karpen, MSC, became the chief of the Sanitary Engineering Section. The optometry slot was not filled. The surgeon general had personally rejected the first board's choice, and, with just a few optometrists in the Army, the second board had little to choose from.[30]

All three assistant chiefs were assigned to the Surgeon General's Office where, in accordance with the board's recommendation, they handled corps responsibilities as an additional duty. Karpen noted that the assistant chiefs of the corps "became excellent tight rope walkers" as they balanced the demands of their full-time positions with the additional duty of planning for their specialty areas. Colonel Goriup also relied on the Medical Service Corps Advisory Council, established in March 1948, for policy recommendations, but the body fell into disuse under subsequent chiefs and was ineffective.[31]

Excitement over the establishment of the corps was punctured by the reality of the hard work facing the chief's office. As Major Benade put it, "we had the legislation, but now what?"[32] Postwar demands on the Army and concomitant requirements for medical support meant that the new corps must grow. An essential task was determining how to achieve that growth. Goriup and Benade undertook the lengthy process of establishing position requirements for MSC officers in the Army's manning documents.[33]

The job of pulling disparate specialties into a cohesive whole was made more difficult by various vocal interest groups. In December 1947 Goriup was invited to speak at the annual meeting of the Association of Military Surgeons of the United States, representing quick acceptance of the new corps by a well-estab-

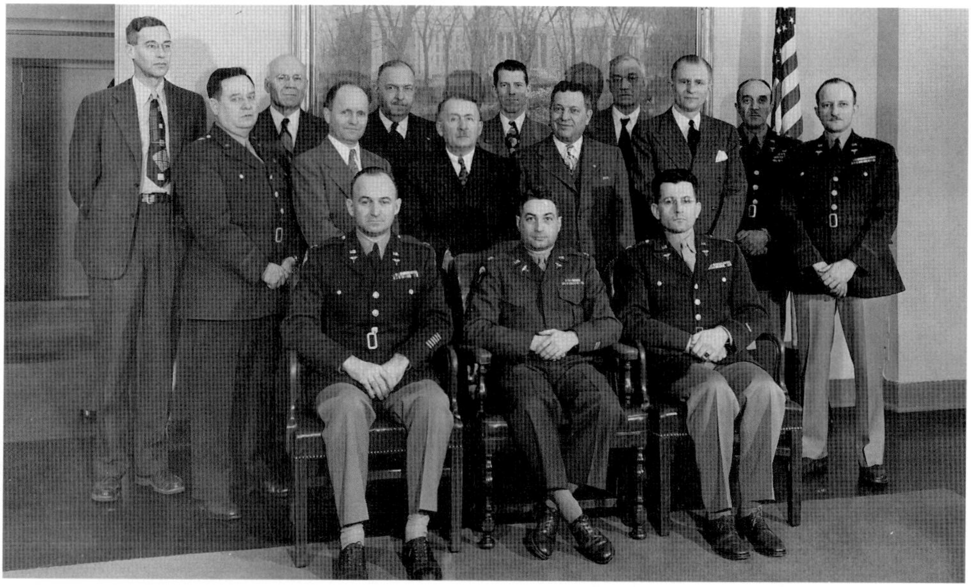

Colonels Karpen and Gersoni and Major Painter (seated, left to right) *after being sworn in, March 1949. General Armstrong is standing second from right.*

lished group.[34] But such instant acquiescence was unusual, and Goriup found himself on the road for his first two years in office, mending fences and performing "constant missionary work." In the end, he believed that the effort was successful, welding "the numerous professional groups of the Medical Service Corps into one harmonious whole."[35]

One of the early problems the chief faced was an artifact of the 1947 legislation, which had unintentionally created a promotion inequity. As a result of a quirk in the law, about forty MSC officers who had been integrated into the Regular Army in 1947 became junior in permanent grade to other officers whom they outranked in their active duty temporary grade, creating a great deal of resentment. That imbalance was corrected in 1949 by special legislation.

The 2 percent cap on colonels was an irritant from the outset, and Colonel Goriup explored ways to seek relief from the inequity almost immediately after assuming office. He floated a proposal for a legislative remedy in 1949, but his effort was not fully embraced by the Medical Department's leaders. Brig. Gen. Silas B. Hays, chief of the Surgeon General's Supply Division, for example, disagreed strongly. Although proclaiming himself "a strong booster of the MSC," Hays believed the department should proceed slowly over a three- to four-year period before lifting the promotion cap. During that time it could create more slots for MSC colonels while it gradually groomed officers for promotion to colonel by placing them in more responsible jobs.[36]

In 1947 General Bliss instituted daily meetings with his key staff, who were encouraged "to let their hair down."[37] They did, and the typed summaries of those morning meetings, prepared over the next twenty-two years by Arlyne Fransway,

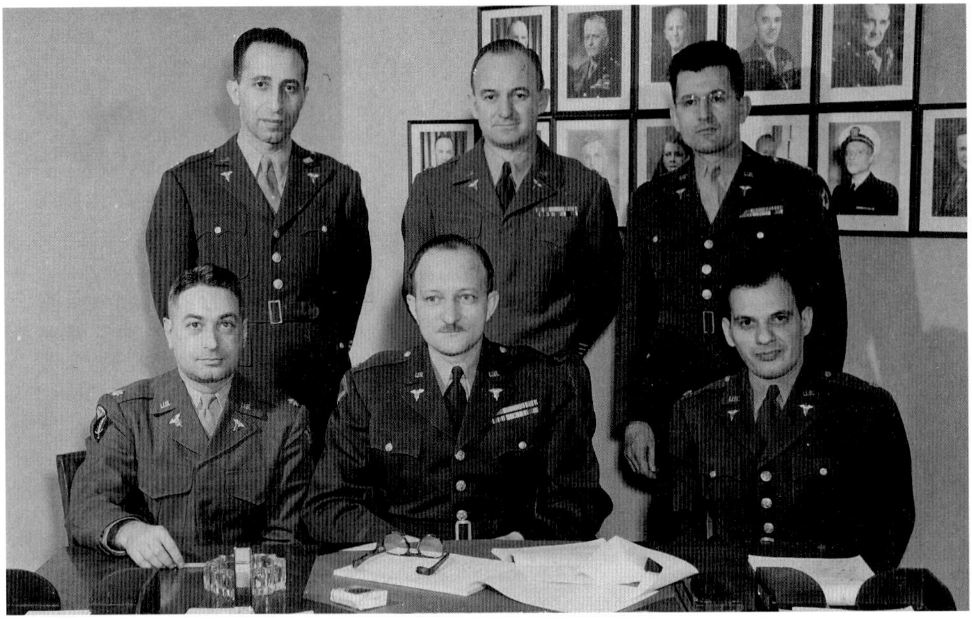

Colonel Goriup (seated, center) *and staff. Major Benade is seated at right.*

the surgeon general's secretary, are an invaluable historical resource. The proper role of the MSC was a frequent topic of discussion. General Bliss made it clear he desired that the four assistant corps chiefs should be "dual-hatted" with a full-time assignment in their specialty, while performing their corps responsibilities as an additional duty. The exception would be Colonel Goriup, who worked full time in the Office of the Surgeon General.[38]

The demand for MSC officers quickly accelerated. As usual, the shortage of Army physicians was a major incentive. In February 1948 the Regular Army Medical Corps was authorized 3,000 officers, but only 1,200 were on active duty. The pressure to free up physicians for clinical duties became so intense that at one point Goriup listed the replacement of physicians as the sole mission of the Medical Service Corps. The urgency of the physician shortage was so great that in March 1948 the Army authorized a recall to active duty of 300 Medical Service Corps officers, a number that was raised to 800 in September. But at mid-month it had recalled only 165 officers, and the department was advertising vacancies for 500 lieutenants and captains in administrative and scientific specialties.[39]

Recruiting of physicians continued to lag significantly behind MSC recruitment, and some positions that legitimately required officers with medical training were of necessity filled by MSCs. Examples in 1948 were Maj. Gary C. Hill, MSC, division surgeon of the 7th Infantry Division, and Capt. William H. Thornt, MSC, division surgeon of the 6th Infantry Division.[40] Some MSC officers assumed dispensary medical duties akin to the sick call responsibilities of battalion surgeon's assistants. This assumption of clinical duties was necessitated by the physician shortage and because many Medical Corps officers were dissatisfied with dispensary duty. Col. Paul I. Robinson, MC, chief of the Surgeon General's Personnel Division, suggested assigning MSC pharmacy officers to dispensaries where they would provide routine medical care. This, he argued, would make pharmacists happier, while relieving the physicians of "tedious work."[41] General Bliss rejected Robinson's idea because the use of MSCs to conduct military sick call was tantamount to "poor house" medical care for soldiers.[42]

The department was scrutinized in a succession of probes. Physician manpower was a major issue each time, and the constant refrain was to use physicians only in positions that required medical training. The Committee on Medical and Hospital Services of the Armed Forces was typical in this regard. Called the Hawley Committee for its chairman, Maj. Gen. Paul Hawley, MC, USA, Ret. (chief surgeon of the European Theater of Operations in World War II), its report demanded the "full use of non-professional officers in administrative positions in peace and in war."[43] A 1952 survey of 2,359 Medical Corps officers had a 75 percent response rate with an unequivocal message. Physicians assigned to field medical units—all in a peacetime garrison status—were overwhelmingly dissatisfied; 90 percent believed they had insufficient opportunity to use their medical training. The study recommended expanded utilization of MSC officers.[44]

Yet there were not even enough MSCs to fill all the positions opened by the policy of replacement and substitution of Medical Corps officers. As an example, sixteen MSCs at Fort Knox had diminished to eight, which prevented the release of physicians from administrative duties. "Now MCs will do everything *but* professional work," said a member of the surgeon general's staff.[45] The department also considered adding chiropody to its commissioned specialties as a means of easing the demand for physicians. By the fall of 1947 there was agreement within the Medical Department's senior leadership that chiropodists would be acceptable for commissioning in the MSC. However, that would not actually occur for another decade.[46]

To complicate matters, the surgeon general's staff gave Colonel Goriup conflicting guidance on the problem of increasing the number of active duty MSC officers. Some said the department should "lower its sights" in selecting officers for recall to active duty if it were to succeed in obtaining the number required.[47] Others suggested it should be more selective. General Bliss, for one, cautioned that he had begun to hear disparaging remarks about MSC officers, a sentiment that was echoed by Maj. Gen. Paul H. Streit, MC, commander of Walter Reed General Hospital. Streit said he had some very ineffective MSC officers assigned to his command. "Colonel Goriup should be informed to watch his corps most carefully and hand-pick his officers if possible."[48]

In fact, Colonel Goriup had been extremely attentive to the concerns of the surgeon general and others about the need to improve the quality of MSC officers. At one point characterizing portions of the early corps as "an army of gas station attendants and ex-shoe clerks,"[49] he was determined to reverse that situation, selecting only 349 of nearly 2,000 applicants for MSC commissions from 1949 to 1950. Colonel Goriup and Major Benade thus elected to remain selective while trying to improve opportunities in the corps so as to make MSC careers more attractive to high-quality officers. Due to their attention, pharmacy ROTC programs were established in July 1948 at four universities: California, Wisconsin, Minnesota, and Ohio State, and nine distinguished military graduates from ROTC programs were appointed in the MSC in 1949.[50]

Goriup believed that education and training were the best route to improving the recruitment and retention of the best officers. He took great pride in the establishment of opportunities for graduate training, which opened in 1949 for a wide variety of areas, particularly entomology, bacteriology, clinical psychology, public health, and other sciences. Eleven MSCs entered graduate programs that year, and by 1950 there were thirty-seven officers pursuing university training in fields ranging from hospital administration to radiochemistry, and two officers were in a training-in-industry program.

They also paid attention to the opportunities for military schooling. In 1950, a representative year, four officers attended the regular course of both the Armed Forces Staff College and the Command and General Staff College. One was Lt. Col. Floyd Berry, MSC, the first sanitary engineer to attend the Fort Leavenworth course. At the Medical Field Service School another eighty-five MSC officers attended various military courses in 1950, including a 26-week Officer Basic Course and a new Hospital Administration Course.[51]

The efforts in recruiting and retention paid off in rapid growth. In December 1948 there were only 1,022 MSC officers on active duty. By June 1950 the corps had more than doubled to 2,715, of which 588 were Regular Army officers. At the end of 1951 there were 4,976 officers on active duty, a number that included 70 Women's Army Corps officers detailed to the MSC and 621 Regular Army officers.[52]

The department was determined to have an insignia for MSC officers distinctly different from members of the Medical, Dental, and Veterinary Corps, all of whom could be called "doctor"—even though some MSCs held doctoral degrees. The idea was that members of the Medical Administrative Corps, Sanitary Corps, and Pharmacy Corps were sometimes mistakenly addressed as "doctor" because of their gold caduceus. Some physicians had the notion that this could prove embarrassing when someone unfamiliar with Army insignia asked medical questions.[53]

In fact, the Surgeon General's Office had broached the matter of an insignia with the War Department Staff while Congress was still considering the establishment of the MSC. The Quartermaster General's Office suggested using the same caduceus for both the Medical Service Corps and the Women's Medical Specialist Corps by superimposing an "M" on the insignia in one case and a "W" for the other. The Surgeon General's Office rejected the idea out of hand and proposed other designs. One was a black cross of Malta and a thunderbolt on a round shield. Another was a gold cross of Malta on a silver caduceus for the Medical Service Corps and a round shield with a thunderbolt on a silver caduceus for the Women's Medical Specialist Corps. The Quartermaster General's Office rejected those alternatives and fell back to its original proposal, which was the one finally approved on 11 December 1947.[54] The MSC insignia became black enamel letters "MS" superimposed on a silver caduceus. It was identical to the Women's Medical Specialist Corps with the exception of inverting the "M" to form a "W."[55]

The story of the insignia did not end there, because the silver versus gold controversy persisted for years. Colonel Goriup, while on a visit to Letterman General Hospital in San Francisco, California, had an argument over it with the hospital commander, Brig. Gen. Leonard D. Heaton. The MSC chief raised Heaton's hackles when he brought up the subject of a single caduceus for all the corps of the Medical Department. "I really got upset about it," said Heaton, "and let him know in no uncertain language that I would fight him to the finish if he proposed such a thing as that because we would never, never acquiesce to wearing the same insignia that the Medical Service Corps wore because that was downgrading the Medical Corps."[56]

The Army-Baylor Program

A desire to improve the training of officers of all Medical Department officer corps, especially the Medical Service Corps, for management positions in Army hospitals led to the founding of the Hospital Administration Course in 1947 at the Medical Field Service School. The course, which in 1951 became the Army–Baylor University Program in Hospital Administration, was the twelfth such program established in the United States and one of ten formed in the rapid expansion of graduate programs in hospital administration between World War II and the Korean War.[57]

The Army-Baylor Program provided immediate returns to the Medical Department and served the Army well in the years that followed. It was championed by Maj. Gen. Joseph I. Martin, MC, commandant of the Medical Field Service School. Martin's wartime experience as the Fifth Army surgeon in Italy had convinced him of the need for trained administrators, and he persuaded the surgeon general to support establishing a course. Col. Byron L. Steger, MC, who had served with Martin in the Far East, was an important ally as chief of the Surgeon General's Education and Training Division.

The three-month-long Hospital Administration Course was organized according to a program of instruction developed by Lt. Col. James T. Richards, MSC. Richards had completed a master's in hospital administration at Northwestern University in 1947 and returned to San Antonio where he joined other MSC graduate hospital administrators such as Lt. Cols. Gordon McCleary, Howard Scroggs, and Sam Edwards to form a core faculty for the Hospital Administration Course.[58]

The first class began in November 1947 with 40 students: 1 Canadian, 25 Army Nurse Corps, and 14 MSC officers. The staff of eight officers and one civilian employee was headed by Col. Dale L. Thompson, MSC, the first director. The second class entered in 1948, when Richards replaced Thompson as the director. The third and fourth classes entered in 1949, the fifth in 1950, and one class entered annually thereafter. The course was lengthened several times: to 20 weeks in 1949, to 33 weeks in 1950, and to 39 weeks in 1951. The weekly course schedule was based upon eight hours of classes per day for five days a week; the class size ranged from thirty-six to sixty students. The curriculum covered academic subjects such as statistics and accounting as well as military medicine. Army Nurse

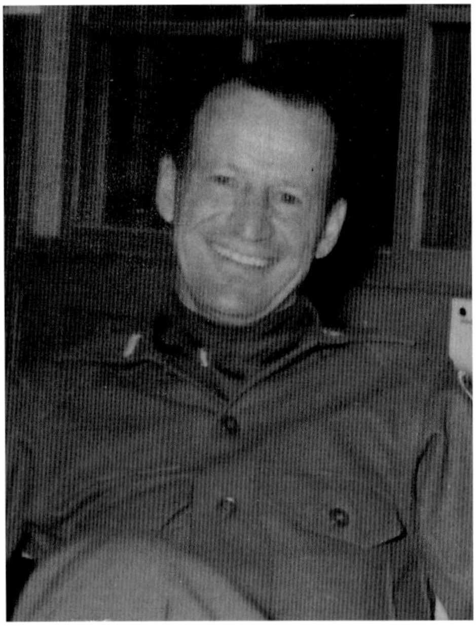

Colonel Richards

Corps officers made up 61 percent of the 178 students in the first four classes, and a separate nursing administration course to accommodate their special requirements began in 1950. Although the Medical Department also sent Medical Corps officers to civilian hospital administration programs after the war, including four officers in 1949, physicians subsequently attended the Army-Baylor Program.[59]

Initially, no students in the Hospital Administration Course possessed a baccalaureate degree, and not until 1950 were any officers enrolled who were eligible for academic recognition at the graduate level. Yet its supporters believed the course would have to affiliate with a university if it was to play an influential role in establishing the profession of hospital administration in the Army. Colonel Richards' desire for affiliation was facilitated by a friend of his, Professor Hardy A. Kemp, M.D., a bacteriologist who had wartime service in the Medical Corps and was a member of the Loyal Order of the Boar. During a chance meeting in the summer of 1949, Kemp, then the director of graduate studies of Baylor University's College of Medicine, suggested that Richards try to affiliate the course with Baylor. Richards discussed the idea with General Martin, who supported it, and in August 1950 he presented the proposal to the executive council of Baylor University's Graduate School.

Richards was assisted by Maj. Harry Panhorst, MSC. Panhorst, a military intelligence officer in World War II, was then associate director of the Washington University Program in Hospital Administration and a reservist on a three-week active duty tour at Brooke Army Medical Center. He provided the council a favorable report he had prepared on behalf of Malcolm T. MacEachern, M.D., who had been Richards' program director at Northwestern. MacEachern was a pioneer in hospital administration and a member of the Association of University Programs in Hospital Administration, and his sponsorship of the Army-Baylor Program carried a great deal of weight. The Baylor Executive Council voted its unanimous support, and the proposal then went to the Office of the Surgeon General for submission to the Army Staff. However, in a surprising setback, the Surgeon General's Office refused to forward the proposal because it believed the request would need a stronger justification in order to gain approval.[60]

The reversal was greatly disappointing to Colonel Goriup. "To say this job of mine has been fraught with heartaches would be a further understatement. The action on Baylor affiliation is the greatest heartache of them all." He told Richards

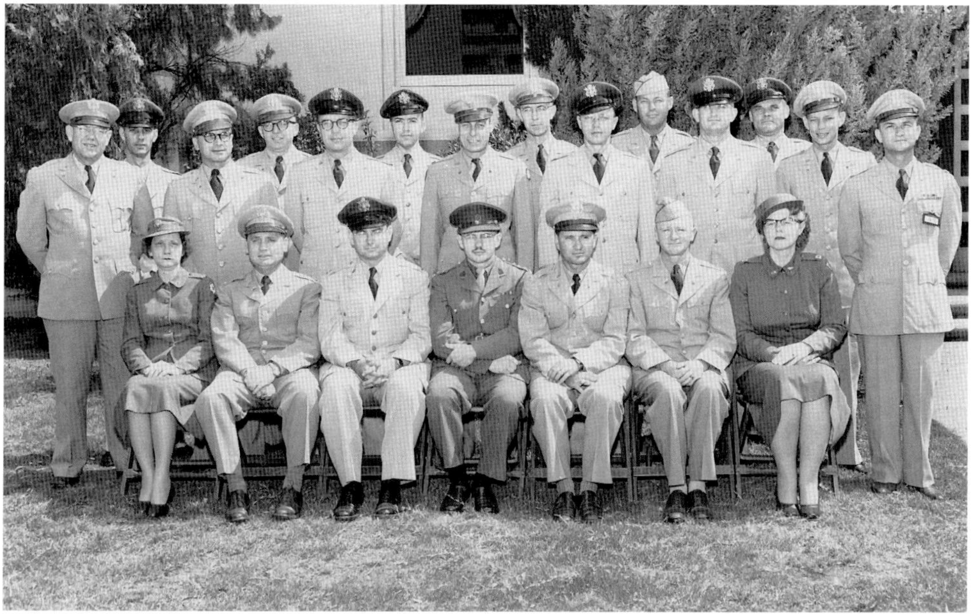

Officer graduates of the Hospital Administration Course, Medical Field Service School, May 1953

to wait for the right time to reopen the issue, and in the meantime to be patient. "Please bear with us a little longer, Tommy. I can't but feel that we must charge our *temporary* setback off to growing pains."[61]

General Martin provided a strengthened justification in September, and Colonel Steger submitted the proposal to the Army Staff, where it was disapproved. This time Martin called on friends in the Army Staff for help. He also asked for assistance from Fred A. McNamara, chief of the Hospital Branch of the Bureau of the Budget (forerunner of the Office of Management and Budget). McNamara, "an unusually gifted man," was an important influence on the Medical Department. He had been instrumental the year before in establishing another pioneering course, the Inter-Agency Institute of Hospital Administrators, later renamed the Interagency Institute for Federal Health Care Executives.[62]

Martin's efforts produced results. The Army Staff withdrew its objection in March 1951, but with a stipulation that prohibited any formal affiliation with Baylor of a contractual nature, including any appointments of the program's instructors to unremunerated Baylor faculty positions. The assistant chief of staff, G–3, harbored reservations over entanglements with universities, principally due to concerns over legal implications, and had turned down similar requests (including one from the Army War College) for affiliation with civilian universities. There was also a concern that the Army must pursue training with military requirements in mind and not fund graduate training for the personal benefit of officers who could enhance their civilian job opportunities at the Army's expense. Baylor accepted the affiliation on the Army's terms in September 1951.[63]

The connection with a respected university was an important step in the Army-Baylor Program's maturation. Richards was determined that the course be academically respectable rather than a diploma mill. That was a view shared by Goriup, who asked Richards if the students were motivated and "striving to do just a little more than is expected and assigned to them."[64] Indeed, one of the concerns over affiliating with Baylor was that most students in the course were not eligible to matriculate in the Baylor Graduate School. So many students were academically deficient that the program had added a thirty-hour remedial reading course, and in 1950 only three students met Baylor's prerequisites for graduate school admission.[65] Students who were not college graduates could enroll for a bachelor of science in business administration. Meanwhile, Baylor appointed Richards as an associate professor of hospital administration. This became the customary pattern for the program's faculty members, in spite of the original stipulations by the Army Staff.

With the program affiliated with Baylor, the next step in ensuring academic respectability was to seek accreditation from the Association of University Programs in Hospital Administration (AUPHA), the national organization that set standards for training in health care administration. Richards undertook an aggressive campaign. A key part of his strategy was the cultivation of prominent leaders in the health care industry, whom he invited to San Antonio as guest speakers in the course. He was assisted in this by Colonel Steger from Steger's position in Washington. Richards was able to use those visits as opportunities for personal diplomacy, and the efforts paid off.[66]

Professor MacEachern agreed to sponsor the program's application for accreditation, and the AUPHA granted provisional accreditation at a special meeting in September 1951. Students who met the prerequisites of Baylor Graduate School were then eligible to work toward an accredited master's degree. Baylor submitted the program for full AUPHA membership the following January, and Colonel Richards and his staff hosted the association's annual meeting that spring in a smoothly organized event at Fort Sam Houston. Richards was pleased. "By now we were 'accepted' and had a group of nation-wide ambassadors of good will." The application was approved and the Army-Baylor Program became a member of the AUPHA. The accreditation by an external agency followed the examples of hospital accreditation surveys and approval of physician residency training programs, a pattern of external certification that became fully accepted throughout the military medical services.[67]

Administrative Specialty Officers

MSC administrative specialty officers continued their service to the Army in the tradition of expanded roles pioneered by their predecessors. The inspector general (IG) position in the general hospitals was one opportunity opened to MSC officers during this period. The prerequisites desired by the Surgeon General's Office for detail to an IG position were high, specifying an officer who was a graduate hospital administrator and had broad experience at all levels of the hospital organization, including a tour as an executive officer.[68]

Another out-of-the-ordinary position opportunity was medical intelligence. Four officers were assigned as assistant attaches to Finland, Iraq, the Soviet Union, and Thailand during this period. Major Aabel was one of those, being assigned to the American embassy in Finland shortly after testifying for the formation of the MSC in 1947. Aabel completed a training and orientation program en route, including the Strategic Intelligence School in Washington, D.C., and reported to Helsinki in March 1948 as the assistant military attache. He held that position until July 1951 when he returned to the United States to attend the Army War College. Fluent in Norwegian and Swedish, Aabel studied Russian while in Finland, where he was quite popular with both the Finns and the Americans. He was praised by the U.S. military attache for having a better understanding of the Finnish people than anyone else in the American legation, and upon his departure he received Finland's Order of the White Rose.[69]

The war had also again demonstrated the necessity for medical control of the medical logistics system, a lesson reaffirmed by the Hoover Commission in 1949.[70] Training opportunities for medical logistics officers in the postwar period included courses for medical supply officers conducted by the St. Louis Medical Depot, Missouri, and the Army-Navy Medical Procurement Office, Brooklyn, New York. Other training was offered by the Industrial College of the Armed Forces (ten months), civilian business schools (six to nine months), and various civilian industry programs (ten to thirty days). Medical equipment maintenance officers could take advantage of the Joint Army-Navy Medical Equipment Repair Course, a six-month course open to officers and enlisted personnel at the St. Louis Medical Depot.[71]

Administrative specialty officers assigned to field medical units maintained the Army's field medical apparatus while in garrison. In Japan Lt. Col. Frederick H. Gibbs, MSC, served as the executive officer and "tower of strength" for Col. James A. Bethea, MC, the chief surgeon of the Far East Command. The shortage of physicians became so acute that Bethea had to assign MSC officers as division surgeons of the 6th and 7th Infantry Divisions, a stopgap measure that worked out very well. The MSC officers were preferred by both division commanders over young, inexperienced medical officers.[72]

Maj. Matthew Kowalsky, MSC, was one of the MSC division surgeons. He served in Korea from 1947 to 1949, both as commander of the 7th Medical Battalion and as the 7th Infantry Division surgeon. In January 1949 the division redeployed to Japan as part of the U.S. withdrawal of forces. There, they were visited by Col. Chauncey E. Dovell, MC, the newly assigned Eighth Army surgeon, who was "completely taken aback" when he learned of Kowalsky's duty position, especially the fact that he supervised four physicians. Colonel Dovell complained about it to the division commander, Maj. Gen. William F. Dean. But Dean would brook no interference, telling Dovell that he would retain Kowalsky as division surgeon as long as he was the commander.[73]

Hospital administration began to mature in the Army as it benefited from the postwar expansion of the health care industry. The field was progressing toward professional recognition in civilian life; more individuals pursued it as their life's work, and hospital trustees and administrators sought individuals qualified as managers. Its numbers grew to meet the increased number of hospitals, a growth fueled by passage of the Hospital Survey and Construction Act of 1946 (Hill-Burton). Another milestone was passed in 1951 when representatives of the American College of Surgeons (ACS), the American College of Physicians, the American Hospital Association, and the American Medical Association formed the Joint Commission on Accreditation of Hospitals (JCAH). The JCAH took over the hospital accreditation program begun by the ACS.[74]

In 1948 the American College of Hospital Administrators (ACHA), then in its fifteenth year, portrayed the profession as a "unique and complex activity" which required the ability to deal with finance, general management, personnel, hospital care of patients, and the interrelationships among professional groups involved in the delivery of health care. Above all, the profession demanded sound judgment and skill in human relations. The shift toward professional administrators was apparent in civilian industry, as nurse and physician hospital superintendents were replaced by graduate hospital administrators. The profession had changed in other ways, from predominantly female to predominantly male. The trend accelerated as Medical Administrative Corps officers were discharged from the Army and sought careers in hospital administration. The ACHA had stimulated their interest during the war by sending a questionnaire on career desires to some ten thousand Medical Administrative Corps officers. About fourteen hundred responded that they were interested in civilian careers. Many took advantage of the GI Bill to go to graduate school. The veterans were a promising market for universities hungry for students, and both hospital administration graduate programs and the ACHA turned to a common goal of providing them the graduate training and professional certification they would need to assume leadership roles in the health care industry.[75]

Scientific Specialty Officers

With the creation of the Pharmacy, Supply, and Administration Section, pharmacy officers had a home in the MSC, an important step in their striving for professional recognition that was saluted by the American Pharmaceutical Association as "among the major achievements of the 80th Congress."[76] In 1948 the surgeon general directed commanders of the general hospitals to appoint MSC pharmacy officers as the chiefs of their pharmacies. The first ninety pharmacy ROTC cadets attended summer camp in 1949 at the Medical Field Service School. MSC pharmacy officers headed the ROTC programs as professors of military science and technology, and Colonel Goriup received good reports on their performance.[77]

Maj. Ludwig R. Kuhn, MSC, chief of the Medical Allied Sciences Section, chaired a meeting at the Pentagon in May 1948 that was important for the future of MSC scientific specialty officers in the Medical Allied Sciences Section. Kuhn called the meeting to address the major issues of the day, principally career planning, promotions, and pay. Officers representing the section's fourteen specialties (*see Appendix E*) were invited as well as representatives of fourteen national organizations (*see Appendix F*). The meeting opened with welcoming remarks by

General Bliss, the surgeon general; Maj. Gen. Malcolm C. Grow, the air surgeon; and Vannevar Bush, D.Eng., chairman of the Research and Development Board of the National Military Establishment. The Pentagon meeting set the tone for the management of Medical Service Corps scientific specialty officers in the postwar era.[78]

Lt. Col. Fred J. Fielding, MC, chief of the Surgeon General's Career Management Branch, described the development of career guidance patterns for all Medical Department officers. Those had been made possible by the War Department action in June 1947 that had assigned career planning responsibility for Medical Department personnel to the surgeon general. The plans were projected on a thirty-year basis. The first five years of an officer's service were a basic training period, followed by fifteen years of specialized training. The period from the twenty-first year until retirement was the "definitive period" in which officers would reach the peak of their specialty.[79]

The conferees raised several controversial issues. Certainly the most dramatic was a proposal for a separate science corps outside the Medical Department. The principal reason was a perception of second-class citizenship for MSC scientific specialty officers. Norman Laffer, Ph.D., representing the American Society of Professional Biologists, expressed some bitterness over the department's treatment of scientists. Laffer and others related demeaning attitudes of physicians toward bioscientists, a complaint that was frequently voiced during the meeting. Such experiences diminished the attractiveness of a military career to such a degree that some found the title Medical *Service* Corps objectionable, seeing in this an implication of subservience.

Many believed there was an institutional bias in the Medical Department against nonphysician scientists that generated career limitations. An example was the inability of MSC laboratory officers to advance beyond the position of assistant laboratory chief, because the Medical Department continued to require a physician as chief. They also believed the bias was manifested in the 2 percent cap on MSC colonels. Additionally, there was a fear that scientists, by being mixed in with MSC administrative specialty officers, would have to serve in administrative assignments in order to be promoted.

Some conferees at the Pentagon meeting stressed the advantage of broader assignment possibilities outside the Medical Department that an Army general science corps would offer. Others expressed dissatisfaction with federal service of any kind. Gilbert F. Otto, Sc.D., a Johns Hopkins University parasitologist, related that whenever he asked graduate students who were veterans if they would consider a government position, their reaction was that they would accept "almost anything else but a federal job. We got fed up with that during the war." The attitude was confirmed by a National Research Council survey of biomedical scientists. As reported to the Pentagon meeting, only 32 percent of the 2,519 World War II veterans who responded had military duties that had required their specialized training.[80]

Others at the meeting were more optimistic. They saw promise in the inclusion of medical scientists within the Medical Service Corps. Gustav J. Dammin, M.D., a Washington University pathologist, recalled the difficult task of Arthur

Stull, Ph.D., the laboratory officer consultant who, as a Sanitary Corps major, had served with Dammin in the Surgeon General's Office during the war. Stull had looked after the fortunes of the laboratory officers, but had been limited in what he could do since there was no formal structure within which he could operate. Now, as the conferees at least agreed, scientific specialty officers were no longer improperly assigned and there was a permanently established mechanism to plan for their appropriate use. Indeed, as Colonel Goriup pointed out, an allied scientist could become chief of the corps. Dr. Stull, for one, saw promise in the corps, telling his fellow scientists that they were in on "the birth of a new organization."[81]

Colonel Goriup emphasized the importance he attached to the Medical Allied Sciences Section. It was a concern so deep that Major Kuhn was the first assistant chief he had appointed, and they had called the Pentagon meeting just six months after the corps was formed. The chief addressed some of their concerns, and further stated that removing the 2 percent cap on colonels was high on his project list and that his "very able assistant," Maj. Leo Benade, MSC, was tasked with drafting legislation to correct that inequity.[82] Promotion opportunity would be maintained for the officers of the Medical Allied Science Section whether they went into administrative positions or not. Promotions would be based on performance in assignments that would follow the career pattern for the scientific specialties, not some other field. Further, the Medical Department would conduct its own promotion boards. That was an additional protection for bioscientists, because the medically dominated boards were expected to have a greater understanding of the duties and responsibilities of MSC scientific specialty officers. In time, he foresaw that MSCs would serve on those boards (as they eventually did), once there were sufficient senior MSC officers to form a pool for board membership. That would be another guarantee that the scientific specialty officers would receive a fair shake.

The department had 62 Regular Army Medical Allied Science officers and was working toward a procurement objective of 300. As the department's representatives pointed out, their assignments included new career opportunities, especially in research. The military medical research establishment had a growth spurt in the postwar era as new funding became available and as civilian consultants to the Surgeon General's Office took on a permanent advisory role.[83]

Col. Rufus L. Holt, MC, commandant of the Army Medical Department Research and Graduate School (formerly the Army Medical School), told of the exciting programs at his institution of about two hundred fifty people. In fact, he was prevented from undertaking some research projects because of a shortage of scientists. In all, he described twenty-five major research areas, including basic research in disease immunity, viral and rickettsial vaccines, dysentery studies, and development of new tests and reagents. Researchers at Brooke General Hospital were conducting a study of Bacitracin, an antibiotic ointment.

A new specialty of nuclear science was emerging as developments in nuclear research were applied to medicine. Lt. Col. Roy D. Maxwell, SnC, a pioneer in the field, had participated in the Bikini atomic bomb tests in 1946 as a radiological safety officer, and in 1947 he began postgraduate work at the Crocker Radiation Laboratory of the University of California at Berkeley. Another research opportunity was at the U.S. Army Prosthetics Research Laboratory, established in 1946 at Walter Reed General Hospital under the directorship of Lt. Col. Maurice J. Fletcher, OD, an Ordnance Corps officer who later transferred to the MSC. It was set up by the Army because the United States had essentially no prosthetic research program but it now had thousands of amputee veterans. The available prosthetic devices were little more than peg legs with crude leather sockets and "simple 'baling' hooks, a la Captain Hook, for hands."[84]

The report of the Medical Allied Science Conference made eight recommendations:

1. Convert the Medical Allied Science Section into a separate Medical Science Corps.
2. Take actions to provide equity in positions, promotions, and pay.
3. Expand research and training opportunity.
4. Carefully delineate initial assignments of scientists.
5. Ensure a supply of trained scientists, including student deferments from the draft.
6. Establish civilian advisory boards for the various scientific specialties.
7. Establish a reserve program for medical allied scientists.
8. Rapidly implement the committee's recommendations.

The report concluded that adoption of the recommendations would preclude the need for establishment of a general science corps in the Army.[85]

The Surgeon General's Office digested the recommendations and took action on some of them. These included initiating a study of position designations in Army organization documents, reviewing personnel management practices, appointing civilian consultants for the MSC scientific specialties, and encouraging research activities and graduate training. As an example of the latter, in 1947 Capts. Philip R. Carlquist, MSC, and Warren C. Eveland, MSC, began doctoral programs in bacteriology at Yale and the University of Maryland, respectively. They were the first two officers in their specialty funded by the Army to attend civilian universities at Army expense.[86]

Other recommendations were rejected. The proposal for a separate corps was not accepted, because the surgeon general believed that establishment of the Medical Allied Science Section along with continued improvements in the management of Medical Department scientists would achieve the aims expressed by the committee. However, proposals for a separate medical science or general science corps would come up again.

Social Work

A larger peacetime Army than in the past and an increasing number of family members produced a day-to-day need for social workers. Brig. Gen. William C. Menninger, MC, the champion of the expanded mental health team, left wartime active duty and returned to the Menninger Clinic in Topeka, Kansas. His replacement, Col. John Caldwell, Jr., MC, carried on his predecessor's initiatives. He established a Psychiatric Social Work Branch in the Surgeon General's Office, and Maj. Daniel E. O'Keefe, MAC, became the first chief. In 1947 Colonel Caldwell arranged for Maj. Elwood Camp, MSC, to return to active duty to replace O'Keefe. Camp, an infantry officer during World War II, became the only Army officer on active duty who possessed a graduate degree in social work.[87]

Major Camp oversaw the establishment of a program to recall qualified officers to active duty as MSC graduate social workers. By May 1948 there were four on active duty and plans for forty. As an additional measure to meet the immediate need, he established a 26-week course to train officers with college degrees as partially trained social workers to work in Army hospitals in a "case aid" role. Two-thirds of the course consisted of classwork, and the remaining third covered the supervision of neuropsychiatric technicians. Several of the first graduates were Women's Army Corps officers who had received Regular Army commissions under the provisions of the Women's Armed Services Integration Act of June 1948. One of those officers was posted to the 82d Airborne Division at Fort Bragg, where her assignment caused "a ruckus."[88]

By the fall of 1947 Camp had arranged to send officers for graduate training in social work and was recruiting reserve officers then in graduate programs for return to active duty. He visited thirty graduate schools for this purpose in the days before commercial jet liners, and at a time when stoicism was a necessity for air travelers. This was illustrated by one of Camp's trips from Washington, D.C., to San Antonio, Texas. His first stop was 100 miles away in Richmond, Virginia. Thirteen stops and two plane changes later he arrived at his destination.

Camp especially sought officers with line experience since he believed that social workers in the Army were most effective when they were fully qualified as Army officers. He also believed that a strong identification with Army life facilitated handling the problems of soldiers and their families. For that reason he expected that social work officers would not neglect their military education and training. Among the officers who met Camp's specifications were a former Army Air Corps fighter pilot, a former infantry company commander, and a former Navy combat pilot.

Camp advertised in professional journals and served in national leadership positions to enhance his recruiting efforts. In 1949 he instituted a program for two-year graduate master's degree training in social work whose graduates were commissioned in the Regular Army. The first officers to benefit from this opportunity were Capt. Fernando Torgerson, MSC, who enrolled at Columbia University, and Capt. Herbert Richek, MSC, who attended the University of Pennsylvania. By 1951 Camp's efforts had resulted in 129 social work officers on active duty, including 7 women. Another 89 officers were in the reserves.[89]

Psychology

Robert M. Yerkes, Ph.D., a Yale University professor who as a Sanitary Corps officer had headed the psychology program in World War I, chaired military psychology planning meetings at the National Research Council in 1944. His committee made recommendations to the secretary of war on psychological services in the postwar Army. Dr. Yerkes cautioned that the Army had failed to capitalize during the interwar years on the progress it had made during World War I, but that it would be difficult to prevent another period of stagnation since very few psychologists planned to stay on active duty after World War II ended. The Army needed a strong research program to overcome that tendency by ensuring that it remained abreast of advances in the field and able to adopt new methods and technology. This would require the retention of talented psychologists, but in order to successfully compete with the civil sector for their services the Army would have to establish a well-defined professional status for the specialty and guarantee research opportunities. Therefore, Yerkes proposed forming a research and development corps to serve as their institutional guardian and advocate.[90]

Yerkes' recommendation for a separate corps made no headway, but his prediction of difficulties in retaining psychologists was borne out in the years after the war. By 1949, although the department had requirements for ninety psychologists, it had only three on active duty. The Medical Department was unable to successfully compete with other federal agencies for the 800 graduates from accredited programs in the United States each year. It tried every means it could, but was unsuccessful in obtaining a single applicant for a tour of duty.[91]

Lt. Col. Charles Gersoni, MSC, the psychology consultant for the surgeon general, developed a proposal to subsidize students in doctoral training. The Army, acting upon his concept, established the Senior Psychology Student Program in August 1949. Selected psychology students who had completed at least two years of their studies were commissioned and allowed to continue in their university program for up to two more years. The students received a second lieutenant's pay and allowances, from which they paid the tuition, fees, and expenses of their third and fourth years of the doctoral programs. They completed an Army internship at Walter Reed, Fitzsimons, or Letterman Hospitals during their third year, and returned to their universities for their fourth year. The program produced about seventy clinical psychologists during the period of its existence that ended in 1954.[92]

Sanitary Engineering

Attention was directed to U.S. capabilities for cold weather operations as tensions increased between the United States and the Soviet Union. The Arctic posed its own special preventive medicine challenges. In 1948 Maj. Raymond J. Karpen, MSC, participated in a survey of environmental conditions in Alaska, Nova Scotia, Greenland, and Iceland. Two years later he contributed to a study that evaluated the operation of an evacuation hospital set up under arctic conditions at Fort Shilo, Manitoba, Canada. Col. Ralph R. Cleland, MSC, headed a team sent to Fort Churchill, Canada, to study the problem of waste disposal in the Arctic. Among other things, Cleland's team found that typhoid organisms remained viable for extended periods under those conditions.[93]

The principal sanitary engineering issue during this period centered around a controversy led by Col. William Hardenbergh, SnC, USA, Ret., over the control of his specialty by the surgeon general rather than the chief of engineers. The demise of the Sanitary Corps still rankled Hardenbergh, and his opposition to the Medical Department's actions became a vitriolic dispute. In October 1948 the retired sanitary engineering chief castigated General Armstrong, now the deputy surgeon general, for rejecting the proposal for an Army science corps. He accused Armstrong of a "doublecross" for not supporting a separate Medical Department corps and assured him that a split would develop between the nonphysician medical professions and the department. Hardenbergh rejected Armstrong's offer to support legislation to remove the 2 percent cap on colonels as a "red herring." He insisted that unless Armstrong could persuade the new surgeon general, Maj. Gen. Raymond W. Bliss, MC, to accept Hardenbergh's position, Hardenbergh would soon make himself unwelcome in the Surgeon General's Office. "I'm sorry, Army, but there she is. I will not bother you with the matter any further."[94]

To the contrary, Hardenbergh bothered Armstrong a great deal after that as the editor of *Public Works Magazine*, a position he assumed following his retirement from the Army. Hardenbergh regularly used his editorial forum to berate the Medical Department. He made charges of broken promises, and he lamented that sound sanitary engineering would be impossible in the Army. He criticized the Medical Department for its lack of leadership and failure to do things his way. He echoed his public pronouncements in his correspondence, voicing a conspiratorial view of the Medical Service Corps' formation, which he said was done to spite him. He fulminated over "an official record of delay and brushoff."[95] Hardenbergh engendered so much emotionalism that Francis B. Elder, the engineering associate of the American Public Health Association, joined the silver versus gold insignia controversy and challenged the use of a symbol of lesser quality.[96]

An exasperated General Armstrong complained that he had wracked his brain to find some way to mollify his critics but without success.[97] However, he did not budge from his basic position. "Sanitary engineers are carving a definite place for themselves on the preventive medicine team. I fail to see how the surgeon general could fulfill his mission without control and outright ownership."[98] Further, he believed that because of the department's actions, sanitary engineers were much better prepared for the department's wartime requirements than their predecessors in the Sanitary Corps had been at the beginning of World War II.

The controversy caught the attention of the National Research Council. In September 1948 the chairman of its Committee on Sanitary Engineering and Environment, Abel Wolman, Ph.D. (who had overseen the Army's use of sanitary engineers in World War II as a director of the Procurement and Assignment Service), invited the surgeon general to present to the committee the concept of career planning for sanitary engineers. They met with a delegation led by Colonel Goriup.[99]

The committee's report, issued in December, criticized the absence of any general officer promotion opportunity for MSCs, an opportunity that they would have in the Corps of Engineers. The Medical Corps had 16 generals out of 3,000 officers; the Dental Corps had 4 generals out of 743 officers; and the Veterinary Corps with just 186 officers had 1 general. The Medical Service Corps, with 1,022 officers, had none. Further, Wolman's committee voiced concern that lines of authority and responsibility for sanitary engineering were not clearly delineated, a situation that could infringe upon professional prerogatives. Having said all that, the committee believed that no action was called for on its part. The members agreed to let the matter rest "for the present."[100]

Optometry

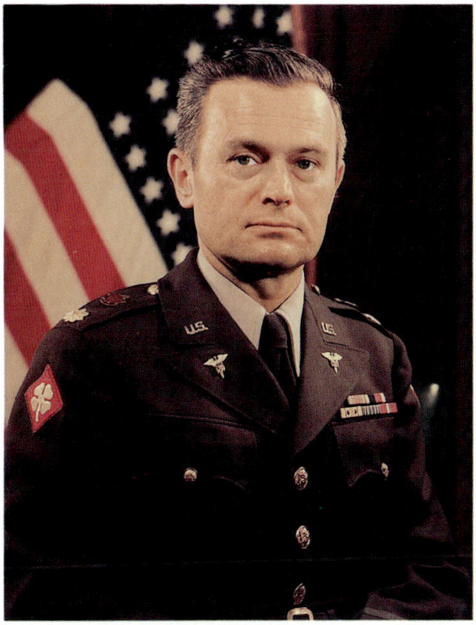

Colonel Sheridan
(Photo taken in 1951.)

Creation of the Medical Service Corps gave the Medical Department a mechanism for commissioning optometrists, and the department began recruiting to fill the Regular Army authorization of twenty optometrists. Capt. John W. Sheridan, MSC, an Ordnance Corps officer in World War II, became in September 1947 the first optometrist commissioned in the MSC.[101] Sheridan was "tickled pink" with his assignment to Walter Reed General Hospital where he was joined by Capt. Milton A. Lewis, MSC. All optometrists brought on active duty were temporarily placed with Sheridan for initial training prior to reporting to their duty stations. Many of the newly appointed officers were veterans like Sheridan; others were recent graduates of optometry schools. Organized optometry was so pleased with the new corps, the commissioning opportunities, and the opportunity for military careers that several associations provided flowers for an MSC anniversary dinner dance held in Washington in 1950.

Summary

A lot happened very quickly after the war. Within two years the MSC was formed, a permanent office organized, career programs established, and a blueprint of sorts sketched for the future of scientific specialty officers. Formation of the corps was both a culminating and a beginning point for the Medical Department's administrative and scientific specialties. It culminated three-quarters of a century of precursor organizations since Letterman's ambulance corps in the Army of the Potomac. It was the beginning of a permanent organization that would nurture those officers in peacetime as well as wartime.

Military medicine had become much more complicated, and the Medical Department had to have a permanent source for the specialties included in the MSC if it was to meet its new combination of responsibilities. The peacetime mission, in both the wartime readiness and peacetime operating aspects, was much larger than before the war. Emergence of the United States as the leading world power gave the Medical Department global requirements, including a standing research and development effort. This was accompanied by an expanded day-to-day health care mission in a larger Army that increasingly assumed responsibility for the care of family members and retired military personnel.

There was another factor to consider. The United States, acting upon the insistent recommendations of its wartime leaders, had unified its military establishment into the Department of Defense. Military medicine was caught up in the movement to unify U.S. air, naval, and ground forces, along with concomitant concerns for efficiency and effectiveness. The Medical Department's peacetime mission, and to a lesser extent planning for wartime medical support, were subject for the first time to the scrutiny of a higher medical authority, the DOD Office of Medical Services. The old ways of doing business had changed for good, and with those changes had come new requirements for greater sophistication in the management of the military medical enterprise. The surgeon general needed talented MSC officers to stay even, for the game demanded players of great administrative and organizational ability.

Unlike the period after World War I, the post–World War II period did not release the Army Medical Department from the pressures it had been under in wartime to ensure the appropriate use of physicians. The ending of the draft and the small number of physicians interested in joining the Army dried up the medical manpower pool at the same time that the demand for health care was increasing. The department turned to the MSC for replacement of and substitution for physicians as it scrambled to fill voids left by shortages in the Medical Corps.

Tension between Medical Service Corps and Medical Corps officers was inevitable, but it was much less significant than the teamwork that went on between the groups. A mutual respect had contributed to the formation of the corps. It was often expressed through close personal bonds between MSC and MC officers, ties that had been forged during difficult assignments together. Medical Corps officers in key positions were influential in forming the MSC and in opening up training, position, and promotion opportunities for its members. They were instrumental in improving the quality of the Medical Service Corps.

At the same time there were tensions internal to the MSC. The formation of a permanently constituted corps for both the administrative and scientific specialties was accompanied by some friction between the groups, the origins of which predated the formation of the corps. Scientific specialty officers now had a permanent place on the Regular Army team, but they did not participate without some misgivings and they would continue to have second thoughts. Proposals for a separate bioscience corps or secession from the Medical Department had an irresistible allure for some, both then and later.

Internal tensions were both transmitted to and shaped by groups external to the Army. The opposition of a retired sanitary engineer, Col. William Hardenbergh, was the most pronounced manifestation of that, as well as an example of how the corps and the Medical Department could be affected by external pressures. The influence of outside groups was at work throughout the formation of the corps and during its early developmental period. The representatives of the guilds who testified at the congressional hearings were midwives to its birth; the spokesmen for the associations who attended the Pentagon meeting of the Medical Allied Sciences Section represented the attending staff. Moderating the dissatisfaction of those groups was high on the list of concerns of Col. Othmar Goriup, the first chief of the corps, and it occupied much of his time. External associations would remain keenly interested in the affairs of their individual specialty groups as the youthful corps stepped off into an uncertain future. They were both blessing and bane to the chiefs of the corps.

Of the three measures of opportunity—position, promotion, and education—education took the largest strides in this period. Graduate training opened, and a major step was the formation of the Army–Baylor University Program in Hospital Administration. It was an important influence in the maturation of hospital administration within the Army, as well as in the Navy, Air Force, Public Health Service, and Veterans Administration. The Army-Baylor Program expanded opportunity for MSC officers and, perhaps more important, provided an intellectual center for the specialty within the Army. It represented a pioneering affiliation between the Army and a university and set a precedent for later affiliations. The program was so successful that the label "Baylor graduate" would become a source of envy within the corps.

The question of the future of the Medical Department's administrative and scientific specialty officers after World War II was answered in a much more satisfying way than it was after World War I. This time there would be a place in the peacetime Medical Department for MSCs. There would be opportunities for attending both military and civilian schools, and there would be opportunities to serve in meaningful positions. Nonetheless, those opportunities were abridged. There was schooling, but there was no opportunity for senior service college, the *sine qua non* of military education. There was opportunity for substantive positions, but the highest positions remained blocked. Promotion opportunity was available, but opportunity to become colonel was capped at 2 percent of the MSC Regular Army strength. The abridgment of opportunity both caused and manifested underlying tensions that would carry forward into future years.

Notes

[1] Medical demobilization: Eli Ginzberg, "Federal Hospitalization; II—Current Trends," *Modern Hospital* 73 (August 1949): 73. Quoted words: Weigley, *History of the United States Army*, p. 501.

[2] Unification: See Richard V. N. Ginn, "Organization of the Military Health Care System," *Military Medicine* 151 (June 1986): 300–302; Ginn, "Of Purple Suits and Other Things; An Army Officer Looks at Unification of Defense Medical Services," *Military Medicine* 143 (January 1978): 18; U.S. Congress, Senate, *National Defense Establishment—Unification of the Armed Services*, 80th Cong., 1st sess., 18 April 1947, pp. 400–408; Department of Defense, *Telephone Directory*, 1949, copies in USACMH; Kendrick, *Blood Program in World War II*, pp. 715–16.

[3] Challenges: It was a "rugged" period according to a principal staff member who was there. See Interv, Nepthune Fogelberg, Comptroller, OTSG, with Samuel Milner, THU, OTSG, 23 Oct 63, MSC-USACMH.

[4] Economic pressures: Ginzberg, "There's a Place in the Sun for Federal Hospitals," *Modern Hospital* 73 (December 1949): 47.

[5] Regular Army (RA) integration: WDSO 255, 25 Oct 45, and WD Cir 392, 29 Dec 45, both in PL; McMinn and Levin, *Personnel in World War II*, pp. 505–09.

[6] RA integration: Maj William V. Davis, MSC, Technical Liaison Office (TLO), OTSG, folder 238, box 15/18, MSC-USACMH. Williams' comments: Interv, Col Louis F. Williams, MSC, Ret., with Lt Col Richard V. N. Ginn, MSC, Clearwater, Fla., 15 Nov 84, MSC history files, DASG-MS. Kanaya: Col Jimmie Kanaya, MSC, Ret., to Ginn, 12 Oct 84, DASG-MS. Gott: Interv, William E. Gott with Samuel Milner, THU, OTSG, 15 Mar 67, USACMH.

[7] Quoted words: Voorhees, "A Lawyer Among Army Doctors," p. 240.

[8] Personnel authority: WD Cir 143, 5 Jun 47, PL; Memo, Maj Gen George E. Armstrong, Deputy Surgeon General, for CSA, sub: Medical Service for the Army and the Air Force, 28 Jun 48, MSC-USACMH. Weakening of the surgeon general's authority in World War II had complicated management of the medical support system. See Interv, Maj Gen Raymond W. Bliss, MC, TSG, Ret., with Samuel Milner, THU, OTSG, 14–16 Jul 63, USACMH; Eli Ginzberg, "Army Hospitalization, Retrospect and Prospect," *Medical Bulletin* (January 1948): 39; Samuel Milner, draft chapter, sub: World War II Leaves a Legacy, in CMH project, The U.S. Army Medical Service in the Post–World War II and Korean Eras, undated (1965), box 1/18, MSC-USACMH. Quoted words: Armstrong to CSA, 28 Jun 48.

[9] Quoted words: Bliss, Milner Interv, USACMH.

[10] Physician training: 1958 MSC History Project; Maj Gen George E. Armstrong, Israeloff Interv, 12 Mar 76, MSC-USACMH; WD Cir 392, 1945. MC substitutions: Brig Gen Floyd L. Wergeland, MC, in 1958 MSC History Project.

[11] MFSS: Medical Field Service School, Historical Rpt, 1946, folder 141, box 9/18, MSC-USACMH; Rpt, 1st Lt France F. Jordan, MSC, sub: A History of the Medical Field Service School at Carlisle Barracks, 1920–1946, 24 Apr 51, DASG-MS. The school had outgrown the limited space at Carlisle, and Fort Sam Houston offered more facilities and space. It moved into four permanent Spanish-style buildings of the former 9th Infantry quadrangle, supplemented by other buildings at Fort Sam Houston. Lt. Col. Allen J. Blake, MSC, was commander of the student detachment. The school used a large, nearby training area, Camp Bullis, for field exercises and demonstrations where the newcomers found that "biting and stinging insects abound, including chiggers, mosquitoes, ticks, spiders, and scorpions."

[12] Quoted words: Silas B. Hays, "The Army Medical Service," *U.S. Armed Forces Medical Journal* 4 (February 1983): 170. The noted economist Eli Ginzberg, Ph.D., served in OTSG as an influential civilian adviser during the war as head of the Facilities Utilization Branch, later the Resources and Analysis Division. He agreed with Hays. "Experience disclosed in this war the need for throwing as much medical means and talent into the forward areas as possible." Memo, Ginzberg for Dir, Hist Div, OTSG, 25 Sep 45, MSC-USACMH.

[13] Medical doctrine: The discussion is based on Hays, "The Army Medical Service," pp. 167–74; Cowdrey, *The Medics' War*, pp. 133–37, 149–54, 197–207, 213–17, 257–60; Joseph R. Darnall, "Medical Evacuation System in a Theater of War," *Military Surgeon* 105 (September 1949): 191–95; W. H. Thornton, "The 24th Division Medical Battalion in Korea," *Military Surgeon* 109 (July

1951): 13; *Military Medical Manual*, p. 471; OTSG (Secretary to TSG), Surgeon General's Early Morning Conference Notes, 6 Oct 52 (hereafter referred to as SG Conference plus the date); Interv, Col Gene Quinn, MSC, with Samuel Milner, THU, OTSG, 28 Oct 63; Interv, Col John W. Wisearson, MSC, with Samuel Milner, THU, OTSG, 22 Sep 66; Interv, Lt Col Raymond E. Adams, MSC, with Samuel Milner, THU, OTSG, 16 Jun 65, all in USACMH; Rpt, 25th Medical Bn, 25th Inf Div, sub: Transmittal of Command Report, 1 Oct 1951, RG 407, Entry 429, Box 3870, NARA-WNRC.

[14] PSH: Portable Surgical Hospital, T/O 8–572S, *Military Medical Manual*, pp. 643–44. The ETO General Board said it was essential for support of division clearing stations. ETO, Rpt no. 89, p. 27.

[15] Air ambulances: Tierney and Montgomery, *The Army Aviation Story*, pp. 206–07; Richard P. Weinert, Jr., *A History of Army Aviation—1950–1962* (Fort Monroe, Va.: Training and Doctrine Command, 1991), pp. 210–11; David M. Lam, "From Balloon to Black Hawk: World War II," pt. 2, *U.S. Army Aviation Digest* 27 (July 1981): 47–48. The tests were by an Army board at Fort Bragg, North Carolina, with the 82d Airborne Division.

[16] Numbers, 1 January 1947: Sec War to Sen Elbert O. Thomas, Chm, Committee on Military Affairs, U.S. Senate, 1 Aug 47, box 3/18, MSC-USACMH.

[17] Early proposal: Memo, TSG for ACS, G–1, ASF, sub: Establishment of Post War Medical Service Corps as Part of the Medical Department, 8 Oct 45, MSC-USACMH. Kirk: "Proposed Postwar Medical Department Plan," *Medical Bulletin* (January 1946): 43–47. MSC requirements: Staff study, OTSG, sub: The Procurement of Medical Officers, 1 Jul 46, MSC-USACMH. MSC consolidation: Robert L. Black, "The Army's Medical Service Corps," *Military Surgeon* 115 (July 1954): 11–13.

[18] Blueprint: Rpt, Arthur H. Einbeck, Chm, Committee on Status of Pharmacists in Government Service, sub: A Blue Print: The Pharmacy Corps of the United States Regular Army, 14 Jun 46, folder 78, box 6/18, and Paper, Maj Einbeck, MSC, USAR, sub: The History of the Pharmacy Corps, 29 Feb 56, folder 72, box 6/18, both MSC-USACMH.

[19] Quoted words: Arthur H. Einbeck, Report of Steering Committee, 20 Nov 46; Kirk to Einbeck, 14 Jun 46, folder 78, box 6/18, MSC-USACMH.

[20] Hearings on MSC: U.S. Congress, House, Committee on Armed Services, Hearings on H.R. 1982, "To Establish a Permanent Medical Service Corps in the Medical Department of the Regular Army," beginning February 20, 1947, and hearings on H.R. 1361 and H.R. 1603, Navy Hospital Corps and Navy Medical Associated Sciences Corps, 80th Cong., 1st sess. All three bills were considered at the same time by the committee as H.R. 3215, "The Army-Navy Medical Services Act of 1947," and are hereafter cited as House, MSC Hearings. Name: A proposal to name it the "Medical Auxiliary Corps" was rejected because it would make it "too much like a ladies' branch of this outfit." 1958 MSC History Project. Army and Navy approaches: Interv, Rear Adm Clifford A. Swanson, Surg Gen, USN, with Samuel Milner, THU, OTSG, 14 Nov 67, USACMH.

[21] Testimony: Arthur H. Einbeck, Chm of the American Pharmaceutical Association's (APA) Committee on Pharmacists in Government Service; Robert P. Fischelis, Pharm.D., APA Secretary; Robert L. Swain, Pharm.D., Editor of *Drug Topics*; and Andrew G. Du Mez, Ph.D., Dean of the University of Maryland School of Pharmacy, House, MSC Hearings. See also Armstrong, Israeloff Interv, USACMH. Agreement: Rpt, Col Robert L. Black et al., sub: Committee Study: Pharmacy in the Army, OTSG, 9 Mar 55, citing Ltr, Kirk to Chairman of Committee on Status of Pharmacy in Government Service, 9 May 47, folder 78, box 6/18, MSC-USACMH.

[22] Testimony: Chick testified on 26 February, Ezell testified on 27 February, and Walsh submitted a written statement that was read to the committee on 12 March. House, MSC Hearings.

[23] Criticism: Statement by a group of officers at Seventh Service Command headquarters, with memo routing slip, Capt Allen, Nutrition Branch, ASF, to Lt Col Regan, Sanitation Division, SGO, ASF, 29 Mar 46; Memo, Col William A. Hardenbergh, SnC, for Ch, Pers Svc, OTSG, sub: Personnel Plans for the Sanitary Corps of the Medical Department of the Post-War Army, 19 Oct 44, and Memo for Brig Gen Simmons, sub: Recommendations Pertaining to Sanitary Engineers and Other Technical Men in the Postwar Regular Army, 15 Nov 45, all in folder 89, box 6/18, MSC-USACMH; Hardenbergh, "Sanitary Corps Functions and Organization," *Military Surgeon* 100 (March 1947): 224.

[24] Quoted words: House, MSC Hearings, 12 Mar 47.

[25] Law: 61 Stat. 134, 4 August 1947.

[26] 2 percent cap: 61 Stat. 734, 4 August 1947; Col. Othmar F. Goriup, the first chief, would soon be writing the surgeon general complaining of this injustice in terms of "equity and merit." See Col Othmar F. Goriup, Chief, Medical Service Corps, to Brig Gen Armstrong, 4 Feb 48, Lend Lease file, folder 42, box 4/18, MSC-USACMH.

[27] WMSC: 61 Stat. 41, 16 April 1947; Col. Robert S. Anderson, MC, ed., *Army Medical Specialist Corps* (Washington, D.C.: Office of the Surgeon General, Department of the Army, 1968), pp. 1–9, 309, 344, 402; Gibbs, Milner Interv, 8 Nov 63, USACMH; Maj Walter F. Robbins, MSC, draft chapter, sub: Reconditioning, THU, OTSG, 1958 MSC History Project, p. 76.

[28] Air Force MSC: Jack Buel, "Recent Contributions of the Medical Service Corps to Military Medicine," *Military Surgeon* 114 (February 1954): 115. The first chief of the AF MSC, Col. Philip G. Fleetwood, was not appointed until 1953. Special projects: SG Conference, 1 Jun 49. This branch, called variously the Personnel Projects or Personnel Policy Division, attracted uniquely talented officers until it was abolished in a 1985 reorganization. It was later resurrected under another name.

[29] Goriup appointment: George A. Armstrong, "Your Profession in the Army," *Journal of the American Pharmaceutical Association* 9 (January 1948): 33. Goriup: Goriup obituary, *Washington Post*, 3 August 1980; Roderick M. Engert, USACMH, Biography of Col. Othmar Frank Goriup, MSC, May 81; Goriup, Standard Form 57, Application for Federal Service, 30 Dec 61; and Biographical summary, THU, OTSG, 30 Sep 60, all in DASG-MS. Quoted words: Goriup in 1958 MSC History Project.

[30] Selections: Memo, Cols Paul I. Robinson, MC; Tom F. Whayne, MC; and Othmar F. Goriup, MSC, for Maj Gen Bliss, sub: Chiefs of the Medical Service Corps, 19 Dec 47 (as amended), folder 41, box 4/18; Rpt, Robinson, Whayne, Goriup, sub: Minutes of the Board of Officers, 7 May 48, folder 158, box 10/18, all MSC-USACMH. The first board recommended Capt. John W. Sheridan, MSC, as chief of the Optometry Section. It is not clear why Bliss rejected the nomination. A likely reason could be that when the first board convened, Sheridan had been an MSC for just one month and there was only one other MSC optometrist on active duty. Bliss may have decided that, with such a limited field and a junior officer nominee, it would be better to wait awhile.

[31] Assistant chiefs: Memo, Goriup for Chief, Hist Div, OTSG, sub: Report of Activities, MSC Division, 2d half Fiscal Year 1949, 26 Sep 49, DASG-MS. See also *Medical Bulletin* (May 1949): 446. Quoted words: Karpen to Israeloff, 14 Apr 76, MSC-USACMH. Advisory council: Memo, Goriup for Chief, Hist Div, 26 Sep 49, MSC-USACMH; THU, draft chapter, sub: Establishment of the Medical Service Corps, in 1965 MSC History Project.

[32] Quoted words: Benade, Ginn Interv, 25 Jan 84, DASG-MS.

[33] Manning requirements: Interv, Lt Gen Leo Benade with Samuel Milner, THU, OTSG, 5 Nov 63, USACMH.

[34] Resistance: Goriup in 1958 MSC History Project. Also see Goriup, Annotation of Ltr, Col William A. Hamrick, MSC, to Goriup, 3 May 66, DASG-MS. AMSUS: Goriup, "The Medical Service Corps," *Military Surgeon* 100 (May 1949): 362.

[35] Quoted words: Speech, Goriup, sub: The Role of the Optometrist in the Army Medical Department, New Jersey Optometric Association, 15 Oct 47, DASG-MS. See also Col James T. Richards, USA, Ret., to Ginn, 28 Feb 86, DASG-MS.

[36] Promotion inequity: Goriup, "Realignment of the Medical Service Corps Promotion List," *Medical Bulletin* (November 1949): 898, 913. 2 percent cap: MSC Historical Rpt, 1st half FY 1948, folder 234, box 14/18, MSC-USACMH; Goriup to Brig Gen Armstrong, sub: Recommendations for Internal Organization of the Medical Service Corps Division, SGO, 4 Feb 48, folder 42, box 4/18, MSC-USACMH. Quoted words: MSC Historical Rpt, 1st half FY 1950, Post WWII file, box 2/18, MSC-USACMH. Hays' position: Brig Gen Silas B. Hays, MC, Chief, Supply Div, OTSG, Comment (Cmt) 2, 18 Aug 49, to DF, Chief, Medical Plans & Operations Div, OTSG, sub: Possible Legislation Affecting the Medical Service Corps, 11 Aug 49, folder 156, box 10/18, MSC-USACMH.

[37] Quoted words: Bliss, Milner Interv, 14 Jul 63, USACMH.

[38] Quoted words: SG Conference, 28 Aug 48.

[39] MC strength: George E. Armstrong, "Current Personnel Problems," *Military Surgeon* 101 (February 1948): 100. The Army unleashed an advertising barrage of ten thousand radio releases and two million pieces of literature. Paul I. Robinson, "About the Medical Department Public Information Program," *Medical Bulletin* (November 1948): 861. Use of MSCs: Memo, Brig Gen George E. Armstrong, DSG, for CSA, sub: Medical Service for the Army and the Air Force, 28 Jun 48, MSC-USACMH. Goriup wrote that the MSC mission was "to augment, supplement and replace the medical officer within the Medical Department whenever and wherever possible." Goriup to Armstrong, sub: Recommendations for Internal Organization of the Medical Service Corps Division, SGO, 4 Feb 48, folder 42, box 4/18, MSC-USACMH. MSC recall: SG Conference, 8 Mar 48; *Medical Bulletin* (June 1948): 419–20 and (October 1948): 821. 800 officers: 250 laboratory officers, 65 psychologists, 45 social workers, 45 pharmacists, 25 optometrists, 40 sanitary engineers, 20 physical reconditioning officers, and 310 administrative specialty officers. Goriup to Pers Div, SGO, sub: Rejection Boards, 21 Sep 48, folder 158, box 10/18, MSC-USACMH. 500 vacancies: "Medical Service Corps Vacancies," *Medical Bulletin* (September 1948): 672.

[40] Division surgeons: The 7th Infantry Division assistant division surgeon from 1947 to 1948 was also an MSC. Dwight Oland, draft Ms, 1973 MSC History Project, citing from 7th and 6th Divisions' medical historical rpts, 1947–48, folder 234, box 14/18, MSC-USACMH. In both cases the medical battalion commander was an MSC.

[41] Quoted words: SG Conference, 5 May 48.

[42] Quoted words: SG Conference, 24 Nov 48.

[43] Quoted words: Hawley Committee. Hawley became chief medical director of the Veterans Administration after the war.

[44] MC survey: Rpt, DOD and Human Resources Research Office, George Washington University (GWU), sub: Medical Officers' Opinions on Professional and Personal Problems of Army Service, in Memo, Don Calahan, HRRO, GWU, for Lt. Col. Z. A. Zehrer, OTSG, 28 Jul 53, MSC-USACMH.

[45] Quoted words: SG Conference, 6 Jan 48.

[46] Chiropody: SG Conference, 17 Nov 47.

[47] Quoted words: SG Conference, 14 Sep 48.

[48] Bliss and Streit: SG Conference, 10 May 48 (including quoted words).

[49] Quoted words: Cited in Intervs, Col Vernon McKenzie, MSC, Ret., PDASD (HA), with Ginn, the Pentagon, 17 May 84 and 20 Jun 84, DASG-MS.

[50] Applicants: 1,440 were applicants for direct appointment, 288 for transfer into the MSC, and 158 for recall to active duty. MSC Historical Rpts, 2d half FY 1949 and 2d half FY 1950, Post WWII file, box 2/18, MSC-USACMH. ROTC: MSC Historical Rpt, 2d half FY 1948, Post WWII file, box 2/18, MSC-USACMH. Appointments in 1949: MSC Historical Rpt, 1st half FY 1949, Post WWII file, box 2/18, MSC-USACMH.

[51] Training: Goriup, Standard Form (SF) 57, 30 Dec 61, DASG-MS; Historical Rpt, 1st half FY 1950, 26 Sep 50, Post WWII file, box 2/18, MSC-USACMH. 1950: Andrew J. Colyer, "Career Management for the Medical Service Corps," *US Armed Forces Medical Journal* 1 (June 1950): 710; Weidenkopf, Sanitary Engineering, 1958 MSC History Project, p. 76. Thirty officers were in civilian programs in 1949. MSC Historical Rpt, 2d half FY 1949.

[52] Numbers: (1948) National Research Council, Committee on Sanitary Engineering and Environment, sub: Minutes of Twelfth Meeting, 21 Dec 48, DASG-MS; (1950) Colyer, "Career Management for the Medical Service Corps," p. 709; (1951) MSC Historical Rpt, 1st half FY 1952, 31 Jan 52, Post WWII file, box 2/18, MSC-USACMH.

[53] Insignia: DF, Army-Navy General Hospital, to TSG, sub: Proposed Insignia for the Medical Service Corps, 15 Aug 47, recapitulated in Memo for Record (MFR) of Ltr, TSG to Quartermaster General (QMG), 4th Ind to Ltr, sub: Insignia for Women's Medical Specialist Corps, 2 Oct 47, and subsequent correspondence on insignia, in RG 112, Entry 64A–2161, Box 103/162, NARA-WNRC.

[54] Insignia alternatives: SG Conference, 19 Aug 47. TSG request: TSG to QMG, sub: Insignia for the Women's Medical Specialist Corps, 9 May 47, with 1st Ind, Brig Gen W. H. Middleswart, QMC, Military Planning Div, QMG, to TSG, 18 Jun 47; 2d Ind, TSG to QMG, 24 Jun 47; 3d Ind, QMG to TSG, 30 Jul 47; 4th Ind, TSG to QMG, 2 Oct 47, all in RG 112, Entry 64A–2161,

Box 103/162, NARA-WNRC; SG Conference, 19 Aug 47. The Quartermaster General said the best idea was something totally different—use the same insignia for all corps of the Medical Department.

[55] Insignia authorized: DA Cir 67, 11 Dec 47. When the Women's Medical Specialist Corps was renamed the Army Medical Specialist Corps in 1955, its insignia was changed to a black "S" superimposed on a gold caduceus, formerly the insignia of the Sanitary Corps and the design originally preferred by the Women's Medical Specialist Corps in 1947. The name change was occasioned by congressional action that provided authority for the commissioning of male nurses and medical specialists in the formerly all-female ANC and WMSC. Goriup on rationale: Goriup to Dr. E. R. Serles, Dean of Pharmacy, University of Illinois, 21 Feb 43, RG 112, Entry 64A–2161, Box 103/162, NARA-WNRC.

[56] Quoted words: Interv, Lt Gen Leonard D. Heaton, MC, Ret., with Col Robert D. McLean, MC, U.S. Army War College and USAMHI Senior Officer Oral History Program, 7 Dec 78, USAMHI.

[57] HCAD course: Discussion principally drawn from Rpt, MFSS, sub: History of the Hospital Administration Course, undated, MSC-USACMH, hereafter cited as MFSS, History of the Hospital Administration Course; and AHS, Baylor File, a collection of documents assembled in 1986 by the Army-Baylor Program, in DASG-MS. Several documents in the Baylor File by Col. James T. Richards, USA, Ret., are particularly useful, including Richards to Ginn, "Here's My Story," 28 February 1986, and Richards to James P. Cooney, "Dear Jimmy," 30 April 1954. Early programs: Neuhauser, *Coming of Age*, p. 93. Nine years separated the founding of the second program at Northwestern University in 1943 and the first program at the University of Chicago in 1934.

[58] Establishment: See also Maj Gen Joseph I. Martin to James P. Cooney, 27 Sep 54, and Col Melvin A. Modderman, MSC, Dir, Army-Baylor Program, to Ginn, 23 Apr 87, both DASG-MS.

[59] Physicians: Armstrong, "Current Personnel Problems," p. 101.

[60] Baylor affiliation: Col James T. Richards to Byron Steger, 18 Aug 50; Hardy A. Kemp to Bliss, 5 Sep 50 and 1 Nov 50, all in DASG-MS.

[61] Heartache: Goriup to Richards, 10 Oct 50, DASG-MS.

[62] Affiliation approval: Martin to TSG, sub: Affiliation of Hospital Administration Program with Baylor University, 14 Sep 50; TSG to Martin, same sub, 27 Sep 50; Fred A. McNamara, Bureau of the Budget, Executive Office of the President, to Richards, 8 Mar 51; DF, Col Raymond E. Duke, MC, Asst Commandant (Cmdt), Army Medical Service School (AMSS), to Dir, Dept of Admin, AMSS, sub: Extract of TELECON from AMSS to SGO—1430 hrs—25 Jun 1956, DASG-MS; DF, Lt Col Willard E. Thompson, MSC, Ch, Operations Div, AMSS, to Dir, Dept of Admin, AMSS, sub: Baylor University and AMSS Agreement Relative to 8–0–6 Course, 22 Jun 56, including Msg, OTSG R 201330Z to CG, Brooke Army Medical Center (BAMC), all in DASG-MS. Quoted words: "Citation for Fred A. McNamara," *ACHA News* 15 (October–November 1952): 13. Institute: Federal Health Care Executives Institute Alumni Association *Newsletter*, January 1986, DASG-MS; SG Conference, 8 May 50.

[63] Affiliation: TSG to CG, BAMC, sub: Affiliation of Hospital Administration Program with Baylor University, 3 Apr 51, including quotation from Asst C of S, G–3, Comment to TSG, 16 March 1951. Baylor accepted the arrangement in: Wilby T. Gooch, Administrative Vice President, Baylor University, to Martin, 13 Sep 51 (Responding to 6 Sep 51, Martin to Gooch), both in DASG-MS. Queries in 1956 revealed that the program continued five years later without formal affiliation, and the program director was still looking for a copy of a formal agreement in 1962. Msg, OTSG, 201330 to CG, BAMC, and DF, Col Raymond E. Duke, MC, to Dir, Dept of Admin, BAMC, 25 Jun 56; Jefferson D. Bragg, Dean, Baylor University Graduate School, to Col Sam A. Edwards, BAMC, 4 May 62, all in DASG-MS. Appointments: W. T. Gooch, Dean, Baylor Graduate School, to Richards, 13 Sep 51, DASG-MS.

[64] Concerns: Goriup to Richards, 10 Oct 50 (including quoted words); Richards to Steger, 18 Aug 50; Richards to Lt Col Francis C. Nelson, Ch, Technical Information Office, OTSG, 19 Feb 52; Memo, Col Frederick H. Gibbs, MSC, 7 Nov 52, all in DASG-MS. Richards did not want it to be a "laughing stock" (Richards, "Here's My Story").

[65] Remedial course: MFSS, History of the Hospital Administration Course.

[66] Accreditation: MacEachern to Martin, 25 Aug 50, and Martin to Gooch, 6 Sep 51, both in DASG-MS; SG Conference, 21 Sep 51 and 25 Oct 51.

[67] AUPHA membership: Wilby T. Gooch to Dr. John Gorrell, Dept of Hospital Administration, Columbia University, 22 Jan 52, DASG-MS; Rpt, AUPHA, sub: The Development of the Association of University Programs in Hospital Administration, 1958, Simpson Library (SL), Academy of Health Sciences, U.S. Army, Fort Sam Houston, Tex.

[68] IGs: Memo, Lt Col Fred J. Fielding, MC, Asst Ch, Pers Div, OTSG, for Ch, Pers Div, 12 Nov 48. Also see Col H. W. Glattly, Inspector General Department (IGD), to TSG, sub: Replacement of MSC Officers Detailed in IGD, and Memo, Goriup for Asst Ch, Pers Div, OTSG, 5 Nov 48, all in folder 133, box 9/18, MSC-USACMH.

[69] Attaches: Col. Bernard Aabel, Finland; Lt. Col. Raymond J. Creamer, Iraq; Lt. Col. James W. Dean, USSR; and Maj. Kenneth L. Hoffman, Thailand. Raymond Creamer, draft chapter, sub: Intelligence, 1958 MSC History Project. Aabel: Rpt, Norman D. Moore, THU, OTSG, sub: Curriculum Vitae of Colonel Bernard Aabel, May 1968, DASG-MS.

[70] Hoover Commission: See U.S. Commission on Organization of the Executive Branch of Government, *The Hoover Commission Report* (New York: McGraw Hill, 1949), ch. 7. Also see SG Conference, 12 Mar 54, for discussion of the second Hoover Commission, which had the same finding.

[71] Medical supply: "Supply Training of Medical Service Corps Officers," *Medical Bulletin* (December 1947): 998; "Training of Medical Equipment Maintenance Officers," *Medical Bulletin* (August 1948): 665.

[72] Substitutions: Interv, Maj Gen James A. Bethea with Samuel Milner, THU, OTSG, 15 Nov 63, USACMH.

[73] Kowalsky: Interv, Col Matthew Kowalsky, MSC, with Samuel Milner, THU, OTSG, 29 May 66.

[74] JCAH: George W. Stephenson, "The College's Role in Hospital Standardization," *Bulletin of the American College of Surgeons* (February 1981): 28.

[75] Hospital administration: Monograph, American College of Hospital Administrators, *Hospital Administration: A Life's Profession* (Chicago: American Hospital Association, 1948), p. 7; Neuhauser, *Coming of Age*, pp. 41–42, 69. MAC impact: Notes from Interv, Weir Richard Kirk, Director of Developmental Credentialling Programs, ACHA, with Ginn, Chicago, 12 Feb 85, DASG-MS. Survey of officers: Dean Conley, "Professional Education in Hospital Administration," *Higher Education* 9 (1 May 1953): 195; Neuhauser, *Coming of Age*, p. 69. Merging of missions: Editorial, James O. Hepner, "A Lifelong Hunger," *Health Care Executive* 5 (March–April 1990): 5.

[76] Quoted words: "At the 93d A.Ph.A. Convention," *Journal of the American Pharmaceutical Association* 8 (October 1947): 493.

[77] Pharmacy: Editorials, Robert P. Fischelis, Secretary, APA, "Pharmacy in the Armed Services," *Journal of the American Pharmaceutical Association* 8 (May 1947) and "Army Pharmacy Takes on New Significance," *Journal of the American Pharmaceutical Association* 8 (Sep 1947). George E. Armstrong, "Your Profession in the U.S. Army," *Journal of the American Pharmaceutical Association* 9 (January 1948): 32–35; Memo, Goriup, sub: Report of Activities, FY 1949, MSC-USACMH; Henry D. Roth, "Utilization and Training of Pharmacists in the Army Medical Service," *Military Surgeon* 115 (July 1954): 43–45.

[78] MAS meeting: Discussion is based on Memo, OTSG, sub: Agenda for Conference on the Medical Allied Sciences Section of the Medical Service Corps, 27–28 May 1948, and Rpt, OTSG, sub: Transcript of the Medical Service Corps Conference, Medical Allied Sciences Section, 27–28 May 1948, hereafter cited as OTSG, Medical Allied Science Meeting, 1948, both in DASG-MS. See also Memo, Goriup for Hist Div, SGO, sub: Report of Activities, Service Corps Division, 2d half of FY 1949, 26 Sep 49, MSC-USACMH.

[79] TSG responsibility: WD Cir 143, 5 Jun 47, PL.

[80] Quoted words: OTSG, Medical Allied Science Meeting, 1948. Survey results: Ibid.

[81] Quoted words: Ibid.

[82] Quoted words: Ibid.

[83] Research funds: Eli Ginzberg, Milner Interv, 10 Sep 63, USACMH.

[84] Maxwell: TLO, OTSG, Biography of Col. Roy D. Maxwell, MSC, Feb 1962; and Rpt, Col Charles R. Angel, MSC, sub: Development of Nuclear Science Within the MSC, undated (1976), both in DASG-MS. Prosthetics: Col Maurice J. Fletcher, MSC, draft section, sub: Prosthetics, 1958 MSC History Project. Col. Robert S. Allen, who lost an arm as the G–2 of Patton's Third Army, led the fight that resulted in formation of the laboratory.

[85] Science corps: The same idea resurfaced periodically in subsequent years.

[86] First students: Lt Col Charles A. Pendlyshok, MSC, to Lt Col John P. Ransom, MSC, 29 May 60, box 19/18, MSC-USACMH.

[87] Social work: Elwood H. Camp, "The Army's Psychiatric Social Work Program," *Social Work Journal*: 29 (April 1948): 76–77, 78, 86; Rpt, Camp, sub: As I Remember Army Social Work from April 1947 to June 1951, in Ltr to Ginn, 20 Sep 84, DASG-MS, hereafter cited as Camp, As I Remember Social Work; MSC Newsletter, October 1960; Camp, "Psychiatric Social Work in the Army Today," in Henry S. Maas, ed., *Adventures in Mental Health* (New York: Columbia University Press, 1951), pp. 203–20; Lecture, Camp, Notes for Presentation at the Army Social Work Meeting, National Conference of Social Work, Atlantic City, New Jersey, May 1951, DASG-MS; WD SO 50, 12 Mar 47, DASG-MS; "Clinical Psychology and Psychiatric Social Work," *Medical Bulletin* (September 1947): 755–56; "Psychiatric Social Worker's Program," *Medical Bulletin* (January 1948): 22; Col Henry W. Adams, MSC, and Lt Col Ralph W. Morgan, MSC, draft chapter, sub: Social Work, in 1958 MSC History Project.

[88] Women: Camp, As I Remember Army Social Work.

[89] Social work graduate program: SR 605–60–42, 2 Sep 49, PL. Camp was assigned to Fitzsimons from 1951 to 1954 as chief of social work. He later entered hospital administration and served as the executive officer of Tripler Army Hospital in Hawaii from 1955 to 1958.

[90] Yerkes: Robert M. Yerkes, "Post-War Psychological Services in the Armed Forces," *Psychological Bulletin* 42 (1945): 396–97.

[91] Recruiting failure: Maj Gen R. W. Bliss, TSG, to Lt Col E. E. Beauchamp, Dir Programs and Analysis, sub: Regular Army Procurement and Specialty Training of Medical Service Corps Officers, 12 Apr 49, folder 160, box 11/18, MSC-USACMH.

[92] Psychology graduate program: SR 605–60–40, 16 May 49, PL; "The U.S. Army's Senior Psychology Student Program," *American Psychologist* 4 (1949): 424–25; Bliss to Beauchamp, 12 Apr 49. Number: Paper, Harold D. Rosenheim, "A History of the Uniformed Clinical Psychologist in the U.S. Army," presented to the American Psychological Association, Montreal, Canada, 2 Sep 80, DASG-MS.

[93] Cold weather: Col Raymond J. Karpen, MSC, to Israeloff, 14 Apr 76; OTSG, Travel Orders, 14 Jul 48 and 19 Jan 50; App B to Rpt of Subcommittee on Waste Disposal, National Research Council, 6 Oct 49, all in Karpen Files, DASG-MS.

[94] Hardenbergh's opposition: Hardenbergh to Karpen, 21 Oct 48, and Ltr, Karpen to Col Earl Herndon, MSC, 7 Nov 83, both in DASG-MS; also see Rpt, Col George W. Hunter III, MSC, sub: Reminiscences, 1971, MSC-USACMH. Quoted words: Hardenbergh to Armstrong, 15 Oct 48, DASG-MS.

[95] Complaints: Hardenbergh, "What's Wrong with Army Engineering?" *Public Works Magazine* 79 (October 1948): 7; Hardenbergh, "I've Had Enough," *Public Works Magazine* 79 (December 1948): 7; "For Your Information and Amusement," *Public Works Magazine* 81 (October 1950): 14; Hardenbergh to Karpen, 12 May 49, and Hardenbergh to Col Tom Whayne, 19 Aug 59, both DASG-MS; Editorial, Hardenbergh, "The Army Reserve," *Public Works Magazine* 79 (December 1948): 14.

[96] Elder: Armstrong to Francis B. Elder, 17 Aug 50, responding to Elder's 14 Aug 50 letter, DASG-MS.

[97] Quoted words: Armstrong to Hardenbergh, 19 Jun 50, DASG-MS.

[98] Quoted words: Memo, Goriup for Armstrong, 15 Jun 50, DASG-MS.

[99] Wolman: Abel Wolman to Lt Col Fred F. Fielding, Ch, Career Management Br, Pers Div, OTSG, 27 Sep 48; Karpen to Herbert M. Bosch, Environmental Sanitation Div, Minnesota Dept of Health, 24 Nov 48, both in DASG-MS. Wolman died in 1989 at the age of ninety-six. He had pioneered the use of chlorine in water purification and advised fifty nations on their water systems. *U.S. News and World Report* 113 (6 March 1989): 16.

[100] Quoted words: National Academy of Sciences–National Research Council, Committee on Sanitary Engineering and Environment, sub: Minutes of Meeting, 21 Dec 48, DASG-MS.

[101] Optometrists: Speech, Goriup, sub: The Role of the Optometrist in the Army Medical Department, New Jersey Optometric Association, 15 Oct 47; Speech, Lt Col John W. Sheridan, MSC, Ch, MSC Optometry Sec, sub: Military Optometry, undated (late 1950s), both in DASG-MS; Goriup to Andrew F. Fisch, O.D., Secretary, New Jersey Optometric Association, 11 Aug 50, folder 39, box 4/18; OTSG, Biography of Lt Col John W. Sheridan, MSC, 1958, folder 55, box 5/18, both in MSC-USACMH. Sheridan received his O.D. from Ohio State in 1935 and was commissioned from the Ordnance OCS in 1942. Not all optometrists were pleased, such as those who were over thirty years old and thus ineligible for a Regular Army commission. See Ltr to editor, Elmer S. Friedberg, "Optometric Progress in Army Medical Service Corps Questioned," *Optical Journal-Review* 85 (15 February 1948): 50.

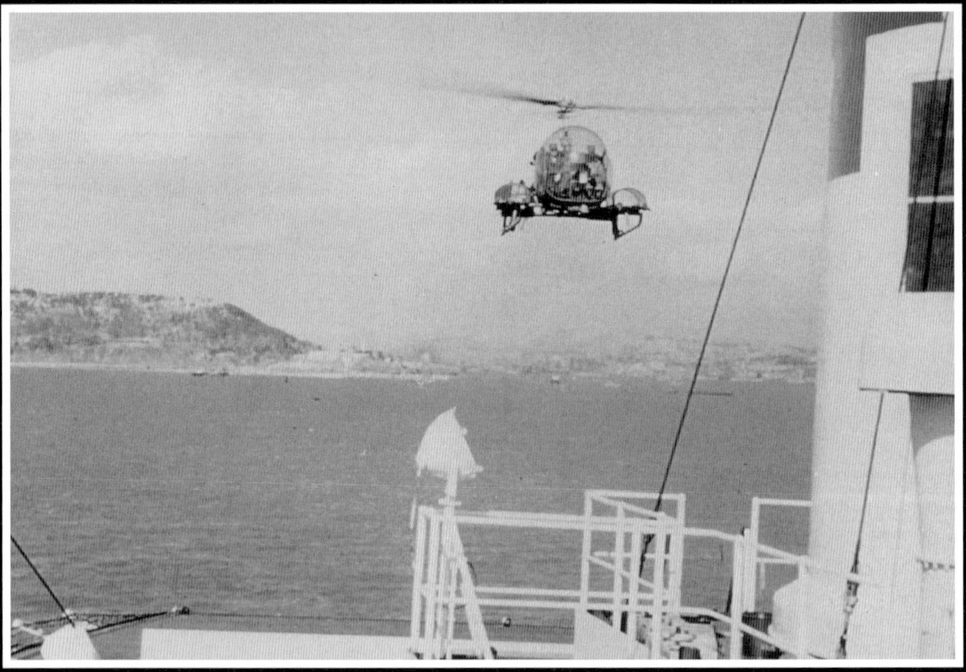

Helicopter landing on the deck of the Haven

8

KOREA

In June 1950 the Army was organized, at least on paper, into ten divisions plus nine separate regimental combat teams and the division-size European Constabulary. With a total strength of under six hundred thousand soldiers, it was a force that was insufficient to meet the nation's commitments, which had grown with the onset of the Cold War and the creation of the North Atlantic Treaty Organization in 1949. Combat units were frequently manned at half strength—divisions were short a brigade, brigades short a battalion, and battalions short a company.[1]

One point where Soviet and American power touched was the Asian peninsula of Korea. Soviet forces had entered Korea in August 1945, established a Communist government in the north, and as relations with the United States deteriorated they had fortified the frontier at the 38th Parallel. In this way a supposedly temporary division between two zones of occupation became a permanent division into two nations: the Democratic People's Republic of Korea in the north, and the Republic of Korea (ROK) in the south. Increasing antagonism between North and South Korea resulted in incidents of armed conflict. In June 1949 the United States withdrew from Korea, as the Soviets had done previously. The 500 American military advisers left behind reported to General of the Army Douglas MacArthur's Eighth Army in Japan.

The North Korean Army (NKA) was a Soviet-trained force of seven divisions and five separate brigades supported by Soviet-made tanks and aircraft. South Korea, with a weak army supported by an unprepared American ally, could mount little resistance when the North Korean Army crossed the 38th Parallel without warning on Sunday morning, 25 June 1950. Premier Kim Il Sung ordered his commanders to conquer the south by 15 August. He would have succeeded if it had it not been for the quick reaction of U.S. President Harry S. Truman, who ordered naval and air support for the ROK on 27 June and requested action by the United Nations (U.N.) Security Council. The South Korean capital of Seoul fell on the twenty-sixth, and two days later Truman committed American ground forces. U.N. forces deployed rapidly, but within a month the Communists had pushed them southeast into a 200-square-mile area around the port city of Pusan. The defenders were now no farther than fifty miles from the sea. Less than two months after the invasion, the United States had sustained over ten thousand casualties, including 543 killed. A 24th Infantry Division medic summed it up: "We were outmanned, outgunned, outtanked and outflanked."[2]

For two months Americans led a growing international army in defense of the Pusan perimeter. Then, on 15 September, General MacArthur staged a classic amphibious assault, landing at Inchon on the northwest side of Korea. He maneuvered east, recaptured Seoul on 26 September, severed NKA lines of communication, crossed the 38th Parallel, and pushed on to the Yalu River, North Korea's border with China. But on 25 November the war took on a dramatically new dimension when 180,000 Chinese attacked MacArthur's widely separated forces. By the end of January 1951 Seoul had again fallen, and U.N. forces had been pushed back to the 37th Parallel. In April Truman relieved MacArthur, the climax of a deep rift between the old general and the president.

General Matthew B. Ridgway replaced MacArthur and by June 1951 led the U.N. forces back to the 38th Parallel. Here the battle lines stabilized, and the conflict changed from a war of movement to a positional war. Battles of attrition on Heartbreak Ridge, Old Baldy, and Pork Chop Hill made headlines. The North Koreans dragged out truce negotiations, which began in July 1951, until the armistice was finally signed two years later. The Army maintained an average strength of 208,000 soldiers in Korea during the war. Military forces of twenty-two allied nations saw combat there, and over one million people died.[3] The United States had 54,260 deaths, including 33,643 battle deaths.

The MSC Contribution

MSC officers, like personnel of all branches, were immediately affected by the United States redeployment to Korea, often responding to a 72-hour alert notification.[4] The Eighth Army surgeon, Col. Chauncey E. Dovell, MC, moved to Korea from Japan with a small staff as part of the advance section of the Eighth Army headquarters. Dovell, described as burly and a bully, was one of the more colorful characters of the war.[5] He arrived in Korea on 12 July 1950, accompanied by Lt. Col. Charles A. McAllister, MSC, his executive officer, and his key staff, nearly all MSC officers. They set up operation in an old schoolhouse at Taegu, north of Pusan. They were at the right place to participate in one of the most desperately convoluted military actions in American history.[6] Colonel Goriup wrote in the fall of 1950 that the reports of MSC officers in Korea were "enough to warm the 'cockles of one's heart.'" Twenty MSCs received Silver Stars in the first year of the war.[7]

Lt. Col. William A. Hamrick, MSC, on leave, was en route to Japan when the war broke out. Diverted to Korea as Colonel Dovell's personnel officer, he reported to Taegu in July only to join an evacuation of the headquarters back to Pusan. Hamrick and most of the other staff officers returned to Pusan by boxcar, sleeping on the floor. Later, when they returned to Taegu, they quickly settled in to a round-the-clock operation. Capt. Paul M. Levesque, MSC, an operations officer, worked from 0700 to 2400 seven days a week. Some of the staff would sleep in the office each night to take advantage of clear phone lines for calls from hospital commanders and division surgeons throughout Korea.[8]

Regimental Medical Service

Each Korean War division had thirty-eight MSCs, more than any other corps except the infantry and artillery.[9] They were essential components of the regimental and division levels of medical service, beginning with the medical platoons of the maneuver battalions. One of the first heroes of the war was 1st Lt. Raymond (Bodie) E. Adams, MSC, battalion surgeon's assistant of the 1st Battalion, 21st Infantry, 24th Infantry Division. His platoon was part of a task force of two reinforced rifle companies commanded by infantry Lt. Col. Charles B. Smith. Maj. Gen. William F. Dean's orders to Smith were to go to Pusan and head for Taejon, south of Seoul, to "block the main road as far north as possible." While other division elements followed by sea, Task Force Smith flew to Korea on a perilous mission intended to provide a show of force to deter the North Koreans.[10]

The unit landed on a muddy airstrip in Pusan on 1 July, arrived in Taejon by train the next morning, and moved north. At 0300 on 5 July, Smith's men dug in to form a roadblock straddling a ridge north of Osan about eighty miles from Taejon. That was as far as they got, because a column of about thirty T34 tanks rolled through five hours later, followed an hour after that by trucks loaded with North Korean infantry who dismounted and began encircling the Americans. They were lead elements of a column estimated to be six miles long.

Adams and the battalion surgeon, Capt. Edward L. Overholt, MC, located their aid station within the defensive perimeter in a twelve-foot-square hole dug five feet into the ground. There, the medics did the best they could to keep their patients alive. As the day went on North Korean attacks (controlled by voice and bugle) became more intense as they surrounded the defenders, who were running out of ammunition.

Smith eventually ordered his command to withdraw in groups back to friendly lines, and they took off in several directions. Only 185 of the more than 400 soldiers made it back safely. The medical platoon, the second group to leave, left two medics behind to care for the patients that were unable to move. Adams led a group of about seventy-five soldiers, including walking wounded, south to the American positions. As they began to pull out they were held up by a North Korean machine gunner, whom Adams, the pitcher for the regimental baseball team, took out with a hand grenade. (Later Smith jested that he had always thought more of Adams' pitching than his medical knowledge.) None in Adams' group were lost in the escape, and Adams and Overholt received Silver Stars for their valor. For his part, Adams said Task Force Smith was "an example of what a few can do when esprit, commitment, and leadership all come together in a cause you believe in."[11]

Medical units encountered overwhelming casualty loads. At one point in November 1950, after the Chinese attack, one of the 25th Medical Battalion's clearing stations had 750 patients, with more coming all the time. In the 7th Division, Sgt. Donald E. Wagoner's medical platoon at Hargaru-ri had nearly four hundred patients when they were ordered to "make a break for it" at the end of November. The battalion surgeon, wounded and unable to walk, was one of the patients. Leading the platoon's vehicles in column, Wagoner, who received an MSC battlefield commission, came upon a Chinese soldier armed with a potato-masher hand grenade at a roadblock. Wagoner shot the soldier with his pistol at such close range that he could watch the North Korean's "look of stunned surprise."[12]

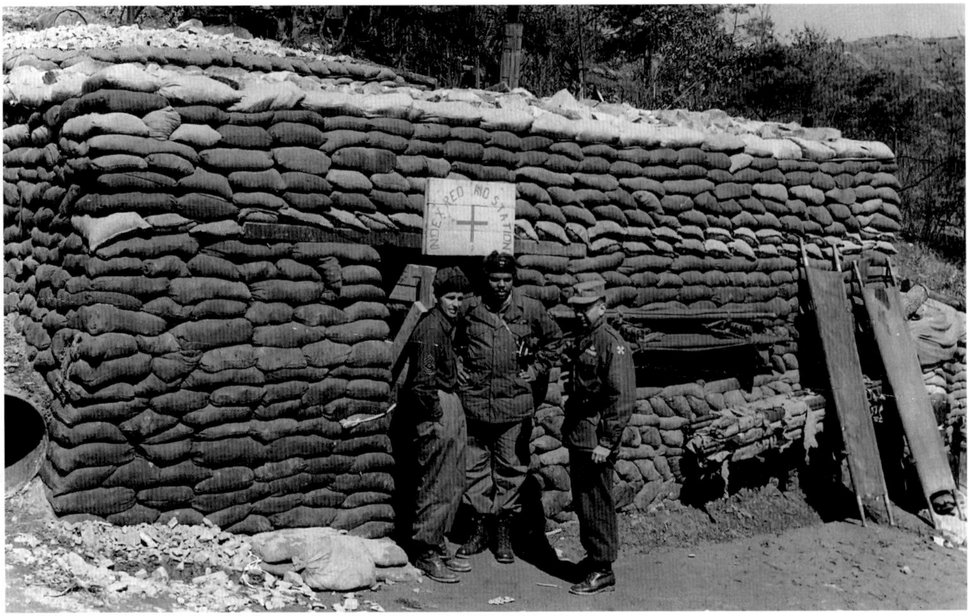

1st Battalion ,9th Infantry Regiment, aid station

Combat support units were staffed at little more than a fourth of their authorized manning levels. Medical Corps officers were at about half strength. There were not enough physicians to assign one to each maneuver battalion, and some MSC battalion surgeon's assistants became battalion surgeons. Some divisions substituted MSCs for the battalion surgeon in all but the infantry battalions. The 7th Infantry Division, for example, consolidated as many of its physicians as it could into the medical companies. It depended upon MSC battalion surgeon's assistants as the only medical officers in engineer, tank, and artillery battalions (and reported "no impairment of essential medical activities").[13]

The engineer battalion surgeon was 1st Lt. Robert Levi, MSC, and 1st Lt. Robert N. Gilliam, MSC, was the tank battalion surgeon when the 2d Infantry Division deployed from Fort Lewis, Washington, in August 1950. The division received more physicians in the spring of 1951, but both battalion commanders declined the offer of replacing their MSCs. One week before the invasion of Korea 1st Lt. Paul A. Lavault, MSC, arrived in Japan and was assigned to the 1st Cavalry Division as a battalion surgeon's assistant, becoming the battalion surgeon since there was no physician assigned to his battalion. Lavault remained in that capacity for the movement to Korea, the defense of Pusan, and the Inchon landing.[14]

The movement phase of the Korean War tested the mobility of medical units at all levels of the combat zone, and MSC battalion surgeon's assistants learned that things did not always go smoothly. Lieutenant Lavault found his platoon's ability to keep up with its battalion severely compromised when the battalion operations officer would occasionally fail to tell him that the battalion was relocating. Consequently Lavault's aid station would end up stranded in enemy territory. A battalion surgeon's assistant in the 3d Infantry Division, 1st Lt. Rudolph A. Sarka, MSC, established a forward battalion aid station in December 1950 on a ridge west of Hamung, while the battalion surgeon established the principal aid station farther back with the battalion trains. Sarka was located within a few yards of the battalion's riflemen. He was authorized to administer plasma and blood and to call for helicopter evacuation from his forward position.[15]

Division Medical Service

Medical companies also had to be able to keep up with the units they supported. The principal duties of Capt. Lewis H. Huggins, MSC, executive officer of a 25th Infantry Division clearing company, included site selection for the clearing stations and coordination with the battalion aid stations so as to maintain an uninterrupted evacuation flow. Standard operating procedures dictated that the two clearing platoons of each clearing company would leapfrog each other to keep up with the tempo of battle. As one platoon set up and operated a clearing station the other would displace to a new location, and, when the second was operational, the first platoon would shut down and relocate. This was an exhausting regimen. The company operated in shifts whenever it was able to reassemble and operate a single clearing station. Then the soldiers could get some rest.[16]

In some cases medical units engaged in direct combat. In May 1951 a Chinese unit was bypassed by U.S. elements and stumbled into the hillside location where the 21st Medical Company of the 24th Infantry Division had set up for the night about three hundred yards from the regimental command post. The chance encounter turned into a general melee in which the lightly armed medical company killed twenty-three enemy soldiers and took fifty-eight prisoners. The medical company had one killed and ten wounded, and 1st Lt. John Atkins, MSC, received the Silver Star for his valor. In the same month, 1st Lt. William W. Cook, MSC, was killed in action when his 38th Regimental Combat Team battalion aid station was cut off by North Korean Army forces. In another case, Capt. Clarence L. Anderson, MSC, a battalion surgeon's assistant, along with his battalion surgeon, Capt. Alexander M. Boyson, MC, were captured at Chochiwon. They spent three years in North Korean hands.[17]

Because of the Medical Corps shortages, MSCs filled administrative positions, such as command of medical battalions, that were designated as physician assignments. Consequently, when those units deployed to Korea, they remained under the command of their Medical Service Corps commanders. By 1951 Medical Service Corps officers commanded four of the six division medical battalions in Korea. The 24th Infantry Division reported in 1953 that its medical battalion was under MSC command nearly the entire year, and the arrangement was successful.[18] When the 7th Medical Battalion redeployed to Korea from Japan, it did so under the command of Maj. Oren C. Atchley, MSC. His battalion covered the Inchon landing and then provided evacuation over a 230-mile route in temperatures as low as -24° F. In November an ambulance with five patients was lost. Major Atchley led a search party, which was ambushed; the survivors included one soldier whose feet were so severely frostbitten his toenails

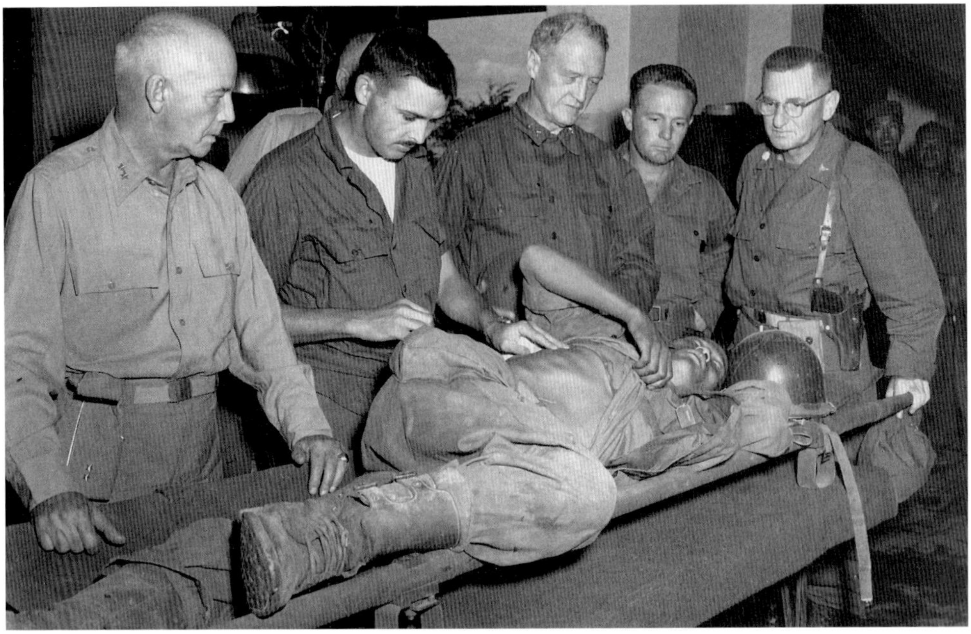

*Major Walker (*second from right*) with a Chinese POW in a clearing station of the 25th Medical Battalion, September 1950. Maj. Gen. Raymond W. Bliss, the Surgeon General, is at left.*

were dropping off. Atchley became separated from the group, was listed as missing in action, and later presumed killed.[19]

Maj. Herman A. Walker, MSC, was commanding the medical battalion of the 25th Infantry Division in Japan at the time of the invasion of South Korea. Walker deployed his battalion to Pusan on 10 July and moved north. The battalion received its first patient on 12 July and by the end of the month had cared for almost eleven hundred patients. Over nine hundred had to be further evacuated, but since the Eighth Army was unable to provide casualty evacuation support, the battalion assembled rail cars to move patients to the rear. Not unlike other medical units at that time, Walker's unit was one-third understrength. The personnel situation became so critical that one of his clearing companies had to be augmented by fifteen soldiers from the division band. As Walker summed up his battalion's actions, "we were too busy to worry."[20]

Command opportunities extended to other positions normally reserved for physicians. For example, Capt. Herman Richards, MSC, commanded a medical company in the 7th Infantry Division that deployed from Yokohama, Japan, for the Inchon landing. His unit moved to the Pujon Reservoir where it provided medical support to the regiment in an area so cold that Richards wrapped his feet first in toilet paper and then multiple layers of socks for warmth. Soldiers in Richards' company received nineteen Silver Stars for their heroism.[21]

Operations in Korea taught that medical operational planning must account for refugees, enemy prisoners of war, and support for allied forces—missions that can utterly swamp a medical unit. After the Inchon landing Captain Richards' company discovered that although the division's aid stations and clearing stations had their hands full with the American wounded, "it was clear something would have to be done for the civilian casualties who were streaming to the rear piggyback, on wheelbarrows, and some even crawling." Richards put 2,500 patients in a three-story rice warehouse on the banks of the Han River near one of the battalion aid stations. Major Walker's battalion also encountered refugees streaming through the American lines during the winter of 1950–51. His medics found the South Korean hospital at Sangju so low on medical supplies that its surgeons were performing amputations without anesthesia.[22]

Field Army Medical Service

Mobile Army Surgical Hospitals (MASH), operating under tents close to the divisions they supported, proved their worth in casualty resuscitation and stabilization. The staff of the 8055th MASH, the model for the 4077th MASH of movie and television fame, routinely worked twelve-hour shifts, the standard practice for medical units in combat. President-elect Dwight D. Eisenhower visited the hospital in December 1952 and thought it was too cold. Later the medical supply officer was able to cite presidential authority as justification for space heaters.[23]

Rail lines came close to the front lines in Korea, and trains became workhorses for the United Nations units. As a result, some MSCs got into railroading. Colonel Dovell, the Eighth Army surgeon, gave Maj. Matt Kowalsky, MSC, now an operations officer on his staff, the mission of putting together hospital trains to move patients from Taegu south to the hospitals in Pusan and, after the Inchon landing, from Seoul to Pusan. Kowalsky located some Korean coaches; shingled the roofs with flattened gas cans; covered the windows with sheet metal and wood; put in 55-gallon drums for heat, water, and fruit juice; and placed the trains in service, using Korean crews. Litter patients were loaded into the cars through the windows and placed across the seat backs or on the floors.[24]

The trains were continually subjected to ambushes and sniper attacks. Kowalsky put sandbagged flatcars mounted with heavy machine guns on the front and rear of the trains and loaded patients at night so as to reach Pusan by daylight. He also had his share of excitement. After the capture of Pyongyang he set up a train between that city and the port of Chinnamp'o. On one run the MSC major had the feeling that something was amiss. He stopped the train, interrogated the crew at pistol point, and found it included two North Korean infiltrators who planned to drive the train into the sea with all aboard.

The United States shipped some hospital trains to Korea. They were too big for the Korean railbed and tunnels, so Kowalsky had to rig a system of jacks and pulleys to get cars back on the track when they derailed. One figure-eight tunnel was much too small, and the cars would scrape the sides as they went through. It made a perfect ambush site, and there were about twenty-five attacks at that spot. On one of those occasions Colonel Dovell was on the train when it came under fire from front, rear, and both sides. The flatcar weapons kept the North Koreans pinned down while Kowalsky called for a 7th Division patrol to clear out the

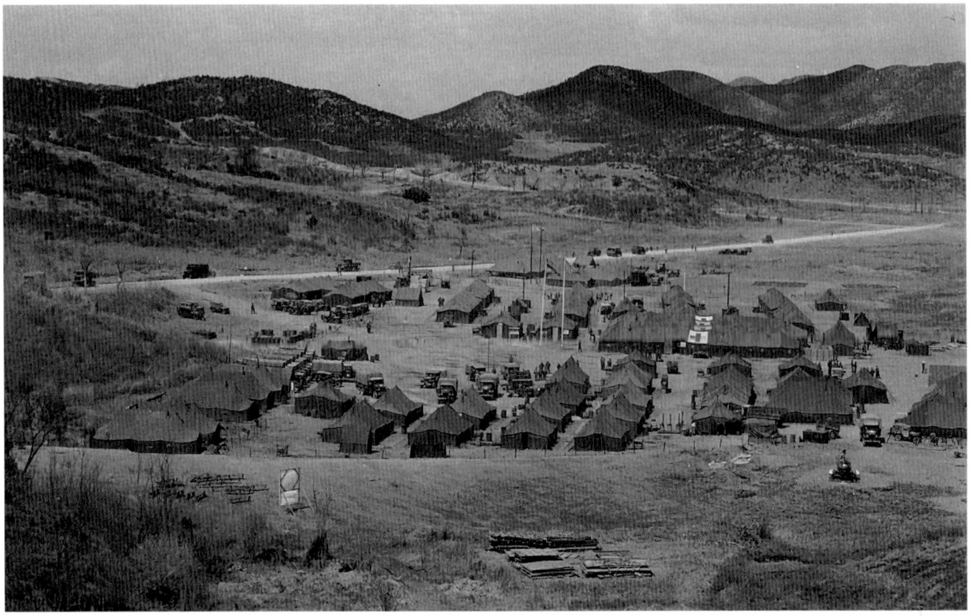

45th Mobile Army Surgical Hospital (MASH)

enemy positions. Dovell characteristically braved enemy fire, crawled under the last car, and fired at the enemy soldiers. Kowalsky went forward to get the train moving after the action ended, and a North Korean soldier jumped him. He was able to lay his attacker out with a single blow to the head.[25]

Other MSCs had a taste of hospital command, even though it was officially not possible. The 64th Field Hospital, commanded by Lt. Col. Joseph Bornstein, MC, left San Francisco in August 1950 and set up in Pusan, a city described by the hospital's executive officer, Maj. Rudolph P. Czaja, MSC, as "a dirty, filthy place, full of refugees and a health hazard itself." Bornstein split the 64th into two hospital units, taking one unit forward to relieve Major Walker's battalion and leaving the other at Pusan under Major Czaja.[26]

After the Inchon landing, the United Nations forces began establishing prisoner of war camps around Pusan, and Czaja's Hospitalization Unit 1 began receiving POW patients. Within ten days his hospital had 2,000 POWs, a population he supported with 3 physicians, 2 MSC officers (including himself), 10 nurses, and 2 dentists. In October, Czaja's unit was relieved by the 14th Field Hospital, and he took his unit north to rejoin the rest of the 64th, which had reassembled in the Pyongyang area.

When the Chinese attacked, the 64th Field Hospital commander went to Inchon to find a relocation site while Czaja remained behind. The situation worsened, and after some time had elapsed Czaja began to feel that they had been forgotten in the confusion of the Eighth Army withdrawal. He called the switchboard (before it also left) and found that no one left in Pyongyang had the authority to order the 64th's withdrawal.

Deciding that he was not going to let his unit be captured, Czaja moved 1,200 patients to safety in twenty-four hours through the Pyongyang airfield, dispatched the unit's vehicles and equipment south under the command of a dental officer, and sent most of the hospital cadre by rail to Seoul. He placed himself and the physicians in two rail cars attached to a train that evacuated the Turkish Brigade. Czaja said that Colonel Dovell later told him the 64th had been given up as lost. The exhausted unit returned to Japan for refitting.[27]

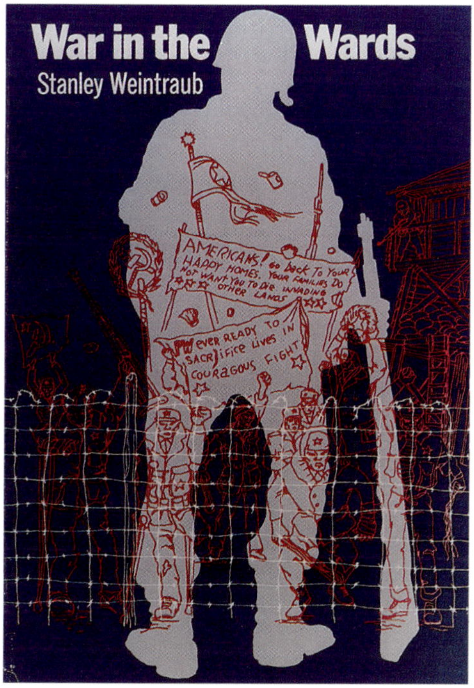

War in the Wards *cover*

Prisoners of war were another challenge. Stanley Weintraub, MSC, a first lieutenant, was stationed in Pusan as the patient administration officer of the 1st POW Field Hospital (Provisional), a unit formed from the 3d and 14th Field Hospitals. His book, *War in the Wards*, is a hair-raising account of operating a prisoner of war hospital in the face of overwhelming resistance by the prisoners. When Weintraub arrived in the summer of 1951, the hospital was admitting and discharging over a thousand patients a day, and its daily census approached eleven thousand patients. It treated nearly ninety thousand patients during the period of its operation and performed about thirteen thousand operations, all the while fighting a "private little war."[28]

American experience with POWs in World War II had not prepared them for North Korean soldiers who did not stop fighting when captured, even if they were hospitalized. Nor were they prepared for the North Korean government's use of the POW camps for propaganda claims of mistreatment. Weintraub wrote that the Americans could not understand the duplicity of their communist prisoners, nor comprehend "that amputees, tuberculars and the dying could be used as a fighting force" by a disciplined band of fanatics.[29] The patients laid siege to the hospital, rioted, held kangaroo courts, and executed fellow prisoners until the situation was brought under control by an infantry attack.

In Korea, the Army was part of a combined U.N. force. This posed interoperability challenges for some MSCs. In September 1950 Capt. Robert I. Jetland, MSC, was detached from the 1st Cavalry Division and sent to Pusan to head an American liaison unit of thirty-four personnel attached to a Swedish Red Cross hospital. Sweden had agreed to provide the 200-bed unit if the Americans would supply and equip it. About one hundred fifty Swedes under the command of Col. Carl Erik Groth had come to Korea with some international fanfare. Jetland acted as the executive officer, and his detachment provided the administrative functions for the hospital, which expanded to 450 beds and treated over seven thousand patients. Jetland received Sweden's King's Medal for his service.

International staffs produce multilingual communications problems. This was demonstrated when an American officer came to the hospital with an ear problem. The American was greeted by one of Captain Jetland's soldiers, who told one of the Swedish medics that a "full colonel" wished to see a physician. Jetland happened by as the Swedish soldier was taking the colonel by the shoulders and maneuvering him into a small closet. It turned out that full colonel meant a *drunk* colonel to the Swedes, and the physician had directed the medic to place the officer in the closet until they could get to him.[30]

Scientific Specialties

Scientific specialty officers were essential members of the medical team in Korea as they had been in World War I and World War II. Again, diseases that were not significant threats in the United States were militarily significant in a theater of operations. The mission of conserving the fighting strength required the expertise of MSC specialists in preventive medicine, the biosciences, and clinical specialties such as optometry.

Preventive medicine units deployed early in the conflict. One, the 37th Preventive Medicine Company under the command of Maj. Arthur Kidwell, MSC, was activated on 12 August 1950, arrived in Pusan on 30 October, and moved to Seoul to undertake pest control operations. It went into North Korea in November but pulled back when the Chinese invaded. By December it was back in Pusan. There it performed vector control for the POW camps, where over 75 percent of the prisoners were infested with body lice. In less than two weeks the unit twice deloused 150,000 POWs, learning in the process that the Korean body louse was resistant to DDT.[31]

Sanitary Engineering Section officers were important members of the preventive medicine team in Korea. Lt. Col. Stanley J. Weidenkopf, MSC, as the X Corps sanitary engineer concentrated on water supply problems. Some developed from the use of oil and gas tankers—which first had to be cleaned out—to transport water for the Inchon landings. Another was the restoration of public water systems in liberated towns. The shortage of Medical Corps preventive medicine officers necessitated the use of MSC officers in some of those positions, and both Lt. Col. Floyd Berry, MSC, and Maj. Marlo E. Smith, MSC, were assigned as preventive medicine officers in 1952.[32]

Malaria was a constant threat in Korea because of a large civilian reservoir of the disease and the presence of anopheline mosquitoes. There were 311 cases of malaria and 29 deaths among United States troops during 1950. Over 106,000 gallons of insecticide were aerially dispersed the following year as part of the malaria control program. The program highlighted the need for a portable apparatus that could be carried by the Army's light aircraft. Maj. William Wyatt, MSC, developed an improved apparatus for that purpose at Edgewood Arsenal, Maryland.[33]

The importance of optometric support for combat operations was again demonstrated in the Korean War. Soldiers would frequently appear at the hospitals in Korea for replacement spectacles, but without their prescriptions. As in previous wars, they could lose their glasses or the prescriptions unintentionally, but it was also an effective way for a respite from combat. Maj. Anthony J. Zolenas, Jr., MSC, commander of the 8065th Medical Depot, discovered at one point that over two hundred soldiers were at the 8054th MASH waiting for new spectacles. Zolenas dispatched a forward optical platoon and the problem ended.[34]

One of the medical surprises of the war was the outbreak in 1951 of epidemic hemorrhagic fever. Laboratory officers at the 1st Medical Field Laboratory and Hemorrhagic Fever Center in Korea spent countless hours in unsuccessful attempts to identify the etiologic agent. Capt. Eugene D. Shaw, MSC, described his experience.

> The incessant work, the frustration of negative diagnostic tests, the despair of one doctor over his patients' deaths (sometimes four to five per day), the hot Korean summer, the dedicated nurses and members of the unit, the tarpaulin floor of the laboratory tent, the shock of Radio Peking listing us by ranks, names and serial numbers as Bacteriological Warfare Criminals, the rare sojourns back to "civilization" in Seoul, Korea, and the friendships made—each contribute to my memory when the two words "Hemorrhagic Fever" are mentioned.[35]

Aeromedical Evacuation

The existence of functional helicopters at a time when the Army was faced with the inadequate road net and inhospitable terrain of Korea hastened their use as air ambulances. The helicopter was much less punishing to patients than ground vehicles, provided quicker transport time, and was not slowed by roadblocks and destroyed bridges. Initially Air Force, and later Marine and Army, aviators, employing the primitive equipment available to them, used innovation to forge an aeromedical doctrine that would become a sophisticated part of the Army's medical evacuation and treatment system. The helicopters were piloted by officers from a number of branches during the war, some of whom later transferred to the Medical Service Corps.[36] They moved a large number of patients—some estimates run as high as 22,000.[37]

An Air Force unit, the 3d Air-Sea Rescue Squadron, arrived in Korea in July 1950 under the command of Capt. Oscar N. Tibbetts, USAF. There was little air opposition in Korea. Consequently there were few pilots to rescue, and one of the squadron's detachments began responding to evacuation requests for Army casualties. On 3 August Capt. Leonard A. Crosby, MSC, a former Army glider pilot and an operations officer on Colonel Dovell's staff, set up a demonstration for Dovell in the courtyard of Taegu Teachers' College. It was a convincing show, and a week later the Fifth Air Force commander authorized the use of helicopters for frontline evacuations.[38] The marines were also quite active in the use of helicopters for evacuation of casualties, although they did not develop units or aircraft specifically dedicated to this mission. The Marine Corps Sikorsky HRS–1 transport helicopter could carry up to five litter patients inside the aircraft. A Marine observation squadron, VMO–6, flying the more primitive HO3S, evacuated casualties throughout the Inchon-Seoul operation, including the movement of Army casualties, principally from the 1st Cavalry Division.[39]

In October the surgeon general, Maj. Gen. Raymond W. Bliss, visited Korea where he became convinced that the Medical Department needed its own air ambulance helicopters. The deputy surgeon general, Maj. Gen. George E. Armstrong (who succeeded Bliss in 1951), successfully carried the argument to the Army Staff. The Air Force and Army agreed that Army units would provide frontline evacuation and Air Force units would evacuate patients outside the combat zone.[40]

Four helicopter detachments arrived in Korea for assignment to the Eighth Army surgeon beginning in January 1951. Each detachment had four helicopters; two had Bell H–13s, and two had Hiller H–23s. Each helicopter had one pilot and was rigged with two exterior pods for litter patients; one ambulatory patient could be carried at the same time under ideal conditions. One detachment never became operational because its aircraft were diverted to other units immediately upon arrival. The remaining three detachments were each attached to a forward-deployed MASH. On 3 January 1st Lts. Willis G. Strawn, Artillery, and Joseph L. Bowler, Infantry, flew the first mission. Bowler went on to set a record of 824 medical evacuations in ten months.[41] The first detachments were general aviation units, but in November 1952 the 49th Medical Detachment (Air Ambulance), commanded by Capt. John W. Hammett, Artillery, was organized as the first purely medical aviation unit. Hammett, a World War II artillery liaison pilot, later transferred to the MSC.[42]

The helicopters were primitive aircraft. The Army's H–13 had a ten-gallon gas tank with a sixty-mile range, and the pilots had to either carry extra gas cans or refuel en route for longer missions. Because its weak battery system gave no guarantee of restarting the engine, the pilots engaged in "hot refueling." Leaded gas would foul sparkplugs and cause forced landings, so the pilots had to clean the plugs every day. The power transmission systems depended on a series of fan belts, which added more excitement, and with two outboard litters the aircraft would get nose heavy if the fuel ran low. Its gas tank was not self-sealing and the gearbox was exposed to enemy fire. Furthermore, the aviators did not have formal training in casualty care.[43]

Almost any damage from enemy fire was fatal to the helicopters. Therefore, the rules for their use were strict and tightly monitored by the Eighth Army Surgeon's Office. Missions were restricted to serious injuries, and the pilots had a right to refuse any mission that would damage the helicopter. Pickups were supposed to occur only at medical treatment facilities and only in daylight hours. However, the plucky aviators often ignored the rules when there were emergencies. As one put it, they would go to "any spot that was big enough to get the blades into."[44]

The pioneers had to be adept at improvisation. Intravenous bottles would freeze outside. Lieutenant Bowler and Lt. Col. James M. Brown, MC, commander of the 8063d MASH, devised a rig for suspending bottles for infusion of plasma or blood inside the cabin with a tube that ran outside to the litter. The door would pinch off the line to the patient, and Capt. Hubert D. Gaddis, Artillery, devised a notched opening in the fuselage large enough to accommodate the bottle while allowing the tubing to clear the door.[45]

Lieutenant Bowler also rigged covers for the Stokes litters mounted on each side of the helicopter. The cover and the litter were fashioned into a coffin-like

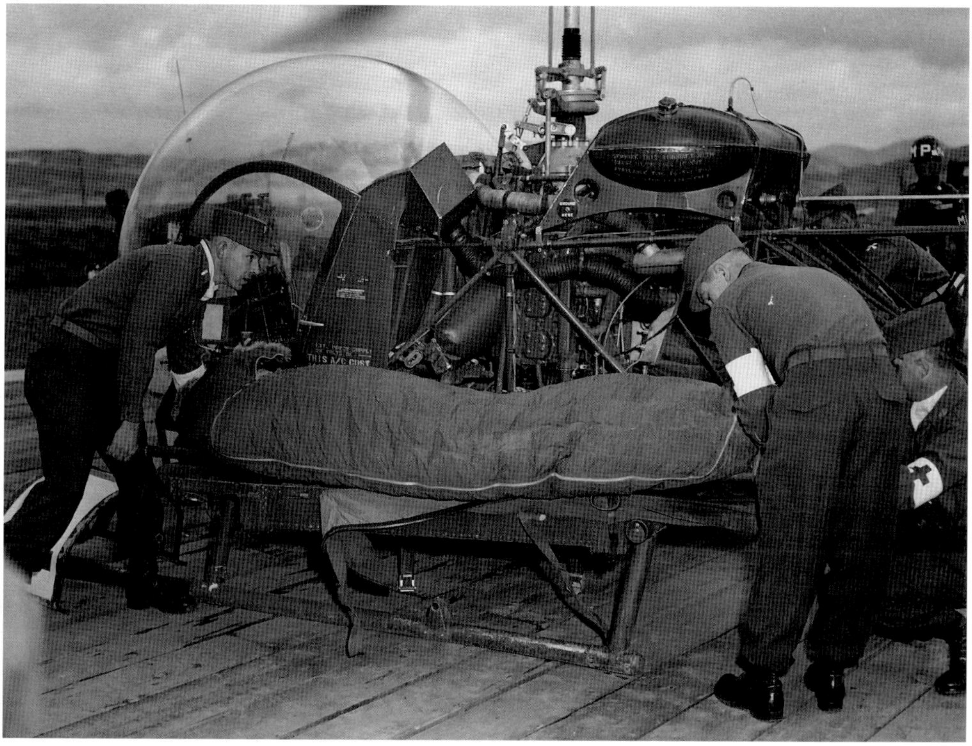

Wounded United Nations POW is loaded into an evacuation helicopter, April 1953.

box that protected the patient from the elements, but few patients were prepared for a flight in the claustrophobic airborne capsules. Colonel Dovell tried it for himself. "By the time I got to Pusan, I was wringing wet and I'm not a fearful individual as my record will show." He directed that the medics would sedate all patients evacuated in this manner.[46]

Developments in the Corps

Colonel Goriup's four-year term as chief of the corps ended in September 1951, and he was replaced with Col. Robert L. Black, MSC (*see Appendix G*). Both chiefs faced the tasks of fielding MSC officers to a theater of operations, meeting added demands for the use of MSCs, responding to concerns over the quality of the corps, expanding incentives, and encouraging developments in the administrative and scientific specialties. Their efforts included initiatives to improve morale and cohesion in the corps. One began in 1953, when Colonel Black attempted a draft of a history of the corps, the first in a series of attempts over the next forty years.[47]

The chief's office was affected by pressures on the Department of the Army and the Surgeon General's Office from the demands of the Korean War and the political developments of the time. The war was not popular, and General Dwight

D. Eisenhower's successful campaign for president was highlighted by his promise to go to Korea and end the fighting. The Cold War was a reality when Eisenhower took office in 1952. Communist hegemony in Eastern Europe as well as the intransigence of the People's Republic of China had created a fear of Communist domination of the world. Senator Joseph McCarthy of Wisconsin fanned the fear of communism into a hysteria.

That tension was part of the milieu surrounding the day-to-day duties of MSC officers in the Surgeon General's Office. For example, Lt. Col. Elwood Camp, MSC, chief of the Social Work Branch, was ordered to terminate the appointment of a civilian consultant whose name had surfaced in one of Senator McCarthy's lists of "known Communists." When the appointee asked why, Camp was allowed only to say: "I am sorry, but I have no comment."[48]

Although the Surgeon General's Personnel Division continued to exercise primary authority in personnel assignments, the corps chief was involved with establishing the governing policies. One was the commissioning of women. Colonel Black served as a member of an ad hoc DOD committee on the utilization of women. There he supported commissioning women in nearly every specialty of the corps. However, he opposed a Medical Department proposal to use second lieutenant MSC authorizations as a vehicle for commissioning medical, dental, and veterinary school students while they were still in school. Nevertheless, this eventually became a common practice.[49]

A major policy issue which concerned the chief was the replacement and substitution of physicians with MSC officers.[50] The physician shortage kept the fire under this problem, along with the continuing scrutiny of the department's use of its Medical Corps officers and strong pressure to replace those in administrative positions with MSCs. A *Washington Star* article on the "extravagant use of medical manpower by the Armed Forces" got the attention of the Surgeon General's staff, as did a telegram to the secretary of defense from Leland S. McKittrick, MD, president of the Massachusetts Medical Society. McKittrick wired that his organization was "deeply disturbed by [the] Army threat to call up medical officers." When the department proposed extending the physician draft in 1952, the American Medical Association proposed ending dependent care instead.[51] The external pressure contributed to a running debate within the department over the proper number of physicians on active duty. Surgeon General Bliss was sensitive to physician overstaffing. "We do not want to repeat the mistake made in World War II; i.e., having doctors idle and, therefore, disgruntled and unhappy." By and large it appears his dictum was followed in Korea.[52]

The shortage of physicians again dictated the substitution of MSCs in patient care roles, for example as battalion surgeons. There was trepidation over this practice. Col. Douglas Lindsey, MC, the Eighth Army surgeon's operations officer in 1953, was an outspoken critic because he believed MSC battalion surgeon's assistants did not receive adequate training for those medical responsibilities.[53]

In fact, there was a renewed debate over the use of MSCs as battalion surgeon's assistants, and in some cases MSCs were replaced by warrant officers. By March 1953 there were forty-three warrant officers assigned to different medical units in Korea, thirteen of whom were serving in divisions as battalion surgeon's

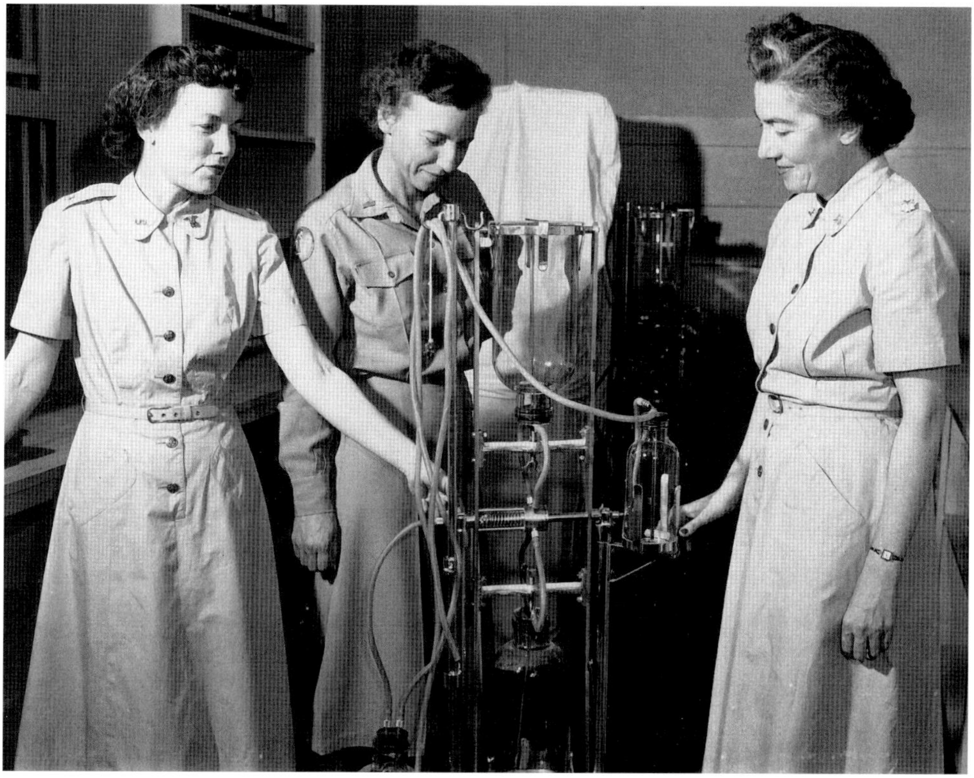

WACs checking a blood machine at the Camp Roberts Army Hospital, California, August 1951

assistants. Brig. Gen. L. Holmes Ginn, Jr., who became Eighth Army surgeon in January 1952, strongly favored this approach, citing insufficient medical training of young MSCs. In fact, Ginn proposed reducing by twenty-six the MSC positions in an infantry division and adding sixteen medical warrant officers. The surgeon general rejected his proposal, reaffirming the department's position that the medical treatment function was a secondary consideration for the utilization of MSC battalion surgeon's assistants. Their primary role was to support the administrative functions for that segment of the first level of the medical evacuation and treatment system. Further, the surgeon general viewed the positions as an excellent first step on a career ladder that "proves of inestimable value to the officer in later years as a result of the experience gained." That philosophy led to changing the administrative MSC specialty title to field medical assistant.[54]

The replacement of physicians in administrative duties included command positions. While command of active medical treatment facilities remained the province of Medical Corps officers, the shortage of physicians continued to prevent the department from always adhering to that doctrine. In 1950 the Surgeon General's Office considered assigning an MSC officer to command the 3,000-bed Philippine Scout Hospital. That did not occur, but there was regular use of MSC officers as medical battalion commanders during the first year of the Korean War, a reality recognized by the surgeon general's staff, which also accepted the assignment of MSC officers in lieu of physicians as medical company commanders.[55]

Personnel policy changes and wartime needs doubled the requirement for MSCs. The strength of the corps had dropped to 2,428 (and only 15 colonels on active duty) just prior to the outbreak of hostilities, a number that included less than 600 Regular Army officers. By 1952 the corps numbered over forty-seven hundred officers on active duty. The Pharmacy, Supply, and Administration Section accounted for 75 percent of the corps; the Medical Allied Sciences Section totaled 20 percent; and the Sanitary Engineering and Optometry Sections rounded out the picture with 3 and 2 percent, respectively. The increased use of MSC officers was evident when compared to the World War II ratio of MSC precursor officers to Medical Corps officers of approximately 1:2. By 1951 it was 3:4.[56]

The Medical Service Corps principally depended upon Reserve Officer Training Corps (ROTC) and officer candidate schools (OCS) for its accessions. A monthly quota of sixty OCS candidates was established for the MSC beginning with the class graduating in July 1952; by the spring of 1953, there were 600 OCS graduates on active duty. Another source was the direct commissioning of noncommissioned officers, and an additional 100 officers had received battlefield appointments at that point.[57]

The Medical Department discarded one option from the outset for, with some exceptions in the scientific specialties, it elected not to recall senior reserve officers to active duty. In the first place, Colonel Black reasoned that the greatest demand in Korea was for junior officers to fill assignments in combat units. Second, there had been no temporary (i.e., accelerated) promotions after World War II for the MSC officers who had remained on active duty, and they had received permanent promotions only. Consequently, they enjoyed no advantage in rank over MSC officers who had returned to civilian life but stayed in the reserves. The chief believed that recalling reservists to active duty would have caused a morale problem for those who had remained on active duty.[58]

There continued to be concerns about the quality of MSC officers, and discussion in the surgeon general's staff meetings on several occasions turned to problems with MSC officers in terms of performance, discipline, attitude, and capability. Those concerns seemed to be supported by the results of interviews with 56 direct-commissioned MSC officers that the Personnel Division conducted at the Medical Field Service School in 1952. They reported that 12 were "good officers," 30 were in a middle category ranging from "indifferent to low grade of satisfactory," and 14 "should have never been commissioned." Colonel Black believed some of the applicants for Regular Army commissions were not academically qualified and had mediocre performance records. Further, the officers who were OCS graduates or direct commissioned did not have college degrees.[59]

Maj. Gen. Joseph I. Martin, MC, commandant of the Medical Field Service School, tackled the issue of quality head-on in a controversial address to a monthly meeting of MSC officers at the Walter Reed Army Medical Center. General

Martin prefaced his remarks by saying that he spoke as a supporter of the MSC and saluted it for the superior performance of its officers in Korea. He complimented the corps on its great improvement since the prewar period when some Medical Administrative Corps officers were "nothing short of criminals."[60]But the general, who said there is "no wisdom like frankness," said he would be candid.

Martin challenged his audience to further improve the quality of MSC officers in terms of performance, dependability, honesty, and loyalty. He called for removing poor performers from active duty, beginning with clock watchers and avoiders of extra work. "You will always be judged by the weakest of your members. Get rid of them." By the same token, he urged the corps to bring in higher quality officers. He suggested raising the education prerequisites for commissioning and recruiting top graduates from the U.S. Military Academy at West Point. He urged the corps to stress generalization in the development of the administrative specialty officers. Martin believed there was too much emphasis on specialization, to which he feared weaker officers escaped as a way to avoid command or leadership positions, duties which required a diverse background.[61]

Perhaps most significantly, General Martin urged complete integration of MSC administrative specialty officers within the Medical Department in such a way as to prevent their removal. To that end, he insisted that MSC officers gain a practical knowledge of medicine, and he praised efforts along those lines at the Medical Field Service School to include basic medical skills in the training of MSC officers. Martin believed that MSCs, especially administrative specialty officers, must internalize the special ethos of the patient care environment. In other words, being a medic *was* different. The department stood to lose its MSC officers if it could not inculcate that distinction.

> Unless good improvement is made in this area you will have to fight off, again and again, the challenge to the specificity of your position by members of the line and by the other administrative service officers who today, in most cases, are equal to you in general administrative background and ability.[62]

He warned that there had already been an attempt to group all Army administrative officers into a single corps, and he predicted that more would follow. General Martin's comments were prescient, and his speech was remembered long after his retirement.[63]

Colonel Black recognized that improving the quality of the corps depended in great measure upon incentives that would attract and retain the highest quality officers. Thus he kept up the initiative begun by Colonel Goriup to remove the 2 percent cap on the number of full colonels. The effort advanced when DOD included a proposal to remove the 2 percent cap in its 1952 legislative program. Fred A. McNamara, chief of the Hospital Branch of the Bureau of the Budget, supported the initiative, introduced in Congress as House Resolution (H.R.) 5509. Black presented the proposal before a Pentagon legislative policy group in September, but he found both the Navy and Air Force lukewarm about a peculiarly Army problem. He lobbied for hearings on H.R. 5509, a proposal he described as "not a promotion bill but, rather, an equality of opportunity bill." Unfortunately the effort would not succeed during the Korean War period.[64]

MSC officers continued to break new ground. In 1951 Lt. Col. Frank K. Lawford became the first MSC in the Office of the Secretary of Defense when he was assigned to the Armed Forces Medical Policy Council. The corps passed an important military training milestone in 1951 when Lt. Col. Bernard Aabel, MSC, returned from attache duty in Finland to attend the Army War College.[65]

The Army-Baylor Program in Hospital Administration was an educational opportunity for MSC officers as well as officers of all the Medical Department corps and other federal agencies. Baylor awarded the first four degrees to Army-Baylor students at commencement exercises on 29 May 1953. Two officers received master's of hospital administration (MHA), a "professional" degree that required completion of course work, a residency year, and a thesis acceptable to the Graduate School. The other two received master's of science in hospital administration (MSHA), an "academic" degree that permitted waiver of the residency year based upon an individual's experience in supervisory positions. The MSHA was especially designed for Army Nurse Corps and Medical Corps officers, but was eventually abandoned.[66]

Students completed the first part of the program at the Medical Field Service School in an academic year of three quarters, which began the first week of September and ended the following June. The second half of the program was a residency year conducted according to the standards of the Association of University Programs in Hospital Administration (AUPHA). It was intended as the field work component of the program, a concept patterned after residency training performed by physicians in medical specialties.[67]

Col. Frederick H. Gibbs, MSC, replaced Colonel Richards in 1953 as the program director. When Gibbs took over, the class had sixty students, of which thirty-eight were "special students," or those ineligible for matriculation in the Baylor Graduate School—a situation that was not looked upon favorably by Baylor—and Colonel Gibbs himself was not a college graduate. Baylor maintained academic pressure on the program, and the percentage of fully eligible graduate students gradually increased.[68]

Gibbs took to task Dean Conley, executive director of the American College of Hospital Administrators, when Conley failed to include the Army-Baylor program in a list of twelve United States graduate programs he published in a 1953 article. Conley "broke out in profuse apologies" and explained that he wrote the article before the AUPHA had accepted the Army-Baylor program into its membership. The slight was so keenly felt that Hardy Kemp, M.D., director of graduate studies for Baylor University's School of Medicine, threatened to pull the program out of the AUPHA. "Here we put in more than three years of work piecing, splicing, stretching, sewing, stitching, and otherwise trying to join these things together . . . it burns the pants off me to be slighted in this way."[69]

Developments in the Administrative Specialties

Growth continued in the different administrative specialty fields. One, medical logistics, was an essential element of the Medical Department's capability in Korea and a specialty dominated by MSCs. The 8065th Army Medical Depot deployed from Yokohama on 8 July 1950. Its commander, Maj. Anthony J. Zolenas, Jr., MSC, said he "bottled every type of diarrhea mixture I could." By September 1951, when Maj. Marvin Ware, MSC, replaced Lt. Col. Carrol C. Barrick, MSC, as the Eighth Army surgeon's medical supply officer, there were base depots at Pusan and Taegu and an advance platoon with each of the three United States corps.[70]

Medical supply officers utilized supply schedules that were marginally useful in Korea because the usage factors did not account for new drugs or the increased use of others. They certainly did not allow for the astronomical rates of pilferage caused by widespread black market activity. Maj. Lynn B. Moore, MSC, in 1953 the Eighth Army medical supply officer, found that military police arrested some black marketeers as many as sixteen times for selling medical supplies. Lt. Col. Edwin D. McMeen, MSC, head of the medical depot at Yongdongpo, and Maj. Samuel Gottry, MSC, commander of the 60th Medical Depot, began using the steel shipping containers that were being tested beginning in 1950 for a container express (CONEX) service to store medical materiel. They found that the reusable CONEX containers, which measured approximately 8 by 6 by 7 feet, were very helpful in preventing pilferage.[71]

Operations and training officers did the hard staff work that made possible the deployment of the field medical support capability to Korea. Some officers served as instructors at the Medical Field Service School and in medical units. There was a sense of urgency in their training responsibilities, especially in preparing physicians for field medical service in Korea. Some observers strongly believed that the department's postwar emphasis on clinical training had gone overboard in correcting clinical deficiencies and failed to keep physicians current with the military side of their duties as Army officers. General Ginn said they had not received "the simple fundamentals of the care of the wounded man, or of the problems involved in the management of battle casualties."[72] Albert E. Cowdrey, author of *The Medics' War*, the definitive study of Army medicine in Korea, said that for the residents and interns quickly pulled from training and sent to Korea, "the general picture was one of innocents in the field."[73] The department benefited from the military training and experience of the MSC officers who coached Medical Corps officers assigned to their first field unit. A representative case was the 2d Infantry Division. Some of its physicians received their initial weapons training by firing off the fantails of ships transporting them to Korea.[74]

A new operations field was aeromedical plans and operations, and in November 1952 Maj. Leonard Crosby, MSC, returned to Washington, D.C., from Korea to head a newly formed Aviation Section in the Surgeon General's Office. Early ideas of training physicians as pilots were discarded as the department specified MSC aviators. In April 1953 the first seven earned their wings. All but one of the officers were assigned to Brooke Army Medical Center where the first United States–based air ambulance detachment, the 53d Medical Detachment (Air Ambulance), was formed. The first MSC aviators reached Korea on 29 August 1953, shortly after the cessation of hostilities.[75]

An out-of-the-ordinary operations job was performed by Maj. Thomas O. Matthews, MSC, who was stationed in Japan as the head of Far East Command's psychological warfare operations. Matthews began daily broadcasting two days after the invasion—initially from Japan and later from Korea—as the Voice of the United Nations Command. At its peak he directed thirty-nine stations broadcasting in Korean and Chinese.[76]

Some officers in the medical registrar specialty served as medical regulators controlling movement of patients along the evacuation chain. Officers, such as Lt. Col. Vincent J. Amato, MSC, medical regulating officer for the Pusan area, had to be fully conversant with each hospital's location, its language capability, bed availability, and specialty mix. Expanded use of air evacuation for overseas movement out of the theater led to the formation of the Armed Services Medical Regulating Office in October 1950, located in Washington, D.C. Maj. Donald E. Domina, MSC, became its first chief. He described it as the agency that matched patients to beds in the United States without regard to branch of service.[77]

MSC officers filled personnel positions at all levels of the Medical Department. In 1951 Maj. Vernon McKenzie, MSC, was assigned to the Surgeon General's Personnel Division where his duties included developing legislation for career incentive pay for physicians and the 1952 extension of the physician draft. In a routine action he authenticated the order promoting a dental officer, Capt. Irving Peress, DC, to major. Peress turned up on one of Senator McCarthy's lists, and the incantation became, "Who promoted Peress?" The answer was, of course, Major McKenzie. A sound truck circled the Pentagon blaring, "Who promoted Major Peress?" The surgeon general was required to furnish a list of all who had been involved with the case. McKenzie had to testify twice before the Senate Permanent Subcommittee on Investigations, and he was investigated by the FBI and the CIA. "I lost about seven or eight months struggling with that case."[78]

Hospital administration was beginning to flourish as a profession. By 1953 there were about six thousand hospitals in the United States with an estimated ten thousand administrator and assistant administrator positions, the two top executive levels in hospital administration. The profession progressed in the Army with the results of Medical Department studies and the maturation of the Army-Baylor program. Yet the emergence of MSC graduate hospital administrators was threatening to traditionalists. One wrote that physicians who denigrated assignments to hospital administration positions were making an error since "every profession has found that it is unsound to turn over top authority to essentially housekeeping personnel."[79]

Lt. Col. Frederick H. Gibbs, MSC, returned from Japan to an assignment in Washington, D.C., as the executive officer of the Surgeon General's Plans and Operations Division. There he played an important role in the modernization of Army hospital administration. Gibbs was instrumental in setting up and later heading the Surgeon General's Hospital Management Improvement Branch, which conducted a number of innovative studies from 1948 to 1952. With the solid backing of General Bliss, the surgeon general, the branch analyzed the organization, structure, and staffing patterns of Army hospitals using the Valley Forge Army Hospital in Pennsylvania as a test site for experiments. It was a remarkably productive period of innovation.[80]

The program established the hospital executive officer as the chief of administration and the principal adviser on management to the commander. It reduced the number of administrative divisions from twenty-two to nine and developed automated hospital procedures using IBM data-processing equipment for supply and medical registrar functions. The team designed an intensity of care measurement for grouping patient care and developed a new food service operation that employed a central kitchen and airline-style carts and trays. Based on its findings, the responsibility for hospital food service was transferred to dietitians of the Women's Medical Specialist Corps.[81]

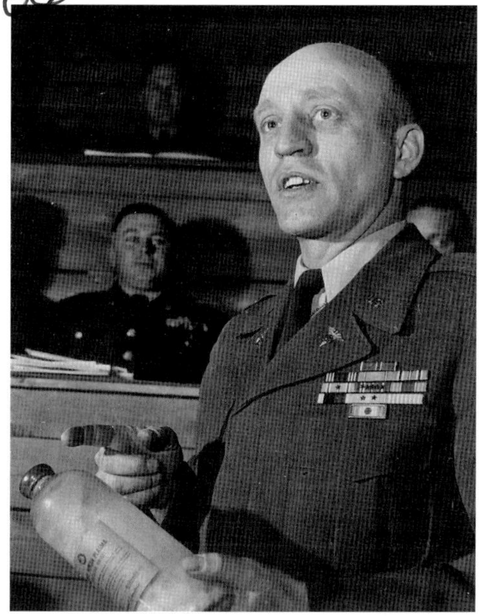

Maj. Edward H. Frick presents medical information at the Seventh Army Commander's Preventive Maintenance Course, November 1952.

The studies also influenced MSC opportunities for hospital administration positions. Gibbs recommended filling all hospital executive officer positions with MSC officers, and General Bliss approved that recommendation in 1949, with the proviso that the second in command, the deputy commander, would always be a physician. The change of the executive officer position was adopted in pilot tests of a revised standard organization for the Class I (or community) hospitals beginning in May 1950.[82] Although the position of hospital commander (in civilian life, the hospital administrator) remained closed, opening the executive officer position (the civilian hospital assistant administrator) to MSCs assured the Army that its hospital executive officers—in effect the chief operating officers—would be trained in hospital administration. Col. William Hamrick, MSC, was one of the first MSCs to benefit from the new policy when he was assigned as the executive officer of Fitzsimons Army Medical Center, Denver, Colorado, upon his return from Korea in 1951.

MSC hospital administrators participated in national professional organizations. Many were active in the American College of Hospital Administrators, which had grown to nearly twenty-five hundred members in the twenty years since its formation. Colonel Gibbs served on the American Hospital Association's Council on Administrative Practices. In 1952 the council established a Committee on Methods Improvement. That group, which Gibbs chaired, gave a national forum for the Medical Department's hospital management developments.[83]

Developments in the Scientific Specialties

In 1952 Lt. Col. Henry D. Roth, MSC, a pharmacy officer and chief of the Pharmacy, Supply, and Administration Section, could point to "great strides" achieved by pharmacy officers over the previous decade.[84] The surgeon general had directed that whenever possible pharmacies would be under the supervision of commissioned pharmacists, and that was the case at the general hospitals and the larger station hospitals. The pharmacy ROTC programs were popular, and by 1951 three of the pharmacy officers assigned as professors of military science and technology had taken advantage of their university assignments to earn master's of science degrees. The fourth had earned a Ph.D. A pharmacy officer, Lt. Col. Ralph D. Arnold, MSC, was chief of the pharmacy technician course at the Medical Field Service School. In addition, commissioned pharmacists had opportunities for positions that went beyond strictly pharmacy duties. Those included medical supply officer, battalion surgeon's assistant, hospital administrator, administrative assistant to major command surgeons, instructor, and medical unit commander.[85]

However, the Medical Department had backtracked from promises made to the American Pharmaceutical Association (APA) when the MSC was formed. General Armstrong, the surgeon general, told the 1952 annual meeting of the APA that although his predecessors, Surgeons General Kirk and Bliss, had both pledged that a pharmacist would always head the MSC, Armstrong was breaking with that policy. He said that pharmacists would always be a minority in the corps and the promises had been unrealistic. However, he assured his audience that a pharmacist would always be chief of the Pharmacy, Supply, and Administration Section.[86] Of course, as time would prove, that too was unrealistic.

In 1951 the Medical Allied Sciences Section included nine specialties: bacteriologist, biochemist, parasitologist, entomologist, serologist, clinical psychologist, research psychologist, and psychiatric social worker. In addition, there were sixty-nine physical reconditioning and six nutrition officers, although those specialties were phasing out of the MSC. The rehabilitation of veterans was now the responsibility of the Veterans Administration, and the last class of the Physical Reconditioning Course graduated in November 1953.[87]

While the specialties of the Medical Allied Science Section were well established within the Medical Department's clinical and research organizations, there were still concerns for their opportunities as MSC officers, and there were further recommendations for establishment of a separate scientific corps, as well as a proposal for a preventive medicine corps.[88] A study by the Surgeon General's Office addressed the problem of MSC officers in narrow specialty fields whose small numbers limited the number of field grade officer positions and constrained their promotion opportunities. The study conclusions provided no pathway through that situation because the positions—in Army force development terms—were characterized by "limited responsibilities and, for the most part, no command responsibilities." The report recommended that the department establish a combination of commissioned and warrant officer spaces and save its commissioned officer authorizations for key positions. Educational status was suggested as a criterion for determining commissioned or warrant appointment. Applicants with doctoral or master's degrees would qualify for commissions, while those with baccalaureate degrees would be appointed as warrant officers. The recommendation was not acted upon.[89]

There were recommendations in the press to commission chiropodists in 1949, and by 1952 the matter was under active consideration. The Armed Forces Medical Policy Council, a triservice group operating under the auspices of the DOD Office of Medical Services, considered a proposal to include chiropodists in the MSC. General Hays, General Armstrong's deputy, opposed this and said the Army was considering a warrant officer option. While chiropody was seen as "a useful medical adjunct," the Medical Department viewed commissioning with disfavor since, among other things, it was believed that osteopaths would then desire recognition comparable to the chiropodists'. The department reversed its position later that year when Surgeon General Armstrong considered formation of a chiropody section, but it went no further.[90]

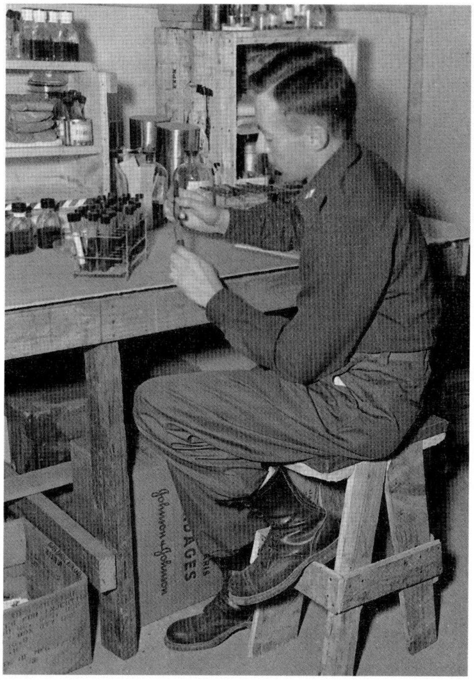

A member of the Medical Research Team, 46th Army Surgical Hospital, performs test in the laboratory, January 1953.

Army medical research provided MSC officers opportunities for worthwhile contributions. Lt. Col. Roy Maxwell, MSC, left the Crocker Radiation Laboratory in 1949 to head the Department of Biophysics at the Army Medical Service Graduate School. Maxwell's team of pioneers in the nuclear medical science specialty investigated the uses of radioactive isotopes in diagnosis and therapy. Capt. Joseph V. Brady, MSC, initiated studies of behavior measurement, later called the Conditioned Emotional Response, a step in the evolution of test systems used in the development of tranquilizers and psychoactive drugs. Another researcher, Lt. Col. Joseph F. Ackroyd, MSC, conducted studies that inaugurated research into platelet immunology.[91]

Col. George W. Hunter III, MSC, gained international recognition for his work with schistosomiasis. United States forces occupying Japan required food handlers to be free of parasites, and Hunter fielded a mobile laboratory outfitted in railroad cars that tested nearly nineteen thousand Japanese over a four-month period in 1949. The researchers found that 93.2 percent of those tested were infected with some form of intestinal parasite. Demand always creates a supply, and the team also found that there was a black market for parasite-free stools.

One of the parasitic diseases was schistosomiasis, a disabling and potentially fatal disease. Hunter concentrated his research effort on that endemic problem, and by 1951 his team had eliminated it in the Nagatoishi district of Kurume City, Japan, using a landmark program of molluscicides to control the snail host. Japan

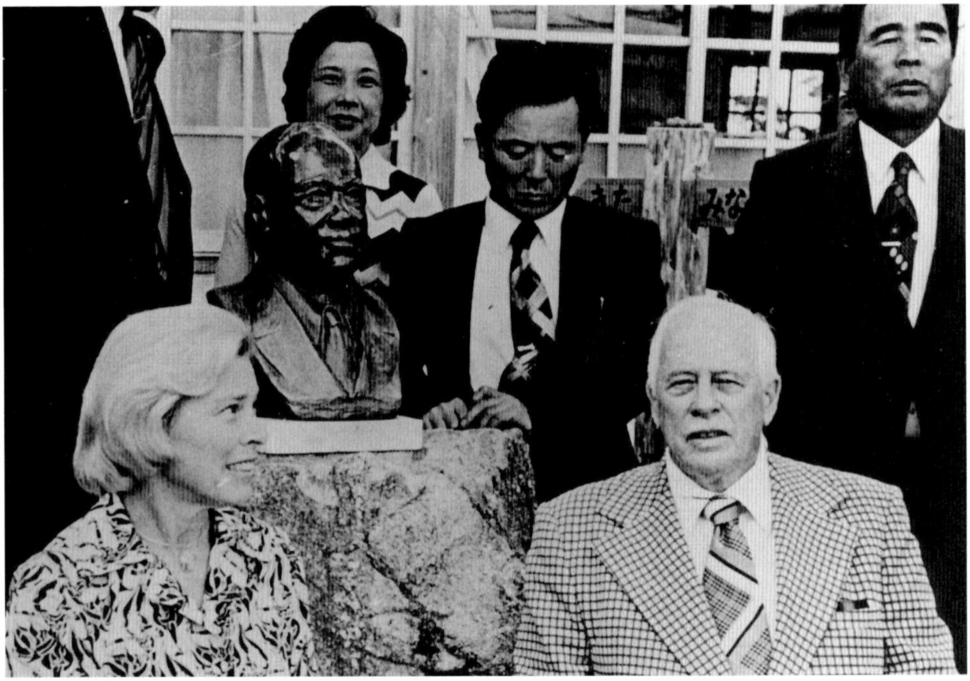

Colonel and Mrs. Hunter on a visit to Japan, April 1976

adopted Hunter's methods and by 1970 had virtually eliminated the disease. Hunter became a public figure in Japan, and in 1952 the townspeople of Kurume erected a bust of him as a permanent tribute to their "great benefactor."[92]

Social work entered a period of rapid growth in March 1950, when General of the Army George C. Marshall, president of the American Red Cross, announced the withdrawal of Red Cross social workers from Army hospitals, a move precipitated by budget cuts. The Medical Department expanded its number of social workers with programs that included commissioning women as reserve officers in the MSC, one of whom, Maj. Barbara B. Hodges, MSC, was appointed head of the Medical Social Work Section of the Surgeon General's Office. By May 1951 there were 129 social work officers on active duty, including 7 women. They served at Army hospitals, mental hygiene consultation services, and Army disciplinary barracks.[93]

Psychologists with a Ph.D. were well established as members of the neuropsychiatric team, although there was frustration that they were not treated as "real doctors." Lack of professional recognition was reflected in the entry grade of first lieutenant, as compared to captain for physicians. In March 1953 there were 56 psychologists on active duty, but the department had identified a requirement for 149.[94]

Col. Frederick A. Zehrer, MSC, an innovator in child psychology and the psychology consultant to the surgeon general, directed the revision of the department's manual for psychologists, *Military Clinical Psychology,* which was published in 1951.[95] It updated a scope of practice for clinical psychologists that was princi-

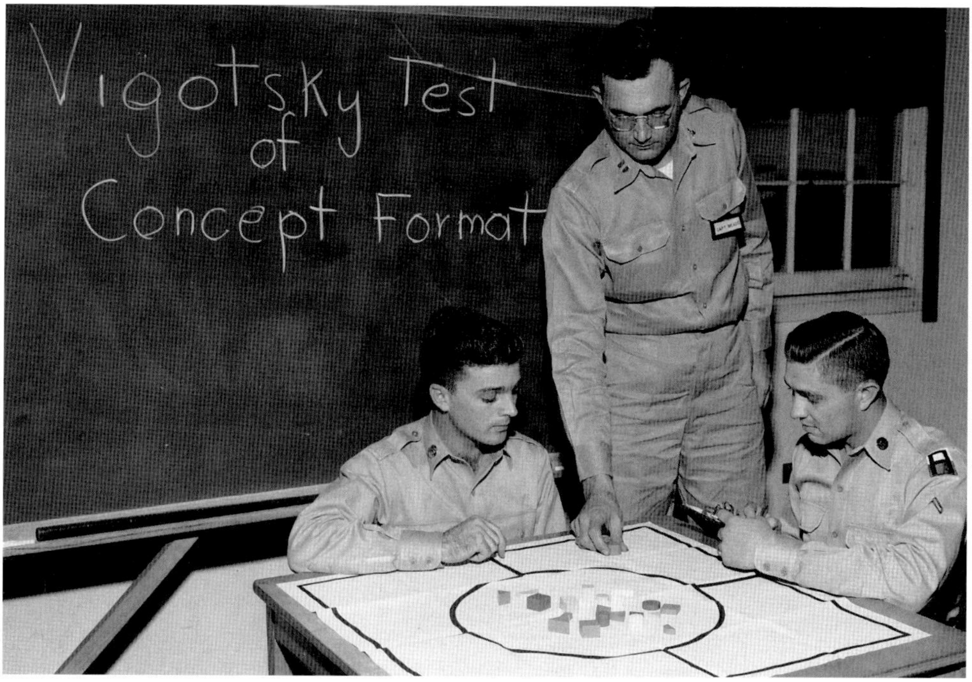

Clinical psychology students demonstrate the Vigotsky Test of Concept Formation at the Medical Field Service School, Brooke Army Medical Center, Fort Sam Houston, Texas, October 1951.

pally confined to diagnostic testing, but with provisions for psychotherapy and clinical research.

There were fifty-two positions for commissioned optometrists, a number insufficient to meet the workload. As a result, some optometrists were drafted and employed as enlisted soldiers in their specialty. An example of this practice was John Herron, O.D., an optometrist serving as an enlisted optician with an optical repair unit who was loaned by his first sergeant to the 121st Evacuation Hospital to perform refractions.[96] Not surprisingly, the Army's return to old habits prompted complaints by the American Optometric Association (AOA). The solution was to increase the authorized positions for commissioned optometrists to match the actual requirement for that specialty. Colonel Black was able to report to the AOA in 1952 regarding efforts to establish optometry positions at all levels of deployable hospitals.[97]

The AOA was convinced that some optometrists were assigned administrative specialty duties, a perception given credence by suspicions on the part of the surgeon general's staff of an "undercover campaign" by optometrists to thwart their utilization in positions not requiring their specialized training. Colonel Black attempted to defuse the controversy with the president of the AOA, an effort made difficult because of the latter's belief that the MSC chief encouraged the assignment of optometrists to administrative positions in field units.[98]

An example of what they were referring to was 1st Lt. Aaron Ryan, MSC, a World War II Navy veteran who completed optometry school on the GI Bill. Unable to obtain a commission as an optometrist, Ryan had received an infantry commission through OCS. He then transferred to the MSC and volunteered for duty as a battalion surgeon's assistant in Korea where he was decorated for valor. Colonel Black said that Ryan's record proved that "a person with a scientific background can ably be put to use in military medical fields other than his profession."[99]

Unfortunately, assignments such as Ryan's did not help make up the department's shortcomings in optometric capability, and that incongruity had piqued the interest of organized optometry. A trade journal article criticized the department for not first filling its requirements for optometry duty, even though it was understandable that some optometrists wished to volunteer for combat duty in administrative positions. What further complicated the matter was a turnabout of the substitution of MSCs for MCs when some physicians were pressed into optometry duties. In 1951 the Eighth Army began using physicians in the division medical battalions to handle eye refractions.[100]

A new regime of occupational vision programs at Army installations created additional demands for optometrists to screen employees for visual defects, to provide protective eye wear, and to analyze jobs for vision requirements and eye hazards. The Occupational Vision Section of the Army Environmental Health Laboratory at Edgewood Arsenal, Maryland, was headed by 1st Lt. Robert J. O'Shea, MSC. His program was based on pilot studies that had shown that approximately 30 percent of the Army's civilian employees had visual deficiencies.[101]

Summary

The Medical Service Corps was an important asset for the Medical Department when a "come-as-you-are" war required deployment of a precariously understaffed and unprepared field medical force. The MSC provided the range of specialty expertise the Army needed to support its combat operations. It also provided officers to substitute for or replace physicians during a period of shortages. Replacement of physicians in administrative positions gave the department the means to prevent the inevitable political fallout from using drafted physicians for nonclinical duties. A reflection of that migration was that nearly all the staff officers of the Eighth U.S. Army Chief Surgeon's Office were MSCs, and at all levels of the evacuation chain they were a repository of the "soldier" skills that had become rusty throughout the Medical Department.

The valor and hard work of MSC officers made a difference in Korea. Lt. Bodie Adams, a battalion surgeon's assistant, was one of the first heroes of the war. Other names come to mind: Maj. Matt Kowalsky, an operations officer running a railroad in combat; Capt. John Atkins, executive officer of a medical company in a firefight; Lt. Col. Stanley Weidenkopf, a sanitary engineer getting clean water supplies to the Inchon landing; Capt. Robert Jetland, executive officer of a Swedish hospital; Capt. Eugene Shaw, a laboratory officer at a hemorrhagic fever laboratory hearing his name broadcast as a war criminal; Lt. Stanley Weintraub, a registrar with a ringside seat for a hospital under attack by its own patients; Maj.

Arthur Kidwell, commander of a preventive medicine company that ranged from Pusan to Inchon, to Seoul, to Pyongyang, and back to Pusan fighting plague; and Maj. Oren Atchley, a medical battalion commander killed in action searching for a lost ambulance crew and its patients.

MSC officers participated in the development of new medical technologies. Col. George Hunter's pioneering medical research in schistosomiasis was memorialized by one of the few statues in Japan erected to the memory of an American. Innovations by Col. Frederick Gibbs led to genuine improvements in Army hospital administration. Some MSCs attended flight school to take over the operation of the Army's fledgling aeromedical evacuation capability. That humanitarian advance had its beginnings in ungainly Korean War helicopters that called to mind the Ford Model T ambulances of the U.S. Army Ambulance Service in World War I. The care and feeding of those machines included careful attention to fan belts and batteries. Intrepid pilots, some of whom later transferred to the MSC, flew patients in coffin-like boxes suspended outboard in a fashion guaranteed to terrify those occupants who remained conscious.[102]

The corps was challenged to improve the quality of its officers, and its first two chiefs looked for ways to provide incentives that would attract and retain good officers. Opportunity for training advanced with the selection of the first MSC to attend the War College. Unfortunately, promotion opportunity remained abridged by the 2 percent ceiling on the number of colonels. Five years' worth of initiatives to turn that aside were not successful, but the corps remained hopeful. There was some advancement in position opportunity as the hospital executive officer was designated for MSC officers, although the senior hospital administrator position, the commander, remained closed.

MSC officers showed that they had the ability, training, and experience to serve in all kinds of leadership positions, including command. The department's actions in Korea demonstrated the tenuousness of its doctrine, which restricted the selection of commanders of operational medical units to physicians. When push came to shove, MSCs commanding medical battalions remained in command of their units. The department was very fortunate to have had those officers available for that duty, but the lesson would fade as the department entered another postwar period. MSCs were unsure what their future would bring. But General Martin had lifted the curtain on one possibility, the potential for efforts to remove some or all of their specialties from the Medical Department.

Notes

[1] Army strength: Weigley, *History of the United States Army*, p. 502. The Army strength was 591,487 in June 1950. The Air Force totaled 411,000 personnel. Korean War: Numbers are based on U.S. Department of Defense, *Defense 86, September/October 1986*, pamphlet (Arlington, Va.: Armed Forces Information Service, 1986), p. 46, and Frank H. Reister, *Battle Casualties and Medical Statistics: U.S. Army Experience in the Korean War* (Washington D.C.: The Surgeon General, Department of the Army, 1972), hereafter cited as Reister, *Battle Casualties*. An essential source is Cowdrey, *The Medics' War*. A good chronology and critique of the war are in T.R. Fehrenbach, *This Kind of War: A Study of Unpreparedness* (New York: Pocket Books, 1964). A helpful bibliographic survey is Terrence J. Gough, *U.S. Army Mobilization and Logistics in the Korean War: A Research Approach* (Washington, D.C.: U.S. Army Center of Military History, 1987).

[2] Quoted words: Sgt. Daniel Cavanaugh, Medical Company (Med Co), 34th Infantry, 24th Infantry Division (Inf Div), in Donald Knox, *The Korean War, Pusan to Chosin: An Oral History* (New York: Harcourt, Brace and Jovanovich, 1985), p. 60.

[3] Forces in Korea: Reister, *Battle Casualties*, p. 1.

[4] Notifications: See intervs, Samuel Milner with Lt Col Robert A. Byrne, MSC, OTSG, 15 Jul 66, and with Maj Edward J. Kelly, MSC, OTSG, 9 Sep 66, interview files, USACMH.

[5] Dovell: Rpt, Charles W. Ellsworth, Jr., THU, OTSG, sub: Biography of Col Chauncey E. Dovell, MC, undated, USACMH; Cowdrey, *The Medics' War*, p. 81. Sixty years old at the outbreak of the Korean War, Dovell was a holder of the Distinguished Service Cross from World War I and had served as a regimental surgeon in World War II. He made it a point to be as far forward as possible. In September 1950 he was personally responsible for the capture of thirteen enemy soldiers, for which he received the Silver Star.

[6] Advance staff: The initial staff was Maj. Sam Hill, MSC, entomologist; Maj. Fenner Whitely, MSC, sanitary engineer; Capt. Harry L. Gans, MSC, supply officer; Capt. Leonard A. Crosby, MSC, operations officer; and 2d Lt. Joseph A. Mikos, administrative assistant. They were soon joined by other officers, including Lt. Col. William Moore, MC, the deputy surgeon. Intervs, Milner with Col Harry L. Gans, MSC, OTSG, 29 May 66; Col Paul M. Levesque, MSC, OTSG, 30 Sep 59; Col William A. Hamrick, MSC, OTSG, 7 Jul 66, all in USACMH; Hamrick to Ginn, 15 Sep 88; Gans to Hamrick, undated (1988); Col Leonard Crosby, MSC, to Hamrick, 14 Mar 88, DASG-MS; Cowdrey, *The Medics' War*, p. 81; Medical Sec, HQ, EUSA, Annual Rpt 1950, extract, box 13/18, MSC-USACMH. Casualties: SG Conference, 14 Aug 50.

[7] Quoted words: Col Othmar F. Goriup, MSC, to Lt Col James T. Richards, MSC, 10 Oct 50, DASG-MS. Awards: Rpt, TLO, OTSG, sub: Army Medical Personnel—Decorations, Aug 51, DASG-MS.

[8] Levesque: Levesque, Milner interv, 30 Sep 59.

[9] Division MSCs: Speech, Col. Bernard Aabel, MSC, Chief, MSC, to Idaho and Oregon state pharmacy conventions, Jun 57, folder 78, box 6/18, MSC-USACMH.

[10] Task Force Smith: Interv, Brig Gen Charles B. Smith, with Milner, 15 Jun 65, USACMH; Cowdrey, *The Medics' War*, pp. 73–74; Michael W. Cannon, "Task Force Smith: A Study in (Un)Preparedness and (Ir)Responsibility," *Military Review* 68 (February 1988): 63–73; Intervs, Lt Col Raymond E. Adams, MSC, with Milner, OTSG, 16 Jun and 22 Jul 65; Milner, draft chapter, sub: North Koreans, in MS, U.S. Army Medical Service in the Post–World War II and Korean Eras, undated (1965), box 1/18, MSC-USACMH.

[11] Smith: Smith, Milner interv, 15 Jun 65. Quoted words: Adams to Ginn, 2 May 86, DASG-MS. Pfc. Max Myers and Cpl. Ernest Fortuna volunteered to stay with the wounded. They were repatriated at Operation Big Switch.

[12] 25th Medical Battalion: Interv, Maj Herman A. Walker, MSC, with Milner, OTSG, 28 May 66, USACMH. Wagoner: Interv, Maj Donald E. Wagoner, MSC, with Milner, OTSG, 5 Oct 65, USACMH. The battalion surgeon was Capt. Vincent J. Nevarre, MC.

[13] Shortages: Cowdrey, *The Medics' War*, pp. 66–68. Utilization: Surgeon, 1st Cav Div, 1952 Annual Rpt; Med Sec, HQ, Far East Command (FEC), 1950 Annual Rpt. The 40th Inf Div surgeon said that MSCs were "of highest caliber." Surgeon, 40th Inf Div, 1952 Annual Rpt. However, the EUSA found that the preparation of battalion surgeon's assistants was uneven and established a

refresher training program in 1952. Surgeon, 3d Inf Div, 1953 Annual Rpt; Med Sec, HQ, EUSA, 1952 Annual Rpt, all from extracts in box 13/18, MSC-USACMH. 7th Inf Div: Surgeon, 7th Inf Div, 1952 Annual Rpt, extract in box 13/18, MSC-USACMH.

14 Levi and Gilliam: Lt Col Andrew J. Colyer, MSC, draft chapter, sub: Medical Field Service, 1958 MSC history project. Lavault: Interv, Lt Col Paul A. Lavault, MSC, with Milner, 14 Jul 66.

15 Lavault: Lavault, Milner interv. Sarka: John G. Westover, *Combat Support in Korea* (Washington, D.C.: Combat Forces Press, 1955), pp. 109–10.

16 Leapfrogging: W.H. Thornton, "The 24th Division Medical Battalion in Korea," *Military Surgeon* 109 (July 1951): 13. Huggins: Interv, Lt Col Lewis H. Huggins, MSC, with Milner, OTSG, 11 Aug 66, USACMH. Huggins' most enduring lesson of the war was the "utter dedication to duty" of his enlisted medics.

17 Atkins: Med Co, 21st Inf Rgt, 24th Inf Div; Surgeon, 24th Inf Div, Annual Rpt, 1951, extract, box 13/18, MSC-USACMH; Cowdrey, *The Medics' War*, pp. 161–62. Cook: Surgeon, 2d Inf Div, Annual Rpt, 1951, extract, box 13/18, MSC-USACMH. Anderson and Boyson: Cowdrey, *The Medics' War*, p. 75.

18 MSC battalion commanders: Cowdrey, *The Medics' War*, p. 142; Surgeon, 24th Inf Div, Annual Rpt, 1953, extract, box 13/18, MSC-USACMH.

19 Atchley: DF, Cdr, 7th Medical Battalion (Med Bn), to Surgeon, 7th Inf Div, sub: MIA Report on Battalion Commander, 7th Med Bn, 28 Nov 50, and encl 1 to Command Rpt, 7th Med Bn, 1 Dec 50, RG 407, entry 529, box 3185, NARA-WNRC.

20 Walker: Walker, Milner interv, 28 May 66; Interv, Col Richard H. Ross, MC, with Milner, OTSG, 28 May 66, USACMH. Quoted words: Annex 11 to 25th Inf Div History, July 1950, RG 407, entry 429, box 3747, NARA-WNRC.

21 Richards: Interv, Lt Col Herman Richards, MSC, Ret., with Milner, OTSG, 19 Aug 66, USACMH. His company was attached to the 32d Infantry.

22 Refugees: Richards, Milner interv, 19 Aug 66; Walker, Milner interv, 28 May 66.

23 8055th MASH: Suzanne Ward, "And Now, Will the Real M–A–S–H Please Stand Up," *AMEDD Spectrum* 1 (1974): 11, copy in JML. Also see Intervs, Milner with Col Kryder E. Van Buskirk, MC, CO, 8076th MASH, OTSG, 7 Jul 66, and Col George Zalkan, MC, CO, 8054th MASH, OTSG, 9 Aug 66, both in USACMH.

24 Hospital trains: Cowdrey, *The Medics' War*, pp. 149–50; Levesque, Milner interv, 30 Sep 59. Kowalsky: Intervs, Milner with Kowalsky, 29 May 66 and with Col Chauncey E. Dovell, MC, Hampton, Va., 21 Sep 66, USACMH.

25 Train ambush: Kowalsky tried unsuccessfully to get an award for Dovell. Yet Maj. Gen. Edgar Erskine Hume, MC, FEC surgeon, who was visiting Korea and was also aboard, received a Silver Star and a Purple Heart. Kowalski could not account for that, because "told to stay out of sight, the General did so." Hume is criticized in several accounts for his love of medals and decorations (Dovell called it "a positive mania"). See intervs, Milner with Kowalsky, 29 May 66; Dovell, 21 Sep 66; Lt Col Richard Stacey, MSC, OTSG, 28 Sep 66, USACMH; and Maj Gen Silas B. Hays, MC, OTSG, 25 Oct 63, USACMH.

26 Quoted words: Interv, Col Rudolph P. Czaja, MSC, with Milner, OTSG, 1 Jul 66, USACMH. 64th Field Hospital: Czaja, Milner interv; Cowdrey, *The Medics' War*, pp. 123–24, 310.

27 Given up for lost: Czaja, Milner interv, 1 Jul 66.

28 POW hospital: Stanley Weintraub, *The War in the Wards: Korea's Unknown Battle in a Prisoner-of-War Hospital Camp* (1964; reprint, California: Presidio Press, 1976), p. 10; Cowdrey, *The Medics' War*, pp. 316–19. After the war Weintraub became an English professor, Guggenheim fellow, and distinguished writer and critic.

29 Quoted words: Weintraub, p. 89.

30 Swedish hospital: Interv, Col Robert I. Jetland, MSC, with Milner, OTSG, 7 Sep 66, USACMH. Colonel Groth said, "One thing I'll always remember about the Americans is how easy they made it for us doctors to practice our profession." Jetland, "Medical Service Corps Duties in Korea," *Military Surgeon* 112 (May 1952): 353; "Featured Retired Alumnus," *The Bear Facts: U.S. Army–Baylor University Alumni Club Newsletter* (Winter 1990), DASG-MS.

31 DDT resistance: Herbert S. Hurlbut, Robert M. Altman, and Carlyle Nibley, Jr., "DDT Resistance in Korean Body Lice," *Science* 115 (4 January 1952): 11; Col Ralph W. Bunn, MSC, and

Col Joseph E. Webb, Jr., MSC, sec. 7, sub: Entomology, of draft chapter 8, sub: Laboratory Specialties, 1958 MSC History Project, pp. 108–09, DASG-MS.

[32] Sanitary engineering: Rpt, Col Raymond J. Karpen, MSC, Ret., to Col Earl J. Herndon, MSC, sub: Preventive Medicine Activities, 1950–53, 7 Nov 83, DASG-MS, hereafter cited as Karpen, Preventive Medicine, 1950–53; Cowdrey, *The Medics' War*, pp. 145–46; Lt Col Sam Hill, FEC, to Lt Col Webb, OTSG, 13 Sep 50, DASG-MS; Interv, Col Stanley J. Weidenkopf, MSC, with Milner, OTSG, 18 Feb 67, USACMH.Preventive medicine officers: Med Sec, HQ, FEC, 1952 Annual Rpt, extract, box 13/18, MSC-USACMH.

[33] Malaria rates: Karpen, Preventive Medicine, 1950–53. Wyatt: Ibid.

[34] Optometry: Memo, Col Howard W. Glattly, MC, Chief, Pers Div, OTSG, for Chief, Med Plans and Operations Div, OTSG, sub: Utilization of Optometrists (including extract from ltr by FEC chief surgeon), 22 Aug 52, DASG-MS; Interv, Col Anthony J. Zolenas, MSC, with Milner, OTSG, 13 Jul 66, USACMH; SG Conferences, 18, 20, and 26 Jun 52; "Army M.S.C. Optometrist Is Cited" *Southern Optometrist* (January 1954): 23–24. Respite from combat: Glattly, FEC extract, DASG-MS.

[35] Shaw's experience: Capt Eugene R. Shaw, MSC, to Lt Col John R. Ransom, 6 Nov 59, cited in Ransom, section, sub: Microbiology, in 1958 MSC history project, folder 253, box 16/18, MSC-USACMH.

[36] Aviation: Intervs, Col Leonard A. Crosby, MSC, OTSG, 25 Aug 66, USACMH; Dovell, 23 Sep 66; Col John D. Davenport, MSC, OTSG, 28 Oct 66, USACMH; and Levesque, 30 Sep 59, all with Milner; Interv, Lt Col John W. Hammett, MSC, with Capt Peter Dorland, MSC, THU, OTSG, undated, USACMH; Ltr, Col Kryder E. Van Buskirk, MC, to Dorland, 24 May 74, USACMH; Richard P. Weinert, Jr., *A History of Army Aviation—1950–1962* (Fort Monroe, Va.: U.S. Army Training and Doctrine Command, 1991), p. 203–04; Robert F. Futrell, Lawson S. Mosley, and Albert F. Simpson, *The United States Air Force in Korea 1950–1953* (New York: Duell, Sloan and Pearce, 1961), pp. 543–46; Lynn Montross, *Cavalry of the Sky* (New York: Harper and Brothers, 1954), pp. 134–35, 154–55; Peter Dorland and James Nanney, *Dust Off: Army Aeromedical Evacuation in Vietnam* (Washington, D.C.: United States Army Center of Military History, 1982), pp. 10–20; Allen D. Smith, "Medical Air Evacuation in Korea and Its Influence on the Future," *Military Medicine* 110 (May 1952): 323–32; Spurgeon H. Neel, Jr., "Helicopter Evacuation in Korea," *U.S. Armed Forces Medical Journal* 6 (May 1955): 691–702; Cowdrey, *The Medics' War*, pp. 163–67; Martin Blumenson, "Helicopter Evacuation," in Westover, *Combat Support in Korea*, pp. 111–13. Air ambulance pilots in Korea were Artillery, Infantry, Signal Corps, Corps of Engineers, and Transportation Corps officers. The first MSC graduates of flight school did not arrive in Korea until after the hostilities had ended.

[37] Number evacuated: Dorland and Nanney put the number evacuated at 17,700. Lt. Gen. Heaton, TSG, cited 20,000 in 1967, and Col. Leonard Crosby put the total at 21,852, based on his records. Remarks, Heaton, sub: Dedication of Kelly Heliport, 7 Apr 67, and Crosby to Hamrick, 14 Mar 88, both DASG-MS. Kelly heliport was the airfield located at Fort Sam Houston, San Antonio, Texas. Lt. Col. Kryder E. Van Buskirk, CO of the 8076th MASH, lauded the benefit of speedy evacuation. "It is not uncommon for casualties to arrive in such excellent shape that they are ready for immediate operations." Van Buskirk, "The Mobile Army Surgical Hospital," *Military Surgeon* 113 (July 1953): 31.

[38] Demonstration: Crosby, Milner interv, 25 Aug 66.

[39] Marines: Lynn Montross, Hubard D. Kuokka, and Norman W. Hicks, *The East-Central Front,* volume in the series U.S. Marine Operations in Korea, 1950–1953 (Washington, D.C.: Headquarters, U.S. Marine Corps, 1962), pp 49, 56, 188–90. VMO–6 evacuated 1,396 casualties in the first six months of 1951. Montross, *Cavalry of the Sky*, p. 155.

[40] TSG requests helicopters: SG Conference, 9 and 13 Oct and 15 Nov 50.

[41] Bowler and Strawn: Tierney and Montgomery, *The Army Aviation Story*, p. 208.

[42] 49th Medical Detachment: Crosby to Hamrick, 14 Mar 88. On 1 June 1953, Hammett's detachment, along with five others, combined to form the 1st Helicopter Ambulance Company (Provisional) under the command of Maj. Rusty Russell, FA.

[43] Need for medical training: Interv, Col Hubert D. Gaddis, MSC, Ret., with Dorland, OTSG, 2 May 74, USACMH.

[44] Quoted words: Hammett, Dorland interv, undated, USACMH.

[45] IV bottle hatch: Gaddis, Dorland interv, 2 May 74; Cowdrey, *The Medics' War*, p. 166.

[46] Quoted words: Dovell, Milner interv, 21 Sep 66.

[47] Draft history: Rpt, Col Robert L. Black, Chief, MSC, OTSG, sub: History of the Medical Service Corps (draft), 1 Jun 53 (32 pp.), DASG-MS.

[48] Quoted words: Elwood Camp, As I Remember Social Work.

[49]Role of chief: Interv, Brig Gen William A. Hamrick, Ret., with Col Ernest J. Sylvester, MSC, San Antonio, Tex., USAMHI Senior Officer Oral History Program, 21 Feb 84, USAMHI; Interv, Louis F. Williams with Ginn, 15 Nov 84, DASG-MS. Women: Memo, 1st Lt M.E. Snyder, MSC, sub: Medical Service Corps Policy Council Meeting, 1000 Hours, 9 Jan 1952, 14 Jan 52, citing Memo, Black for DSG, 2 Jan 52, DASG-MS, hereafter cited as Snyder, 14 Jan 52 Memo; SG Conferences, 26 Jun and 14 Jul 52; Robert S. Anderson, ed. in chief, *Army Medical Specialist Corps* (Washington, D.C.: Office of the Surgeon General, Department of the Army, 1968), pp. 402–04. Opposition to use of spaces: Snyder, 14 Jan 52 Memo.

[50] MSC use: Isaac Cogan, head of TSG's Resources Analysis Division, took the argument a step further and argued that MSCs were performing jobs that should be handled by warrant officers and sergeants (SG Conferences, 26 Mar 51 and 15 May 53). That did not appear to be a concern of TSG.

[51] Quoted words: "Extravagant Use of Medical Manpower by the Armed Forces," *Washington Evening Star*, 24 October 1951; SG Conference, 25 Oct 51. Quoted words: Telegram (Telg), Leland S. McKittrick, M.D., President, Massachusetts Medical Society, and seventy-five representatives of hospitals and medical schools, to Louis Johnson, Sec Def, Stuart Symington, Chm, National Security Resources Board, and Sen Millard E. Tydings, Chm, Senate Armed Services Committee; SG Conference, 25 Aug 50. AMA: Interv, Lt Col Vernon McKenzie, MSC, with Milner, OTSG, 4 Nov 63, USACMH.

[52] MC strength: See Bliss in SG Conferences, 21 Feb 51 and 8 Aug 50; Armstrong in SG Conference, 23 Mar 51. Korea: Col. Harold W. Glattly, MC, chief of the Personnel Division, OTSG, reported after a visit in October 1952 that "not one complaint was received from a medical officer based upon inactivity." Memo, Glattly for TSG, sub: Personnel Survey of Medical Activities and Installations in FECOM and USARPAC, 13 Oct 52, in SG Conference, 13 Oct 52.

[53] MSC substitution: SG Conference, 1 May 51; Lt Col Douglas Lindsey, MC, Dir, Med Research, U.S. Army Chemical Warfare Laboratory, to Col Gene Quinn, MSC, 3 Jun 59, USACMH; Interv, Col Lynn B. Moore, MSC, with Milner, OTSG, 28 Jul 66, USACMH. Lindsey said his opinion was "unprintable." The department's performance was one of its "blackest chapters" because it "lost the lives of 10,000 men in Korea who would have been saved by the Marine Corps medical service in the same war. I lay a lot of the blame for this on the policy of giving, to the MSC assistant battalion surgeon, responsibilities for which he was and always will be totally unprepared."MC shortages: Interv, Col John W. Wisearson, MSC, with Milner, OTSG, 22 Sep 66, USACMH.

[54]WO/MSC debate: Brig Gen L. Holmes Ginn, Jr., Surgeon, EUSA, to Maj Gen George Armstrong, TSG, 8 Mar 53; Lt Col Thomas P. Caito, MSC, Pers Div, OTSG, to Chief, Pers Div, sub: Utilization of Warrant Officers in Lieu of MSC Officers to Staff Divisional Type MOS 3506 Positions, 27 May 53; Col O. Elliot Ursin, MC, Asst Ch, Pers Div, OTSG, to Maj Gen William E. Shambora, MC, Ch Surgeon, U.S. Forces, Far East, 8 Apr 53, all in DASG-MS. Quoted words: Ursin to Shambora, 8 Apr 53.

[55] Company command: SG Conference, 7 Jul 52. Philippine Scout Hospital (10th General Hospital): SG Conference, 16 Sep 49.

[56] MSC:MC ratio: Cowdrey, *The Medics' War*, p. 21. Corps strength: Heaton, Statement Before the Committee on Armed Services, U.S. Senate, 8 Sep 66, DASG-MS; Memo, Lt Col Manley G. Morrison, Pers Div, OTSG, sub: Structure of the Medical Service Corps, 16 Apr 53, file 228–01, box 4/18, USACMH; Andrew J. Colyer, "Career Management for the Medical Service Corps," *U.S. Armed Forces Medical Journal* 1 (June 1950): 709.

[57] OCS: MSC Historical Rpt, 1 July–31 December 1951, file Post World War II, box 2/18, MSC-USACMH. Accessions: SG Conference, 23, 25 Apr 53.

[58] No recall: Robert L. Black, "The Army's Medical Service Corps," *Military Surgeon* 115 (July 1954): 12.

[59] Concerns: Maj Gen Bliss, TSG, and Col Schwichtenberg, MC, SG Conference, 8 Sep 49; Maj Gen Bliss, TSG, SG Conference, 14 Nov 50; Maj Gen Hays, DSG, SG Conference, 7 Sep 51; MFSS Study, SG Conference, 13 Feb 52; Maj Gen Armstrong, TSG, SG Conference, 15 Feb 52; Maj Gen W.E. Shambora, MC, SG Conference, 7 Aug 53; Col. Ursin, MC, SG Conference, 4 Nov 53.

[60] Quoted words: Speech, Maj Gen Joseph I. Martin, MC, sub: Address to Medical Service Corps Officers, MSC Officers Meeting, Walter Reed Army Medical Center (WRAMC), 1953, file 228–5, box 5/18, MSC-USACMH, hereafter cited as Martin, Address to MSC Officers. MSC meetings: SG Conferences, 21 May 50; 10 and 13 Oct 52; and 14 Jan 53. Colonel Goriup started the meetings in 1950 for MSCs stationed in the Washington, D.C., area. General Armstrong said Goriup "gave a most impressive talk" at the first one.

[61] Generalization: See Colyer, "Career Management for the Medical Service Corps," p. 709.

[62] Quoted words: Martin, Address to MSC Officers.

[63] Martin's influence: See quote by Col Caroll C. Barrick, MSC, in Rpt, 549th Hospital Center, sub: Proceedings of the MSC Conference in USAREUR, 2–4 April 59, DASG-MS.

[64] Two percent cap: Snyder, 14 Jan 52 Memo; MSC Historical Rpt, 1 July–31 December 1951, file Post World War II, box 2/18, MSC-USACMH; Memo, Black for Chief, Pers Div, OTSG, 9 Mar 53; Memo, Glattly for Chief, MSC Div, OTSG, 24 Jun 53; Cmt 2, Brig Gen R.E. Chambers, MC, Ch, Professional Div, OTSG, to Memo, Ch, MSC, sub: Position Authorizations for Colonels, MSC, 14 Sep 53, all in DASG-MS.

[65] First OSD: Lt Col Andrew J. Colyer, MSC, draft chapter, sub: Administrative Specialties, 1958 MSC History Project. War College: SG Conference, 18 Jul 51; Interv, Col James T. Richards, MSC, Ret., with Ginn, San Antonio, Tex., 28 Feb 86, DASG-MS.

[66] Degrees: The first degrees were awarded to Lt. Col. Helen Abromoska, ANC (MSHA); Lt. Col. Juanita Costa, ANC (MSHA); Lt. Col. Glenn C. Irving, MSC (MHA); and Maj. Herman Jones, MSC (MHA). "Unique Program Graduates First Class," *ACHA News* 16 (June 1953): 3; Memo, Gibbs, 7 Nov 52; Col Melvin E. Modderman, MSC, Dir, Army-Baylor Program, to Ginn, 23 Apr 87, both in DASG-MS.

[67] Course structure: Ltr, Gibbs to American Council on Education, Washington, D.C., 17 Dec 53; Ltr, Hardy Kemp, M.D., Dir Grad Studies, Baylor College of Medicine, to Maj Gen R.W. Bliss, MC, TSG, 1 Nov 50, both in DASG-MS. It was important to call the practicum year a residency "to have them equated with the senior medical personnel in the hospital, the residents, and certainly not the interns, or clerks, or anything of that variety." Interv, Gary Fillerman, President, AUPHA, with Lewis E. Weeks, American Hospital Association (AHA), Chicago, in McLean, Va., 28 Dec 79, copy in AHA Library, Chicago.

[68] Gibbs: Memo, Gibbs, 7 Jan 53, DASG-MS. Baylor's acceptance of Gibbs was based on his experience in hospital administration, not his academic background. Gibbs earned a baccalaureate degree in 1958, following his retirement from the Army in 1957. Student composition: Dean Conley, "Army Course in Hospital Administration," *Higher Education* 10 (September 1953): 7; Ltr, Maj H.M. Noolf, USAF, Med Svcs Career Control Br, USAF SGO, to Richards, 30 Jun 52, DASG-MS. Objections: Ltr, Wilby Gooch, Baylor Admin VP, to Harvey Kemp, 9 Nov 53, DASG-MS. The mixing of undergraduate and graduate students was "foreign to graduate standards."

[69] Conley's slight: Conley, "Professional Education in Hospital Administration," *Higher Education* 9 (1 May 1953): 193–97; Conley, "Army Course in Hospital Administration," pp 6–7; Kemp to Gibbs, 14 and 22 May 53; Gibbs to Kemp, 18 May 53, all in DASG-MS.

[70] Medical logistics: Cowdrey, *The Medics' War*, p. 136; Intervs, Milner with Col Marvin Ware, MSC, OTSG, 19 May 66; Col Philip L. LaManche, MSC, OTSG, 12 Aug 66; Maj Gen Silas B. Hays, OTSG, 25 Oct 63, all in USACMH. Quoted words: Zolenas, Milner interv, 13 Jul 66, USACMH.

[71] Pilferage: Interv, Col Lynn B. Moore, MSC, with Milner, 28 Jul 66; also see Rpt, Office of Chief of Transportation, DA, sub: CONEX: A Milestone in Utilization, 22 Mar 57, DASG-MS. The surgeon, Brig. Gen. L. Holmes Ginn, refused to use McMeen as his MSO. See DA rpt, above, and Ware, Milner interv, 19 May 66.

[72] Quoted words: Ginn, cited in Cowdrey, *The Medics' War*, p. 191. See Cowdrey's discussion, "How Good Was the Medical Service?" on pp. 187–96. Also see Brig Gen Crawford F. Sams, Chief,

Public Health and Welfare Section, Supreme Commander for the Allied Powers (SCAP), unpublished MS, sub: Medic: An Autobiography, p. 2: 668, USACMH. "None of them had been trained in that basic function of all military medical officers which is the evacuation and care of the sick and wounded."

[73] Quoted words: Cowdrey, *The Medics' War*, p. 140.

[74] Lack of training: Interv, Maj Gen Albert H. Schwichtenberg, USAF, with Milner, 4 Oct 63; SG Conference, 26 Jun 50; Wisearson, Milner interv, 22 Sep 66.

[75] Aviation section: Crosby to Hamrick, 14 Mar 88; Tierney and Montgomery, *The Army Aviation Story*, p. 190. MC pilots: SG Conference, 23 Apr 51; Silas B. Hays, "The Army Medical Service," *U.S. Armed Forces Medical Journal* 4 (February 1953): 172. First pilots: SG Conference, 7 Jul 52; Press Release, OTSG, "1st MSCs Earn Helicopter Wings," 11 April 1953, USACMH. The first MSC pilots graduated at Fort Sill, Oklahoma, on 11 April 1953: 2d Lt. Marian Burroughs, Capt. Warren Garfield, 1st Lt. William R. Knowles, 2d Lt. Frank Mettner, Capt. William R. Schmidt, 1st Lt. Eddie G. Sullivan, and Capt. Richard K. Whitehouse.

[76] Matthews: Brig Gen William A. Hamrick, MSC, Ret., to Ginn, 21 Dec 88 and 23 Mar 89, incl CV, Col. Thomas O. Matthews, MSC, Ret., DASG-MS. Matthews later became the executive producer of the Peabody Award–winning television series "The Big Picture."

[77] Medical regulating: Cowdrey, *The Medics' War*, p. 257.

[78] Peress: Interv, Col Vernon McKenzie, MSC, Ret., with Ginn, Pentagon, 19 May 84, DASG-MS; McKenzie, Milner interv, 4 Nov 63, USACMH; SG Conferences, 3, 4, 8, and 16 Feb 54. Peress left active duty on 2 February 1954. McKenzie said the whole thing was an error to begin with, since Peress should have entered active duty as a major, not as a captain. Quoted words: McKenzie, Ginn interv, 19 May 84.

[79] Hospital administration: Conley, "Professional Education in Hospital Administration," pp. 193–94. Quoted words: Col William S. Stone, MC, Commandant of the Army Medical Service Graduate School. Stone, "Military Medicine as a Career," *Military Medicine Notes* I (1951), p. 3, JML.

[80] Management improvement: Rpt, Lt Col Fernando S. Rojo, MSC, sub: A Historical Account of Organized Methods Improvement Efforts in the United States Army Medical Service, 31 Mar 62, folder 268, box 17/18, MSC-USACMH, hereafter cited as Rojo, Methods Improvement Efforts; Gibbs, Milner intervs, 24 Oct and 8 and 11 Nov 63. The branch was known variously as the Medical Administration Branch, Management Improvement Office, Management Research and Planning Branch, Hospital Methods Improvement Branch, and by various other titles.

[81] Organization: DA Cir, sub: Organization of U.S. Army Hospitals Designated as Class II Installations or Activities, 15 Sep 59; DA SR 40–610–5, sub: Organization Structure for Hospitals in the Continental United States Designated as Other than Class II Activities, 16 Jan 52, both in PL. Valley Forge closure: The experiments were continued in a reduced fashion from 1952 to 1959 by a research unit at Brooke Army Medical Center. Dietitians: Anderson, *Army Medical Specialist Corps*, pp. 515–18.

[82] Executive officer (XO): Memo for Record, Col A.M. Schwichtenberg, MC, Ch, Med Plans and Ops Div, OTSG, sub: Medical Service Corps Officers, 27 Mar 49, folder 133, box 9/18, MSC-USACMH. Gibbs recommended MSC executive officers on 15 March; Hays approved that on 16 March. XO position: Hamrick to Ginn, 1 Sep 88, DASG-MS; DA SR 40–610–5, 16 Jan 52; SG Conference, 17 Mar 49. According to Gibbs, General Bliss, TSG, "very definitely" wanted physicians in the top two administrative positions (commander and deputy commander) "regardless of what their titles might be." Gibbs, Milner intervs, 1 and 11 Nov 63.

[83] AHA leadership: Rojo, Methods Improvement Efforts. ACHA: Col. James T. McGibony, MC, commander of the hospital at Fort Belvoir, Virginia, in 1954 became the first Army officer to advance to ACHA fellowship. *ACHA News* 17 (October–November 1954): 3.

[84] Quoted words: Henry D. Roth, "The U.S. Army," *Bulletin of the American Society of Hospital Pharmacists* (July–August 1952): 264–67. Also see SG Conferences, 3 and 29 Dec 52.

[85] Progress: Speech, Roth, sub: The Role of the Pharmacist in the Medical Service Corps, Philadelphia College of Science and Pharmacy, 21 Feb 52, folder 43, box 4/18, MSC-USACMH.

[86] APA promise: SG Conference, 30 Aug 51.

[87] MAS specialties: Rpt, Lt Col Joseph J. Gilbert, MSC, to Col Thomas F. Whayne, MC, Ch, Prev Med Div, OTSG, 20 Sep 51; Lt Col Robert Ryer, MSC, draft chapter, sub: Nutrition, and

Maj Walter F. Robbins, MSC, draft section, sub: Reconditioning, both 1958 MSC History Project.

[88] Preventive medicine corps: Proposed in report to Col. T.F. Whayne. Gilbert, the World War II assistant to Colonel Hardenbergh, was a reservist on a two-week tour with OTSG tasked with evaluating the status of sanitary engineering.

[89] Utilization study: Memo, Pers Div, OTSG, sub: Problem Incident to the Utilization of Medical Service Corps Officers in Narrow Specialty Fields Upon Attaining Field Grade, 23 Dec 52; Memo, Arthur Stull, Ph.D., Laboratory Consultant, Office of Chief, Pathology and Allied Sciences Consultants, OTSG, for Ch, Prof Div, OTSG, sub: Positions for Colonels, MSC, Medical Laboratory Officers, 1953, both in box 5/18, MSC-USACMH.

[90] Podiatry: SG Conferences, 2 Sep 49 (which also cites Drew Pearson column) and 29 Apr 52; Memos, Capt Charles J. Simpson, MSC, sub: Twenty-Eighth Meeting of the Armed Forces Medical Policy Council, 0900 Hours, 28 April 1952; and 1st Lt B.W. Wingo, MSC, Staff Asst to TSG, sub: Thirty-Sixth Meeting of the Armed Forces Policy Council, 3 November 1952, at 1330 Hours, in SG Conferences of the respective dates.

[91] Medical research: Hays, "The Army Medical Service," p. 167; Berge, Virology and Immunology, pp. 15–16; Rose C. Engleman and Robert J.T. Joy, *Two Hundred Years of Military Medicine*, (Washington, D.C.: The Historical Unit, Office of the Surgeon General, 1975), pp. 32–35; Col Raymond J. Karpen, MSC, Ret., to Col Earl J. Herndon, MSC, 7 Nov 83, DASG-MS; Intervs, Col William H. Meroney, MC, with Milner, OTSG, 26 Aug and 7 Sep 66, USACMH. Maxwell: TLO, OTSG, Biography of Col Roy D. Maxwell, MSC, Feb 62; Rpt, Col Charles R. Angel, MSC, sub: Development of Nuclear Science Within the MSC, undated [1976], both in DASG-MS.

[92] Hunter's team: Speech, Yamashita Kuranosuke, Chief, Construction Committee for Hunter Statue, sub: Congratulatory Address, Kurume City Hall, 15 Jul 52 (translation), DASG-MS; George W. Hunter III et al., "Control of the Snail Host of Schistosomiasis in Japan with Sodium Pentachlorophenate (Santobrite)," *American Journal of Tropical Medicine and Hygiene* 1 (September 1952): 831–47; "Fruitful Result of Cooperation," *Mainichi Shimbun* (Daily News), Japan, 9 August 1968 (translation), DASG-MS; Hunter et al., "Control of Schistosomiasis Japonica in the Nagatoishi Area of Kurume, Japan," *American Journal of Tropical Medicine* 31 (1982): 760–70; Hunter and Muneo Yokogawa, "Control of Schistosomiasis Japonica in Japan: A Review, 1950–1978," *Japanese Journal of Parasitology* 33 (August 1984): 341–51; Notes of telephone interv, Col George W. Hunter III, MSC, Ret., with Ginn, 1 Feb 86, DASG-MS. Hunter headed the Medical Zoology Section of the 406th Medical Laboratory in Tokyo from 1947 to 1951. Schistosomiasis: The team eliminated 99 percent of the snail population over a two-year period beginning in 1949.

[93] Social work: Camp, As I Remember Army Social Work; Camp, "The Army's Psychiatric Social Work Program," *Social Work Journal* 29 (April 1948): 76–78, 86; Camp, "Psychiatric Social Work in the Army Today," in Henry S. Maas, ed., *Adventures in Mental Health* (New York: Columbia University Press, 1951); Memo, Maj Barbara B. Hodges, MSC, Ch, Med Social Work Sec, Social Svcs Br, Prof Div, OTSG, for Ch, Prof Div, sub: Position Utilization for Colonels, MSC, Social Workers, USACMH; Speech, Camp, sub: Notes for Presentation at Army Social Work Meeting, National Conference of Social Work, 78th Annual Meeting, Atlantic City, New Jersey, May 1951, DASG-MS; SG Conference, 9 Nov 50.

[94] Psychology: Memo, Brig Gen R.E. Chambers for Ch, Pers Div, SGO, sub: Report of Structure of MSC, 18 Mar 53, box 5/18, MSC-USACMH; Memo, Lt Col Frederick A. Zehrer, MSC, for Ch, MSC, sub: Grade of Colonel, MSC, for Clinical and Research Psychologists, 1953, MSC-USACMH; Paper, Harold D. Rosenheim, "A History of the Uniformed Clinical Psychologist in the U.S. Army," presented to the American Psychological Association, 2 Sep 80, DASG-MS; DA Technical Manual (TM) 8–242, *Military Clinical Psychology* (Washington, D.C.: Department of the Army and U.S. Air Force, July 1951), copy in USACMH; "The U.S. Army's Senior Psychology Student Program," *American Psychologist* 4 (1949): 424–25; Hays, "The Army Medical Service," p. 169; Col. Charles A. Thomas, Jr., MSC, Ret., "Contributions of and Challenges Faced By AMEDD Psychology: 1950's–1970's," Proceedings of the 1982 AMEDD Psychology Symposium, 14–19 November 1982, Dwight David Eisenhower Army Medical Center, DASG-MS.

[95] Zehrer: Zehrer established the first Army child guidance clinic in 1948 while assigned at Brooke General Hospital. Col Frederick A. Zehrer, MSC, Ch, Off of Educ Svcs, Army Med Svc School, Fort Sam Houston, Tex., to Dir, THU, 8 Feb 60, box 9/18, MSC-USACMH; Arnold B. Schiebel, Zehrer, and Rawley E. Chambers, "The Establishment of a Child Guidance Center in an Army General Hospital," *Medical Bulletin* (June 1949): 449.

[96] Number: MSC Newsletter, September 1956. Enlisted optometrists: Speech, Capt George B. Coyle, MSC, sub: The History of Army Optometry, 8 Nov 65; Col Robert L. Black, MSC, to Fred Niemann, General Counsel, Texas Optometric Association, 23 Nov 51; Leon Hoffman, O.D., to Capt Albert L. Paul, MSC, THU, 2 May 60, all in folder 58, box 5/18, MSC-USACMH. Hoffman enlisted in the Scientific and Professional option. He was the only optometrist at the 25th Evac Hosp at Taegu, Korea, from 1951 to 1952. Dr. Herron: Interv, Maj Francis L. McVeigh, MSC, with Sgt Maj (Ret.) Melvin E. Johnson, in unpublished paper, U.S. Army Command and General Staff College, sub: The History of Army Optometry: The Battles, Triumphs, and Future Challenges, June 1993, DASG-MS.

[97] Positions: Address, Col Robert L. Black to AOA meeting, Miami Beach, Fla., 8–11 Jun 52, folder 63, box 5/18, MSC-USACMH.

[98] Quoted words: SG Conference, 18 Jun 52. AOA: SG Conference, 20 and 26 Jun 52.

[99] Ryan: "Army M.S.C. Optometrist Is Cited," pp. 23–24; News release, OTSG, January 1965.

[100] Use of physicians: Interv, Capt Daniel B. Sullivan, MC, with 1st Lt Martin Blumenson, 3d Historical Detachment, in Westover, *Combat Support in Korea*, pp. 113–14.

[101] Occupational vision: Address, 1st Lt Robert J. O'Shea, MSC, sub: Occupational Vision Program at Army Installations, presented to AOA seminar, 30–31 March 1952, and Pamphlet, Army Environmental Health Laboratory (AEHL), *Essentials of an Occupational Vision Program* (Army Chemical Center, Md.: AEHL, 2 March 1956): 1, both in folder 59, box 5/18, MSC-USACMH.

[102] Helicopter: Armstrong called it "the most humanitarian advance that has been made in the evacuation of the wounded in the past fifty years." Armstrong, "Recent Advances in Military Medicine," *Military Medicine* 114 (January 1954): 31.

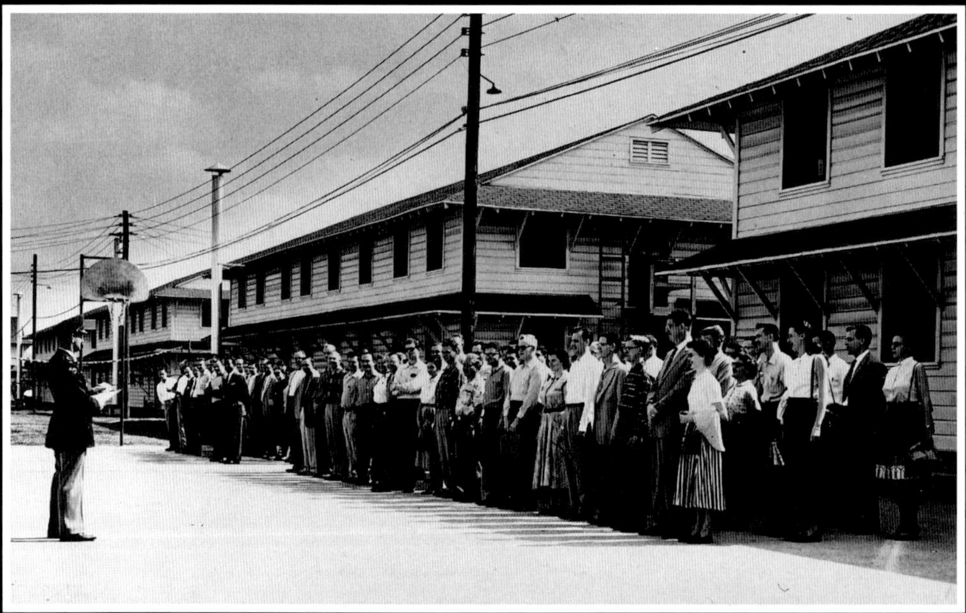

Future health services officers arrive at Fort Sam Houston, Texas, for training.

9

The Post-Korea Era

American soldiers returning from Korea were not treated to the victory parades that awaited soldiers coming home from World War II. Rather, they received at best benign neglect as they resumed lives interrupted by the war. At least Medical Service Corps officers came home to the appreciation of their senior medical leaders. Deputy Surgeon General Maj. Gen. James P. Cooney told them they were "bastions of strength," and Maj. Gen. Alvin Gorby, MC, chief surgeon of the U.S. Army, Europe, asked them to reflect on their contributions: "I wonder if you fully appreciate the gains you have made in this short span of years."[1]

The Army shrank from a Korean War peak of over 1.5 million to under 860,000 by 1961. This was partly accomplished through a reduction in force (RIF) as the Eisenhower administration forced down the strength of the Army by involuntarily separating soldiers from active duty. The reductions were painful, but the number remaining on active duty was considerably more than after World War II due to the continuing Cold War between the United States and the Soviet Union.

Tactical doctrine in the period between the Korean and Vietnam Wars was briefly hinged to nuclear weapons. The Army created a five-sided "pentomic" division consisting of five battle groups armed with tactical nuclear weapons. The idea was that divisions spread out in this formation over a large area could face the enemy simultaneously in all directions, much like a circled wagon train in the Old West. However, no one could eliminate the chance that tactical use of nuclear weapons would lead to all-out nuclear war. Three senior leaders, Generals Matthew Ridgway and Maxwell Taylor and Lt. Gen. James M. Gavin, argued unsuccessfully for flexible deterrence, a strategy that, unlike nuclear massive retaliation, would depend upon an ability to modulate military response to meet varying levels of threat. But the administration of President Dwight D. Eisenhower had committed itself for budgetary reasons to a policy of massive retaliation, or "more bang for the buck," emphasizing nuclear weapons.

Flexible response was adopted by President John F. Kennedy's administration, a change that generated a balance of forces, caused a resurgence of Army fortunes in the 1960s, and renewed attention to conventional weapons and tactics. There were eleven divisions in the active Army when Kennedy took the oath of office in 1961; when he was assassinated almost three years later there were sixteen. The changed climate prompted interest in irregular warfare, and the Special Warfare School at Fort Bragg, North Carolina, flourished when the Kennedy administration greatly increased the size of the Green Berets.

Other changes also affected the Medical Department. A significant milestone had occurred in 1954 when the last black unit was fully integrated. By 1956, 100 of the 500 MSC officers commissioned from the Reserve Officers Training Corps (ROTC) were black.[2] The Medical Department also continued to be affected by changes occurring in American health care, by now a sophisticated industry.[3] Technologically advanced medicine required a modern plant, and the Army undertook an ambitious program of hospital construction. The need to keep current with contemporary medical practice kept the emphasis on clinical medicine and gave the Class II teaching hospitals favored status. That reinforced a perception that the combat medical force took a second seat, and a polarity emerged between fixed facility and field unit proponents. Col. Robert S. Peyton, MC, headed a board that examined the command and control of Army hospitals in 1952. The Peyton Report described a "schism in the household" between "the white-coat group on one hand and the field-jacket group on the other."[4]

The surgeon general's personnel management authority twice survived reorganizations of the Army Staff in the interwar period. The first, in 1954, consolidated personnel management authority under the deputy chief of staff for personnel (DCSPER). The second, in 1962, completed the earlier effort by abolishing the technical services. The Surgeon General, Lt. Gen. Leonard D. Heaton, was convinced the loss of chiefs of the technical services to serve as proponents for those officers "broke their morale." He noted with some pride that the medics and the engineers were the only technical services that did not lose their identity.[5]

The principal development in field medical service was that of an aeromedical evacuation doctrine. Its flavor was captured in an article by Lt. Col. Spurgeon H. Neel, MC, who wrote that the Korean War had taught the necessity of medical control of evacuation and the need for pilots and aircraft dedicated to that mission alone. Field maneuvers after Korea included use of aeromedical evacuation. The department based its doctrine on an air ambulance company of 170 personnel, organized into a headquarters platoon, a maintenance platoon, and three evacuation platoons. Each evacuation platoon supported a corps. The doctrine achieved medical control by placing the company directly under the theater surgeon, and it firmly identified MSC pilots as integral to the system. It established a requirement for medical training of aeromedical aviators, because they were required to supervise the handling of casualties and the medical care provided en route.[6]

The Medical Department needed a suitable helicopter; the H–13 and the later H–19 models were both inadequate. The department was persistent in seeing that the Army develop a new aircraft that would be sufficiently large to carry patients internally and to accommodate their in-flight treatment. This led to a formal requirement in 1952 for a general utility helicopter that would also be suitable for medical evacuation. The effort paid off in a 1955 design competition, won by Bell Corporation's XH–40, which joined the Army as the UH–1 Iroquois. Nicknamed the Huey, the aircraft featured a turbine engine and a first-generation capability of carrying two litter patients, a medical attendant, a crew chief, and two pilots. Lt. Col. John W. Hammet, MSC, who served at the U.S. Army Aviation Board during the Huey's development and accepted the

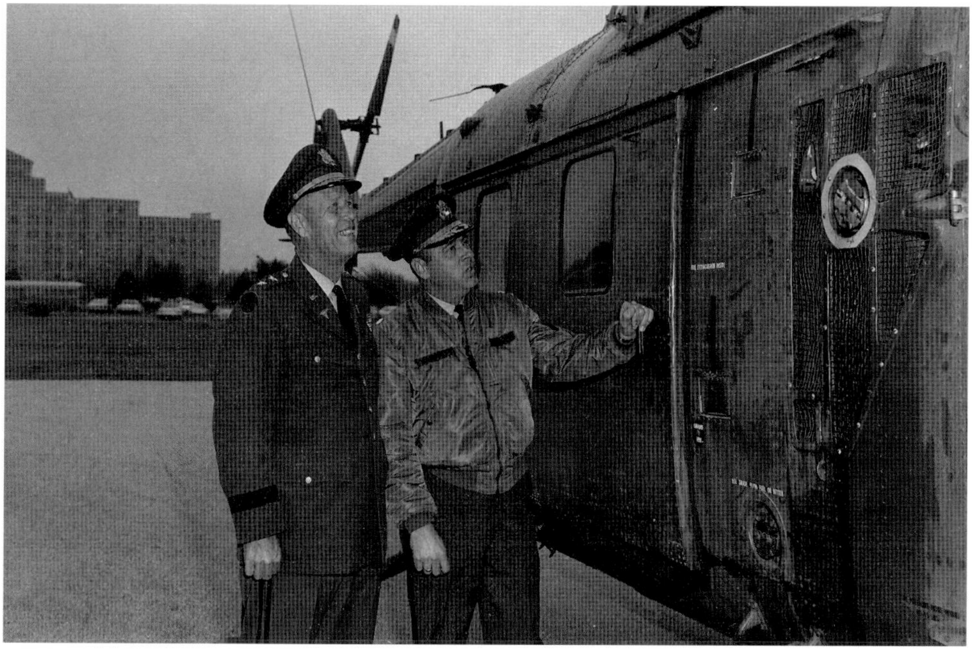

*Maj. Gen. Laurence A. Potter (*left*) and Colonel Hammet with the last H–19 helicopter in Army Medical Department service, February 1969*

first aircraft for the Army, said that without the department's efforts (much of it the hard work of MSC officers) there would not have been an aeromedically capable helicopter.[7]

Developments in the Corps

Colonel Black retired as chief of the Medical Service Corps in 1955. He was succeeded by Col. Bernard Aabel, MSC, who as a major had testified at the hearings on the formation of the corps (*see Appendix G*). Aabel was followed in 1959 by Col. Roy D. Maxwell, MSC, the nuclear medicine pioneer. While chief, Colonel Maxwell was also appointed to an Atomic Energy Commission special project. Those duties occupied him fully beginning in August 1962, and Col. Dale Thompson, MSC, executive officer of the Personnel Division, served as the acting chief in Maxwell's absence. Col. William A. Hamrick, MSC, took office in March 1963 and served as chief of the corps for the next six years.

The job of tying together the "Austro-Hungarian empire" (as Colonel Peyton called the corps) was facilitated in 1962 by increasing the MSC chief's authority over assignments of his officers. A Medical Service Corps and Warrant Officer Branch was established in the 1950s as part of the Surgeon General's Personnel and Training Division. The MSC chief influenced the activities of that office, commonly referred to as "Branch," but had limited authority since it was independent of the chief's office.[8] The chief's influence was enhanced when the surgeon general transferred career management functions for MSC officers from the director of personnel to the MSC chief, who was also designated as chief of the Medical Service Corps and Warrant Officer Branch.[9]

An Army policy change in 1956 eliminated the two MSC warrant officer specialties of field medical assistant and medical supply officer because those were the same titles held by commissioned officers. Warrant officers in those specialties would eventually have to be reclassified into other Army fields, a process that would proceed slowly. The department's request to replace the specialties with two others, medical administrative assistant and medical supply assistant, was turned down. However, an opportunity to create new specialties occurred in 1959, and the department submitted a proposal for 366 MSC warrant officers in five fields: clinical laboratory, dental laboratory, medical equipment repair, optician, and sanitarian. Of that number, only the medical equipment repair technician was adopted. It joined the MSC as the only warrant officer specialty in 1961, replacing the commissioned medical equipment maintenance officer. CWO W. B. "Foxy" King, a medical supply officer, was one of the officers affected by this change. He returned from Korea in 1960 to attend the medical maintenance officer's course in Saint Louis, Missouri, and was reclassified the following year. By the end of 1961 the corps counted eleven warrant officers in the new field and by 1964 there were ninety-six.[10]

MSC quality remained an issue, and Branch sent a few "buck-up" letters each month to officers who had a declining Officer Efficiency Index (OEI). The OEI was calculated from annual efficiency reports in which officers were rated from 0 (unsatisfactory) to 5 (outstanding) in a variety of categories. The reports were the basic document used by promotion boards, and some observers were convinced that MSCs were not treated as generously as they should have been. A comparison of MSC scores with overall Army scores concluded that "medical raters are pikers compared with raters of the combat arms."[11]

The corps declined from a peak of 4,719 officers during the Korean War to a low of 3,499 in June 1959 (including 7 medical and dental students occupying MSC spaces). The number began rebounding (it was 3,832 at the end of 1961—*see Appendix H*), and by 30 September 1964 it had risen to 4,363 as the U.S. involvement in Vietnam increased. In 1961 MSCs served in fifty-eight specialties in eighteen career fields. At that point, 81 percent of the corps was in the Pharmacy, Supply, and Administration Section, an increase from 60 percent in 1947. The Medical Allied Sciences Section dropped from 30 to 12 percent of the corps during the same period. The Sanitary Engineering Section increased slightly from 2 to 3 percent, while the Optometry Section increased its share from 2 to 4 percent.[12]

The Army RIF board listed ninety MSC officers among those it eliminated from active duty in 1953. Over seven hundred MSCs separated during the six-month period beginning in October 1953, 100 of those leaving active duty involuntarily. A RIF that would have separated another 139 in 1958 was canceled when it was apparent that the earlier reductions had created shortages in the MSC.[13] RIF actions were tough on morale, but Colonel Black believed it was to the corps' advantage to remove "weak or blight-tainted individuals." He supported "housecleaning" actions throughout his tenure as chief.[14]

The RIF did not help retention, which was affected by other factors as well. One was frequent moves. The corps found in the spring of 1960 that 97 percent of all MSCs had moved in the previous 24 months. Another was dependence on ROTC as the principal source of officers, because only 2 percent of ROTC graduates remained on active duty beyond their two-year obligation. Few were inclined toward a career in the military, partly due to the uncertainty of military careers.[15]

An accordion effect set in as attempts to reduce and then expand the corps followed in quick succession. The growing peacetime health care mission needed MSCs. Demand was also driven by the need to substitute or replace Medical Corps officers in administrative positions, a pressure heightened by shortages of physicians. From 1953 to 1955, 76 percent of the Medical Corps captains who could leave active duty did, as did 66 percent of the majors. The Army curtailed assignment of physicians to garrisoned field medical units in order to meet the burgeoning health care demand, but that was not enough. The insufficient number of physicians was one of the most pressing problems of Maj. Gen. George E. Armstrong as surgeon general from 1951 to 1955, but he was dismayed that only two-thirds of the Medical Corps was in direct patient care. In fact, there were complaints about the number of physicians in the Surgeon General's Office, a view hardly helped by an embarrassing incident in which one officer, while at home, rushed to assist a neighbor in distress only to discover that his stethoscope wouldn't work.[16]

The loss of veteran MSC officers through RIF, resignation, or retirement had other consequences for the Medical Department. The MSC's "hard core" of reserve officers, a pool of experience gained in two wars, retired as they hit their mandatory twenty-year retirement date. The MSC was becoming an inexperienced corps with slight prospect of the situation's improving. Half of the corps was in the grade of lieutenant in 1954, but only 7 percent of those officers were careerists. This improved by 1959 when 37 percent of the corps was lieutenants, 25 percent of whom were careerists, but was still a discouraging figure.[17]

The double jeopardy of MSC and Medical Corps shortages became so pronounced that the Army filled forty-three Medical Department positions, including medical battalion commanders, with line officers. The shortages of MSCs stiffened the department's resolve to retain MSC officers in medical assignments, and proposals to assign MSCs to nonmedical duties were resisted. The situation was further aggravated by the 1961 Berlin Crisis that created additional demands for MSC officers, especially in the optometry, laboratory sciences, comptroller, operations, sanitary engineering, and pharmacy fields.[18]

Consequently, recruiting followed on the heels of the RIF. Military pensions were a selling point, including the ability to retire after twenty years of active duty service. The Army transferred some officers to the MSC from other branches. For example, 2d Lt. Ernest M. Irons, MSC, was commissioned in the Artillery in 1954, but when he received his Regular Army commission it was in the MSC. He went from a gun platoon to a medical platoon. The department resorted to selecting individuals for direct appointment to the MSC in order to fill the gap. Four hundred were selected from thirteen hundred applicants in 1957. A special program was established for commissioning scientific specialty officers; they incurred a three-year active duty obligation (two years if they held a Ph.D.). Another incentive was a higher entry grade for some specialties. Beginning in 1962 officers who entered active duty with doctoral degrees in the allied sciences, sanitary engineering, optometry, pharmacy, and hospital administration were granted eighteen months' credit for promotion to captain. Colonel Aabel suggested commissioning West Point graduates, but that did not come to pass during this period. However, Colonel Hamrick was pleased with the accession of sixty-one ROTC distinguished military graduates in 1964, and each year more ROTC cadets listed the MSC as their first choice for a branch.[19]

The Medical Service Corps and Warrant Officer Branch, in a project headed by Lt. Col. William J. Clegg, Jr., MSC, refined the career plans initially formulated in 1948, this time including reserve component officers who could now remain on active duty for a twenty-year career. The plans represented a compromise between the specialist and generalist philosophies. Junior officers would concentrate initially on developing a thorough grounding in their basic specialty, and as they matured through the ranks they would develop the broader-based perspectives necessary for senior positions. By 1960 Branch had published plans for eleven specialties and five more were in preparation.[20]

Colonel Aabel was an enthusiastic promotor of ways to enhance esprit de corps. The corps made it to the movies in 1955 with a half-hour show filmed at Fort Sam Houston for the television series "The Big Picture." Aabel instituted a corps newsletter and threw an MSC birthday party in 1958 that impressed the surgeon general's staff with its camaraderie.[21] Colonel Aabel asked the director of the U.S. Army Band to compose a march for the corps. That did not materialize, so John Philip Sousa's "U.S. Army Ambulance Corps March" remained the closest thing. He also sought recommendations for a motto and submitted ten to the U.S. Army Institute of Heraldry for consideration. "Medicine, Service, Country" led the list, its acronym having a nice symmetry to it, followed by "Service Before Self." Other suggestions were equally ponderous and a motto never materialized. Neither did a corps flag, even though Aabel invited several companies to submit proposals.[22]

The gold versus silver controversy continued. This time Colonel Aabel kicked up a storm by suggesting use of the same basic insignia for all corps as a means of promoting teamwork. Aabel regretted the stir he caused. He wrote Capt. Knute A. Tofte-Nielsen, MSC, a junior officer who had recommended a new design, that he shared Tofte-Nielsen's desire for a new insignia and conceded there was agreement that it should be gold. However, Aabel said the subject had become far too controversial and he had dropped the matter.[23]

An effort to designate an official birth date for the corps backfired. A committee recommended 11 March 1864, the date of the law that established the Ambulance Corps. The surgeon general's chief historian agreed, and Colonel Aabel submitted it for approval. However, Maj. Gen. James P. Cooney, the deputy surgeon general, did not agree. Cooney argued that there was not an unbroken continuity between the Civil War Ambulance Corps and the World War I Sanitary Corps, and he convinced the surgeon general to use the formation of the

Sanitary Corps as the birth date. Cooney picked 18 May 1917, the date of the emergency war powers legislation that gave President Wilson the authority for mobilization, rather than the more precise 30 June 1917 date of the general orders that established the Sanitary Corps.[24]

The energy expended in picking a birth date reflected an interest in the MSC heritage, but the effort to write a history of the corps, which began in 1953, did not succeed.[25] Colonel Aabel requested establishment of a formal history project. That was acted upon when the surgeon general appointed the Advisory Editorial Board for the Medical Service Corps History. The board met in November 1958 and organized the book as a multiauthor effort in which thirty-nine officers were designated to write specific sections. Publication was projected for 1962. Col. John B. Coates, Jr., MC, editor-in-chief of the department's series on World War II, advised the board that they were undertaking a very difficult project. It was "not something you can push a button and call a secretary in and get done as you would write a memorandum, or a staff study, or a course directive."[26] Time would certainly prove him right. The multiauthor effort failed, and by the end of the decade the project was adrift (*see Appendix I*).

Opportunity

The existence of a corps chief gave the Medical Department's administrative and scientific specialty officers an accessible spokesman for their aspirations, beginning with their next assignment. In his travels, Colonel Hamrick interviewed officers for that purpose. Capt. Lloyd A. Schlaeppi, MSC, a medical company commander, met the chief in Germany. Schlaeppi told Hamrick that he wanted to go to San Francisco, "because I hear it's a nice place to be." "Well, you're the first person who's been honest today," General Hamrick responded. Schlaeppi got his orders, much to the amazement of his fellow officers.[27]

The chance for a Regular Army career improved. In 1956 only 18 percent of the active duty MSC was in the Regular Army. Congressional increases in the size of the Regular Army expanded the Regular Army MSC from 950 officers in 1956 to 2,000 in 1963. In March 1957 there were 950 applications for 250 openings.[28]

Education and Training

Colonel Aabel was especially proud of improvements in opportunity for education, which "set the pace for the entire Army and has brought about an upsurge in the prestige and status of the corps." Its effect on retention was significant as the department had to compete with the expanding civilian health care industry for MSC officers.[29]

The first task was to improve the number of college graduates. In 1956, 53 percent of Army officers held at least a baccalaureate degree, but only 44 percent of the Medical Service Corps. Aabel believed that all MSCs should be college graduates. He pressured them to complete at least two years of college by enrolling in off-duty programs and encouraged those at the two-year mark to complete their degrees. A final semester plan provided an opportunity for completing degrees in residence, and twelve officers were enrolled by November 1958.[30]

Aabel put teeth in his suggestions by including off-duty education as a criterion for Regular Army selection boards. Branch wrote nearly six hundred letters to officers who fell behind. Capt. Roy S. Church, MSC, stationed in Germany, received one. He had failed to keep off-duty course work posted on his records, and the letter from Branch got his attention. Aabel's pressure worked; by 1959 one-third of all MSCs were enrolled in civilian education courses, and the percentage of baccalaureate degree holders had increased to 53 percent. By 1962, 2,116 of the 3,674 officers on active duty were college graduates.[31]

The corps continued to emphasize graduate training. In 1957 it set a goal of placing up to fifty officers each year in graduate school in order to meet its requirements for officers trained at the master's level or higher. The range of schooling was impressive. Thirty-seven officers were selected in 1958 for graduate training in eight fields. Four years later MSC officers could compete for ten doctoral programs and twenty-six master's degree programs. Educational opportunities expanded to the extent that there were grumbles about MSC officers pursuing education "of no benefit to the military"; in fact, a study some years later found no correlation of advanced degrees with efficiency reports. By 1961, 100 MSCs had doctoral degrees and another 480 were at the master's level; the corps had ten times as many Ph.D.s and two times as many master's degrees as the rest of the Army. Most scientific specialty officers held graduate degrees, and this accounted for much of the exceptional educational level.[32]

The Army-Baylor Program continued to be an important opportunity, and by 1954 it enrolled one class of sixty students annually. In 1956 Colonel Hamrick completed the course and replaced Col. Frederick H. Gibbs as its director. "I guess it's only in the Army that you could be a student one year and the director the next."[33] The average student was thirty-five years old. Eight of the faculty held Baylor appointments.

The program underwent close scrutiny during this period, not all of it favorable. The statistics tell the tale. There were 412 graduates from 1951 to 1959. Of that number, only 184 were able to matriculate in the Baylor Graduate School, and only 145 of those had received the master's degree. In 1952 only 35 percent of the students had a college degree; 5 percent had not graduated from high school.[34]

The Association of University Programs in Hospital Administration periodically surveyed the program as a condition of accreditation. The first survey occurred in 1952. The report said the program was "an eminently practical approach" that had the advantage of older, more experienced students who were motivated toward remaining on active duty. But there was stinging criticism. It was "not truly a graduate level program," and it had students who could not matriculate in the Baylor Graduate School. The surveyors believed Baylor "rubber stamped" actions by the course director. They questioned locating the program in San Antonio, Texas, rather than at the Waco, Texas, campus of Baylor University because that created a remoteness from university life and research facilities. They concluded that the course should cease as a graduate program if it could not bring its standards up to graduate school level.[35]

This was not a happy time for supporters of the course. Colonel Gibbs, while acting on some recommendations, contested others. He cautioned that the accreditation findings had to be taken in context; the surveyors had found weaknesses in all thirteen programs they visited in the United States. He actually believed that the Army-Baylor Program was one of the stronger programs.[36] Unfortunately, the report came at a time when some of the department's senior leaders were having their doubts. The question in Washington was whether they were embarked on a fruitless quest, because it was "doubtful that the majority of the past and present student body are capable of absorbing the hospital administration course."[37]

In the long run, the scrutiny had salutary effects. It concentrated the Medical Department's attention on improving the program, raising standards for admission, and increasing its difficulty. Prerequisites were tightened to include a minimum of a baccalaureate degree and undergraduate courses in statistics, financial management, and management methods, although Baylor Graduate School remained lenient with its 2.5 grade point average requirement for admission. The program set an enrollment age limit of forty because there were complaints that the students were either "old colonels" or "frisky majors."[38] Gibbs, while he believed the students were "a studious, hard-working and serious group," kept the pressure on students who completed the course but failed to write their theses.[39] A faculty committee conducted an oral examination of each student at the end of the academic year, and in February 1955 the option for an undergraduate degree ended, and so did the option for a master of science in hospital administration (MSHA). The only degree offered from then on was the MHA, a step taken to bring the program up to the standard practice of accredited graduate programs in the United States.[40]

The next accreditation survey, in 1955, praised the program for its improvements and congratulated Gibbs for doing "an unusually fine job." The report ranked the course in the upper half of all programs.[41]Another challenge came in 1962 when an Army study of military schools recommended using civilian programs in hospital administration. The Medical Department successfully defended the Army-Baylor Program by arguing that it was tailored to the needs of the military and could not be replicated by civilian programs.[42]

University education was important, but so was military training conducted at the Medical Field Service School. The department considered the Basic Officer Course sufficiently important for MSCs that it increased the length to fourteen weeks (later sixteen) for them while simultaneously decreasing the length for the other corps. Attendance for MSCs was, with few exceptions, mandatory. The Advanced Course, also a mandatory requirement for MSCs, increased from twenty-two to thirty-three weeks in 1963. The full-length version was required for Regular Army officers, but reserve component officers on active duty had the option of either a sixteen-week associate course or a correspondence course. Another option was attendance at the advanced course of other branches, including the Infantry School Advanced Course. In 1958 Col. Joseph Carmack, MAC, Ret., established the Carmack Medal, awarded to the top MSC graduate of the Advanced Course. In June of that year he presented the first award to 1st Lt. Charles B. Counselman, MSC (*see Appendix J*).[43]

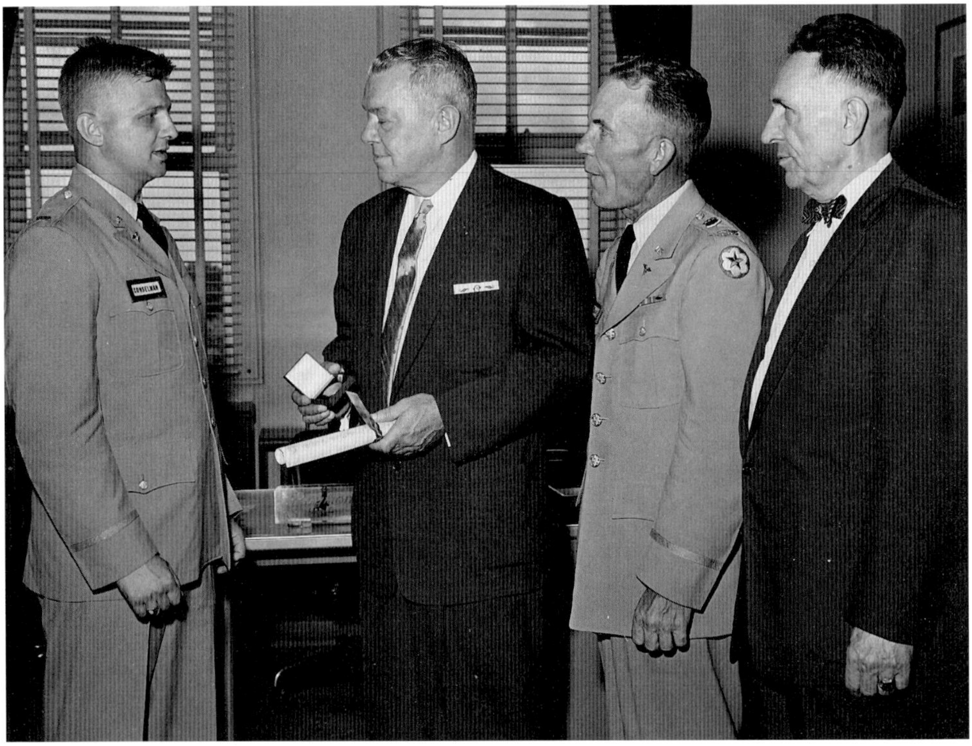

Colonel Carmack (second from left) *presents award to Lieutenant Counselman, June 1958.*

Other courses provided junior officers with their initial training in various administrative specialties. In addition, many of the specialty groups kept their members current with annual institutes (short courses). These were generally five-day meetings held at Walter Reed or Brooke Army Medical Center. Longer courses—for example, preventive medicine—provided training in new skills. In addition, there were meetings of a general nature for all MSCs, and an annual MSC conference in Germany became a tradition.[44]

Colonel Aabel believed there was insufficient opportunity to attend the Regular (resident) Course of the Command and General Staff College at Fort Leavenworth. In 1956 there were seven MSCs selected, but by comparison the comparably sized Signal Corps had twenty-seven. Aabel asked for twenty slots, but lost ground when only three were selected in 1957. The number bounced up to nine the following year, but was still less than half the number desired. By 1961 only sixty-six MSCs were graduates of the Regular Course. Another seventeen were graduates of the Armed Forces Staff College at Norfolk, Virginia, the shorter, tri-service version of military staff college. An additional sixty-nine officers had completed the Associate (correspondence) Course.[45]

Senior service school opportunity was also limited. The corps identified a requirement for seventeen graduates a year in order to fill senior-level positions, but that figure was not reached. In 1956, a typical year, only three MSCs were

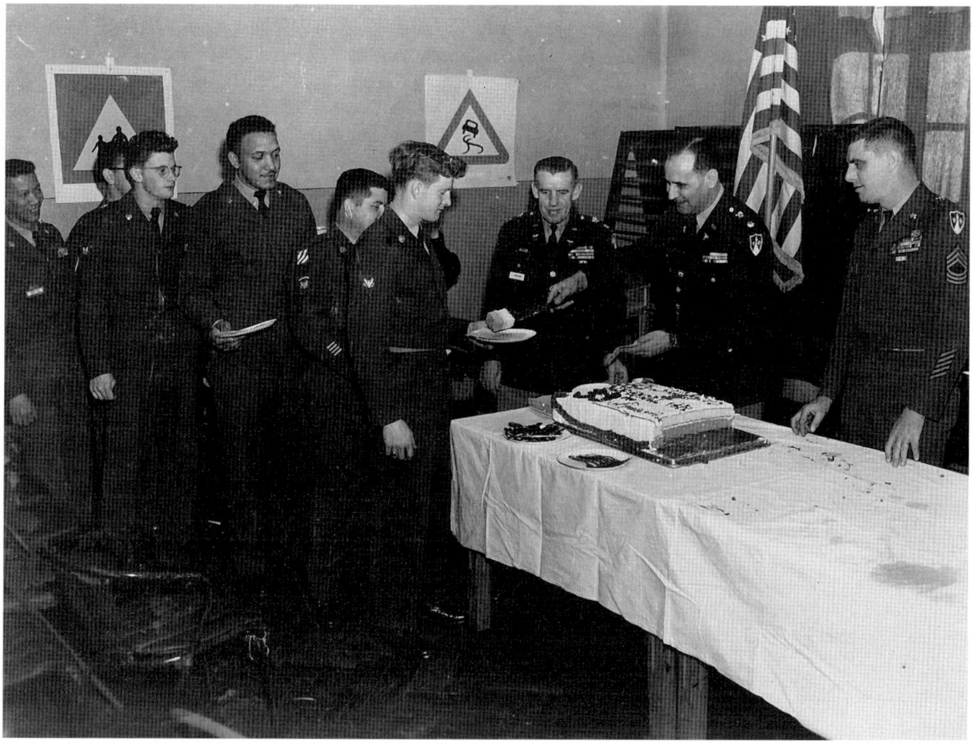

Lt. Col. John Mikuluk cuts the corps anniversary cake in Verdun, France, January 1957.

selected: two for the Army War College and one for the Industrial College of the Armed Forces. By 1961 the corps had only fourteen senior service school graduates on active duty.[46]

Positions

There was a feeling of general pessimism over the prospect of opening the top jobs in the Medical Department to MSCs, Colonel Goriup for one being convinced that there was little potential for this.[47] Some MSC officers found opportunity outside the department in branch-immaterial assignments (positions not requiring a specific branch), especially assignments on the Army Staff. Those appointments opened new doors for talented MSCs and new channels of communication for the department. By 1956 thirty officers were in "prestige assignments" with DCSPER, the deputy chief of staff for logistics (DCSLOG), and others.[48]

MSCs had some command opportunities in the Medical Department. By 1962 MSCs commanded medical research units in Malaya and Panama, the Medical Equipment Development Laboratory at Fort Totten, New York, and the Prosthetics Research Laboratory in Washington, D.C. MSCs commanded the medical supply support activity in Brooklyn, New York, and the Medical Optical and Maintenance Activity, St. Louis, Missouri, as well as medical depots in

Louisville, Kentucky, and overseas in Germany, France, and Korea. MSC officers continued to command medical battalions in a garrison status, and in 1955 Lt. Col. John A. Mikuluk, MSC, assumed command of the 1st Medical Group in Verdun, France, an MSC first. In fact, there were discussions of "responsibility pay" for MSCs in selected positions.[49]

Yet a tension continued to exist in the Army Medical Department over the use of MSCs in command positions beyond a carefully circumscribed few. This was set out in a 1958 change to Army regulations that ratified the policy of allowing MSCs to command medical units only when they were not actively engaged in patient care. When the units assumed patient care responsibilities, the senior Medical Corps officer had to assume command. Any movement toward MSC command of operational medical units was firmly rebuffed. That included command of installations (such as posts) that housed medical activities, in order to avoid situations in which a Medical Corps officer would report to an MSC. Colonel Black was not sanguine about using MSCs to replace Medical Corps officers in administrative positions because he believed physicians were the best candidates for the top jobs. "An M.D. degree unquestionably is a preferential academic background for any medical management or ancillary position in the field of medicine." His view was not unlike that held by some of the department's senior leaders.[50]

The heart of the matter was command of hospitals. General Heaton had strong feelings. "I don't care how large it is or how small it is. The man that can run it and run it well is the physician."[51] In fact, some senior MSCs agreed—Colonel Black for one. "We believe that the command function of medical units and facilities wherein patient care occurs should never be other than Medical or Dental Corps, as the case may be."[52] One MSC colonel insisted that "any aspiring MSC administrator who thinks otherwise should, in my judgment, get his jollies elsewhere than in the Army Medical Department."[53] On the other hand, some senior leaders understood that the real problem was finding MSCs willing to seek the responsibility of command. One senior medical officer believed that MSCs would inevitably command hospitals, but he had great difficulty in finding any eager to assume that burden.[54]

The surgeon general forced the Medical Department's command policy upon the National Guard Bureau, in spite of the Guard's protests that it could not find enough physicians interested in administration to meet its needs. The policy was so firmly held that in 1955 the department chose not to participate in an American Hospital Association (AHA) test of a Civil Defense Emergency Hospital. The AHA had asked the Army to place a trained hospital administrator in command of the test unit and that would have meant use of an MSC commander.[55]

The department's policy came up in the 1952 accreditation survey of the Army-Baylor Program. The report was very critical of the practice of assigning physicians to senior hospital administrator positions—that is, as hospital commanders—but failing to require their training in hospital administration. "Optimal administration of military units is not achieved when subordinate officers are prepared in administration more effectively than superiors whose work is, after all, also administrative in nature."[56] Maj. Gen. Joseph Martin, MC, commander of Brooke Army Medical Center, agreed. "It has always been my contention that we were failing utterly to prepare medical officers for command of hospitals without requiring formal training in hospital administration."[57] The problem remained unresolved. A few physicians attended the Baylor course, but they were an inconsequential minority of those who commanded Army hospitals and none reached the top positions in the department during this period.

The surgeon general would, however, support opening command opportunities for MSCs in nonmedical assignments. By 1960 the law that prohibited Medical Department officers from commanding nonmedical units was interfering with MSC assignments to logistical organizations. General Heaton forwarded a legislative proposal drafted by Maj. Leo Benade, MSC, to allow MSCs to command outside the department. Benade based his rationale on the use of MSCs for branch-immaterial duties in research and development, logistics, intelligence, military assistance advisory groups, military missions, Army aviation, and the Army Staff. Benade's argument was that MSCs, like other Army officers, were qualified for a variety of duties and should have the opportunity for command. The effort succeeded. In August 1961 the law was changed, making MSCs the only Medical Department officers authorized to command nonmedical units.[58]

The Army sent a message that amplified this to an astonishing degree. Not only were MSCs authorized to command outside the Medical Department, but the secretary of the Army could appoint them as commanders of major commands, army groups, armies, corps, divisions, chiefs of service, and heads of Department of the Army staff agencies. Officially, at least, the sky was the limit.[59]

Promotions

Promotions to colonel remained constrained by the 2 percent ceiling. Colonel Black complained that the corps could not survive with such a bottleneck, which formed a detriment to recruitment and a serious morale problem. The Surgeon General's Personnel Division assisted his campaign to remove the cap by identifying MSC positions that should call for a colonel based upon their level of responsibility, and Black used that to support his testimony in hearings on H.R. 5509. The bill, which passed in March 1954, removed the 2 percent limitation on the MSC, allowing the promotion of colonels up to 8 percent of the Regular Army strength of the corps, the same as other branches of the Army. The problem did not end there, because the ability to promote ultimately depended upon the number of positions in the Army for MSC colonels. That number did not expand quickly. In 1961 the Army selected only four of eighty-five lieutenant colonels eligible for promotion to colonel, partly due to the lack of slots.[60]

Not only was there a problem in promotion to colonel, but all promotions slowed so much that Aabel described the outlook as "very ominous."[61] MSCs promoted to captain and major were a year and a half behind their contemporaries, and some MSCs sought transfers to other Army branches where they believed they would have better opportunity for promotion. One alternative was the integration of MSC officers with the Army Promotion List (APL), the promotion list for line officers, in which the much larger aggregate number would provide greater opportunity than considering MSC officers for promotion by themselves. Supporters of this solution argued that the issue was *equality*.[62]

Colonel Aabel actively considered that option. Integration would have ensured promotion equity with line officers, but the surgeon general would lose independence in MSC personnel management, including the ability to "borrow" MSC authorizations for use by other corps, principally the Medical Corps. It would have made MSCs eligible for assignment to an additional range of positions—including command—available only to APL officers, thereby allowing MSCs to venture where other Medical Department officers could not go. Further, it would have made MSCs eligible for promotion to general at the same potential rate as other Army officers.

The department was not willing to accept those consequences, and so MSC officers continued to compete for promotion in separate Medical Department boards. Aabel managed to convince the Army Staff to provide temporary equity with the line by establishing new zones of consideration (eligibility periods) for MSC promotions. As a result, 850 MSC officers of all grades were promoted in fiscal year 1957, including 92 majors promoted to lieutenant colonel in one month alone.

There was not complete agreement on the need for promotion opportunity. General Hays, in a parting shot before retiring as the surgeon general, recommended that the Army transfer MSC colonels out of the Medical Department to positions that genuinely required that grade. He believed that MSCs performed ancillary functions, few of which supported the rank of colonel. Col. Vernon McKenzie, MSC, took Hays to task over this. He told the general that he would have to decide whether he wanted a first- or second-class Medical Service Corps. "If you want the latter then, yes, get rid of all those God-damned uppity colonels MSC and cut it off even lower than that."[63]

General officer stars are the ultimate promise of the Army's promotion system. Unfortunately, the MSC remained the only male corps without general officers, and this nettled its members. As one put it, "to be worth a damn, a person must be ambitious to achieve greater heights, to 'reach for a star.'"[64] A path to stars was available for officers filling branch-immaterial general officer positions, but no MSC was able to capitalize on that approach.[65]

General Armstrong believed the corps should have three generals, and actively pursued that objective with Colonel Black. Black told the surgeon general there were two ways to proceed. One was to seek Army-sponsored legislation, but that would be very slow. The other was to encourage the civilian specialty associations to use their political clout. They chose that route, and in 1955 optometry, pharmacy, and sanitary engineering organizations introduced resolutions for MSC general officers.[66] Colonel Aabel continued the effort as chief of the corps when he replaced Colonel Black. As a result, in 1957 Congressman Carl T. Durham, a pharmacist, introduced H.R. 6801, which proposed establishing one major general and two brigadier generals in the MSC. The Durham bill failed to carry, as did two other bills the following year, because of Army opposition.

The Army did not want to see the number of general officers or specific positions prescribed by law. Its objection was not to MSC generals, but to the secretary of the Army's loss of flexibility in distributing general officer allocations. Benade devised a way around that problem by restating the proposal as a request to include the MSC among those Army branches authorized to have Regular Army general officer rank. Benade's approach obviated linking a star to a specific position, the provision which had been objectionable to the Army Staff. Further, by removing any reference to a specific number, Benade's solution would also have provided the corps the same potential for general officers as any other branch of the Army.[67]

General Heaton chose not to adopt that approach when he placed the corps chief first on the list of general officer requirements he submitted in 1961. Members of the Army Staff still objected to tying the star to a position. In addition, they were convinced that the Medical Department's constraints on MSCs held them to duties of "limited scope and responsibility," something that Heaton said was "simply not true."[68] At least the numbers supported the department's request. The Regular Army MSC of 2,000 officers in 1963 would have supported fifteen generals if the customary Army pattern were applied, but the corps was not included in the Army's computation of general officer allotments. None of the arguments worked, and the corps ended the interwar period without opportunity for promotion to general officer.[69]

Developments in the Administrative Specialties

In 1961, 3,018 MSC administrative specialty officers served in thirty-nine military occupational specialties. Those were aligned within nine career fields: supply, comptroller, personnel, registrar, hospital administration, medical intelligence, operations and training, aviation, warrant officer, and a noncareer field that grouped various specialties together (*see Appendix K*). The three largest career fields were operations and training with 1,343 officers, supply with 428, and personnel with 328. Operations and training included 1,070 officers in the entry-level specialty of field medical assistant, the title for officers assigned as battalion surgeon's assistants and in similar field medical positions. The comptroller field included automated data processing, a specialty added in 1961.[70]

Operations and training officers filled positions at all levels, although the top jobs—for example, chief of the Surgeon General's Medical Plans and Operations Division—remained the province of physicians.[71] Much of the Pentagon battle for aeromedical doctrine was waged by operations officers such as Majs. Kenneth K. Wheatley, MSC, and Robert O. Brumley, MSC, who were able to incorporate the air ambulance company into the force structure. Wheatly exemplified the dedication of "iron major" MSC action officers. "Nothing else mattered—not even family when he locked in on a project. Day, night, dawn, dusk were all the same; bring in something to eat and leave him be—time stands still until the job is done with that man."[72]

Maj. Elliotte J. Williams, MSC, and Capt. Joseph P. Jacobs, MSC, assumed duties in 1959 as staff officers for a new position, special assistant to the surgeon general for combat developments. Another six MSCs formed the initial staff for a Combat Developments Group at Forest Glen, Maryland. In addition, seven officers were serving as assistant professors of military science and tactics at universi-

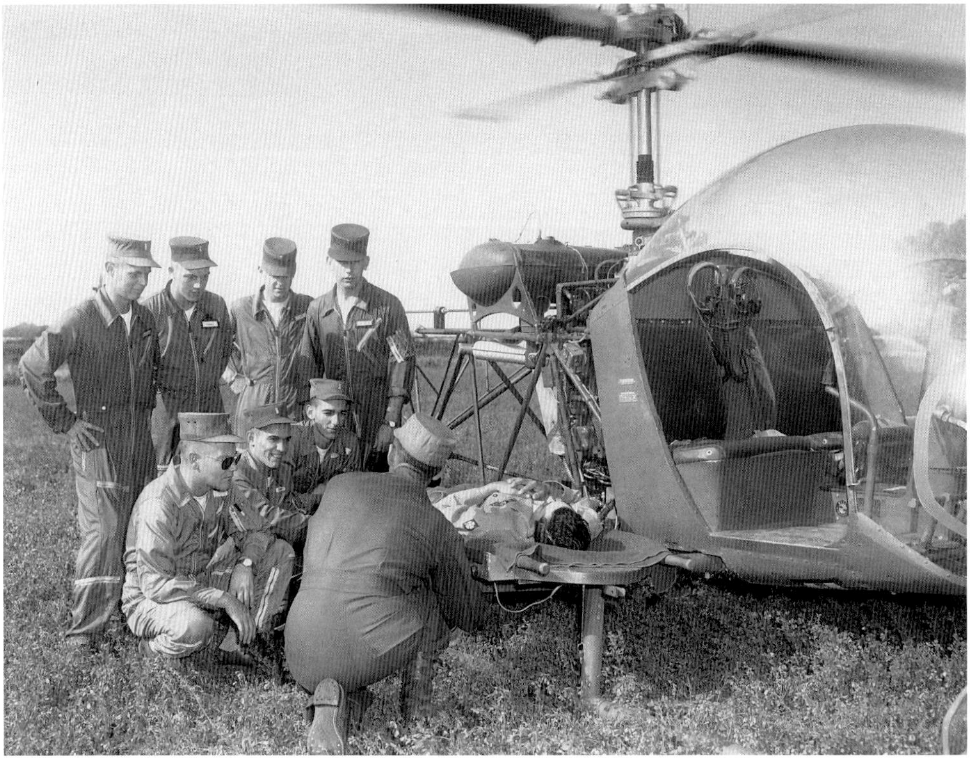

A class of Medical Service Corps officers learns how properly to strap a patient and litter on an H–13 helicopter, October 1954.

ty ROTC programs. There was discussion of a training course for operations officers, but nothing materialized.[73]

Some operations and training officers, along with other MSCs, had the opportunity for overseas assignments with military assistance programs. There were twenty-four MSCs serving with the U.S. advisory effort in Vietnam in 1956. That year Majs. F. W. Sitton, MSC, and Leigh F. Wheeler, MSC, were assigned to a medical troop training team in Germany. By 1959 sixty MSCs were serving with advisory groups in Greece, Turkey, Vietnam, the Ryukyu Islands, Thailand, Iran, Formosa, Peru, Paraguay, Bolivia, Colombia, El Salvador, and Nicaragua.[74]

Lt. Col. Paul F. Austin, MSC, and Maj. Earl Reynolds, MSC, helped the Thai Army organize three medical battalions and three 100-bed field hospitals. They cautioned that officers and their families posted to that part of the world had to be able to cope with poor sanitation as well as an abundance of mosquitos, ants, lizards, and snakes. Lt. Col. Vincent P. Verfuerth, MSC, assisted the Peruvian military plan for a 960-bed military hospital, a job he assumed from Lt. Col. Seth H. Linthicum, MSC.

Maj. James R. Kenney, MSC, found meaningful rewards in his posting to Iran. "Just about the time you're ready to throw in the towel, one of these wonderful Iranians will come up with something that makes you feel like you're sitting on top of the world." Kenney also encountered quite the opposite at times. On one trip he encountered a group of naked men standing near a unit command post in a chilly, remote area. The recently discharged conscripts were being punished for failing to buy any civilian clothes when they were paid.[75]

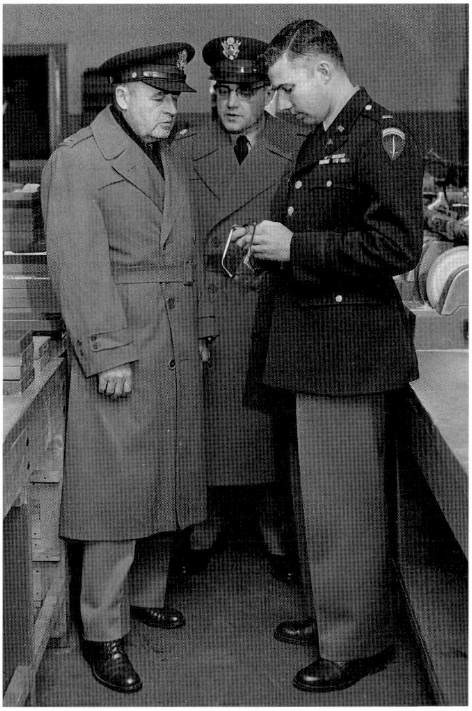

Optical Department, Rhine Medical Depot, Kaiserslautern, Germany, January 1956

Opportunities opened for medical intelligence officers, a field closely associated with operations. A medical intelligence training program began in 1956, and teams of one MSC officer and two enlisted soldiers were dispatched to Korea and Germany. The same year the department consolidated four intelligence elements into a single activity, the Medical Information and Intelligence Agency, and Lt. Col. James W. Dean, MSC, became its first director.[76]

Aviation was a new MSC field. In 1954 there were 98 MSC pilots and another 21 MSCs were in flight school. By 1959 there were 112 MSC aviators, a number that climbed to 181 in 1964 as the United States increased its involvement in Vietnam.[77] The corps needed to provide attractive career opportunities for MSC aviators, but most flying duties called for junior officers. In 1963, 80 percent of the authorized positions were for lieutenants, but 85 percent of MSC aviators were in the grade of captain or higher. This greatly concerned Colonel Hamrick, who assumed the establishment of field grade positions for aviators, either in flying or nonflying duties, as one of his major tasks.[78]

Medical logisticians passed another milestone in 1960 when Col. Renaldo G. Belanger, MSC, became chief of the Surgeon General's Supply Division. He was the first administrative specialty officer to hold that position since Brig. Gen. Edward Reynolds, MAC, seventeen years earlier.[79] By 1961 forty MSCs were in the Army Logistics Program, a specialized program for selected Army logisticians. MSC medical logisticians had a reputation for well-run organizations. In 1955 Col. Louis F. Williams, MSC, assumed command of the Louisville Medical Depot where he installed an IBM data processing system and reduced the staffing from 850 to 450 personnel. General Lyman L. Lemnitzer, the Army Chief of Staff, on a swing through Germany in 1958, said the medical depot at Kaiserslautern was the best organized unit he had seen.[80] DOD established the Defense Supply Agency in 1959, and medical items became the responsibility of a subordinate agency, the Defense Medical Supply Center. MSC officers were in demand to fill key positions within that joint service organization.[81]

Nepthune Fogelberg was appointed in 1952 as the first comptroller for the surgeon general. Fogelberg, a Sanitary Corps major in World War II, had continued as chief of the Surgeon General's Fiscal Division after his release from active duty in 1946. He was a leader in promoting resources management as a career field for Medical Service Corps officers.[82]

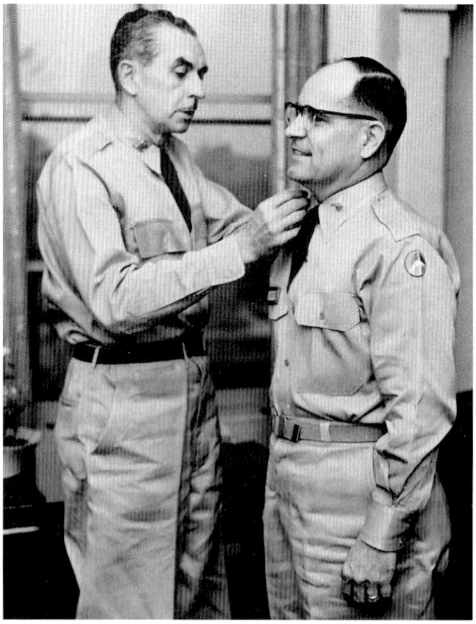

Lt. Col. Jack Houser (right), *Comptroller, Tokyo Army Hospital, during his promotion ceremony, July 1956*

An important step was establishment of a graduate training program for MSC comptrollers. The formation of DOD had been accompanied by new requirements for financial management that created a need for comptrollers throughout the armed services. The Army established the Army Comptrollership Program at Syracuse University, Syracuse, New York, to meet that need. It combined both business and public administration courses in an accelerated program designed to prepare officers and civilian employees for comptroller positions. Capt. David W. Jones attended in 1953 as the first MSC. After 1954 there were an average of three MSCs in each class.[83]

The Peyton Board, while casting a jaundiced eye on "comptrollership," had nevertheless conceded its inevitability and recommended training some officers in the specialty, including physicians. Fogelberg asked the Medical Field Service School to create a course, but the department chose to use other Army courses and civilian graduate programs instead. General Heaton, acting on the Peyton Board recommendation, encouraged physicians to apply for training as comptrollers. Little came of that effort, other than to irritate senior MSCs who understood financial management as an academic field mastered through graduate study in business administration and believed it to be within the province of the MSC. Fogelberg chaired the first meeting of medical comptrollers in 1958, at which time there were 113 MSC positions.[84]

MSCs in the registrar specialty dealt with a more complex environment, for their specialty was complicated by federal, local, and state laws and regulations. They administered medical boards that determined whether soldiers should be retained or released for medical reasons. Accreditation surveys by external agencies kept pressure on the medical records function, along with the associated tasks of transcription and release of medical information.[85]

Lt. Col. Robert G. McCall, MSC, desired to create a medical facilities engineering specialty within his Sanitary Engineering Section because that was the only Medical Department component that required an engineering degree. McCall envisioned a need for eleven officers. Others favored creating the specialty as part of the Pharmacy, Supply, and Administration Section. They believed that making it a sanitary engineering field would block candidates from other equally valid backgrounds. Neither suggestion was acted upon, and health facility planning tasks continued to be handled by MSCs in a variety of specialties.[86]

The changes to the key management team of Army hospitals solidified. A Medical Corps deputy commander headed the clinical services as chief of professional services, and a Medical Service Corps executive officer was chief of administrative services. Both reported to the commander (the hospital administrator). New hospital administration positions for MSCs emerged in both outpatient and inpatient settings. Dispensary administrative officers were an example of the former. Maj. Gen. Silas B. Hays, on a trip to Europe while he was surgeon general, observed that dispensaries with an MSC were performing well but those without had problems. Opportunity in the inpatient side expanded with the use of MSCs as administrative assistants for the chiefs of the larger departments in hospitals. Brig. Gen. Carl W. Tempel, MC, the surgeon general's director of professional services, championed this as a means of freeing physicians for clinical duties.[87]

Not everyone was ecstatic. One physician said MSC hospital administrators were his reason for leaving the Army. He complained that they "gave birth to new positions, new jobs, new offices, new departments, more typewriters, more forms, and these in turn begat more of their kind." Surgeon General Hays called the letter a masterpiece, read it to his staff, and had it distributed throughout the Medical Department.[88] An external advisory committee chaired by Dean A. Clark, M.D., of Massachusetts General Hospital, recommended keeping MSCs at lower-level positions. General Heaton shared that view, and for a while he attempted to block the assignment of MSCs as executive officers of the general hospitals.[89]

Many MSCs continued to contribute to the profession after their retirement from the Army. Col. Anthony J. Zolenas, Jr., retired in 1961 and became the administrator of the Johns Hopkins Hospital in Baltimore, Maryland. Colonel Gibbs became the first full-time director of the Interagency Institute for Federal Health Care Executives in 1956. He continued in that position upon his retirement in 1957. He also completed his baccalaureate and master's degrees and started the George Washington University program in hospital administration, which became one of the country's largest.[90]

Developments in the Scientific Specialties

Tension between the administrative and scientific specialties[91] prompted Colonel Black to suggest reorganizing the corps into an administrative specialties section and a scientific specialties section. Each group would have its own promotion lists, to avoid competing directly against the other. Administrative specialty officers would have primary skill identifiers in just two subspecialties—junior and senior administrative officers. General Armstrong carried this idea a step farther, proposing to create two separate corps, as in the Air Force. Neither proposal gained the momentum necessary for congressional action. There were also unsuccessful proposals to commission chiropractors in the MSC.[92]

Pharmacy became a separate service in the larger hospitals, on a par with other clinical services—a reflection of the sophistication of pharmaceutical technology and the dependence of the clinical staff on pharmacy consultation. In September 1955 Lt. Col. William L. Austin, MSC, became the first full-time pharmacy consultant to the surgeon general. He was responsible for publishing a formulary that provided Army physicians with a pocket-size reference listing all drugs in the medical supply system. Austin followed the example of William Brown, who published the first formulary, the Lititz Pharmacopoeia, during the American Revolution.[93]

Organized pharmacy kept an eye on the department because of its continued use of enlisted and officer graduate pharmacists at a ratio of ten to one. There were 330 enlisted and 36 officer pharmacists on active duty in 1955, the year in which the pharmacy ROTC programs ended.[94] In 1959, 110 graduate pharmacists were still serving as officers in other Army branches in duties unrelated to pharmacy, a carryover of earlier times. Robert P. Fischelis, Pharm.D., of the American Pharmaceutical Association, met with General Hays to discuss commissioning. After his intervention the number of pharmacists serving as MSC officers gradually increased to eighty-nine by 1961.

Very few pharmacists, however, applied for Regular Army status. Colonel Aabel chided them for letting that opportunity go begging after all their long struggle.[95] Those who did pursue a career were encouraged to go to graduate school. Capt. Lewis C. Miner, MSC, and 1st Lt. Douglas J. Silvernale, MSC, in 1959 were the first pharmacy officers to complete master's degrees in hospital pharmacy, and in 1965 Miner was the first to complete a doctoral degree. Graduate training was supplemented in 1960 by establishment of a residency program in the general practice of pharmacy at Brooke Army Medical Center.[96]

In 1961 the Medical Allied Sciences Section had 472 officers on active duty. Two specialties—nuclear medical science and podiatry—had joined the disciplines of psychology, social work, entomology, and laboratory science. Audiology would be added in 1965. In turn, laboratory science encompassed six specialties: bacteriology, biochemistry, parasitology, immunology (virology), physiology, and clinical laboratory officer. The extensive training required for scientific specialties prompted a recommendation, not adopted, for a distinctive insignia to identify officers holding doctorate degrees. Recognition of another sort was afforded when the Medical Department established a system in 1961 for recognizing professional attainment in a series of prefixes added to the specialty codes of officers. Award of the "A" prefix to scientific specialty officers signified the highest level of achievement in their fields. Indeed, the expanding range of medical expertise provided by scientific specialty officers prompted a cautionary note by General Heaton: "We must be very cautious or the fringe people will take over the medical profession."[97]

An Army survey of scientifically trained officers showed that MSCs desired diversification in their assignments. Overall, they believed they were treated as well as or better by the Army than by civilian institutions. Interestingly, the approach of MSCs to education differed from their compatriots in other Army branches. MSCs viewed graduate training as a means for overall growth rather than as a way of enhancing their military careers through "ticket punching." A DOD study concluded that the Medical Service Corps managed scientists better than anyone else in DOD. The study also revealed that MSCs strongly desired to receive the same military training as other Army officers.[98]

Col. Harvey W. Coddington, MSC, was appointed chief of the Medical Allied Sciences Section in 1959. Coddington set a policy that officers in his section would perform only in their specialty, except for courts, boards, duty officer, or similar necessary military duties. He emphasized graduate training and professional certification, for example, encouraging microbiologists to affiliate with the American Board of Microbiology.[99] However, perceptions of second-class treatment persisted. Col. Charles S. Gersoni, MSC, ran into an "undercurrent of bitterness" from senior scientific specialty officers assigned to write articles for the 1958 MSC History Project. Gersoni attributed this to the department's clumsiness in handling MSC scientists and poor relationships between the scientists and military physicians. Not all MSC scientists shared that pessimism. Col. Ludwig R. Kuhn, MSC, a bacteriologist and the first chief of the Medical Allied Sciences Section, praised the research opportunities for MSCs and what he viewed as equitable treatment in promotions. Col. Monroe E. Freeman, MSC, a biochemist, was also optimistic, pointing to improvements in professional status and opportunities for training and research.[100]

Yet the proper utilization of uniformed scientists within the Army's medical research and development program continued to be a vexsome problem. As Lt. Col. John P. Ransom, MSC, a microbiologist, put it, "a completely satisfactory solution to the proper utilization of this group of scientists is yet to be found." Ransom believed that scientific competence demanded a degree of specialization that ran counter to the Army's needs for well-rounded officers, especially at the higher grades. As he pointed out, an unfortunate upshot of this dichotomy could be an officer shorted on both counts, without the opportunity to achieve genuine distinction in science or to compete with other Army officers in terms of military training and experience.[101] Colonel Gersoni believed this situation could be helped by establishing a separate research career program that would be controlled by the chief of the Surgeon General's Research and Development Division. That did not materialize, but a more firmly institutionalized home for MSC researchers was achieved in 1958 when the Army established the U.S. Army Medical Research and Development Command (USAMRDC) as a medical command under the surgeon general. By 1959 USAMRDC employed about one hundred MSCs as researchers and administrators in a broad research program. MSCs headed projects in the Middle East, Southeast Asia, Borneo, Africa, and Central America. Lt. Cols. John Ransom and Avery C. Sanders, MSC, served as staff officers with the Army's chief of research and development. Colonel Freeman headed the European Research Office in Frankfurt, Germany, and Colonel Gersoni headed a similar unit in the Far East.[102]

Capt. Donald L. Price, MSC, completed his Ph.D. in parasitology in June 1959. That August, Price and his wife were assigned to the Belgian Congo where they joined about thirty-five other families of different nationalities at the Institut Pour La Recherche Scientifique en Afrique Centrale (the Institute for Scientific Research in Central Africa). The institute was located about thirty-five miles north of Bukavu within reasonable travel distance of rain forest, savannah, bush country, and the volcanic Mountains of the Moon. Unfortunately, while research opportunities were magnificent, the political situation was unstable. Belgium granted the country its independence in June 1960, much sooner than anticipated, and fighting immediately broke out among competing tribal factions. The situation became perilous, and Mrs. Price left on 15 June. Captain Price departed in the early morning of 22 June after he was warned to leave the night before by the local Belgian commander. He got across the border one hour before it closed driving a truck without any brakes. He made it to Uganda where he continued his research for the next two years at the medical school of the University of Makerere in Kampala.[103]

MSCs contributed to medical advances. Maj. Trygve O. Berge, MSC, and Harvey Kempe, M.D., demonstrated in studies beginning in 1953 that gamma globulin was an effective vaccine against smallpox. Berge headed a team at Fort Ord, California, that in 1954 identified type 7 adenovirus as a new etiologic agent for acute respiratory illness. Col. Warren C. Eveland, MSC, advanced the fluorescent antibody technique for rapid identification of infectious agents. Maj. Harold L. Williams, MSC, conducted early studies in 1959 on the physiological and psychological impact of prolonged sleep deprivation. The expertise of the Prosthetics Research Laboratory under the command of Lt. Col. Maurice J. Fletcher, MSC, enabled over 160 Korean War amputees to be retained on active duty. Lt. Cols. Dan C. Cavanaugh and John D. Marshall, MSC, began a series of studies in 1960 that over the next decade provided major advances in plague research, including its ecology, relation of outbreaks to the impact of weather on the flea vector, and development of a serological test. And in 1960 Berge, then a colonel, headed a research team that fielded a vaccine for Venezuelan equine encephalomyelitis (VEE).[104]

The nuclear age had created requirements for experts in the medical effects of nuclear weapons, the medical management of mass casualties, and the use of nuclear medical techniques in diagnosis and treatment. The development of expertise to meet those requirements that had been marked by the pioneering work of Lt. Col. Roy W. Maxwell, MSC, and others, led to the establishment in 1957 of nuclear medical science as a specialty that encompassed radiation biology, biophysics, and radiological and health physics. It had an initial requirement for thirty-one officers, including ten at the doctoral level. This opportunity for graduate training had produced its first two doctorates by 1960: Majs. Charles R. Angel, MSC, and Ernest D. Jones, MSC. By December 1961 there were twenty officers in the specialty, and Colonel Maxwell, then the assistant for atomic nuclear warfare and casualty studies at the Medical Field Service School, represented their interests as a specialty group.[105]

The chiropody debate was resolved in 1956 with the establishment of nine positions for doctors of surgical chiropody at general hospitals and basic training centers.[106] In 1957 2d Lt. John L. Charlton, Jr., MSC, became the first chiropodist commissioned in the Army in his specialty. Previously, Charlton had been assigned as a noncommissioned officer to the Pentagon dispensary where he established a practice that was popular with a number of general officers. He counted President and Mrs. Eisenhower among his patients. Podiatry became the preferred name for the specialty during this period, and in 1957 the American Podiatry Association cited Lieutenant Charlton for his contributions.[107]

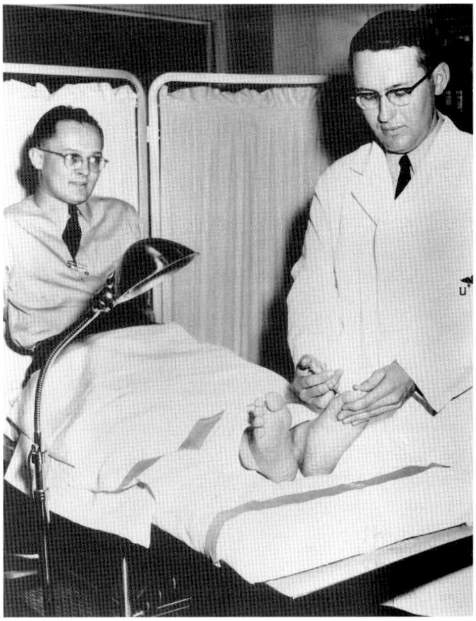

*Lieutenant Charlton (*right*) with patient at Walter Reed Army Hospital*

Hearing loss associated with military service had begun to be a concern in World War II. The Army gradually took an interest in this problem, initially with the clinical needs for audiometric testing, the fitting of hearing aids, and the provision of aural rehabilitation services. That interest assumed a more concrete shape when audiology, another emerging specialty, joined the MSC in 1965 as a career field within the Medical Allied Sciences Section. By December 1966 the Army had commissioned five trained audiologists who were replacing a variety of military personnel in meeting the evolving demands for audiological and hearing preservation services.[108]

In 1954 there were 77 entomologists on active duty, which number dropped to 49 in 1961, a number that included 9 officers with doctorates and 2 enrolled in doctoral programs. DOD established the Armed Forces Pest Control Board in 1956, and entomologists served as its executive secretary on a rotating basis among the Services. There were efforts to move entomology into the Sanitary Engineering Section, the argument being that while entomologists had been at loggerheads previously with sanitary engineers, they were now closely associated in their professional interests. The organization of the preventive medicine company was evidence of that relationship. If the company's mission was mainly entomology, then an entomologist commanded, but if it was principally a sanitary engineering mission, then a sanitary engineer commanded. Those who would realign entomologists argued that as members of a field practice specialty, they were "found more in the mud than in the laboratory." However, entomology remained part of the Medical Allied Sciences Section.[109]

Progress slowed in Army psychology. The scope of practice remained limited, retention was poor, and most psychologists on active duty were junior officers with a two-year military obligation. The graduate student program expired in 1954, but restarted in 1957, and the situation was further helped by a Regular Army augmentation in 1958. One of those officers, 2d Lt. Jimmy L. Hatfield, MSC, became the department's liaison with Project Adam, an Army project at Huntsville,

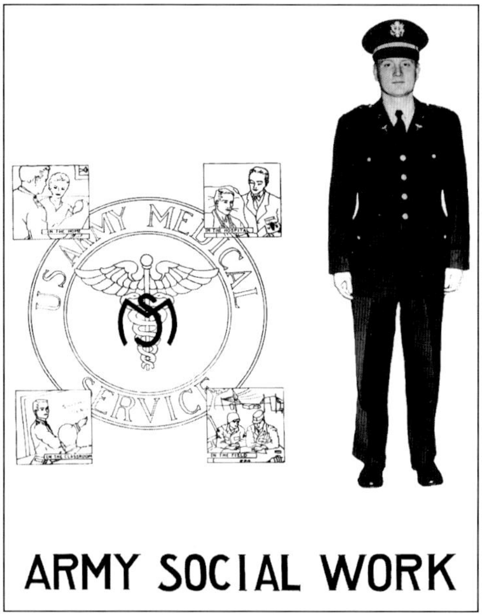

Social work recruiting poster, January 1960

Alabama, that was one of the earliest phases of the U.S. space program. Retention difficulties compelled the Army to commission some psychologists at the master's level, even though the doctorate had become the U.S. standard.[110]

There were only eighty-eight psychologists on active duty in 1961, and ten of those were in training. Lt. Col. James Hedlund, MSC, became the psychology consultant in 1963. He believed the number of psychologists was inadequate for the Army's needs, and he predicted the demise of Army psychology if it continued on the same course. Hedlund was able to get his position reinstated on a full-time basis, he expanded contacts with the civil sector, and he expanded the student program to a three-year course of study.[111]

The Army authorized the addition of an MSC social worker to each division, and in 1961 there were 116 social workers on active duty. Lt. Col. William S. Rooney, MSC, the social work consultant to the surgeon general from 1962 to 1965, was able to negotiate the establishment of social work as a separate service in the larger hospitals. This removed social workers from the direct supervision of psychiatry but more important, in Rooney's view, it "enabled social workers to provide services to all patients in the hospital on an equal basis."[112]

Conflict between sanitary engineering and the Medical Department ended, and Lt. Col. Stanley J. Weidenkopf, MSC, chief of the section, gave an upbeat assessment in 1954 to a National Academy of Sciences panel. There were 99 sanitary engineers on active duty in 1961, with another 175 officers in the active reserves. They were expanding their expertise into industrial hygiene, radiation protection, and research and development, and eight officers became founding members of the American Academy of Sanitary Engineers. Another accomplishment was fielding new equipment, including a portable kit for rapid bacterial testing of water.[113]

In 1954 some of the worst floods in the history of East Pakistan drove ten million people from their homes. Cholera was endemic, and the potential for epidemics of typhoid and cholera was very high. In August the 37th Medical Company (Preventive Medicine), commanded by a sanitary engineer, 1st Lt. Alfred D. Kneessy, MSC, boarded five U.S. Air Force C–124s in Dacca thirty-three hours after being alerted. When they left Pakistan thirty-nine days later, they had administered nearly one million inoculations, a mission complicated by cultural prohibitions against women being touched by strange men. The governor of East Bengal cabled the U.S. secretary of state that their efficiency had been

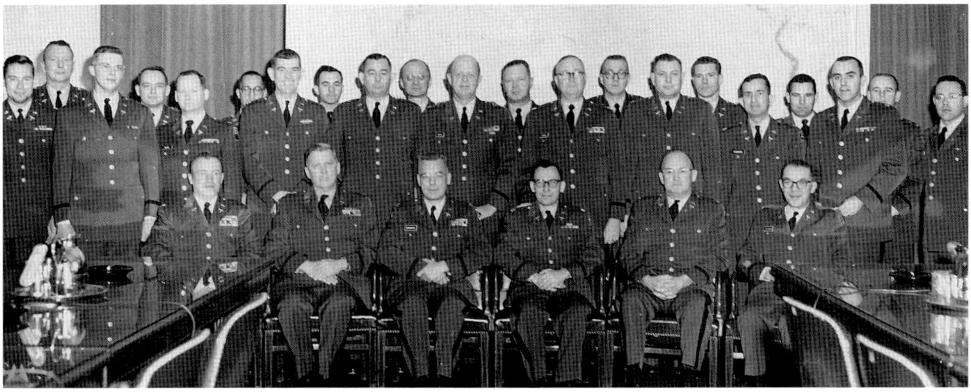

Sanitary engineers meet at Walter Reed in 1959.

an "eye opener." Kneessy's company had used every conceivable conveyance to reach the population, including river steamers and small boats. Shots were sometimes given by medics in one boat to people in another.[114]

The issue of scientific duties versus Army officer duties surfaced at a meeting of sanitary engineers in 1959. Lt. Col. Marlo E. Smith, MSC, argued that they should concentrate on their specialty and not seek positions typically held by administrative specialty officers. There was agreement with his point, but that did not mean scientific specialty officers were excused from learning how to be Army officers. Col. Floyd Berry, MSC, "probably the oldest sanitary engineer present," counseled that they had to be proficient both as engineers and as officers. "If we are going to become prima donnas and go around in a sloppy butcher's coat and cry that we need recognition like the Ph.D.s, then we are not improving our status." Capt. Hunter G. Taft, Jr., MSC, seconded Colonel Berry. He said they were Army officers first, MSCs second, and sanitary engineers third. "We are either 'on the team' or we get off it."[115]

The Medical Department continued to use enlisted optometrists. One was Sgt. David Johnson, assigned to Fort Sill, Oklahoma, where he found his enlisted status galling when he was required to perform the medic's nemesis, bedpan drill. Lt. Col. John W. Sheridan, MSC, chief of the Optometry Section from 1951 to 1960, said it was tantamount to employing enlisted and officer dentists for neighboring chairs in a dental clinic.[116] The American Optometric Association cried foul. It insisted that the intent of Congress was to commission optometrists. If they were not commissioned, then the Army could enlist them, but not for duty as optometrists. The practice of employing enlisted optometrists ended in 1957; from then on the Army used commissioned optometrists only.[117]

The Army's decision to commission optometrists encountered criticism from the American Medical Association. General Hays dismissed it as carping by a small minority. He conceded that the scope of practice for MSC optometrists surpassed that of their civilian colleagues, but he reminded critics that they worked under the supervision of ophthalmologists. He was in no way concerned about the quality of their work, and he pledged his continued support of their expanded employment.[118]

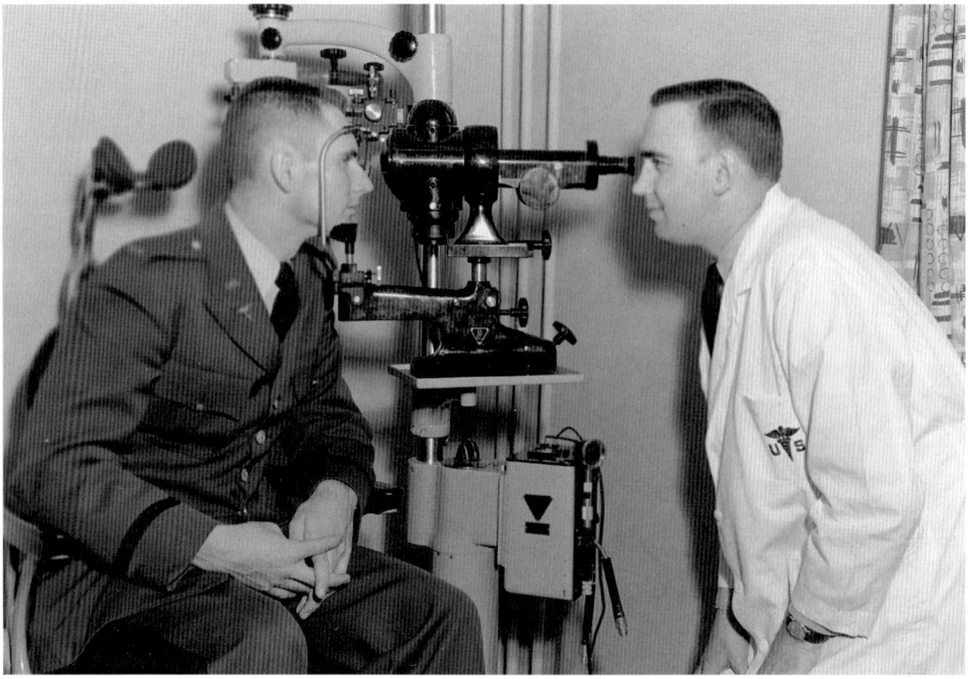

Optometry officer checks a patient at the EENT Clinic, U.S. Army Hospital, Fort Campbell, Kentucky, February 1959.

Demand for optometry had not abated. The department estimated that one-third of soldiers wore glasses, but because of the shortage of optometrists they were waiting up to three months for an appointment in 1954. Colonel Sheridan began visiting the ten U.S. colleges of optometry each year to recruit from the 300 members of the graduating classes. Sheridan's effort paid off as the number of Optometry Section officers on active duty went to 125 in 1958 and 154 in 1961. The first annual meeting for Army optometrists was held in 1963 under the direction of Sheridan's successor, Lt. Col. Billy C. Greene, MSC.[119]

Summary

The author of the Peyton Report disparaged the Medical Service Corps as an "Austro-Hungarian sort of empire" composed of heterogeneous elements.[120] Colonel Peyton's characterization was apt, but not in the way he intended. The diversity of the MSC, while a weakness, was also a considerable strength for the Medical Department. If nothing else, its collection of officers in widely differing specialties made for interesting bedfellows and a synergy not otherwise possible. Administrative and scientific specialty officers were at least compelled to listen to each other.

The success of the corps chiefs in building a vision for the MSC generally shared by its members was a substantial achievement for such a diverse group.

That was especially true given the diffuseness of the surgeon general's power, even in a period in which the Surgeon General's Office enjoyed a high degree of control over all medical personnel in the Army. Efforts to build cohesion with the various devices of group identity—insignia, music, travels by the chief, a birth date, and a history project—were not inconsequential actions. The initiative of setting up a permanent corps and improving the quality of its officers was paying off. Old-timers believed the Medical Service Corps of the 1960s was "a far cry" from the Medical Administrative Corps of the 1920s.[121]

The use of MSCs to substitute for and replace military physicians continued with persistent shortages of Medical Corps officers, but this remained upsetting to some. Colonel Peyton said that substituting MSCs for Medical Corps officers was an inane effort to "put all the 'doctors' in white coats and anchor them in the hospitals."[122] Others shared his view.

Scientific specialty officers had to be technically proficient in a way that encouraged specialization. However, the large number of MSC administrative specialties encouraged overspecialization. Colonel Aabel cautioned against that tendency, especially as it tended to channel the experience and capabilities of administrative officers exclusively into either the fixed facility or field settings. For example, he said that hospital-based officers, particularly registrars, would be lost in field assignments if they had not kept up with field medicine. Operations and training officers, on the other hand, needed familiarity with hospital-based specialties in order to fully comprehend the nature of the department's health care mission. Scientific specialty officers also tended to become isolated in their specific areas. The tug between specialization and generalization was pretty much a draw.[123]

The tension described in the Peyton Report between the fixed and field facility components of the department was present as well in the MSC as a division between "house cats" and "alley cats," which was manifested to a degree in the underlying tension between the administrative and scientific specialties. Officers in field units sometimes felt themselves disadvantaged in their career aspirations. The problem was recognized by the corps leadership at the end of the decade. They realized it was important to make field assignments "so attractive that they will be sought and not shunned."[124] Education and training were kept at the forefront of corps interest, and there was a general upgrading in educational levels, including the standards of the Army-Baylor Program. The assignment of MSCs to General Staff, Army logistics, and other positions outside the Medical Department represented new opportunities and was also indicative of their abilities. Promotion opportunities waxed and waned and waxed again. An initiative to create general officer opportunity did not succeed. Unfortunately, General Heaton's request for a star constrained the corps to proposals for one general officer and the greater potential in Maj. Leo Benade's proposal was lost.

Position opportunity ran up against the larger issue of command. Command of Army units demands the selection of individuals who meet the most stringent requirements for ability—personality, character, training, and experience. The department supported an array of command opportunities for MSCs, including command of nonoperational medical units or medical supporting units, as well as command at all levels of the Army. But it would not accept MSCs in command of its operational hospitals. Perhaps the most insidious side of that policy was the breeding of generations of MSCs who did not seek this level of responsibility or who believed they would never be tested in that way.

In 1953 Maj. Gen. James T. McGibony, MC, a retired deputy surgeon general, interjected a balanced viewpoint into the sometimes acrimonious debate. McGibony recognized the difficulty of interesting the best physicians in administration. However, unlike other nations, the United States had developed graduate programs in hospital administration, and in America some physicians were actually attracted to the specialty.[125] He urged the continued search for top-flight physicians and others who had prepared themselves through a broad general background and management training to enter hospital administration. At the same time, he gave short shrift to those who would argue that only physicians could handle the top hospital administration positions. "It is as foolish to think that the non-medical man cannot develop the concept of medical care as to feel that the acquisition of an M.D. degree automatically removes all administrative ability."[126]

Career opportunity in the Army begins with the education and training that prepare officers for good positions. Solid performance at each level of the hierarchy results in promotions and higher-level positions, but that progression is stunted when there are constraints. Opportunities for MSCs in education, positions, and promotions improved to some degree in the period between the Korean and Vietnam Wars, but not as much as was desired. Their vistas remained limited by actions of the Medical Department.

Notes

[1] Interwar period: See Weigley, *History of the United States Army*, pp. 525–26. Quoted words: James L. Cooney, "Some Notes on the Historical Development of the Medical Service Corps," *U.S. Armed Forces Medical Journal* 8 (February 1957): 254–63; Speech, Maj Gen Alvin L. Gorby, MC, sub: The MSC as a Member of the Army Medical Service Team, in Rpt, 459th Hospital Center, sub: Proceedings of the Medical Service Corps Institute, Garmisch, Germany, 2–4 April 1959, DASG-MS.

[2] Integration: SG Conference, 2 Apr 56.

[3] Changes: See Paul Starr, *The Social Transformation of American Medicine* (New York: Basic Books, 1982), pp. 338–78.

[4] Quoted words: Rpt, Col Robert E. Peyton, MC, President, Army Medical Service Board, OTSG, sub: Report of Study, 17 Sep 56, copy in DASG-MS, hereafter cited as Peyton Report.

[5] DCSPER: Memo, Col Harold W. Glattly, MC, Ch, Pers Div, OTSG, for Armstrong, sub: Consolidation of All Personnel Activities Within the Department of the Army, 29 Jan 54, and DF, Hayes, to G–4, same sub and date, in SG Conference, 29 Jan 54, USACMH. TSG had found "by bitter experience" the need for this authority. Memo, Glattly, 29 Jan 54. OTSG believed TSG was in charge of "*all* Army medical personnel, world-wide" (SG Conference, 14 Jul 59). Technical services: SG Conferences, 3 Apr, 31 Jul, and 11 Dec 64. See Hewes, *From Root to McNamara*, pp. 316–65. Quoted words: SG Conference, 3 Apr 64. Heaton's signature block added a capital "T" (*T*he Surgeon General) as he took office in June 1959. This convention first appeared about March 1959 and was in regular use that summer. The historical title of the department was changed to Medical Service with an Army decree that there could be only one department, *the* Department of the Army. It changed back before the decade was over.

[6] Lessons: Spurgeon H. Neel, Jr., "Helicopter Evacuation in Korea," *U.S. Armed Forces Medical Journal* 6 (May 1955): 695–700. Doctrine: CMT 4, Col Bryan C.T. Fenton, MC, XO, OTSG (drafted by Maj James D. Davenport, MSC, Acting Ch, Aviation Br), to DCSLOG, sub: Branches Authorized Army Aviation, 10 Jan 58, folder 280, box 18/18, MSC-USACMH; Dorland and Nanney, *Dust-Off*, pp. 19–20; Ltr, Col Bernard Aabel, Ch, MSC, to senior MSCs, sub: The Army Medical Service Corps, December 1956, hereafter cited as MSC Newsletter (Colonel Aabel instituted this communication method, and it was used by all his successors). MSC newsletters from 1956 to 1961 are in RG 112, accession 64P–2161, Box 103, and 1963 is in RG 112, accession 66C–3260, Box 35, NARA-WNRC. Also see Maj William R. Knowles, MSC, Asst Ch, Avn Br, OTSG, to Capt John Temperilli, Jr., MSC (in Vietnam), 3 Oct 62, MSC-USACMH.

[7] Huey: Interv, Lt Col John W. Hammett, MSC, Ret., with Capt Dorland, MSC, THU, OTSG, Oct 75, interview files, USACMH; Interv, Lt Col Kenneth K. Wheatley, MSC, Ret., with Dorland, Oct 75, USACMH; Weinert, Jr., *A History of Army Aviation*, pp. 203–04; David M. Lam, "From Balloon to Black Hawk: Vietnam," part 4 of series, *U.S. Army Aviation Digest* 27 (July 1981): 45.

[8] MSC Branch: MSC Newsletters, December 1956 and October 1963; OTSG, DA, Special Orders 10, 23 Mar 63, DASG-MS; Col Dale E. Thompson, MSC, Actg Ch, MSC, to Deputy Surgeon General (DSG), sub: Reorganization of Medical Service Corps Functions, 27 Aug 62; Thompson, Policy no. 45, same sub, 15 Oct 62 (implementing OTSG Memo, 20 Aug 62), DASG-MS; William J. Clegg, "Medical Service Corps Career Planning," *Military Medicine* 125 (November 1960): 757.

[9] Changes: Memo, Col Dale L. Thompson, Actg Ch, MSC, for TSG, sub: Reorganization of MSC Functions, 14 Aug 62, and Col Lawrence A. Potter, MC, XO, OTSG, to Thompson, same sub: 20 Aug 62; OTSG, SO 10, 25 Mar 63, all in folder 127, box 9/18, MSC-USACMH; MSC Newsletter, October 1963, DASG-MS. The Personnel and Training (P&T) Division XO was also made an assistant to the MSC chief.

[10] Warrant officers: DA Cir 611–6, 14 Jun 56, PL; MSC Newsletter, January 1959; Rpt, P&T Div, OTSG, sub: The Army Medical Service Corps and Warrant Officer Career Planning Program, FY 1961, 1 Jun 60, hereafter cited as MSC Career Planning Program, FY 1961; Rpt, Manpower Control Div, OTSG, sub: Fiscal Year Reports, Medical Service Corps, FY 1959–67, hereafter cited as MSC Manpower and dates; Notes of telephone interv, CW4 W.B. King, Ret., with Ginn, 8 Feb 92, all in DASG-MS.

[11] Ratings: Ch, MSC, policy, sub: Release of Information, 30 Aug 62, DASG-MS. Report scores were translated into an Officer Efficiency Index (OEI) based upon the expected statistical distribution. OEIs were averaged into an Annual Efficiency Index (AEI), and officers could compare their OEI with the AEI for an idea of how they were doing. Quoted words: Rpt, Lt Col Charles J. Cowgill, MSC, XO, Med Div, 549th Hosp Ctr, USAREUR, sub: Proceedings of the MSC Institute, Berchtesgaden, Germany, June 1958, MSC-USACMH.

[12] Statistics: MSC Manpower, FY 1959–67; Joseph Israeloff, "The Emerging Role of the Medical Service Corps Officer in the Evolution of the Army Medical Service," *Military Medicine* 125 (April 1960): 273, hereafter cited as Israeloff, "The Emerging Role"; Col Leo F. Benade, MSC, Special Projects Office, OTSG, summary sheet for TSG signature, sub: Proposed Legislation for 1962 Legislative Session, DASG-MS, hereafter cited as Benade, 1962 Legislative Session. Senior medical and dental student programs were established in 1956 to increase MC and DC (and later VC) accessions by commissioning junior and senior medical and dental students as MSC second lieutenants and assigning them to U.S. Army Reserve (USAR) units where they were paid at the rate of one day per week while in school. Specialties: CMT 2, Maxwell, Ch, MSC, to Ch, Medical Plans and Operations (MP&O) Div, OTSG, sub: Consolidation of ARs and SRs, 19 Nov 59, folder 139, box 9/18, MSC-USACMH.

[13] RIF: SG Conferences, 1 Sep 53 and 22 Aug 55; Office Memo, OTSG, sub: Notes, October 1953, copy in JML; MSC Newsletter, February 1958. The 1958 RIF affected ninety commissioned officers and forty-nine warrant officers.

[14] Quoted words: Address to USAREUR and USAF MSC officers, Col Robert L. Black, Ch, MSC, sub: Problems of the Medical Service Corps, April 1954, folder 40, box 4/18, MSC-USACMH, hereafter cited as Black, Problems of the MSC.

[15] Retention: MSC Newsletters, June 1959 and December 1961; SG Conferences, 28 Jan 57, 6 May 60, and 27 Mar 64.

[16] MC: SG Conferences, 1 Sep and 18 Dec 53, 26 Apr 54, 19 Nov 56, 10 Sep and 5 Dec 58, and 2 Jan 59; MSC Newsletters, February 1957 and February 1958; Hamrick to Ginn, 21 Sep 88, DASG-MS. Armstrong: SG Conference, 18 Dec 53.Stethoscope: SG Conference, 25 Jan 57.

[17] Shortages: SG Conferences, 1 Sep 53, 26 Apr 54; MSC Newsletters, February 1957 and February 1958, DASG-MS; Address, Aabel to MSC monthly meeting at Walter Reed Army Medical Center (WRAMC), sub: Today's Army Medical Service Corps, 21 Nov 56, folder 43, box 4/18, MSC-USACMH, hereafter cited as Aabel, Today's MSC. Quoted words: MSC Newsletter, November 1958; SG Conference, 18 Dec 59. Percentages: MSC Newsletter, June 1959.

[18] Substitution of MSCs: SG Conference, 19 Nov 56. Shortages in 1961: MSC Newsletter, December 1961.

[19] Accessions: SG Conferences, 3 Feb 54, 9 Jul 56, and 26 Jun 64; MSC Newsletter, November 1958; Ltr, TAGO, sub: Staffing, Authorization and Utilization of Medical Service Commissioned Personnel in TOE (General Reserve) Units, 16 Mar 56; DF, Col Laurence A. Potter, MC, XO, OTSG, to Dir, P&T Div, sub: Policy of MSC Personnel Holding Ph.D. Degrees, 24 Sep 62, MSC-USACMH. 2d Lt. Irons: OTSG, Rpt of WRAMC conference, sub: Current Trends in the Army Medical Department, 1966, MSC-USACMH.

[20] Career plans: Rpt, MSC&WO Sec, P&T Div, OTSG, sub: Status of Major Projects in Career Management Section, June 1960, DASG-MS; Lt Col William J. Clegg, Jr., draft section, sub: Career Planning, 1958 MSC History Project, hereafter cited as Clegg, Career Planning, 1961; Col Clegg, Ch, Pers Div, 549th Hosp Ctr, Germany, to Lt Col Matthew Ginalick, MSC, Ch, Spec Proj Br, THU, 13 Sep 61, all in folder 246, box 15/18; Lt Col Charles A. Pendlyshok, MSC, to Clegg, MSC, 15 Feb 60, box 19/18, all in MSC-USACMH.

[21] Movie: MSC Historical Rpt, FY 1955, file Post World War II, box 2/18, hereafter cited as MSC FY 1955 Rpt; Maj William V. Davis, MSC, TLO, MSC Historian Materials File, 1956, folder 238, box 15/18, MSC-USACMH. OTSG allocated funds for a Technicolor procurement film in 1956; the author could not locate it. Newsletter: See note 6, this chapter.Party: SG Conference, 19 May 58. The esprit transcended the Services. In 1957 Army, Navy, and Air Force MSC officers formed the MSC Association, headed by Lt. Col. John A. MacCartney, MSC, USAF. *Medical Service Corps Association Newsletter*, November–December 1958, MSC-USACMH.

[22] March: Aabel to Capt Samuel Loboda, U.S. Army Band, Fort Myer, Va., 7 Jul 58. Follow-up with the U.S. Army Band in 1984 and 1985 revealed no record of an MSC march, and Col. Robert I. Jetland, Aabel's assistant, confirmed that none materialized. Jetland to Ginn, 7 Nov 87, DASG-MS. Motto and flag: Aabel to Ch, Heraldic Br, QMG, sub: Establishment of a Motto for the Medical Service Corps, 10 Jul 58; B.W. Dano, Technical Liaison Div, OTSG, to Ch, Heraldic Br, QMG, 11 Feb 59; OTSG, Off of Ch, MSC, file #605–02, sub: MSC Flag and Insignia File, 1963, all in RG 112, accession 64A–2161, Box 103/162, NARA-WNRC.

[23] Insignia: DF, Aabel to Ch, P&O Div, OTSG, sub: Questionnaire on AMEDS [Army Medical Service] Insignia, 9 Jul 56; Aabel to Capt Knute A. Tofte-Nielsen, 14 Feb 57, RG 112, accession 64A–2161, Box 103/162, NARA-WNRC. Aabel proposed a gold snake on a silver staff with letters superimposed for each corps; his alternative was to change the MSC to a gold caduceus, the same as the other corps, with a superimposed "S." Tofte-Nielsen's design was a five-pointed gold star centered on a gold caduceus.

[24] Birth date: Draft rpt, Capt James K. Arima, MSC, Recorder, Lt Col Robert I. Jetland, MSC, and Lt Col Charles A. Pendlyshok, MSC, Chm, sub: Staff Study on Anniversary of the Origin of the Medical Service Corps, November 1956, signed by Aabel and Col John B. Coates, MC, Dir, Historical Unit, AMEDS, 26 Nov 56, with note by Maj Gen Cooney on DD95 routing slip, approved by Maj Gen Hays, 13 Feb 57, folder 37, box 4/18, MSC-USACMH; MSC Newsletters, September 1956 and April 1957; Memo, Hays, TSG, for OTSG Officers and Society of Consultants to Armed Forces, 31 Mar 57, MSC-USACMH. Either Letterman's order of 2 August 1862 or the 11 March 1864 date would have been better. The department cannot point to an unbroken thread either, but no one seriously argues against using 1775 for its formation as "an Hospital."

[25] Project failure: MSC FY 1955 Rpt.

[26] Quoted words: THU, AEB for 1958 MSC History Project.

[27] Quoted words: Notes of discussion, Col Lloyd A. Schlaeppi, MSC, with Lt Col Richard V.N. Ginn, Washington, D.C., 16 May 84, DASG-MS.

[28] Regular Army: SG Conferences, 21 Mar and 1 Apr 56 and 28 Jan 57; MSC Newsletters, September 1956, May 1958, and June 1959; Statement, Heaton, sub: Statement Before the Committee on Armed Services, U.S. Senate, 8 September 1966, DASG-MS.

[29] Quoted words: MSC Newsletter, June 1959. Education: MSC Newsletter, April 1957 and May 1958.

[30] Baccalaureate degrees: MSC FY 1955 Rpt; MSC Newsletters, August 1958 and January 1959; SG Conferences, 25 Nov 57 and 24 Mar 58; Interv, Col Roy S. Church, MSC, Ret., with Ginn, Fort McPherson, Ga., 9–10 Nov 83, DASG-MS.

[31] Letters: Church said that without action his career "was almost at a standstill." Numbers: MSC Newsletter, June 1959; MSC Manpower, 31 December 1961.

[32] Graduate programs: MSC Newsletters, April 1957, June 1959, and July 1961 (FY 1963 programs); MSC Manpower, 31 December 1961. Quoted words: SG Conference, 4 Aug 59. Study: John W. Bullard, "A Study of the Relationship Between Graduate Civil Schooling and Career Advancement of the United States Army Medical Service Corps Officer," Ph.D. dissertation, American University, Washington, D.C., 1971, JML.

[33] Quoted words: Hamrick, Sylvester interv, 21 Feb 84, USAMHI. In 1958 Hamrick organized the Alumni Association of the Army-Baylor Program.

[34] Army-Baylor: Rpt, MFSS, Brooke Army Medical Center (BAMC), sub: Report on the Baylor Army Program in Hospital Administration, 1961, DASG-MS. There were 343 officers by June 1954: 201 MSC, 113 ANC, 8 MC, 2 WMSC, 1 WAC, and 18 foreign officers. MFSS, History of the Hospital Admin Course, undated, MSC-USACMH. Also see Rpt, Lt Col David G. Dougherty, MSC, ADJ, BAMC, sub: Proceedings of the DA Board To Review Army Officer Schools, 5 Sep 65, RG 112, accession 69A–2602, Box 40/81, NARA-WNRC.

[35] Report: Rpt, John M. Nicklas and Herluf V. Olsen, Commission on University Education in Hospital Administration, sub: Report on the Program in Hospital Administration, 1952, DASG-MS, hereafter cited as Accreditation Report, 1952. The survey was sponsored by the Kellogg Foundation and the AUPHA.

[36] Response: DF, Gibbs, Dir, Dept of Admin, MFSS, BAMC, sub: Confidential Report—Army Program in Hospital Administration, 28 Sep 54; Brig Gen James P. Cooney, MC, Commandant,

MFSS, to Herluf V. Olsen, Ph.D., Dir, Committee on University Education in Hospital Administration, undated (1953), including quoted words, DASG-MS.

[37] Quoted words: SG Conference, 10 Dec 52.

[38] Quoted words: Col R.G. Prentiss, Jr., in SG Conference, 15 Feb 54. Attention to weaknesses and changes: DF, Gibbs to Col Snyder, sub: Quality of Students Sent to MFSS, 8 Oct 54; Gibbs to Hardy Kemp, M.D., 4 Feb 55, DASG-MS; Also see SG Conference, 2 Apr 53, and series of 13 memos in 1955, principally by Gibbs. For discussion of continued maturation see: MSC Newsletters, December 1956, November 1958, 1959, and December 1959; Col Glenn K. Smith, Dir, Dept of Admin, MFSS, to Col Millard C. Monnen, MSC, P&T Div, OTSG, 1 Mar 61; SG Conference, 21 Nov 61; Edwards to Hamrick, sub: Baylor-Army Program, 3 Mar 58, DASG-MS; Rpt, AUPHA, sub: The Development of the Association of University Programs of Hospital Administration, 1958, Stimson Library (SL).

[39] Quoted words: Gibbs to Snyder, 8 Oct 54, DASG-MS.

[40] MHA degree: Memo for the record (MFR), Gibbs, 17 Feb 55, DASG-MS.

[41] Quoted words: Olsen to Gibbs, 10 Feb 55. Olsen also noted that the program had assistance from Leonard Duce, Ph.D., of Baylor University and later dean of the Trinity University Graduate School, San Antonio, Texas. Duce maintained a lasting relationship with the program.

[42] Defended: CMT 2, Edwards, Dir, Dept of Admin, MFSS, to Ch, Ops Div, MFSS, sub: Army School System Study, 22 Jan 62, including Msg, USCONARC AT-SCHED 700702, 16 Jan 62, DASG-MS.

[43] Courses: SG Conferences, 8 Sep 54 and 7 May 58; MSC Newsletters, May 1958 and October 1963; Rpt, Army Medical Service School, BAMC, sub: Recommendations of Program of Instruction Conference, 21 Aug 57, MSC-USACMH; Ch, Education and Training Div, OTSG, 7 May 58, in SG Conference, 7 May 58. Carmack Medal: Ltr, Hays to Col Joseph Carmack, USA, Ret., 24 Feb 58, RG 112, accession 64A–2161, Box 103/162, NARA-WNRC; Press releases, Public Information Office (PIO), BAMC, 23 Mar and 9 Jun 58, SL; Carmack to Maj Gen William E. Shambora, MC, CG, BAMC, 10 Jan 58, SL. Carmack was one of the first MACs promoted to colonel.

[44] Courses: MSC Newsletter, November 1958 (see DA Cir 621–21, 9 Jul 58) and October 1963. Meetings in 1958/59 included personnel, comptroller, supply, psychology, entomology, and laboratory.

[45] Staff college: SG Conference, Jan 56; MSC Newsletter, July 1957; Aabel, Status of MSC, 1961; Aabel, Today's MSC; Clegg, Career Planning, 1961, all MSC-USACMH.

[46] Senior Service College (SSC): MSC Manpower, 31 December 1961; Rpt, P&T Div, OTSG, sub: Study—Increase of Officer Quotas, AMEDS, for Military and Civilian Schools, 15 Apr 54, DASG-MS; Aabel, Today's MSC.

[47] Pessimism: Memo, Lt Col Robert C. Miller, MSC, sub: Minutes of Second Meeting of Ad Hoc Committee To Inquire into the Feasibility and Desirability for Integration of the Medical Service Corps Promotion List into the Army Promotion List, 10 Jul 56, MSC-USACMH, hereafter cited as 1956 Ad Hoc Committee.

[48] Outside assignments: SG Conference, 13 Feb 56; MSC Newsletter, December 1956; CMT 3, Col Byron L. Steger, MC, Ch, P&T Div, OTSG, sub: Utilization of Senior Medical Service Corps Officers, 6 Oct 58, to DF, Aabel, same sub, 17 Sep 58, DASG-MS, hereafter cited as Steger, 6 Oct 58 comment.

[49] Command assignments: SG Conference, 1 Feb 54; DF, Heaton to Asst Sec Army (Manpower and Reserve Forces), drafted by Benade, MSC, P&T Div, OTSG, sub: Legislative Proposal for Inclusion in the DOD FY 1961 Program, 10 Aug 60, DASG-MS, hereafter cited as Heaton, FY 1961 Program; Col John A. Mikuluk, MSC, Ret., to Ginn, 26 Jan 84, DASG-MS. Pay: SG Conferences, 7 Oct and 8 Nov 60.

[50] Command assignments: Change 1 to AR 40–2, "Army Medical Treatment Facilities," 7 Apr 58, PL; MSC Newsletter, May 1958; THU, AEB for 1958 MSC History Project; Speech, Clegg, sub: The Army Medical Service Corps and Warrant Officer Career Planning Program, Current and Projected, 1959, DASG-MS; SG Conference, 4 Aug 59. Quoted words: Black, draft section, sub: Achievement and Looking Ahead, 1958 MSC History Project, file 259, box 16/18, MSC-USACMH.

[51] Quoted words: Interv, Heaton with Col Robert B. McLean, MC, Pinehurst, N.C., 7 Dec 78, Senior Officer Oral History Program, USAMHI.

[52] Quoted words: Black, "The Army's Medical Service Corps," *Military Surgeon* 115 (July 1954): 12, hereafter cited as Black, "The Army's MSC"; also see Address, Black, sub: Utilization of the Medical Service Corps, Hosp Admin Class, BAMC, 1 Dec 53, MSC-USACMH.

[53] Quoted words: Richards to Ginn, 28 Feb 86, DASG-MS.

[54] Command responsibilities: Speech, Col Joseph T. Caples, MC, Med Div, HQ, USACOMZEUR, sub: Past, Present and Future of the Medical Service Corps, undated (1964), folder 264, box 17/18, MSC-USACMH.

[55] National Guard: SG Conference, 7 Sep 56. Civil defense: Val Paterson, Federal Civil Defense Administrator, to Charles E. Wilson, Sec Def, sub: Civil Defense Emergency Hospital, 25 Nov 55, in SG Conference, 7 Dec 55.

[56] Quoted words: Accreditation Rpt, 1952.

[57] Quoted words: Maj Gen Joseph Martin, Cdr, BAMC, to Brig Gen James P. Cooney, Cmdt, MFSS, 27 Sep 54, DASG-MS. See also SG Conferences, 10 Sep 58, 2 Jan and 7 Jul 59, and 21 Nov 61.

[58] Command: SG Conference, 23 Mar 59; MSC Newsletter, December 1961; 75 Stat. 364, 17 August 1961. Heaton's request: Heaton, FY 1961 Program.

[59] Appointments: Msg, DA DCSPER 58203, 28 Nov 61, cited in MSC Newsletter, December 1961.

[60] 2 percent: Army-Navy Medical Service Corps Act of 1947—Per Centum of Colonels, 61 Stat. 734, 23 March 1954; Black, "The Army's MSC," p. 13; Rpt, THU, sub: Outline, the U.S. Army Medical Service Corps, 1957, folder 259, box 16/18; Black, Statement Before the Subcommittee of the Committee on Armed Services, House of Representatives, on H.R. 5509, 83d Cong., 1st sess., July 1953, folder 13, box 3/18, both in MSC-USACMH; U.S. Senate Rpt no. 1030, sub: Army-Navy Medical Service Corps Act of 1947—Per Centum of Colonels, 25 February 1954; SG Conferences, 29 Sep 52 and 22 Jun 53. The 8 percent provision allowed for 76 colonels based on the RA strength of 945 officers at the time. OTSG had identified 183 positions for MSC colonels. Follow-on problems: Steger, 6 Oct 58 comment.

[61] Quoted words: SG Conference, 15 Jul 57.

[62] APL: SG Conference, 14 May 56; 1956 Ad Hoc Committee; MFR, Lt Col Samuel A. Plemmons, MSC, Pers Div, OTSG, sub: Integration of the Medical Service Corps and Army Promotion Lists, 1956, MSC-USACMH; MSC Newsletter, September 1956.

[63] Hays' plan: Rpt, Hays, sub: Informal Report to General Magruder on Completion of Tour as Surgeon General, in SG Conference, 19 May 59.Quoted words: Interv, Col Vernon McKenzie, MSC, Ret., Principal Dep to Asst Sec Def (Health Affairs), with Ginn, the Pentagon, 20 Jun 84, DASG-MS. Colonel Black said Hays wanted MSC medical logisticians to move on so as to avoid "invading Medical Corps responsibility areas." Black to Coates, 11 May 60, box 19/81, MSC-USACMH.

[64] Quoted words: Col James T. Richards, MSC, Ret., to Ginn, 28 Feb 76, DASG-MS.

[65] Options: Maj William V. Davis, MSC, Historical Material File, 1956, folder 235, box 15/18, MSC-USACMH.

[66] Resolutions: MSC FY 1955 Rpt.

[67] Stars: Memo, Black, sub: Establishment by Law, on an Incumbency Basis of the Grade of Brigadier General for the Chief of the Medical Service Corps, for Armstrong, TSG, 4 Oct 54 (and annotated by Hays, DSG, 8 Oct 54), DASG-MS; MSC FY 1955 Rpt; MSC Newsletters, July 1957 and July 1961; DF, Heaton to DCSPER, sub: H.R. 10905, 'A Bill To Authorize the Grades of Maj. Gen. and Brigadier General in the Medical Service Corps of the Regular Army and for Other Purposes,' 11 Apr 62; DF, Doan to DCSPER, sub: H.R. 11649, 24 May 62; Cyrus R. Vance, Sec Army, to Rep Carl Vinson, Chm, House Armed Services Committee (HASC), 8 Aug 62; Benade, 1962 Legislative Session; Col James T. Richards to Ginn, 28 Feb 76; Benade, Ginn interv, 25 Jan 84; all documents in DASG-MS; Armstrong, Israeloff interv, 12 Mar 76.

[68] Quoted words: DF, Heaton to DCSPER, 11 Apr 62, MSC-USACMH; also see Benade, 1962 Legislative Session.

[69] General officers: Pamphlet, Clegg, "The Army Medical Service Corps and Warrant Officer Career Planning Program, Current and Projected, 1959."

[70] Support: Heaton briefed the Office of Management and Budget in 1961 that the quality of administrative support made good clinical management possible. Brig Gen Manley Morrison, MSC, Ret., to Ginn, 4 Sep 88, DASG-MS. Administration: MSC Manpower, FY 1959–67; Fact Sheet, OTSG, sub: Army MSC: Knowledge of Special Advantage, 1957, both in DASG-MS.

[71] Operations: MSC Newsletters, December 1956 and January and June 1959; Israeloff, "The Emerging Role," p. 273; Aabel, Today's MSC.

[72] "Iron majors": Richard Halloran, "Of Paper Tigers Whose Joy in Life Is Red Stripes," *New York Times* (25 October 1984). Quoted words: Col John Lada, MSC, Dir, THU, OTSG, annotation to Wheatley, Dorland interv, Oct 75.

[73] Course: THU, AEB for 1958 MSC History Project.

[74] Overseas: MSC Newsletter, January 1959.

[75] Quoted words: Ibid.

[76] Medical Intelligence: MSC Newsletter, December 1956; Lt Col Raymond J. Creamer, MSC, draft chapter, sub: Intelligence, 1958 MSC History Project, folder 248, box 16/18, MSC-USACMH.

[77] Aviators: SG Conferences, 26 Jan 53, 11 Oct 54, and 1 May 57; MSC Newsletter, January 1959; MSC Manpower, FY 1959–67.

[78] Promotion problems: MSC Newsletter, October 1963; Rpt, OTSG, sub: Management Improvement Plan (draft) FY 63, 1963, both in RG 112, accession 66C–3260, Box 35, NARA-WNRC.

[79] Belanger: Col R.L. Parker, MSC, draft chapter, sub: Administrative Medical Supply Officer, 1958 MSC History Project, folder 244, box 15/18, MSC-USACMH.

[80] Louisville: Williams, Ginn interv, 15 Nov 84. Lemnitzer: SG Conference, 12 May 58.

[81] DOD: Rose C. Engelman, *A Decade of Progress: The United States Army Medical Department, 1959–1969* (Washington, D.C.: Office of The Surgeon General, Department of the Army, 1971), pp. 151–54. Logistics program: MSC Newsletter, February 1961.

[82] Fogelberg: Rpt, OTSG, sub: Current Trends Conference, 1966, USACMH; Bio data card, THU, OTSG, undated, USACMH.

[83] Syracuse: Rpt, Syracuse University, sub: Army Comptrollership Program, 1991; Fact sheets, Syracuse, sub: What Is the Army Comptrollership Program? and Synopsis of the ACP (draft), 1990, all in DASG-MS.

[84] Comptrollers: Peyton Board; MFR, Col Manley Morrison, sub: The Medical Service Corps, 22 Mar 62, DASG-MS, hereafter cited as Morrison, The MSC; SG Conference, 19 Jun 57; MSC Newsletter, February 1958.

[85] Registrar: Maj John J. Ward, MSC, draft section, sub: Registrar, 1958 MSC History Project, box 15/18, MSC-USACMH.

[86] Facilities: Rpt, Lt Col Robert G. McCall, MSC, sub: Staff Study on Medical Facilities Engineering, 16 May 60 (result of Walter Reed Army Institute of Research [WRAIR] meeting, 30 Nov–5 Dec 59), 30 Aug 60, DASG-MS. Counter: CMT 4, Col James T. McGibony, MC, Ch, Plans and Ops Div, 30 Aug 60, in McCall, 16 May 60, DASG-MS.

[87] Hospital administration: File, Plans and Ops Div, OTSG, sub: Improvement of Organization Structure (change to SR 40–610–5), 5 Oct 54, Maj James W. Reiber, MSC, to Lt Col David C. Clark, MSC, Hosp Mgmt Engineering Br, OTSG, and other correspondence updating AR 40–22, in RG 112, accession 68H–3359, Box 57/75; OTSG, file 204–01, revision of ASR 40–22, final revised draft 1 Oct 63, RG 112, accession 66C–3260, Box 35, all in NARA-WNRC; SG Conference, 21 Oct 55; AR 40–27, "Organization of Class I U.S. Army Hospitals," 29 Apr 55, PL.

[88] Resignation: Maj Vol K. Philips, MC, to TSG, sub: Reasons for My Resignation from the Medical Corps, in SG Conference, 23 Nov 55; Office Memo, OTSG, 27 Jan 56; also see Maxwell to Col Allen Pappas, MSC, Ch, Log Div, BAMC, 10 Aug 61, MSC-USACMH. Pappas, an MSC, did not like administrative officers either.

[89] Keep MSCs down: Rpt, National Academy of Sciences–National Research Council (NAS-NRC), sub: Report of Committee on Army Medical Education, chaired by Dean A. Clark, M.D., Washington, D.C., Jan 56, JML. MC XOs: Heaton to Col Knox Dunlap, MC, Surg, First U.S. Army, 22 Aug 61 (refers to AR 600–20 and AR 40–2); Morrison, The MSC.

[90] Zolenas: Zolenas, Milner interv, 13 Jul 66, USACMH. Gibbs: Interv, George Bugbee with Lewis E. Weeks, AHA, Chicago, 31 May and 19 Jul 78, American Hospital Association Library; SG Conference, 29 Mar 57. In 1990 James O. Hepner, Ph.D., American College of Hospital Administrators chairman, listed Gibbs as one of the ten most influential pioneers in the field. Editorial, Hepner, in *Healthcare Executive* 4 (March–April 1990): 5.

[91] MSC differences: Col. Anthony C. Tucker, MSC, surveyed 300 administrative officers with the Strong Vocational Interest questionnaire. They were strikingly different from physicians and scientific specialty MSCs, but quite similar to other Army officers. Tucker, "Vocational Interests of Medical Administrative Officers," *Armed Forces Medical Journal* 5 (May 1955): 685–90. Also see Edward K. Strong, Jr., and Tucker, *The Use of Vocational Interest Scales in Planning a Military Career*, APA monograph no. 341 (Washington, D.C.: American Psychological Association, 1952).

[92] Separation: SG Conference, 2 Feb 53; Black, "Problems of the MSC." The AF had an MSC and a Bioscience Corps. Chiropractic: SG Conferences, 18 Mar 57 and 25 Apr 61.

[93] Pharmacy: SG Conferences, 16 and 19 Mar 55; Memo, Black for Ch, Plans and Ops Div, OTSG, sub: Proposed Changes to AR 40–615, 24 Sep 54, RG 112, accession 68A–3359, Box 57, NARA-WNRC; Henry D. Roth, "Utilization and Training of Pharmacists in the Army Medical Service," *Military Surgeon* 115 (July 1954): 43–45; Address, Aabel, sub: The Medical Service Corps, Department of the Army, 22 Jun 55, MSC-USACMH, hereafter cited as Aabel, The MSC; MSC Manpower, FY 1959–67; MSC Newsletters, November 1958, January 1959, and December 1961; Lt Col Alfred W. Gill, MSC, Pharmacy Br, Academy of Health Sciences Lesson Plan 37–365–320, sub: History and Traditions of Army Pharmacy, 1986; MSC Career Planning Program, FY 1961; MSC Newsletters, November 1958 and January 1959; MSC FY 1955 Rpt. Formulary: Edward Kremers, "The Lititz Pharmacopoeia," *Badger Pharmacist* (June–December 1938): 1–70.

[94] ROTC: The University of Wisconsin converted to an MSC ROTC. MSC FY 1955 Rpt.

[95] Regular Army: Speech, Aabel, sub: Utilization of Pharmacists in the Army, presented to the Idaho and Oregon state pharmacy conventions, Jun 57, folder 78, box 6/18; Rpt, Black et al., sub: Committee Study: Pharmacy in the Army, OTSG, 9 Mar 55, citing Ltr, TSG to Chm, Committee on Status of Pharmacy in Government Service, 9 May 47, folder 78, box 6/18, MSC-USACMH. Also see Aabel, The MSC.

[96] Residency program: Maj. Douglas J. Silvernale, MSC, was preceptor for 1st Lt. Robert P. McMahon, MSC, the first resident.

[97] MAS: MSC Newsletter, February 1961; MSC Manpower, 31 December 1961. Insignia: Aabel, Today's MSC. "A" prefix: Unpublished paper, Col John N. Albertson, MSC, sub: History of the Medical Service Corps Contributions to Medical Research and Development, 24 Sep 84, DASG-MS, hereafter cited as Albertson, MSCs in Research and Development. Quoted words: SG Conference, 11 Jul 61.

[98] Army survey: Summary of staff study, Maj Stephen E. Akers, MSC, Asst Ch, Career Planning Sec, MSC and WO Br, OTSG, sub: Utilization of Scientifically Trained Officers, 2 May 60, Clegg file, box 18/18, MSC-USACMH; 109 MSCs responded to the survey. DOD study: Rpt, Col H.A. Ferguson, MSC, P&T Div, OTSG, sub: Final Report on Review of Medical and Biological Programs within the Department of Defense, 12 Oct 62, DASG-MS.

[99] Coddington: MSC Newsletter, October 1963. Utilization: DF, Col Harvey Coddington, MSC, Ch, MAS Sec, to Actg Ch, MSC, sub: The Utilization of Medical Service Corps Officers, 5 Oct 62, with CMT 2, Col Dale L. Thompson, MSC, 15 Oct 62, MSC-USACMH. Coddington was the first nonphysician curator of the Armed Forces Institute of Pathology (AFIP) Medical Museum.

[100] Gersoni: Col Charles S. Gersoni, MSC, Cdr, U.S. Army R&D Group (Far East), to Lt Col Matthew Ginalick, THU, 15 Dec 60, box 19/18, MSC-USACMH. Kuhn: Col Ludwig R. Kuhn, MSC, draft section, sub: Laboratory Specialties. Freeman: Col Monroe E. Freeman, draft section, sub: Biochemistry, all in 1958 MSC History Project, folder 253, box 16/18, MSC-USACMH.

[101] Quoted words: Lt Col John R. Ransom, MSC, draft section, sub: Microbiology, hereafter cited as Ransom, Microbiology.

[102] Gersoni proposal: Memo, Gersoni, Ch, Human Resources Br, R&D Div, OTSG, for Ch, R&D Div, sub: Career Patterns for Research Procurement, Selection, Classification and Management, 4 Dec 56, MSC-USACMH. USAMRDC: DAGO 31, 23 Aug 58, PL; MSC

Newsletter, January 1959; Col Fred W. Timmerman, MC, Ret., to Col William V. Davis, MSC, XO, USAMRDC, 1 Jun 71, DASG-MS; Written interv, Col William C. Luehrs, MSC, Ret., with Ginn, 5 Nov 84, DASG-MS. Major Luehrs worked with Colonel Timmerman, Deputy Chief, R&D Division, OTSG, as the project officer. They formed the command in one day, then worked for months to sort out the details, with Luehrs serving as chief of the support division.

[103] Price: MSC Newsletter, April 1959; Telephone interv, Col. Donald L. Price, MSC, Ret., with Ginn, 28 Sep 91, author's notes; Price to Ginn, 31 Oct 91, DASG-MS.

[104] Research: Engelman and Joy, *Two Hundred Years of Military Medicine*; Fact sheet, THU, OTSG, sub: Chronology: U.S. Army Contributions to Civilian Medicine, 1971; Col Trygve O. Berge, MSC, draft section, sub: Virology and Immunology, 1958 MSC History Project, box 16/18, MSC-USACMH. Gamma globulin: C. Henry Kempe, Berge, and Beatrice England, "Hyperimmune Vaccine Gamma Globulin: Source, Evaluation and Use in Prophylaxis and Therapy," *Pediatrics* 17 (1956): 184. Adenovirus: Berge et al., "Etiology of Acute Respiratory Diseases Among Service Personnel at Fort Ord, California," *American Journal of Hygiene* 62 (1955): 294. Fluorescent antibody: Ransom, Microbiology. Plague: Dan C. Cavanaugh, "Specific Effects of Temperature Upon Transmission of the Plague Bacillus by the Oriental Rat Flea, *Xenopsylla Cheopis*," *American Journal of Tropical Medicine and Hygiene* 20 (March 1971): 264–73, hereafter cited as Cavanaugh, "Specific Effects of Temperature"; Cavanaugh et al., "Plague," chapter in Andre J. Ognibene and O'Neill Barrett, Jr., *General Medicine and Infectious Diseases* in the series Internal Medicine in Vietnam (Washington, D.C.: Office of the Surgeon General and Center of Military History, U.S. Army, 1982), pp. 167–97. Prosthetics: Col Maurice J. Fletcher, MSC, draft section, sub: Prosthetics, 1958 MSC History Project, MSC-USACMH.

[105] Nuclear Medicine: MSC Newsletter, April 1959; Rpt, OTSG, sub: Sanitary Engineering, Report of Conference Conducted at the Walter Reed Army Institute of Research (WRAIR), Washington, D.C., 30 November–5 December 1959, hereafter cited as 1959 Sanitary Engineering Rpt; Memo, Clegg, sub: Conference, Nuclear Medical Officer, 3304, and Nuclear Science Officer, 3308, Career Planning Program, 26 Jan 59; OTSG, MSC Career Planning Program, 1959; Rpt, Col Charles R. Angel, MSC, Ch, MAS, MSC, sub: Development of Nuclear Science Within the MSC, undated (1976), DASG-MS.

[106] Chiropody: MSC Newsletters, November 1958 and April 1959; THU, AEB for 1958 MSC History Project; SG Conferences, 19 Mar and 30 Jul 56 and 28 Mar 61; C.R. Brantingham, "Military Chiropody Today," *Military Medicine* 121 (July 1956): 33.

[107] First podiatrist: "Balm for Sore Feet," *Army-Navy Register* 78 (9 March 1957): 6; 1st Lt J.C. Charlton, Jr., MSC, draft section, sub: Podiatry, 1958 MSC History Project, MSC-USACMH.

[108] Audiology: Fact sheet, OTSG, sub: Audiologists and the United States Army, Jul 71, MSC-USACMH. Numbers: DASG-RMM, Fiscal Year Rpts, FY 1959–1967, DASG-MS.

[109] Entomology: THU, AEB for 1958 MSC History Project; Rpt, MSC, sub: Educational Status of Entomologists, 15 Jun 54; MSC Newsletter, June 1962; Col Ralph W. Bunn, MSC, and Col Joseph E. Webb, Jr., MSC, draft section, sub: Entomology, 1958 MSC History Project, DASG-MS.

[110] Psychology: MSC Newsletter, December 1961; SG Conference, 4 Mar 57; Unpublished paper, Harold D. Rosenheim, Ph.D., sub: A History of the Uniformed Clinical Psychologist in the U.S. Army, presented at the American Psychological Association meeting in Montreal, 2 Sep 80, hereafter cited as Rosenheim, History of the Uniformed Psychologist, and Rosenheim to Ginn, 18 Sep 84; Address, Col Charles A. Thomas, MSC, Ret., sub: Contributions of and Challenges Faced by AMEDD Psychology: 1950's–1970's, 1982 AMEDD Psychology Symposium, 14–19 November 1982, Dwight David Eisenhower Army Medical Center, hereafter cited as Thomas, Contributions by AMEDD Psychology, all in DASG-MS. Hatfield: SG Conference, 16 April 58. Graduate program: "Psychology Students Sought by the Army," *Army-Navy Register* 77 (28 July 1956): 4.

[111] Hedlund: Rosenheim, History of the Uniformed Psychologist; Thomas, Contributions by AMEDD Psychology.

[112] Social work: Col Harry W. Adams, MSC, and Lt Col Ralph W. Morgan, MSC, draft chapter, sub: Social Work, 1958 MSC History Project, MSC-USACMH; MSC Newsletters, April 1959, October 1960, and July 1961. Quoted words: Lt Col William S. Rooney, MSC, Ret., to Ginn, 22 Feb 85, DASG-MS.

[113] Sanitary engineers: Address, Lt Col Stanley J. Weidenkopf, MSC, Prev Med Div, OTSG, sub: Sanitary Engineers in the Army Medical Service, to the Subcommittee on Personnel and Training, Sanitary Engineering and Environment, NAS-NRC, Washington, D.C., 18 May 54, DASG-MS; MSC Manpower, 31 December 1961; MSC Newsletters, 16 October 1963 and January 1959, DASG-MS; OTSG, draft Administrative Letter 1–15, sub: Management Improvement, 17 Aug 62, RG 112, accession 66C–3260, Box 35, NARA-WNRC; SG Conference, 10 Jan 64. Founders: Cols. Ralph R. Cleland, Raymond J. Karpen, Fenner H. Whitely, and Stanley J. Weidenkopf; Lt. Cols. Floyd L. Berry, Robert G. McCall, and Marlo E. Smith; and Maj. John Redmond, MSC.

[114] Pakistan: Rpt, 1st Lt Alfred D. Kneessy, MSC, sub: East Pakistan Relief Action, 37th Med Co (Preventive Medicine) (Separate), EUSA, Korea, Aug–Sep 54; Kneessy to Col Earl J. Herndon, MSC, 16 Aug 83, DASG-MS; Robert Littell, "Air Lift Against Disaster," *Readers Digest* (January 1955): 7–10; THU, "A Challenge to the Army Medical Service, Medical Technicians Manual Supplement," *U.S. Armed Forces Medical Journal* 6 (July–August 1955): 139–42; Cable, Iskander Mirza to Sec State, 30 Sep 54, DASG-MS.

[115] Meeting: 1959 Sanitary Engineering Rpt, p. 176, quoted words, pp. 25, 30.

[116] Enlisted optometrists: Lt Col Robert T. Gmelin, MSC, Ret., to Ginn, 31 Jul 85, and phone conversation with Ginn, 23 Dec 85; Col John T. Leddy, MSC, Ch, Optometry Sec, to Ginn, 12 Feb 88; Speech, Lt Col John W. Sheridan, MSC, Ch, Optometry Sec, sub: Military Optometry, undated (late 1950s), all in DASG-MS.

[117] Commissioning: SG Conferences, 14 Feb 55 and 2 Jul 56; DA Cir 600–12; DF, Black to TSG, sub: Status of Optometrists, 14 Feb 55, hereafter cited as Black, Optometrists, 1955; Chronological rpt, OTSG, sub: Brief History of Optometrists as Commissioned Officers, undated (1971), folder 63, box 5/18, MSC-USACMH.

[118] Hays' views: SG Conference, 22 Jan 58.

[119] Optometry: Black, Optometrists, 1955; SG Conferences, 19 May 58 and 22 Aug 61; Rpt, Office of the Quartermaster General, sub: In Process Review on Eye Protection, 15 Nov 62, RG 112, accession 69A–0127, Box 10/32, NARA-WNRC; MSC Newsletters, September 1956 and October 1963; MSC Manpower, 31 December 1961; Speech, Capt George B. Coyle, MSC, sub: The History of Army Optometry, 8 Nov 65, folder 58, box 5/18, MSC-USACMH. Meeting: Rpt, WRAIR, sub: Current Trends in Military Optometry, June 63, folder 57, box 5/18, MSC-USACMH.

[120] Quoted words: Peyton to Col Gene Quinn, MSC, 26 May 59, MSC-USACMH.

[121] MSC success: Col Seth O. Croft, MSC, Ret., Battle Creek, Mich., to Hamrick, 6 Sep 60, MSC-USACMH.

[122] Quoted words: Peyton to Quinn, MSC, 26 May 59, MSC-USACMH.

[123] Generalization: Aabel, Today's MSC.

[124] Quoted words: Col Roy Maxwell, MSC, in MSC Newsletter, July 1961.

[125] Physicians: A point made by Paul Starr in *The Social Transformation of American Medicine*, p. 178.

[126] Administrators: James R. McGibony, "Medical Administration: Quo Vadis?" *Military Surgeon* 112 (May 1953): 325–27.

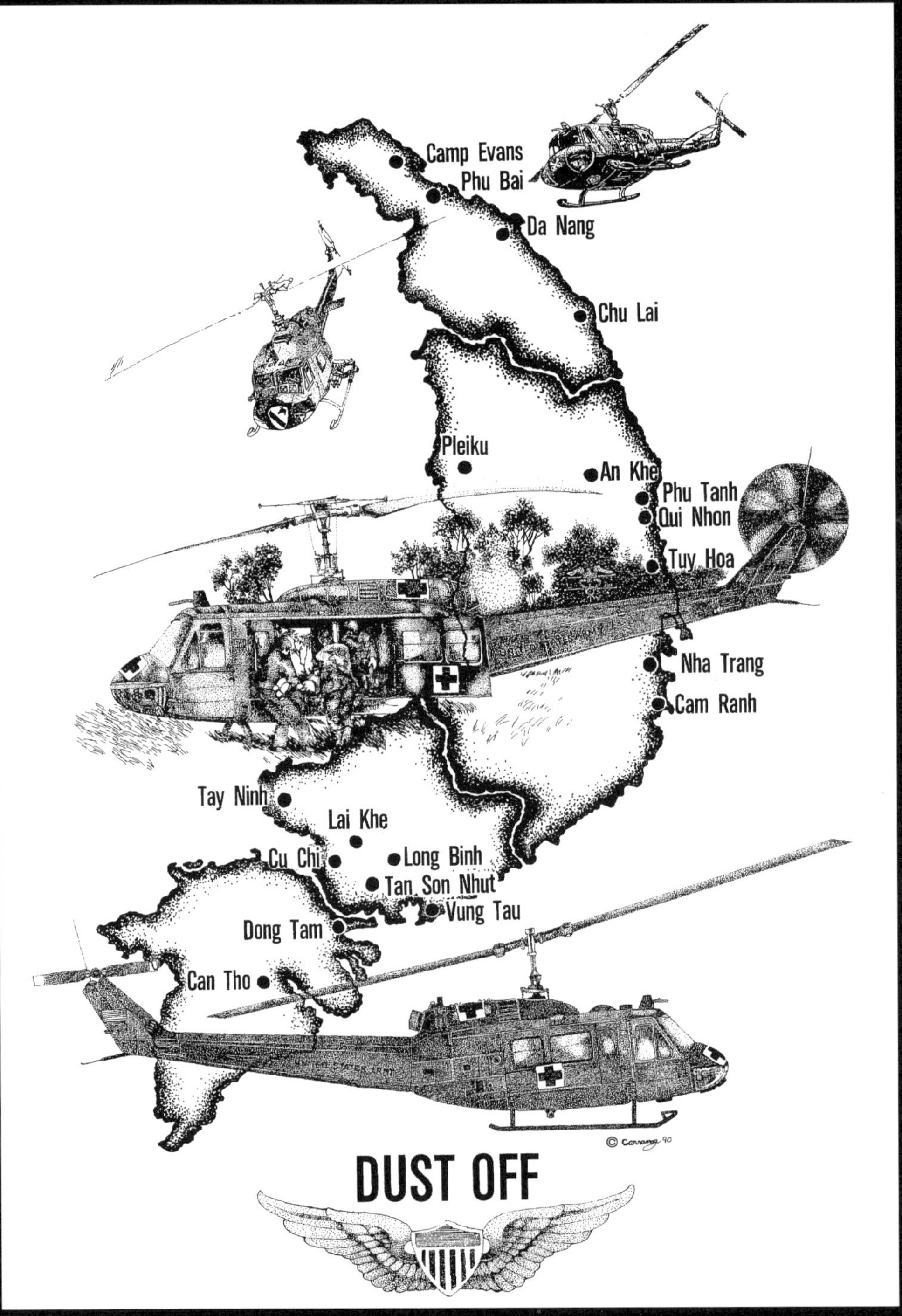

Dust Off *by Luis P. Carranza*

10

Medical Service Corps Officers in Vietnam

Vietnam was a country torn by war long before Americans became involved in the fighting. French domination was interrupted by the Japanese occupation in World War II, during which Communist leader Ho Chi Minh formed his Viet Minh organization and began guerrilla operations against both occupying powers. The Viet Minh came to power when Japan fell, and the French Indochina War began in 1946 as France attempted to regain control over its colony. The war ended in May 1954 when the Viet Minh mauled the French in the Battle of Dien Bien Phu. The Geneva Accords then divided the country into North and South Vietnam.

Ho Chi Minh took power in North Vietnam and one million refugees fled south. The United States became involved in the defense of South Vietnam as guerrilla activity by Communist-led insurgents intensified. The first Americans were killed in 1959. There were 342 advisers in Vietnam in January 1960, but after John F. Kennedy's inauguration as president in 1961 the number rose rapidly to 11,000. Lyndon B. Johnson, made president upon Kennedy's assassination in November 1963, ordered the first air strikes against North Vietnam the following August. Escalation was rapid once the 1964 elections were over. General William C. Westmoreland assumed command of the U.S. Military Assistance Command, Vietnam (MACV), as well as of the U.S. Army, Vietnam (USARV), formed in 1964.

Johnson ordered a major troop buildup in 1965, and on 5 May the 173d Airborne Brigade redeployed from Okinawa as the first Army combat unit in Vietnam. By the end of the year there were 154,000 military personnel in Vietnam, and over sixteen hundred combat deaths had already been recorded. American troop strength reached 536,000 in December 1968. By that time South Vietnamese armed forces totaled 826,500, and allied forces included 50,000 troops from South Korea, over 7,500 from Australia, and smaller groups from the Philippines, Thailand, and New Zealand.

The Communists lost an estimated forty-five thousand killed in a militarily disastrous Tet (lunar new year) offensive in January 1968; the allies lost about fifty-five hundred. However, Tet turned American opinion against the war; peace talks began in Paris, and General Creighton W. Abrams replaced Westmoreland. President Richard M. Nixon was inaugurated in 1969 with pledges to end the war with honor. Although American forces reached their peak of 543,482 in April, reductions began almost immediately thereafter. Nevertheless, domestic U.S.

opposition to the war continued as 500,000 protesters marched in Washington on 4 April 1970. A cease-fire was signed in January 1973, and the final pullout occurred on 7 May 1975. In all, 8,744,000 Americans served in Vietnam, and 47,312 died in combat.[1]

It was a strange, contradictory conflict. The United States fought a high-technology war against adversaries who had only the bare necessities for fighting, moving, and living.[2] American soldiers faced a determined enemy without the support of Congress and with an ambivalent public. The military reflected the tensions of a society undergoing extraordinary turmoil. At home, racial conflict peaked and quickly invaded the Army. One example was racial demonstrations in the form of sit-ins in the commanding general's office at Walter Reed Army Medical Center.[3] The Army was also affected by the burgeoning drug culture in American society. By 1970 a variety of illicit drugs was readily available in Vietnam, including amphetamines, marijuana, and heroin.[4] The tragedies engendered by the war did not end with the fighting.

The Medical Department in Vietnam

Medical Department doctrine listed the same five echelons of the evacuation and treatment chain as in Korea—the unit, division, field army, communications zone, and zone of the interior levels of medical support. (The Army had replaced the regiment with the brigade, and because of this the department had renamed the regimental level of medical support the unit level.) The department's doctrinal evolution after Korea had added a medical brigade commanded by a brigadier general for command and control of corps-level medical groups and battalions, and a medical command headed by a major general for command and control of medical units in the communications zone.[5] The Army activated the 44th Medical Brigade to assume command and control of the nondivisional medical units in Vietnam. The brigade commander and the surgeon, USARV, were separate positions until they were combined in 1967; in 1970 both staffs merged into the United States Army Medical Command, Vietnam. Two subordinate medical groups controlled the activities of eight evacuation hospitals, four surgical hospitals, three field hospitals, and one convalescent center.[6]

Among the changes that affected medical operations in Vietnam was the replacement of the tents and equipment of the sixty-bed Mobile Army Surgical Hospital (MASH) with Medical Unit, Self-contained, Transportable (MUST), equipment. MUST featured inflatable double-walled fabric shelters for wards and turbine engine power packages, called utility packs, which provided electrical power and air-conditioning and maintained the internal pressure of the shelters. The sixty-bed MASH, commonly referred to as a surgical hospital, could augment its capacity with additional MUST sets, and some of the MASH units were converted to 200-bed combat support hospitals as the MUST sets were issued.[7]

Aeromedical capability remained under the theater surgeon's control. The doctrine for air ambulance organizations evolved into two principal units: a 25-helicopter medical air ambulance company allocated on the basis of one per field army, and a helicopter ambulance detachment of six helicopters allocated on the basis of two detachments per division. There were 10 air ambulance helicopters in Vietnam at the end of 1965, 55 by 1966, and 140 by 1969, at which point the air ambulances had moved over 206,000 patients.[8]

The normal chain of evacuation was frequently altered in Vietnam since the helicopter could bypass aid and clearing stations and take casualties directly to the nearest appropriate hospital. The change was necessitated by the absence of a road net and made possible by the presence of helicopters and the absence of an enemy air capability. However, bypassing unit-level facilities was not a universal practice. The 173d Airborne Brigade, for example, evacuated its casualties throughout the war to battalion aid stations or the brigade clearing station before further movement to a supporting hospital.[9]

All of Vietnam was declared a combat zone and Japan, with 3,500 hospital beds, became the communications zone, although some of the hospitals in Vietnam actually performed as station hospitals. There were 110 hospital beds in Vietnam at the beginning of 1965; the rapid buildup resulted in 1,600 beds by December. Capacity peaked in early 1969 with over 5,200 beds. The percentage of casualties who died after reaching a hospital was the same as in Korea, 2.5 percent, but this included the more seriously wounded who were able to be moved because of the capability of the air ambulance system.[10]

While the United States originally sought to quell an internal insurgent movement, the growing commitment of regular combat units from North Vietnam and the size of the American military involvement gave the Vietnam War the predominate characteristics of a conventional war. Most MSCs were assigned to medical units supporting conventional combat operations, but some had a taste of special operations. Although MSCs held command positions, those were generally limited to ground and air ambulance units and hospital enlisted detachments. For the first time, MSC officers commanded battalion-size ambulance units when the Medical Department formed two evacuation battalions to test new air-ground evacuation organizations. In 1970 Lt. Col. Francis A. Copeland, MSC, took command of the first of these, the 55th Evacuation Battalion at Qui Nhon, followed by Lt. Col. Henry P. Capozzi, MSC, who headed the 58th Evacuation Battalion at Long Binh.[11] Nonetheless, the Medical Department policy still required physician commanders for all medical units in the evacuation chain, including medical detachments, clearing companies, hospitals, battalions, groups, the medical brigade, and, later, the medical command. The relatively prolonged buildup, the lengthy period of United States involvement in Vietnam, and a large physician draft enabled the department to hold to this rule, as it had not been able to do in Korea.

Col. Frederick W. Timmerman, MC, deputy commander of the 44th Medical Brigade, later pointed out that most Medical Corps officers in Vietnam had essentially no military training and, as a result of their years of clinical experience, thought of themselves as specialists first. A physician commanding the 58th Medical Battalion agreed, regarding his medical expertise as wasted in his assignment. The old problems of World War II and Korea were thus submerged rather than resolved.[12]

Dissatisfaction extended to the use of physicians as battalion surgeons. Lt. Col. Quinn H. Becker, MC, division surgeon of the 1st Cavalry Division, found his battalion surgeons unanimous in the view that they were not needed at the unit level of medical support. Becker declared that battalion surgeons were never asked anything an advanced medic (military occupational specialty 91C) or an MSC couldn't answer. Capt. William Shucart, MC, battalion surgeon of the 1st Cavalry's 2d Battalion, 7th Infantry, and survivor of the deadly fighting in the Ia Drang Valley in November 1965, said that it was misutilization of a physician and "a total waste of time. They don't need a medical doctor in that job. I figured the major thing I did was morale support, not medical support." Some units pulled physicians from those slots in order to pool them in clearing stations or hospitals. The 25th Infantry Division, for example, reduced the number of physicians assigned to it from thirty-four to nineteen in this way. It removed them from the maneuver battalions, used 91C medics in the battalion aid stations, increased the number of physicians in the brigade clearing stations, and redeployed to Cambodia in the spring of 1970 in that configuration.[13]

MSC Officers in the Theater of Operations

In 1966 there were 642 MSC officers in Vietnam. Corps policy dictated that, as a rule, the first assignment of junior officers should be to field units. Brig. Gen. Manley G. Morrison, the MSC chief from 1969 to 1973, stressed the importance of that experience in an officer's development: "Everything else being equal, my vote is going to the officer who has good, solid field medical unit experience during his early developmental years."[14]

MSCs were key members of Army medical organizations at all levels of medical support. At the unit level, MSC second lieutenants were assigned to the medical platoons of maneuver battalions as the medical operations assistant (formerly the battalion surgeon's assistant) and expected to act as the medical platoon leader, even though the physician battalion surgeon was the platoon commander. These lieutenants completed the Battalion Surgeon's Assistant Course at the Medical Field Service School, Fort Sam Houston, Texas, prior to their assignments to Vietnam. Some also completed Ranger School at Fort Benning, Georgia, or the Jungle Operations Course at Fort Sherman, Panama. Those who went to airborne or Special Forces units completed Airborne School at Fort Benning.

The medical operations assistant for the medical platoon of the 2d Battalion, 7th Cavalry, 1st Cavalry Division, in November 1965 was 2d Lt. John R. Howard, MSC. His battalion was chopped to pieces by North Vietnam's 33d and 66th Regiments in the Ia Drang Valley of the Central Highlands. Howard (who was himself wounded), a wounded sergeant, and four other soldiers were cut off from their battalion on the seventeenth during the savage attack. They found themselves in a no-man's-land between the opposing forces. In actions for which he would receive the Silver Star, Howard led his group to safety with a nighttime escape and evasion, arriving at a 1st Cavalry Division artillery base before daybreak the next day. As they crawled through the elephant grass they could hear the

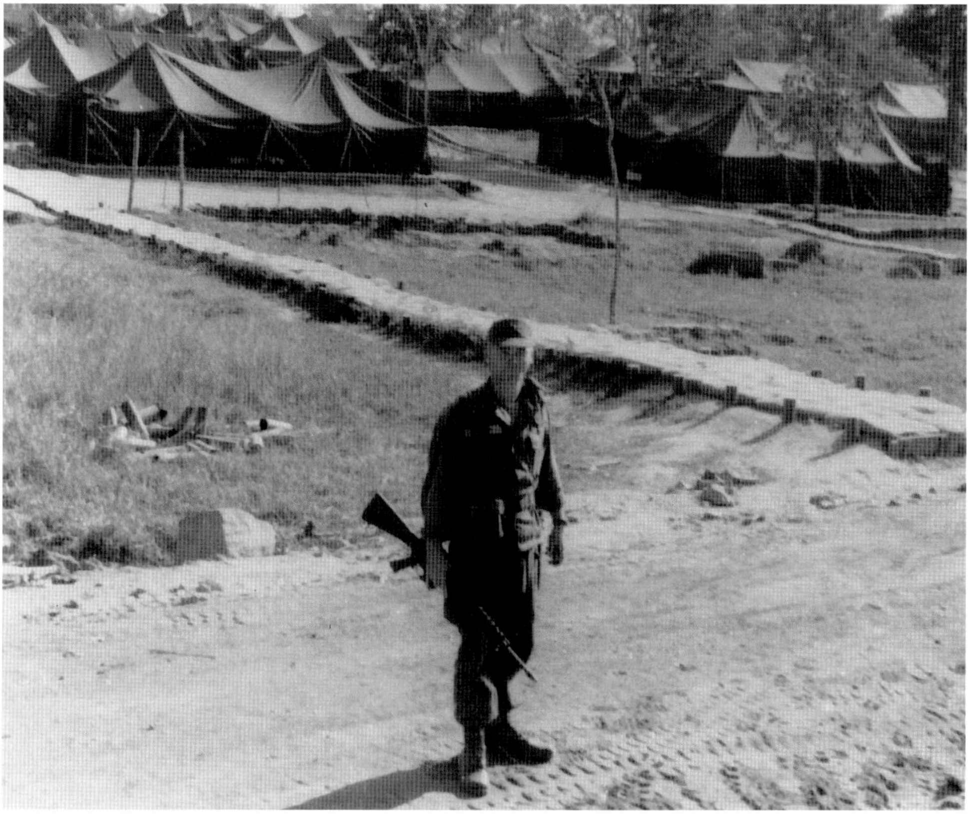

Lieutenant Howard at An Khe, December 1965

voices of the North Vietnamese and realized that the enemy soldiers were signaling to each other by tapping the wooden stocks of their AK–47 rifles.[15]

At the division level of medical support, MSCs filled the administrative positions of the operating medical clearing companies (with the exception of the company commander, which they filled only when the company was in garrison). While MSCs commanded the ambulance units, the highest position open to them in the operational treatment units at that level was the executive officer of the medical company. Capt. George H. Kelling, MSC, was the executive officer of the medical company of the 3d Brigade, 1st Cavalry Division, during the Ia Drang battle in November 1965. Set up in tents, his company was in a race for time to handle the rush of casualties. "We threw caution to the winds and often gave a patient four cutdowns (intravenous tubes tied directly to blood vessels) with four corpsmen squeezing the blood bags as hard as they could. It was not unusual for the patient to shiver and quake and lose body temperature from the rapid transfusion of so much blood—but the alternative was to let him die." Capt. Webb Olliphant, Jr., MSC, was the executive officer of Company D, 25th Medical Battalion, 25th Infantry Division. His clearing station, located at Tay Ninh, received nearly 650 casualties and used four tons of medical supplies in a two-month period beginning

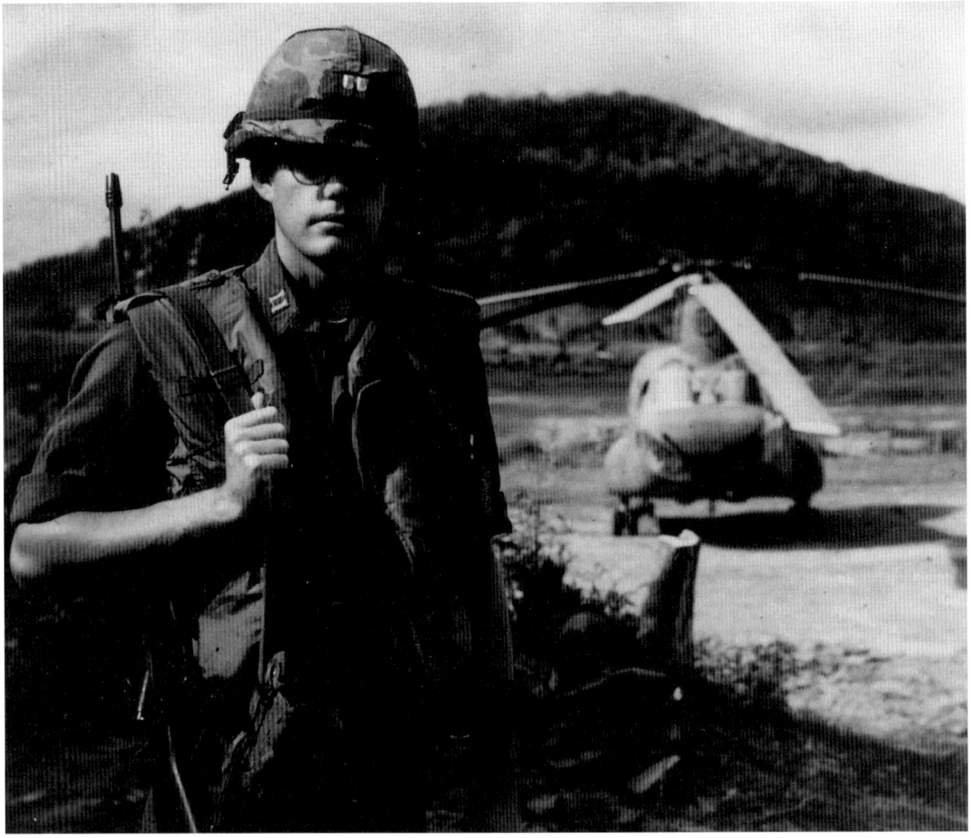

Captain Kelling prepares to leave for the Ia Drang battle from the Camp Holloway airstrip, November 1965.

8 December 1967; at one point the station was hit by mortar and recoilless rifle fire that destroyed twenty of twenty-four cots in one tent. The experience persuaded Olliphant to place his facilities into bunkers, a practice that became common in Vietnam. The medical company of the 173d Airborne Brigade, for example, worked in both underground and aboveground bunkers.[16]

There were new shapes to field medical service as well. Capt. David M. Watt, MSC, served as the executive officer of a medical company supporting the Mobile Riverine Force, a joint Army and Navy command that conducted combat operations in the Mekong River Delta area. The medical platoons of the rifle battalions used converted landing craft (LCM–6) equipped with helicopter landing pads as medical aid boats. Watt's company operated a clearing station aboard a Self Propelled Barracks Ship (APB), itself a converted Landing Ship, Tank (LST).[17]

The combat support and combat service support units of the divisions were organized into division support commands (DISCOM), an element of which was the medical battalion. The highest position open to MSCs in the medical battalions was the executive officer. Maj. John W. Lowe, MSC, was the executive officer of the 15th Medical Battalion, and he represented the DISCOM at the 1st Cavalry Division operations briefing in April 1970 for the invasion of Cambodia. Lowe oversaw the staff planning and the execution of the operational plan for the movement of elements of the medical battalion in the first deployments of the division on the first of May.[18]

Some MSCs served in the surgical and evacuation hospitals of the field army level of medical support. At times they faced mass casualty situations. An example was the 71st Evacuation Hospital at Pleiku during the battle of Dak To in 1967, a fierce engagement fought in the Central Highlands near the Cambodian border. Wounded soldiers began arriving on the third day of November, and for three weeks Maj. Gordon K. Dowery, MSC, the executive officer, led the hospital's administrative staff in an exhausting effort as they treated over seven hundred wounded and nearly a thousand sick and injured soldiers. Casualties were so heavy that the six operating rooms were overwhelmed, and the hospital required over forty tons of medical supplies. The hospital commander reported that Major Dowery expertly handled extraordinary demands caused by the sustained peak load.[19]

The new MUST sets were a technological improvement over the sets they replaced. A distinct advantage was the provision of a clean environment whose temperature and humidity could be controlled to the advantage of both patients and staff in a way not possible with the tents of the old hospital sets. Equipment had also been improved. However, the more complex assemblages posed difficult challenges for the MSC officers charged with their initial fielding and subsequent operations and maintenance.

The logistical demands could be a nightmare.[20] Lt. Col. John O. Williams, MSC, had his hands full as the project officer for fielding the sets in Vietnam, beginning with the 45th Surgical Hospital, which became operational in November 1966 (and whose commander, Maj. Gary P. Wratten, MC, was killed by a mortar round shortly thereafter). The fuel requirements were extraordinary. Williams found that the MUST-equipped hospitals required 2,400 gallons of aviation fuel (JP4) a day, and some needed more, depending on their size and operational requirements. Fragments from mortar attacks collapsed the inflatable shelters, and they required concrete pads or they would float in the mud during heavy rains.[21]

Maj. John P. Jones, MSC, executive officer of the 2d Surgical Hospital, supervised that unit's conversion to MUST in 1969, dealing with the problems of fuel supply, made more difficult because the hospital was not authorized a fuel truck. He had to depend on his local support unit to keep the fuel bladder filled daily. "After running out once or twice they began refueling every day." The utility packs were another source of trouble because their maintenance was a constant aggravation. Further, the connecting sections of the MUST assemblage had to be perfectly aligned even though the hospital had no forklifts or heavy-duty wreckers in its equipment. While the hospital was supposed to be able to move within seventy-two hours, Major Jones believed that seven to nine days was more likely. Such problems prompted Brig. Gen. David E. Thomas, MC, the theater Army surgeon, to suggest it would be best to "forget the MUST and start all over again" once the war was over.[22]

Some officers served as advisers to medical units of the Republic of Vietnam Armed Forces. Maj. Robert F. Elliott, MSC, was one of two officers in 1971 who provided administrative assistance and training support for South Vietnam's Military Medical School in Saigon. This school, originally founded in Hanoi, had moved to Saigon when Vietnam was partitioned.[23]

Other MSCs supported unconventional warfare operations. Green Beret MSCs of the 5th Special Forces Group were considered essential for the administration, training, and logistics aspects of the unconventional warfare medical mission. Capt. George D. Baker, MSC, went to Vietnam in October 1964 when the 5th Special Forces Group deployed from Fort Bragg, North Carolina. Initially assigned as the group's medical supply officer, he soon discovered that someone had overordered kaolinpectate; his detachment had 10,000 one-gallon bottles of the stuff. Baker spent months figuring out ways to use it. One was to mix it with petroleum jelly as a treatment for rashes. Another was to mix antibiotic into each bottle and issue it to the Special Forces detachments as a treatment for diarrhea. "We would sit around shaking those bottles of kaolinpectate. We had enough kaolinpectate to stop up every a-- in Vietnam."[24]

Commanding a Special Forces A Team was not an assignment that MSC officers had been prepared to undertake, but in July 1965 Baker assumed command of Detachment A–212, located at Plei Mrong in the Central Highlands about twenty miles northwest of Pleiku. He later remembered flying to the Green Beret camp thinking that as a medic, "I really did not have a background for this sort of thing." But Baker received the Combat Infantryman's Badge, although he continued to wear his MSC insignia. Another Special Forces MSC, Capt. Joseph Krawczyk, MSC, the intelligence officer for a B Team, changed to infantry brass, but the accoutrement was not entirely helpful when he was interviewed by the chief of the Medical Service Corps. Maj. Sigurd Bue, MSC, ended up with so much Special Forces experience that he requested a transfer to the Infantry (the request was denied). While indicative of their enthusiastic spirit, the use of MSC officers in nonmedical roles during the early years left medical jobs vacant in the 5th Special Forces, and the practice ended.[25]

The small hospitals operated by the Special Forces teams provided the only medical support for Montagnard tribesmen, the nomadic hill people of Vietnam, who supported the U.S. war effort. Organized into militia-like Civilian Irregular Defense Group (CIDG) units, the Montagnards had little affinity with the ethnic Vietnamese on either side. At their peak, the Special Forces hospitals handled over seventy-five thousand outpatient visits a month. Capt. James N. Williams, MSC, worked with perhaps the most unusual situation, the CIDG hospital at Kontum. There, Pat Smith, M.D., a civilian physician from Seattle, Washington, ran a 200-bed facility until the 1968 Tet offensive made it impossible for her to continue. Smith was frustrated by her inability to get medical supplies, so the Special Forces stepped in and assisted.[26]

Capt. John F. Reed, Jr., MSC, was assigned in 1969 to Detachment B–23 at Ban Me Thuot, a Special Forces B Team that operated a CIDG hospital and provided rural health nurse training. Reed was very proud of their medical support for the Vietnamese. Reed's replacement, 1st Lt. Arthur F. Steinberg, MSC, was particularly appreciative of the way the specially trained Special Forces medics developed close rapport with the local population, who were also an invaluable source of intelligence.[27]

Scientific Specialties

The expertise and skill of MSC scientific specialty officers provided commanders at all levels in Vietnam significant assets for the maintenance of a healthy fighting force. The prolonged period of U.S. involvement in this Asian country provided opportunities for MSC scientists to conduct research that had direct application to the soldiers in the field. As in previous wars, unforeseen challenges emerged that required the immediate harnessing of medical scientific expertise to solve pressing medical problems that were degrading combat operations. MSCs in clinical roles encountered the demands of operating in a challenging setting. Preventive medicine remained a very important Medical Department function during the war, prompting the fielding of a new MSC specialty.

In 1964 Lt. Col. Dan C. Cavanaugh, MSC, went to Vietnam as part of a Walter Reed Army Institute of Research (WRAIR) team that worked in Saigon jointly with the Pasteur Institute to establish the only plague research laboratory in Southeast Asia. Their research supported plague control efforts of the U.S. military and the Vietnamese Ministry of Health.[28]

By 1971 four social work officers were serving with divisions or separate brigades and another three were assigned to medical command units. Their service continued after the U.S. withdrawal when some served on Operation HOMECOMING teams set up to handle the U.S. prisoners of war repatriated from Vietnam in 1973.[29]

The contributions of entomologists were also important in Vietnam, where tropical diseases, such as malaria, were endemic. There they designed vector control operations that included aerial dispersal of insecticides. An unusual Field Epidemiological Survey Team formed by the 5th Special Forces provided an aggressive survey capability under combat conditions. Capt. Wayne F. Hockmeyer, MSC, the team's entomologist, reported that it took advantage of combat-seasoned soldiers as team members since these soldiers could take care of themselves under austere conditions.[30]

A new preventive medicine specialty deployed to a theater of operations when the first seven sanitarians (later called environmental science officers) reported to Vietnam in November 1968. Receiving good marks for their contributions in that theater of operations, they were judged more effective at the division level for day-to-day preventive medicine activities than the Medical Corps preventive medicine officers they replaced. The USARV surgeon, Brig. Gen. Hal B. Jennings, praised the innovation, and Col. Ralph J. Walsh, Jr., MSC, the USARV sanitary engineer, described them as "eminently successful."[31]

A drafted optometrist, 1st Lt. Donald D. Schmidt, MSC, was assigned in September 1967 to the 93d Evacuation Hospital, Long Binh, which supported the 1st Infantry Division. Soldiers easily lose or break glasses, but Schmidt found that it took about thirty days to fill eyeglass prescriptions during this period before

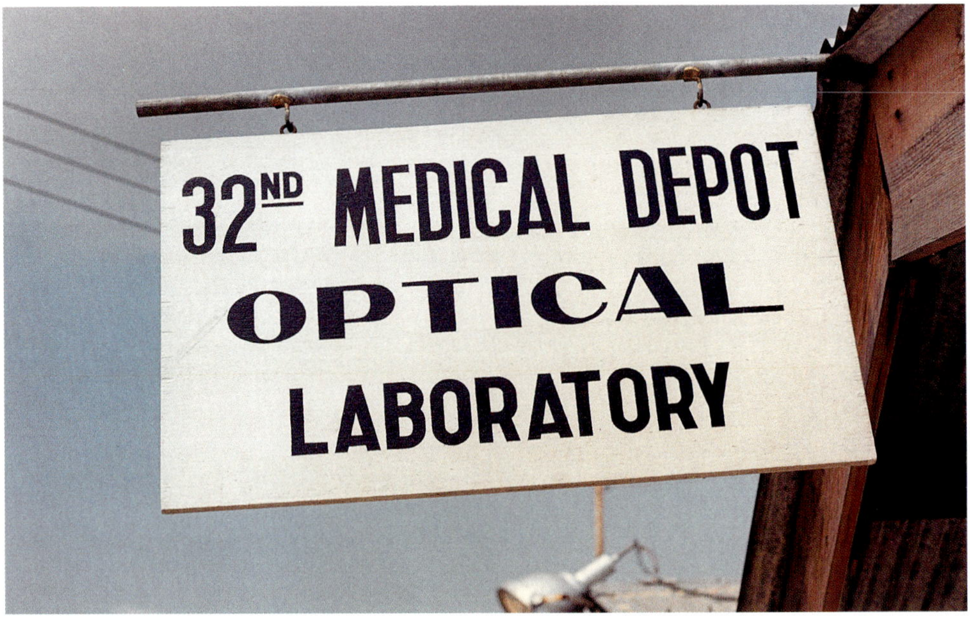

32d Medical Depot Optical Laboratory

the Army established a fabrication capability within Vietnam. Since division policy was that soldiers with uncorrected acuity greater that 20/200 could not be placed on alert status, Schmidt would travel by helicopter to the various units in the division several days a week to perform eye examinations and to deliver new glasses directly to the battalions.[32]

Schmidt was irritated by additional duty requirements, especially administrative officer of the day, a task assigned as a rotating duty. Other additional duties included those typically required of Army officers, such as special services officer and pay officer. Later assigned to the 36th Evacuation Hospital at Vung Tau, he found his administrative responsibilities took on a different meaning during the Tet offensive in 1968. The military situation curtailed routine optometric services. Schmidt and other MSC officers led patrols of their perimeters, accounted for the personal effects of casualties, assisted as litter bearers, acted as Dustoff dispatchers, and handled the disposition of remains. His experience supported General Hamrick's position that optometry officers, just as all MSC officers, must be qualified both in their specialty and "in the application and techniques of the combat arms."[33]

In 1967 the Army authorized placing optometrists directly in the combat divisions, a step that greatly pleased General Thomas, the theater Army surgeon. Bringing them forward was "one of the smart moves in this conflict."[34] The first optometrist was assigned to a division in September 1968, and in twelve months the number of optometrists in Vietnam went from seven to twenty-eight.

The optometrists who filled the divisional positions benefited from their experience. Capt. Jeffrey Halopin, MSC, assigned to the 25th Division, noted that his close working relationship with field units and their commanders afforded "more personal satisfaction than in any other area of military optometry."[35] Capt. O. Howard Smalling, MSC, of the Americal Division, noticed very few eyeglasses among the villagers in his area, and those he did observe, such as a man wearing a woman's glasses, were of marginal utility. Smalling set up an "OPCAP"—an Optometric Civic Action Program—to meet this need, using spectacle frames donated by the Kiwanis Club of Augusta, Georgia.[36]

Maj. Albert Reinke, MSC, the USARV optometry consultant, estimated that only about 18 percent of the soldiers reporting to Vietnam in 1969 arrived with the required number of spectacles. Meeting that demand, as well as filling routine prescriptions, produced a considerable requirement for optical fabrication within the theater of operations. The Optical Section of the 32d Medical Depot fabricated about 75 percent of the eyeglasses made in Vietnam, while division optometry sections made the other 25 percent. In 1969 the combined output of the depot and the division sections was 270,000 pairs, of which the depot accounted for 165,000. Some of the production was for special aviator glasses, an item that became quite fashionable. Lt. Col. Arthur R. Giroux, MSC, assigned as the USARV optometry consultant in 1970, found that requests for those prized items greatly exceeded the valid requirements and that special controls were required to prevent abuse.[37]

Some scientific specialty officers became engaged in a second front during the war, the battle with drug abuse. This problem began to assume visible proportions in 1968, and by the summer of 1971 it was quite apparent that the Army was facing a drug abuse epidemic among its soldiers in Vietnam. In June President Nixon ordered the Services to conduct heroin testing, a program that was later expanded to include amphetamines and barbiturates. A team led by Col. Charles R. Angel, MSC, chief of the Division of Biochemistry of the Walter Reed Army Institute of Research, and his deputy, Lt. Col. Douglas J. Beach, MSC, developed the first large-scale urinalysis screening laboratories for heroin detection. It was the initial stage of Operation GOLDENFLOW, the United States government's war on drug abuse.

Colonel Angel arrived in Vietnam on 19 June to set up laboratories at Long Binh and Cam Ranh Bay. His prototype equipment used free radical assay techniques and thin layer and gas liquid chromatography to screen for opiates, amphetamines, and barbiturates. The 90th Replacement Battalion in Long Binh was tasked with collecting samples, and the GIs quickly tagged the building used for this purpose "The Pee House of the August Moon." The samples were sent to Angel's laboratories, which processed 60,000 specimens by 21 August 1971, of which about 5 percent were positive; soldiers who tested positive were hospitalized at the 9th Convalescent Center at Cam Ranh Bay. Just as Colonel Hunter's schistosomiasis work in Japan had created a market for parasite-free stool specimens, a market developed in Vietnam for clean urine. The going price was $25 per ounce.[38]

The testing program expanded to four military laboratories in Vietnam, as well as commercial laboratories in the United States and Germany. Unfortunately, by October there were problems with erroneous results from the U.S. contract laboratories, and this quickly became a sensitive political issue. Colonel Angel's division set up a quality control section to test the work of the civilian laboratories on an interim basis until a central agency could be established for that purpose. His

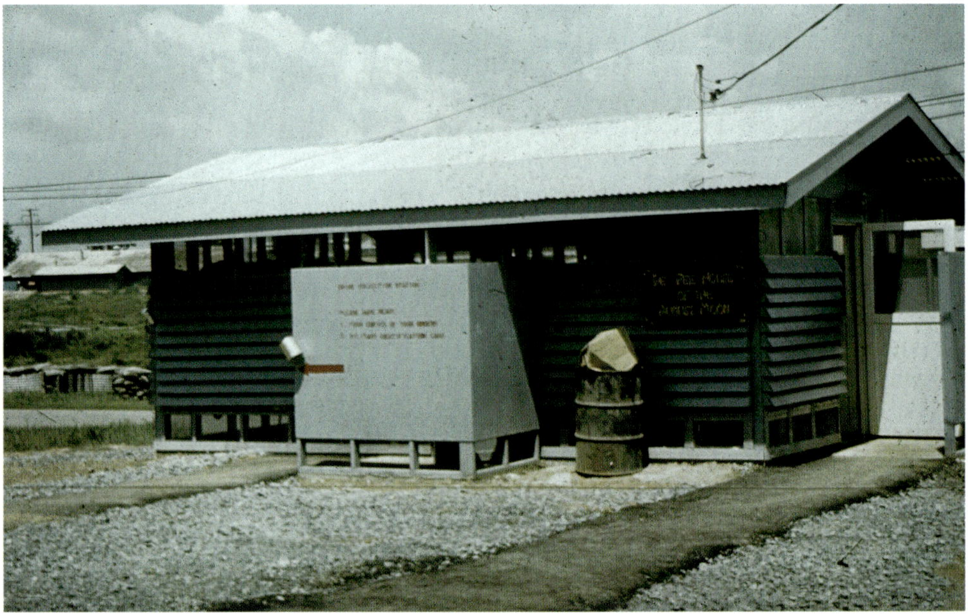

"The Pee House of the August Moon" at Long Binh, 1972

work enabled Brig. Gen. Richard R. Taylor, MC, commander of the U.S. Army Medical Research and Development Command, to report successful corrective action in congressional testimony in February 1972.[39]

Soldiers with positive results who were hospitalized at the 6th Convalescent Center had to demonstrate negative urinalysis test results before they were allowed to leave Vietnam, just as venereal disease patients had to be declared free of disease to leave Europe after World War I. Prior to Operation GOLDENFLOW the center had cared for soldiers with medical and surgical convalescent care conditions (principally malaria and hepatitis) who could be returned to duty within the thirty-day evacuation policy. When Capt. Barry R. Mintzer, MSC, the executive officer, was notified that the center would become a detoxification center for heroin users, he was given seventy-two hours to prepare for the new mission. His preparation included putting a fence around his compound "to keep the heroin out, not keep the patients in."

Mintzer's unit expanded from 300 to 500 beds, was augmented by a military police platoon, and began receiving patients on 19 June. There were no guidelines for running a detoxification center, and the staff received "one hell of an education." Patients were a constant source of disciplinary problems. Many did not want to be helped, and some would break into the mess halls at night for food because they became very hungry from drug withdrawal. The fence did not work because there were not enough military police to keep patients from going under the wire. To make matters worse, the sensationalism of the unique program assured a constant stream of VIP visitors. Mintzer said his commander nearly "reached his wits' end."[40]

Medical Logistics

A wall poster popular with the medical logisticians during the Vietnam War listed twenty requirements for the ideal medical supply officer, including "the smile of a baby" and "the patience of a burro." Someone else designed a fanciful badge. Its colors included silver for "the silver-tongued oratory of those who call supply easy."[41]

Officers in the medical logistics specialty, now called health services materiel, had every right to some humor, given the challenges they faced in support of military operations in Vietnam. The first challenge during the early days of the war came when the Army ignored the wartime lesson that the medical logistics system must reside under medical control. The Army's amnesia was manifested in 1965 when it established the Army Pacific Materiel Management Agency as the central funnel for all supply requisitions, including medical, from Korea, Hawaii, Okinawa, and Vietnam, and set up a computer-supported inventory control point in Hawaii. The arrangement failed. The inventory control point quickly became a bottleneck, and the Medical Department's ability to perform its expanding mission in Vietnam was held hostage by an external agency.[42]

Surgeon General Lt. Gen. Leonard B. Heaton became livid as the situation deteriorated:

> It seems incredible that a mismanaged organization can continue to flourish and do more harm than good. When they meddle with medical supplies, they are playing with life and death and nothing could be more serious. Medical supplies should and must remain in medical channels and not logistical channels.[43]

The Medical Department was essentially the only user of medical items, a situation unlike other categories of supply that had multiple users. It made no sense to divorce the user from the commodity, but that was the situation MSC medical logisticians faced.[44]

Further, the general supply system was unable to cope with the Medical Department's dependence on nonstandard items (materiel not yet incorporated into the federal supply catalog due to the rapidity of technological change). To illustrate, the 32d Medical Depot in Vietnam stocked 1,200 nonstandard items (excluding repair parts) that were very important for medical units. The inability to fill orders for those items from the medical units anguished MSC supply officers who were compelled to rely on the failing general supply system. As Lt. Col. Richard S. Rand, MSC, the 32d's commander explained, the significance of medical supply was not the tonnage involved but its high percentage of critical items. For example, Colonel Rand was enormously frustrated by his inability to provide the Fogarty catheter, a critical nonstandard item used in acute care, to surgeons who were losing patients because it was unavailable.[45]

By the fall of 1965 the Pacific Materiel Management Agency's demand satisfaction rate for medical requisitions (the percentage of requests for stocked items that it filled at 100 percent) was only 79 percent. This was against a medical standard of 95 percent. The deterioration of the medical supply situation came to the attention of Vice Chief of Staff General Creighton Abrams, who directed

General Heaton to "leave no stone unturned" until the problem was corrected.[46] General Heaton immediately asked the Army Staff to return the medical supply system in the Pacific to medical control. A series of fact-finding trips and much bureaucratic jousting ensued as the situation continued to deteriorate. Demand satisfaction dropped to 50 percent in April 1966 and plummeted to a dismal 12 percent in May, horrifying the medical logisticians in Vietnam. Heaton's patience was exhausted by the inaction of the Department of the Army and Pacific headquarters. He told the Chief of Staff, General Harold K. Johnson, that the situation remained unsatisfactory and asked for immediate action.[47]

He got it. The chief of staff transferred medical materiel responsibility for Vietnam to the 70th Medical Depot, stationed in Okinawa. The 70th was instructed to order supplies directly through the U.S. Army Medical Materiel Agency in Phoenixville, Pennsylvania (it later moved to Fort Detrick, Maryland), to the Defense Personnel Support Center in Philadelphia. The subsequent recovery of medical supply was remarkable with the reinstatement of medical control as MSC medical logisticians again assumed responsibility for its operation. Demand satisfaction jumped to 81 percent in June, hit 91 percent in July, and by September had leveled off at 95 percent. At this point the surgeon general's staff concluded the system was working perfectly.[48]

It came none too soon. Ground forces in Vietnam desperately needed a fully responsive medical supply system as the tempo of combat accelerated. Medical logisticians supporting combat operations at the operating unit level had their hands full. For example, over a three-week period during the Battle of Dak To, the 71st Evacuation Hospital used more than forty tons of medical supplies, including 3,300 bottles of Ringers lactate, 1,500 bottles of dextrose solution, 975 units of blood, and more than 600 patient litters. Transporting the supplies to the hospitals was also a challenge. The enemy's interdiction of the main supply roads during the Tet offensive of 1968 put the 32d Medical Depot "in a real jam" and forced the use of fixed-wing aircraft and helicopters to resupply supported units.[49]

The same recovery took place in Korea in 1967 with transfer of medical supply operations to the 6th Medical Depot. In three months demand satisfaction went from 50 to 90 percent. An identical transfer took place in Europe. When it was all over, the result of the resumption of medical supply operations by MSCs at all levels was called a "magnificent accomplishment."[50]

Some MSCs routinely handled medical logistics requirements that went beyond strictly combat support. Maj. Malachi B. Jones, MSC, was assigned to the Military Equipment Delivery Team in Cambodia, another country caught up in the turmoil of the Vietnam War. From 1973 to 1974 Jones directed operations that included distributing over 40,000 tons of rice monthly. In addition, his duties required him to furnish medical intelligence reports to the Army.[51]

Dustoff

Our kind of flying ain't no fun
Dustoff choppers ain't got no guns.
But now and then a medic will say
A machine gun would just get in the way.[52]

Aeromedical evacuation became a routine part of the Medical Department's evacuation system in Vietnam. It was universally referred to as "Dustoff," a radio call sign adopted in 1963. MSC commissioned officer and warrant officer pilots and the enlisted members of the Dustoff crews were heirs to the Letterman legacy. A measure of their devotion is gleaned from the statistics. The Medical Department lost 199 helicopters in Vietnam, and a third of the 1,400 Dustoff pilots were killed or wounded. The memorial book of the Dustoff Association recorded 90 commissioned and warrant officers killed in Vietnam, and another 380 pilots were wounded or injured as a result of hostile fire or crashes. Casualties among crew chiefs and flight medics included 121 killed and 545 wounded or injured.[53]

The air ambulances used a crew of four: aircraft commander (pilot), copilot, medic, and crew chief (who handled the helicopter's preventive maintenance). They flew UH–1 "Hueys" from the early "A" model to the "H" model in use at the end of the war, with a capacity for six litter patients. The pilots and copilots were graduates of a special course for Dustoff pilots, although some warrant officers lacked any specialized training. Close teamwork was a keynote from the beginning.[54]

Aeromedical evacuation became routine in Vietnam. Over sixty-four thousand patients were moved by medical helicopters in 1966, and by 1967 there were sixty-one helicopters providing Dustoff support. Yet, as Col. Joseph P. Madrano, MSC, who had been with the 498th Medical Company (Air Ambulance) in Vietnam, later emphasized, the important story was not in the glamour of air evacuation but in its establishment as a routine part of a larger evacuation and treatment system. Certainly the Dustoff crews approached their duties in a straightforward way. As one pilot put it, "I'm not the hero type, just pulled a mission when called, got the poor guy out, took no chances but never turned one down either."[55]

The early aeromedical system went through growing pains and its doctrine was refined under combat conditions. Capt. John J. Temperilli, MSC, commander of the 57th Medical Detachment (Helicopter Ambulance) stationed at Fort Meade, Maryland, was alerted for movement to Vietnam in February 1962. His detachment arrived in April with five "A" model Hueys. They were handicapped by difficulties in obtaining logistical support, particularly for fuel problems and spare parts (including main rotors).[56] Even the size of the red cross on the helicopter was debated—for some pilots it was a case of the bigger the better. In some cases nonmedical helicopters on a battle scene would extract casualties rather than call for Dustoff, but this entailed the usual "scoop and run" risks for the patients. "Some of these guys died because they didn't have somebody to stop the bleeding. They were just thrown on." However, reliance on the Dustoff system was to the advantage of commanders and their soldiers. Its provision of a medically trained crew and a sufficiently large helicopter enabled the treatment of casualties in flight. The experience of Capt. Terry Woolever, MSC, whose crew routinely performed life-saving care, was typical. On at least one occasion his medic successfully performed cardiac resuscitation by injecting adrenalin with a thoracic needle directly into a soldier's heart while they were airborne.[57]

The greatest problem in the early years was resolution of the ownership of the helicopters. The doctrine of medical control over all elements of the evacuation system was challenged in Vietnam by those who coveted the new Hueys of the medics, and the 57th had to fend off officers with designs on the aircraft. One of the pilots, Capt. Robert D. McWilliams, MSC, was routinely pestered by a colonel who wanted the detachment to fly him to different sites. McWilliams finally told the colonel he would have first priority on a ride by becoming a casualty; until then he had none.[58]

The controversy heated up in 1963 when Col. John Klingenhagen, Transportation Corps, the commander of the U.S. Army Support Command, Vietnam, found out that Temperilli's helicopters were not flying as often as some of Klingenhagen's administrative ships. He proposed painting over the red crosses and using the aircraft as general purpose helicopters that would be on call for air evacuation missions; a removable red cross could be reaffixed to the helicopter when it was on a medical mission. Adopting the same logic, the 57th countered with a suggestion that since there was a shortage of fuel trucks in Vietnam, the Army should use fire trucks as general purpose trucks and fill them with aviation fuel. In case of a fire, the fire truck could be emptied out and filled with water. Told that this was unacceptable because the trucks could never respond in time, the medics responded that the same was true for air ambulances.

Klingenhagen's philosophy, as later recalled by Maj. Gen. Spurgeon Neel, was that "aeromedical evacuation is an aviation operation which entails the movement of patients," not Neel's version of "a medical operation which entails the use of aircraft."[59] Brig. Gen. Joseph W. Stilwell, commander of the Army Support Group, Vietnam, became convinced that Klingenhagen was right, and he attempted to remove the 57th from the theater surgeon's control. Temperilli found himself on the defensive. Meeting personally with General Stilwell, he was able to at least temporarily squash the transfer proposal, but efforts to gain control over aeromedical assets did not cease. When Stilwell left Vietnam in June 1964, Maj. Charles L. Kelly, MSC, then the commander of the 57th, presented Stilwell with a farewell memento that symbolized the struggle. The medics had mounted five red crosses and the tail numbers of the five aircraft on a wooden plaque. "Here General," said Kelly, "you wanted my God-damned red crosses, take them."[60]

It took Kelly's death on the first of July to settle the matter of aeromedical control. Kelly, a World War II veteran, flamboyant, profane, and irrepressible, was the first MSC killed in Vietnam. As he touched down to evacuate an American sergeant his ship came under a hail of small arms fire. The American adviser on the ground shouted over the radio: "Get out, Dustoff, get out." Kelly replied: "When I have your wounded," and then was fatally wounded himself. Stilwell reportedly cried when he heard the news.[61]

Kelly became a legend, revered for his aggressive leadership and fearlessness in evacuating casualties. Ironically, his loss ensured that the Army's aeromedical operations would use his mold, one characterized by unarmed single ships operated without escort aircraft by aviators who, like Kelly, were experienced in night flying. In fact, the flying skills of Dustoff crews were such that some general aviation pilots believed there was a special school to teach their flying techniques. Kelly was posthumously awarded the Distinguished Service Cross, and in 1967 General Heaton dedicated the Kelly Heliport at Fort Sam Houston, Texas.[62]

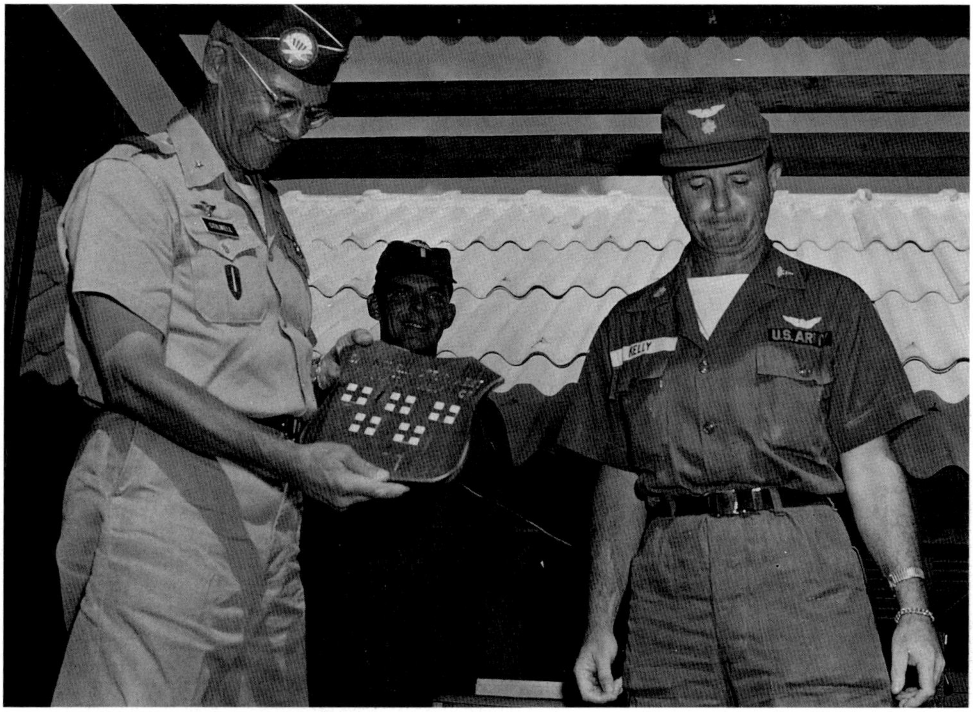

*Major Kelly (*right*) presents a memento to General Stilwell, June 1964.*

After Kelly's death the staff of the 44th Medical Brigade continued to wage a battle over the issue of medical control of the evacuation system, even though overt efforts to seize the aircraft were minimized. Among other things, there was a need for medical control to prevent patients from becoming hitchhikers.[63] The medical aviation capability was also important for its routine ability to rapidly and precisely move life-saving medical supplies, especially whole blood. If that entailed redundancy, then that was a small price to pay for operating a support mission that could leave nothing to chance.[64]

Warrant officer Dustoff pilots were a vital part of the aeromedical system, and three received Distinguished Service Crosses for their valor: WO2 Robert L. Horst, CW2 Warren G. Jackson, and WO1 Stephen R. Purchase. MSCs respected their aviator teammates. Lt. Col. William E. Knowles, MSC, who served as commander of the 498th Medical Company and later as operations officer for the 44th Medical Brigade, found them invaluable. Lt. Col. Eugene Lail, an MSC aviator, praised them for their performance, as did another MSC aviator, Maj. Douglas E. Moore, himself a holder of the Distinguished Service Cross, who called them "super heroes."[65]

Officers such as CW4 Michael J. Novosel were representative of the warrant officer Dustoff pilots. Novosel had originally enlisted in 1941, completed flight school, and as an Army Air Corps captain commanding a squadron in the Marianas had flown in the covering force for General MacArthur's plane as it

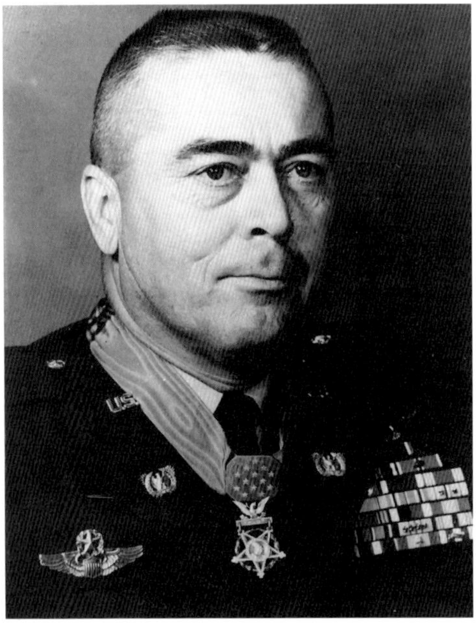

Chief Warrant Officer Novosel

landed in Japan. He was recalled to active duty as an Air Force major in Korea and again returned to civilian life when that war ended. At the time of the early buildup in Vietnam he was flying for Southern Airways and held an Air Force Reserve commission as a lieutenant colonel. Prevented by age from returning to active duty in the Air Force, Novosel came into the Army in 1964 as a warrant officer Dustoff pilot.[66]

By 1969 the 48-year-old aviator was on his second tour in Vietnam. On the afternoon of 2 October CW4 Novosel and his crew responded to a Dustoff request from ARVN units pinned down in an enemy training camp west of Saigon near the Cambodian border. Novosel was forced out of the area by enemy action a half dozen times, and each time came back on another approach. After several such pickups and eleven hours of flying, Novosel—himself wounded at point-blank range by an enemy soldier—managed to evacuate twenty-nine wounded soldiers. President Nixon presented the Medal of Honor to Novosel in 1971 while his son, Michael Novosel, Jr., also a Dustoff warrant officer, looked on. The younger Novosel had joined his father in the same unit at the end of 1969, and from January to April 1970 they flew together.[67]

Flying hours mounted for Dustoff crews. CW2 Michael A. Yourous of the 498th Medical Company described support of the 173d Airborne Brigade as six to eight hours of flying each day, missions that ranged from "hot" pickups to routine "backhauls" when the helicopters returned to the brigade's landing zone in Bong Son after delivering their patients to the 67th Evacuation Hospital in Qui Nhon. There were initially no graves registration units assigned to combat units, and Dustoff crews had the task of flying the remains of American soldiers to the Air Force mortuary at Tan Son Nhut Air Force Base. The crew members stuffed Vicks Vaporub in their nostrils to overcome the stench.[68]

Because the thick vegetation of the 200-foot triple canopy jungles in Vietnam hampered helicopter evacuations, the Army developed a hoist mechanism for lifting casualties out by a cable while the helicopter remained at a hover. The hoist employed an electric winch, and different rigs, including a modified Stokes litter, were attached to a 250-foot cable with varying degrees of success. The preferred device for the less seriously wounded was a folding seat called "the jungle penetrator," a three-foot-tall, bullet-shaped device. Once the penetrator was at ground level the seat pods were opened and the wounded were strapped into the device with chest belts.[69]

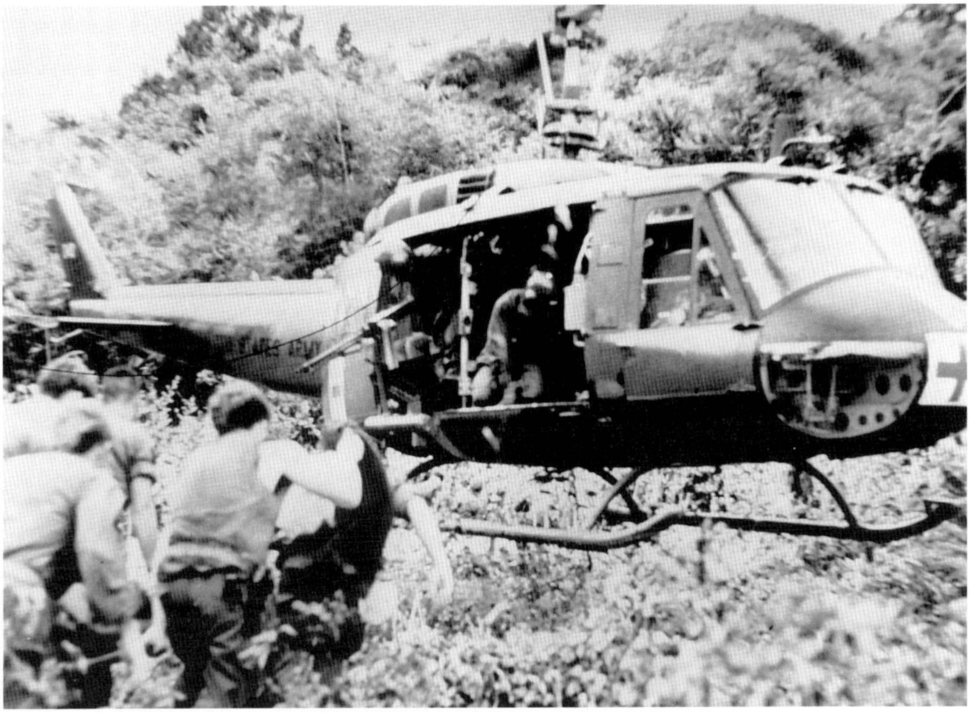

Lieutenant Tuell and Capt. Howard Elliott pilot a helicopter in Dustoff operation, May 1970.

Hoist missions required Dustoff crews to hover the aircraft at treetop level, where they were highly vulnerable to ground fire. In November 1966 Capt. James E. Lombard, MSC, and 1st Lt. Melvin J. Ruiz, MSC, while evacuating casualties near Saigon, became the first crew shot down on a hoist mission. As Lombard hovered and began lowering the cable, they came under fire, and he broke off the hover. With hydraulics gone and the transmission growling, they headed to a clear zone a few minutes away. After traveling 150 meters the engine quit, forcing Lombard to autorotate the burning ship to the ground. Fortunately, the crew was met by friendly forces and got out of the area safely. But two days later Lombard was again shot up on another hoist mission.[70]

Dustoff hoist missions became commonplace, but never dull. One officer, 1st Lt. Henry O. Tuell III, MSC, began a log of his missions, but after ten months he had passed 300 and quit counting. On one mission in Cambodia his copilot, CW2 Greg Simpson, was sick and vomited as they were positioning the helicopter. Nevertheless, they lifted one patient up and were going for a second when a rocket-propelled grenade hit a tree about five feet away and spun the helicopter around. Machine-gun fire hit the fuel tank and ripped through the center console between the pilots, wiping out everything, including their radios and navigational aids. As Tuell said, "we were finally out of aircraft and out of ideas." Tuell and his crew and patients were rescued by another Dustoff ship.[71]

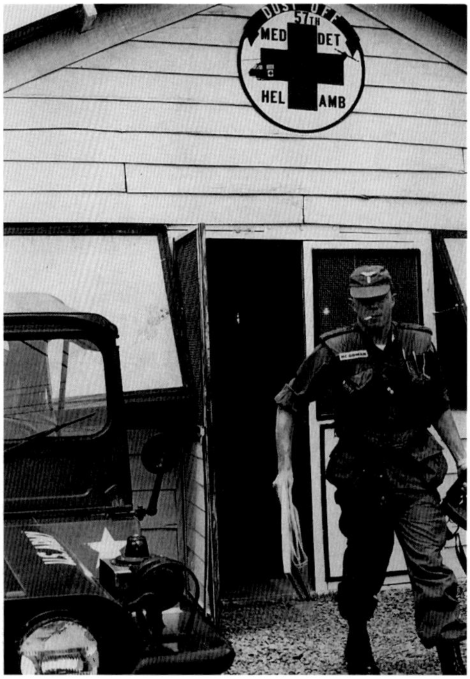

Lieutenant McGowan at Tan Son Nhut Air Base, Saigon

Dustoff crews were often not sure whom they were evacuating in the early days when communications were poor and allegiances of those on the ground not clear. Most night evacuations for South Vietnamese units occurred at locations where there were no American units. Capt. Douglas E. Moore, MSC, found "there probably isn't a more harrowing experience than landing in a rice paddy in the wee hours of the morning and have eight to ten heavily armed men in black pajamas approach the ship." In December 1964 Moore, 1st Lt. James McGowan, MSC, and their crew attempted a pickup of South Vietnamese casualties, but the American adviser on the ground repeatedly radioed the Dustoff ship to back off because of incoming mortar rounds. Finally Moore and McGowan heard, "Dustoff, come back. We have many wounded." This was followed shortly by, "Dustoff, you come back and we will kill you," and laughter.[72]

On the lighter side, Col. Thomas C. Scofield, MSC, remembered the trials of one of his fellow pilots during a night mortar attack on their base camp. Awakened by the commotion, the aviator took off running and hit a center pole in their building. This disoriented him and he ran out the wrong door. A short time later Scofield's crew chief came and told him he had better see something and led Scofield outside. The crew chief shined his flashlight on the pilot, who was gasping for breath, lying in his underwear flat on his back in the deep end of a partially completed swimming pool the Dustoff crew had been digging.[73]

The crews also competed for the record number carried at one time in a Huey, a contest reminiscent of college students stuffing themselves into phone booths. Capt. Thomas L. Christie, MSC, and his crew put nineteen adults and children in a B model Huey at Phuoc Vinh, but, not to be outdone, Col. Lloyd E. Spencer, MSC, claimed the B model record with twenty-two. "If the doors had come off, people would have popped out like popcorn."[74] Pickups from hot landing zones were stressful, and sometimes the medics became overexuberant. Capt. Kenneth M. Radebaugh, MSC, recalled one medic who literally threw patients into the open door of the helicopter. "The first time he was so vigorous that the patient continued through the aircraft and out the other door."[75]

President Nixon presented the Medal of Honor in October 1969 to Maj. Patrick H. Brady, MSC, the first Medical Service Corps officer to receive the nation's highest honor and the only Medical Department officer to win the award in Vietnam. (Years later, Brady would transfer as a colonel to the Aviation Branch, and he was promoted to major general in 1989.) Brady was honored for his heroism on 6 January 1968 during his second tour in Vietnam when he evacuated fifty-one casualties in a series of missions in the mountainous region near Chu Lai. His penchant for the technical aspects of flying figured prominently in his incredible actions during a day in which he had to use three different helicopters.[76]

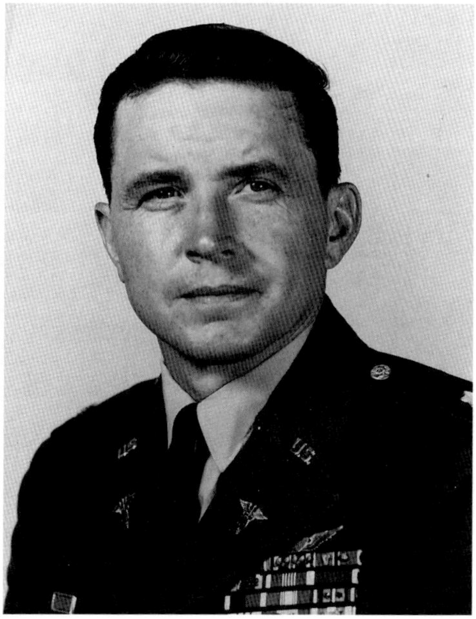

Major Brady

On the first mission that day Brady and his crew evacuated two wounded South Vietnamese soldiers while under fire in a heavily fogged-in valley. This was after an attempt by another Dustoff crew had failed. Brady tipped the helicopter over at an angle so that the rotor would blow the fog away in front of the ship enough so his crew could make out the trail. Meanwhile he flew sideways so he could see more clearly out the open side window. On the second mission Brady responded to a call from a company of the 23d (Americal) Division that was trapped in a minefield in the Hiep Duc Valley where the soldiers were pinned down by six North Vietnamese companies supported from the surrounding hills by mortars, rockets, and antiaircraft weapons. Again, a previous Dustoff attempt had failed. Brady required four flights to extract the casualties, which were within fifty meters of enemy soldiers at a site where two helicopters had already been shot down.[77] The brigade commander had tried to dissuade Brady from returning after he had delivered the first load of casualties to the fire support base overlooking the valley. Soldiers there had witnessed the entire panorama. They cheered as Brady landed, while the division surgeon who met the ship, Lt. Col. William S. Augerson, MC, saluted.[78]

On Brady's third mission he picked up casualties from an American unit surrounded southeast of Chu Lai. He approached the pickup by flying backwards to protect the cockpit from enemy fire, but the helicopter was badly damaged by gunfire. The controls were partially shot away and he had to get another aircraft. For the fourth mission he volunteered to pick up casualties in another minefield. A mine exploded during the pickup, wounding two of his crew and damaging yet another helicopter, but six casualties were successfully evacuated. He changed helicopters again and completed two more urgent missions before the day was over.

In 1972 Capt. Kenneth Ledford, Jr., MSC, received the Navy Cross for actions on 15 September 1970. While flying a Dustoff mission accompanied by

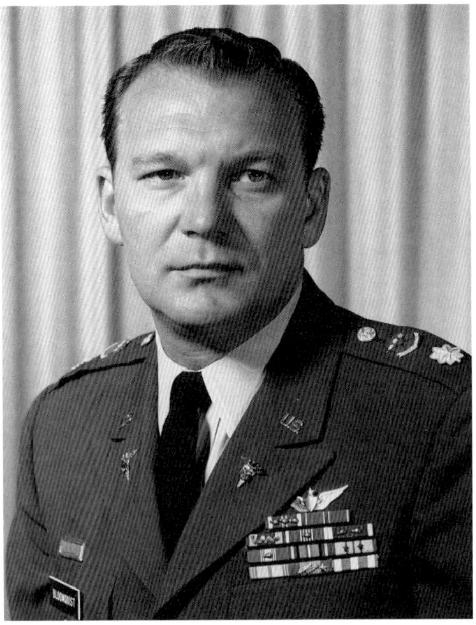

Colonel Bloomquist
(Photo taken in 1966.)

four armed Navy helicopters, two of Ledford's escorts were downed by enemy fire, a third was disabled, and the fourth damaged. Ledford was still able to evacuate six casualties.[79]

In May of the same year a series of three explosions rocked the main entrance to the U.S. Army's V Corps headquarters and the officers open mess in Frankfurt, Germany. A bomb placed in a flowerpot at the entrance to the club was detonated by terrorists of the Baader-Meinhoff gang, wounding thirteen people. Lt. Col. Paul A. Bloomquist, MSC, who was walking into the club at the time, was killed. The attack took the life of an energetic, forceful, and personable officer who was the veteran of two tours as a Dustoff pilot in Vietnam. In 1980 the headquarters of the 68th Medical Group at Ziegenberg, West Germany, was named in his honor as Camp Paul Bloomquist.[80]

Bloomquist, an Infantry OCS graduate, had been honored as the Army Aviator of the Year in 1965 and the following year was the only Army officer selected by the U.S. Chamber of Commerce as an outstanding young American. His nickname, "Big Ugly Bear," used in a *Time* magazine article, was actually the result of some of Bloomquist's mischievous Dustoff comrades who were having fun with a reporter. His fellow pilots had made up stories for the benefit of an impressionable correspondent, insisting that Bloomquist loved war and would lie awake at night thinking of ways to improve his flying. A friend, Capt. Edward J. Taylor, MSC, coined the name on the spot for the benefit of the reporter.[81]

The Dustoff crews possessed the same indomitable spirit as their predecessors in earlier wars. For their part, the crews were unstinting in their respect and compassion for the soldiers they pledged their lives to support. In the early days Capt. Roger Hula II, MSC, had responded to a Dustoff call for a first sergeant. The gravely wounded noncommissioned officer had given one of his squad leaders a present of a day off by taking the man's place in combat. "With tears in his eyes, my medic carried the first sergeant to the helicopter, cradling him in his arms." The memory never faded for Hula. "After twenty long years, my heart still goes out to the family of that man who gave his life on Christmas day of 1965."[82]

Summary

MSC scientific specialty officers demonstrated their importance during the Vietnam War as a quickly deployable medical asset. Col. Dan Cavanaugh's plague team that went to Vietnam in 1964 and Col. Bob Angel's team that set up the drug testing laboratories in 1971 illustrated their significance as a national resource for employment by the United States government in crisis situations.[83] The listing of various scientific specialties as critical shortages during the war and the drafting of optometrists were testimony to the value of those MSCs.

Through the eloquence of their actions the courageous Dustoff crews had also made the point that they were integral to the Medical Department—no different from their predecessor ambulance crews in the Civil War, World War I, World War II, and Korea—and attempts to dislodge them from medical control were doomed to failure. Maj. Pat Brady believed that Maj. Charles Kelly had inculcated a uniquely *medical* orientation to Dustoff that made it fundamentally different from general aviation. "It was more to us than a kind of operation, it was an attitude, an emotion, a way of life that sprang from the heart of one man and seeded in the hearts of others."[84]

Kelly's death had sealed a tradition of intense pride by Dustoff crews in their humanitarian mission. Aeromedical evacuation was firmly established in the day-to-day support of combat operations in Vietnam. Air ambulance ships were forward-deployed into operational areas with no discussion about their use for other missions. The business about hanging removable red crosses on general purpose helicopters—as was actually done in some cases—had ended, at least for the duration of the war in Vietnam.

Yet the end of the war quickly brought new challenges. The Vietnam War's impact on American society continued long after the United States withdrew its forces. American soldiers had returned home from Korea to benign neglect. Their sons and daughters returned home from Vietnam to overt hostility. The MSC officers who remained in the Army's active and reserve components undertook the challenge of rebuilding the Army, refining the Medical Department's doctrine, and improving medical readiness to respond to future national and international emergencies. They had a large task in front of them.

Notes

[1] Casualties: U.S. strength dropped to 335,794 by the end of 1970 and fell to 24,000 at the end of 1972. About 4,368,000 Army personnel served in Vietnam; 30,899 were killed (U.S. deaths are from 1 January 1961). Pamphlet, U.S. Department of Defense, *Defense 86* (Arlington, Va.: Armed Forces Information Service, September/October 1986), p. 46; Brig Gen James L. Collins, Chief of Military History, DA, to Walter B. Edgar, 11 Sep 78, sub: Inclusive Dates of Vietnam Conflict, DASG-MS. *Defense 86* uses 4 August 1964 to 27 January 1973 as the dates for the Vietnam War.

[2] Amenities: In some places the living accommodations included "hot and cold running water, television and movie entertainment, and many other amenities." Vincent Davis, "Americans and War: Crisis and Action," *SAIS Review* 4 (Summer–Fall 1984): 34. Ammunition shipments averaged about a million tons a year from 1969 to 1971, while post exchange (PX) supplies averaged 800,000 tons. Lt. Gen. Walter J. Woolwine, "A Logistics Perspective," *Army Logistician* (March–April 1975): 2–7, 43–44. Col. Harry Summers, Infantry, observed that "the sybaritic lifestyle of the headquarters always differed from the Spartan existence in the field." Harry G. Summers, Jr., *On Strategy: The Vietnam War in Context* (Carlisle Barracks, Pa.: U.S. Army War College, 1981), p. 98.

[3] Racial discord: Underground newsletter, *U-BAD, United Blacks Against Discrimination*, 1 (1972), WRAMC, DASG-MS.

[4] Problems: James Webb, "Viet Vets Didn't Kill Babies and They Aren't Suicidal," *Washington Post*, 6 April 1986.

[5] Doctrine: Leonard B. Heaton, "Medical Support in Vietnam," *Army* 16 (October 1966): 125–28; Medical Field Service School, *Introduction to the Army Medical Department*, Study Guide no. 1, BAMC, May 1971, SL; Academy of Health Sciences, U.S. Army (AHS), Fort Sam Houston, *Medical Support of a Corps*, Study Guide no. 478, July 1974, SL; Interv, Lt Col Ralph W. Parkinson, MSC, XO, 44th Surg Hosp, Republic of Vietnam (RVN), with Maj Daniel G. McPherson, MSC, 27th Military History Detachment, Vietnam, 6 Jun 67, USACMH; Draft MS, Jeffrey Greenhut, sub: I Have Your Wounded: The Medical Department in Vietnam, USACMH, 1986, hereafter cited as Greenhut, Vietnam MS; Dorland and Nanney, *Dust Off*, pp. 115–23; Andre J. Ognibene, "Full Scale Operations," in Ognibene and Barrett, *General Medicine and Infectious Diseases*, pp. 39–71.

[6] Consolidation: Ltr, Heaton (drafted by Lt Col James J. DeFrates, MSC, Ops Div, OTSG), to Col E.S. Chapman, MC, Surg, USAREUR, 12 Jan 66, RG 112, accession 69A–2604, Box 17/38, NARA-WNRC. Brig. Gen. David E. Thomas, appointed brigade commander in May 1969, said he was proud of "getting rid of the 44th Medical Brigade and organizing the U.S. Army Medical Command, Vietnam." Interv, Brig Gen David E. Thomas, CG, BAMC, with Lt Col Charles Simpson, MSC, THU, OTSG, undated (1971), USACMH.

[7] MUST: Spurgeon Neel, *Medical Support of the U.S. Army in Vietnam, 1965–1970* (Washington, D.C.: Department of the Army, 1973), pp. 65–68; Engelman, *A Decade of Progress*, pp. 178–79. The sets were developed upon the recommendation of a DOD committee in 1961 in a project initially headed by Lt. Col. Forest L. Neal, MSC. A MUST demonstration at Fort Sam Houston on 24 February 1965 greatly pleased Heaton, who said "the publicity on TV was great." One viewer was Senator Richard Russell, chairman of the Senate Armed Services Committee and a patient on Ward 8 at BAMC. Russell told Heaton he wanted the equipment in Vietnam "without further delay." SG Conference, 2 Mar 65.

[8] Aviation: Also see AHS, *Aeromedical Evacuation*, Study Guide no. 453, March 1974, SL; Heaton, "Medical Support in Vietnam," p. 126; David M. Lam, "From Balloon to Black Hawk: Vietnam," p. 47. A third unit was the medical evacuation platoon of the airmobile division. With twelve aircraft, it was essentially two detachments.

[9] Evacuation: Bypassing medical units was achieved under "a special set of conditions and may not be subject to extrapolation for world-wide doctrinal requirements." lst Ind, Maj Gen Glenn T. Collins, Acting TSG, to Asst Chief of Staff for Force Development (ACSFOR), 28 Oct 68, RG 112, accession 71A–3154, Box 9/48, NARA-WNRC. For example, in the battle of Dak To nearly all casualties came through the clearing stations of the 4th Infantry Division, 1st Cavalry Division, and 173d Airborne Brigade, where they were stabilized for movement to the 71st Evacuation Hospital.

[10] Statistics: Leonard B. Heaton, "Medical Support of the Soldier: A Team Effort in Saving Lives," *Army* 19 (October 1969): 85–86; Heaton, "Medical Support in Vietnam," pp. 125–26; Rpt, Brig Gen Hal B. Jennings, Jr., CG, 44th Med Bde, sub: Senior Officer Debriefing Report, 1 February 1969–3 June 1969, USACMH; Neel, *Medical Support of the U.S. Army in Vietnam*, pp. 75–76; Dorland and Nanney, *Dust-Off*, pp. 115–17; Weir, McPherson interv, 17 Jun 67. Weir reported the hospital mortality rate as 2.7 percent for November 1965 to December 1966.

[11] Command: Interv, Lt Gen Leonard B. Heaton, USA, Ret., with Col Robert B. McLean, MC, Pinehurst, N.C., Dec 78, U.S. Army War College and USAMHI Senior Officer Oral History Program, USAMHI; Interv, Col Robert D. Pillsbury, MC, Dep Cdr, 44th Med Bde, with Maj Donald A. Lacey, MSC, Cdr, 27th Mil Hist Det, Vietnam, 30 Apr and 1 May 69, USACMH; Lt Col Henry P. Capozzi, USA, Ret., to Capt Peter G. Dorland, MSC, THU, OTSG, 18 Aug 75, USACMH.

[12] Vietnam experience: Interv, Col Frederick W. Timmerman, MC, Deputy Cdr, 44th Med Bde, and Dir Med Svcs, 1st Log Cmd, with Maj Norbert O. Picha, MSC, Cdr, 27th Mil Hist Det, Vietnam, 3 May 68, and interv, Lt Col Anthony J. Trucskowski, MC, Cdr, 58th Med Bn, with Maj William R. Tuten, MSC, Cdr, 27th Mil Hist Det, Vietnam, 20 Dec 69, both USACMH.

[13] Battalion surgeons: See Wier, McPherson interv, Vietnam, 17 Jun 65; Neel, *Medical Support of the U.S. Army in Vietnam*, p. 177; OTSG Lessons Learned Interv, Lt Col Foster H. Taft, MC, 7–8 Mar 86; OTSG Lessons Learned Interv, Lt Col James W. Ransome, MC, former division surgeon, 1st Cav Div (Airmobile), 30 Nov 67; Thomas, Simpson interv, 1971; OTSG Lessons Learned Interv, Lt Col Quinn H. Becker, MC, Cdr, 15th Med Bn, 2 Mar 71, all in USACMH. Quoted words: Harold G. Moore and Joseph L. Galloway, *We Were Soldiers Once . . . And Young* (New York: Harper Perennial, 1993), p. 258. 25th Inf Div: Thomas, Simpson interv, 1971.

[14] Quoted words: Manley G. Morrison, "Medical Service Corps," *Medical Bulletin* (October 1970): 19.

[15] Lieutenant Howard: Moore and Galloway, *We Were Soldiers Once*, pp. xviii, 286–87, 315–18, 416. Lt. Col. (later, Lt. Gen.) Harold Moore commanded the 1st Battalion, 7th Cavalry, which was surrounded by 2,000 North Vietnamese soldiers three days before his sister unit, the 2d Battalion, 7th Cavalry, was ambushed. The 1st Cavalry Division had 234 killed in action in a four-day period, more than were killed in the entire Persian Gulf War in 1993.

[16] Quoted words: Moore and Galloway, *We Were Soldiers Once*, p. 160. Silver Star: U.S. Total Army Personnel Command, Permanent Orders 228–24, 15 Aug 96. Olliphant: Interv, Capt Webb Olliphant, Jr., MSC, with Lacey, Vietnam, 18 Oct 68; Rpt, Company D (Med), 25th Med Bn, sub: After Action Report, Operation Yellowstone, 11 Mar 68, both in USACMH. Surgical hospitals were also sandbagged for protection from mortar rounds and in some cases had earthen roofs. Brig Gen Andre J. Ognibene, MC, Ret., to Ginn, 28 Jul 88, DASG-MS.

[17] Riverine force: Daniel M. Watt, "Medical Support of the Mobile Riverine Force, Vietnam," *Military Medicine* 135 (November 1970): 987–90. The command was composed of the 2d Brigade, 9th Infantry Division, and the U.S. Navy River Assault Flotilla One, Task Force 117.

[18] Cambodia: Interv, Lt Col John W. Lowe, MSC, with Capt Peter G. Dorland, MSC, OTSG, 11 Jan 77, USACMH.

[19] Field support: After Action Rpt, 1st Lt R.M. Cook, MSC, Historical Officer, 71st Evac Hosp, 1967, Appendix III, sub: Dak To, 1 Dec 67, USACMH, hereafter cited as Cook, Dak To After Action Rpt; Dorland and Nanney, *Dust Off*, pp. 59–61, 122. Work demands: Cook, Dak To After Action Rpt.

[20] Logistics: One commander called it "a hair-raising operation." Interv, Col W.R. LeBourdais, MC, with Lacey, Vietnam, 1969, USACMH.

[21] MUST problems: OTSG Lessons Learned interv, Lt Col John O. Williams, MSC, MUST Project Officer for Vietnam, 17 Sep 67; OTSG Lessons Learned interv, Lt Col Foster H. Taft, MC, Surgeon, 9th Inf Div, 7–8 Mar 68; Interv, Lt Col Robert G. Stanek, MC, Cdr, 22d Surg Hosp, with 22d Mil Hist Det, undated (1968); Interv, Maj John P. Jones, MSC, XO, 2d Surg Hosp, with 27th Mil Hist Det, 1969; Thomas, USARV Senior Officer Debrief, 21 Nov 70; Neel, USARV Senior Officer Debrief, 1 Feb 69; OTSG Lessons Learned interv, Ransome, 30 Nov 67, all in USACMH; Greenhut, Vietnam MS, 3: 20–29; Neel, *Medical Support of the U.S Army in Vietnam*, pp. 65–68. Also see Rpt, Brig Gen Robert E. Blount, Spec Asst R&D, OTSG, sub: Inprocess Review, Medical Unit, Self-Contained, Transportable (MUST), 4 Jan 64, RG 112, accession 72C–3503, Box 14/38,

NARA-WNRC; Brig Gen William A. Hamrick, MSC, Ret., to Ginn, 22 Aug 88, DASG-MS. Fuel: Some units reported rates higher than 2,400 gallons per day. Jones said the 2d Surgical Hospital used 3,800 gallons per day; Williams said the 45th Surgical Hospital required a 15,000-gallon fuel truck every other day before it deployed to Vietnam. Stanek reported 2,500 gallons per day for the 22d Surgical Hospital. "We would not become operational until we were assured that we would receive that much fuel on a daily basis. That I would say necessitated delaying becoming operational for a week."

[22] 2d Surgical Hospital: Jones, 1969 interv, including quoted words; Neel, *Medical Support of the U.S. Army in Vietnam*, p. 67. Quoted words: Thomas, USARV Senior Officer Debrief.

[23] Advisers: Rpt, Maj Robert F. Elliott, MSC, Senior Adviser, RVNAF Mil Med School, sub: The Military Medical School, in MFR, sub: Goals and Objectives for RVNAF Military Medical School, 29 Sep 71, DASG-MS.

[24] Quoted words: Interv, Maj George D. Baker with Maj Louis Darogi, MSC, THU, 6 Apr 76, USACMH.

[25] Special Forces: Darogi intervs, sub: Special Forces Oral History, THU, with Lt Col Stanley C. Allison, MC, Surg, 5th Special Forces Group (SFG) (June 1968–69), 20 Dec 76; Maj George D. Baker, MSC, 6 Apr 76; Col Sigurd Bue, MSC, Ret., 22 Mar 77; Maj John F. Erskine, MSC, 11 Jan 77; Maj Robert F. Fechner, MSC, 6 Jan 76; Maj Joseph Krawczyk, MSC, undated; Maj John F. Reed, Jr., MSC, 6 Apr 76; Capt Arthur F. Steinberg, MSC, 19 Dec 76; Maj Demetrious G. Tsoulos, MC, Surg, 5th SFG (July 1966–May 1968), undated; Capt James N. Williams, MSC, 1976, all in USACMH. MSCs as commanders: Darogi intervs with Baker (including quoted words), Erskine, and Fechner.

[26] Montagnard support: Darogi intervs with Reed, Steinberg, and Williams. The nomadic hill people consisted of several ethnic groups totaling over three million people. A 1979 census put the figure at 3.4 million. See Draft article, Judith Banister, sub: Vietnam: Population Dynamics and Prospects, June 1991, Center for International Research, U.S. Bureau of the Census, DASG-MS. Pat Smith: Williams, Darogi interv.

[27] Rapport: Steinberg, Darogi interv.

[28] WRAIR team: Rpt, Col John N. Albertson, Jr., MSC, sub: History of the Medical Service Corps Contributions to Medical Research and Development, 24 Sep 84, DASG-MS, hereafter cited as Albertson, MSCs in Medical Research and Development.

[29] Social work: Rpt, Col Richard H. Ross, MC, Cdr, USMEDCOMV, and Maj William L. Posey, MSC, Command Historian, sub: Army Medical Services Activity Report, CY 71, USACMH, hereafter cited as Ross, AMSAR CY 71.

[30] Entomology: Interv, Capt Wayne T. Hackmeyer, MSC, with Darogi, THU, 28 Apr 76, USACMH.

[31] Sanitarians (ESOs): Senior Officer Debrief, Brig Gen Hal B. Jennings, MC, USARV 25 Jun 69, USACMH; OTSG Lessons Learned interv, Lt Col Joseph J. Smith, MC, Cdr, 20th Prev Med Unit, 23 Oct 68, USACMH. Quoted words: DF, Col Ralph J. Walsh, MSC, HQ, USARV, sub: End of Tour Report, 20 Nov 69, USACMH.

[32] Schmidt: Donald D. Schmidt, O.D., to Ginn, 20 Feb 86, DASG-MS.

[33] Quoted words: Hamrick quoted in "Military Optometry," *Journal of the American Optometric Association* 37 (April 1966): 337.

[34] Quoted words: Thomas, USARV Senior Officer Debrief.

[35] Quoted words: In Rpt, Lt Col Arthur R. Giroux, MSC, Optometry Consultant, USARV, sub: Optometric Activities, CY 1970, Jan 71, hereafter cited as Giroux, 1971 Rpt.

[36] OPCAP: "Optometrists Go Mobile," *Army Reporter* [U.S Army, Vietnam] 5 (24 March 1969), DASG-MS; "Optometrist in Field to Provide Eye Care," *Southern Cross* [Americal Division] 2 (11 May 1969), DASG-MS.

[37] Optical workload: SG Conference, 3 Nov 67; Col Robert W. Green, MC, Acting XO, OTSG, to ACSFOR, sub: USACDC Study, Area Optometric Support of Non-Divisional Units, 7 Nov 68, RG 112, accession 71A–3154, Box 9/48, NARA-WNRC; Giroux, 1971 Rpt; Rpt, Maj Albert R. Reinke, MSC, Optometry Consultant, USARV, sub: End of Tour Report, 12 Aug 69; Unpublished paper, Lt Col Robert J. Bryant, MSC, sub: Optimum Employment of the Division Optometry Section in Combat, March 1972, all in DASG-MS.

[38] Drug problem: Presentation, Col Ronald Blanck, MC, Cdr, 97th General Hospital, Frankfurt, Germany, to the Office of the Inspector General, 7th MEDCOM, Heidelberg, 4 May 90, author's notes, DASG-MS. Urinalysis testing: Ross, AMSAR CY 71, USACMH; Thomas, USARV Senior Officer Debrief; DF, Brig Gen Kenneth R. Dirks, MC, Cdr, USAMRDC, sub: Brief Chronological Report, History of the USAMRDC, 17 Aug 73; Rpt, Col Charles R. Angel, MSC, sub: Drug Detection and the Screening of Military Populations for Illicit Drug Use in Vietnam, undated (1976); Lt Col Douglas J. Beach, MSC, DD Forms 1498, Research and Technology Work Unit Summaries, 1970–74, all in DASG-MS; Greenhut, Vietnam MS, 10: 1–33; William E. Campbell and Charles R. Connell III, "The Pee House of the August Moon," *Army* (June 1987): 68.

[39] Taylor: Testimony, Brig. Gen. Richard R. Taylor, MC, Cdr, USAMRDC, Before the Senate Armed Services Committee (SASC), Drug Abuse Subcommittee, 29 February 1972, DASG-MS.

[40] 6th Convalescent Center: Interv, Capt Barry R. Mintzer, MSC, XO, 6th Conv Ctr, 15 Aug 71, Vietnam, typed 3 Jun 74, USACMH; Neel, *Medical Support of the U.S. Army in Vietnam*, p. 68; Campbell and Connell, "The Pee House of the August Moon," pp. 67–68.

[41] "Burro": 8" x 10" poster (photograph), "What Is an MSO," 1972, DASG-MS. "Silver-Tongued": "MSO Badge" drawing and inscription, undated, DASG-MS.

[42] Logistics: SG Conferences: 9 Nov 65; 15 Apr, 17 May, 8 Jul, 22 Jul, 29 Jul, 30 Sep, and 14 Oct 66; 27 Jan, 17 Feb, 17 Mar, and 4 Aug 67; Thomas, Simpson interv; OTSG Lessons Learned interv, Lt Col Richard S. Rand, MSC, 13 Jun 68, USACMH; Col Campbell, XO, OTSG to ACSFOR, sub: Operational Report, Lessons Learned, 3 Jan 67, RG 112, accession 70A–2772, Box 12/43, NARA-WNRC; Summary sheet, Heaton for CSA, sub: Medical Materiel Logistics Structure for Support of Vietnam, Thailand, and Ryukyu Islands, 15 Apr 66; Msg, DA DCSLOG/DS-SPPD to CINCUSARPAC, 102210Z, Feb 67, sub: Army Logistic System in the Pacific Command in Support of Forces in South Vietnam, all in DASG-MS; Engelman, *A Decade of Progress*, pp. 151–54; Greenhut, Vietnam MS, 5: 32–35, 49; Thomas E. Kistler, "A Case for the Separate Medical Logistics System," *Medical Bulletin* (December 1985): 5–10; Richard V.N. Ginn, "Medical Logistics: A Lesson From Vietnam," *Army Logistician* (November/December 1993): 36–38.

[43] Quoted words: SG Conference, 15 Apr 66.

[44] Supply channel: Notes of discussion, Wilbur J. Balderson, Supply Div, OTSG, with Ginn, 5 Sep 84, DASG-MS.

[45] Losing lives: Rand, OTSG interv.

[46] Critical items: Rand, OTSG interv. Quoted words: SG Conference, 9 Nov 65.

[47] Unsatisfactory supply: Heaton, summary sheet, 15 Apr 66.

[48] Improvements: SG Conference, 30 Sep 66. Heaton said, "At long last we will control our medical supplies." SG Conference, 17 May 66.

[49] Logistics experience: CMT 2 with incls, TSG to ACSFOR, 16 Mar 67; Rpt, Lt Col Theodore R. Sadler, Jr., MC, Cdr, 68th Med Grp, sub: Operational Report, Lessons Learned, for Quarterly Period Ending 31 October 1966, 15 Nov 66, RG 112, accession 70A–2772, Box 12/43, NARA-WNRC; Rand, OTSG interv; Greenhut, Vietnam MS, 3: 15–16. Dak To: Cook, Dak To After Action Rpt, USACMH. Quoted words: Rand, OTSG interv, USACMH.

[50] Quoted words: SG Conference, 17 Feb 76. General Abrams was pleased with what he saw on a visit to Korea. SG Conference, 27 Jan 67.

[51] Foreign aid: Rpt, ASD (I&L), sub: Logistic Support in Vietnam, App. D to monograph no. 4, sub: Common Medical Supply System, 1970, pp. D3–D4, LD no. 25408H, Defense Logistics Studies and Information Exchange (DELSIE), hereafter cited as Besson Board; Lt Col Malachai B. Jones, MSC, Fort Sill MEDDAC, to Ginn, 9 Nov 83, DASG-MS.

[52] Verse: "Ballad of Dustoff," by Maj James B. Fisher, MSC, Capt Herbert L. Halstead, MSC, and Capt Joanne C. Dinga, ANC, 1966, copy furnished by Joseph M. "Doc" Kralich, Dustoff Association Historian, 3 Mar 92, DASG-MS. "Charlie" is a reference to the Viet Cong (VC)—Victor Charlie in the phonetic alphabet.

[53] Call sign: Dorland and Nanney, *Dust Off*, pp. 28–29. "And regardless of the name they gave us we always reverted to dust-off." Lt Col Paul A. Bloomquist, MSC, Cdr, 45th Med Bn, to Lt Col Richard H. Scott, MSC, Asst Ch, Avn Br, OTSG, 1 Feb 71, DASG-MS. Killed: Rpt, Joseph M. Kralich, sub: Dustoff Vietnam—Memorial Book, Mar 92, DASG-MS. Kralich's detailed report lists 108 pilots killed in action as a result of hostile fire and another 103 killed as a result of crashes, many

of which occurred in bad weather or at night. Injured: Dorland and Nanney, *Dust Off*, p. 117; Greenhut, Vietnam MS, 6: 47.

[54] Course: Interv, CW2 David Anderson with Tuten, Vietnam, 25 Nov 69, USACMH. Anderson thought the course was beneficial. Teamwork: Interv, Maj Douglas E. Moore, MSC, with Dorland, THU, 12 Sep 75, USACMH.

[55] Routine: Notes of discussion, Col Joseph Madrano, MSC, Ret., with Ginn, 28 Feb 86, and Madrano, bio data sheet, same date, DASG-MS. He was a bomber pilot in World War II and MSC battalion surgeon's assistant in Korea. Quoted words: Lt Col James E. Bizer, MSC, USA Hosp, Augsburg, to Dorland, THU, OTSG, 20 Aug 73.

[56] 57th: Interv, Lt Col John J. Temperilli, Jr., MSC, with Dorland, THU, 15 Jun 74; Dorland and Nanney, *Dust Off*, pp. 27–32; Notes of discussion, Temperilli with Ginn, 28 Feb 86, DASG-MS. The deployment included MSC Capts. Donald L. Naylor, Robert D. McWilliams, William Balenger, and William Hawkins and Lts. Ernie Collins and Thomas C. Jackson.

[57] Red Cross: Interv, Capt Roger P. Hula II, MSC, with Dorland, THU, 4 Mar 74. Quoted words: Interv, Maj Orson J. Hosley, MSC, with Dorland, THU, undated. In-flight care: Interv, Capt Terry Woolever, MSC, with Dorland, THU, 14 Oct 76.

[58] Control: Temperilli, Dorland interv, 15 Jun 74; Bizer to Dorland, 20 Aug 73, both in USACMH; Dorland and Nanney, *Dust Off*, p. 27.

[59] Klingenhagen: Also see Moore to Ginn, 8 Sep 88. Quoted words: Interv, Maj Gen Neel, USA, Ret., with Lt Col Anthony F. Gaudino, AD, USAWC and USAMHI Senior Officer Oral History Program, 26 Apr 85, USAMHI.

[60] Quoted words: Interv, Lt Col Patrick H. Brady, MSC, with Dorland, THU, 3 Jul 74; Moore to Ginn, 22 Aug 88, DASG-MS.

[61] Kelly's death: Address, Heaton, sub: Dedication Ceremony, Charles L. Kelly Army Heliport, Brooke Army Medical Center, Fort Sam Houston, Texas, 7 Apr 67, DASG-MS; Brady, Dorland interv, THU, 3 Jul 74; Interv, Maj Ernest J. Sylvester, MSC, with Dorland, THU, 12 Jun 74; Speech, Moore, sub: DUSTOFFer, 7th Annual Meeting of the Dustoff Association, San Antonio, Texas, 1 Mar 86, author's notes, DASG-MS; Moore to Ginn, 22 Aug 88; Hamrick to Ginn, 22 Aug 88, DASG-MS; General William C. Westmoreland, Ltr to editor in "A Gift of Love," *McCalls* (December 1966): 72–75; SG Conference, 7 Jul 64.

[62] Special school: Brady, Dorland interv, 3 Jul 74. Brady believed Kelly's death saved Dustoff.

[63] Medical control: SG Conference, 22 Jul 66; Hammett, Dorland interv, Oct 75; Maj William R. Knowles, MSC, Asst Ch, Avn Br, OTSG, to Temperilli, 3 Oct 62, USACMH; Neel, Gaudino interv; 1st Ind, Neel, USARV Surg, to ACSFOR, 1 Nov 68, RG 112, accession 71A–3154, Box 9/48, NARA-WNRC. Heaton continually emphasized his desire to preserve the Medical Department as the Dustoff system's "functional operator." Heaton to Lt Gen Harry W.O. Kinnard, CG, U.S. Army Combat Development Command, 27 Dec 68, RG 112, accession 71A–3154, Box 9/48, NARA-WNRC. Hitchhikers: Brady, "Dust-Off Operations," *Army Logistician* 5 (July–August 1973): 19.

[64] Redundancy: Neel, Gaudino interv.

[65] Distinguished Service Crosses: Joseph Kralich to Ginn, 4 Jan 93, DASG-MS. Value of warrant officers: Interv, Lt Col William R. Knowles, MSC, with McPherson, Vietnam, 7 Jun 67; Interv, Lt Col Eugene Lail, MSC, with Dorland, THU, undated, both in USACMH. Quoted words: Moore, Dorland interv.

[66] Novosel: Interv, CW4 Michael J. Novosel with Dorland, THU, 19 Jun 74; Dorland and Nanney, *Dust Off*, pp. 96–98; Notes of intervs, CW4 Michael Novosel, Jr., with Ginn, 28 Feb and 2 Mar 86, DASG-MS; Boston Publishing Company, *Above and Beyond: A History of the Medal of Honor from the Civil War to Vietnam* (Boston: Boston Publishing Co., 1985), pp. 299–300, hereafter cited as Boston, *Above and Beyond.*

[67] Novosel: When he retired in 1985, the elder Novosel had forty-four years of military service and was the last World War II aviator still on active duty. Reflecting upon his Vietnam experience he said, "It is a strange thing to be part of a war and honestly say you have not killed anyone." Novosel, Dorland interv.

[68] Daily routine: Moore, Dorland interv; Interv, CW2 Michael A. Yourous with Dorland, THU, undated; "The Gamest Bastards of All," *Time* 86 (2 July 1965): 21.

[69] Hoists: Interv, Maj James E. Lombard, MSC, with Dorland, undated; Interv, Capt Henry O. Tuell, MSC, with Dorland, THU, 29 Dec 76; Greenhut, Vietnam MS, 6: 19.

[70] Lombard: Lombard, Dorland interv.

[71] Quoted words: Tuell, Dorland interv.

[72] Quoted words: Moore, Dorland interv; Moore to Ginn, 22 Aug 88, DASG-MS.

[73] Swimming pool: Notes of discussion, Ginn with Col Thomas C. Scofield, MSC, Dustoff Meeting, San Antonio, Tex., 1 Mar 86, DASG-MS.

[74] Quoted words: Interv, Col Lloyd E. Spencer, MSC, with Dorland, THU, 10 Jun 74.

[75] Quoted words: Capt Kenneth M. Radebaugh, MSC, Ops Off, 63d Med Det (RA), to Dorland, 22 May 74, USACMH.

[76]Brady: Brady, "Solo Missions," *U.S. Army Aviation Digest* 12 (July 1966): 2–6; Brady, "Instruments and Flares," *U.S. Army Aviation Digest* 15 (January 1969): 12–13; Brady, "Dust-off Operations," pp. 18–23; Lt Col Robert D. McWilliams, MSC, Cdr, 54th Med Det (Helicopter Ambulance [HA]), "Recommendation for Valor," 22 Jun 68; News release, OTSG, "MSC Officer Wins Medal of Honor," 9 Oct 69; Brady, Dorland interv, 3 Jul 74; "Medal of Honor Awarded Maj. Patrick Brady, MSC," *Service Stripe*, WRAMC, 23 October 1969, all in MSC-USACMH; SG Rpt, 1970, pp. 107–08; Dorland and Nanney, *Dust Off*, pp. 63–66; Nick Adde, "Real American Heroes," *Army Times* (11 April 1988): 41–46; Boston, *Above and Beyond*, pp. 300–301; Hamrick to Ginn, 22 Aug 88, DASG-MS.

[77] Pickup site: Capt. (later Maj. Gen.) Michael J. Scotti, MC, battalion surgeon of the 4th Battalion, 31st Infantry, 196th Light Infantry Brigade, was on the first flight. Ltrs, Joseph M. Kralich to Ginn, 18 Feb 92 and 2 Apr 92, DASG-MS.

[78] Salute: Augerson's salute meant a great deal to Brady. "For some reason that has remained with me and will always be a pleasure to recall." Brady, Dorland interv.

[79] Ledford: MSC Newsletter, 1970–73.

[80] Bloomquist: USAREUR, HQ, V Corps, GO 495, 30 May 72; Rpt, Frankfurt Resident Agency, 2d Region, U.S. Army Criminal Investigation Command, sub: Criminal Investigation Division (CID) Report of Investigation, 16 Nov 72; Eulogy for Bloomquist, Brig Gen James A. Young, MSC, (drafted by Lt. Col. Robert F. Elliott, MSC, XO, 68th Med Group), 16 Jun 80; Lt Col Paul A. Bloomquist, Cdr, 45th Med Bn, to Lt Col Richard H. Scott, MSC, Asst Ch, Avn Br, OTSG, 1 Feb 71; Lt Col Edward J. Taylor, Jr., MSC, to Elliott, 9 Jun 80, all in DASG-MS; Interv, Maj Ernest J. Sylvester, MSC, with Dorland, THU, 12 Jun 74, USACMH; SG Conference, 22 Jul 66.

[81] "Big Bear": "The Gamest Bastards of All," *Time* 86 (2 July 1965): 21; Moore, Dorland interv.

[82] First sergeant: Ltr to the editor, Lt. Col. Roger P. Hula II, MSC, Ret., "The Joy and the Grief," *Army* 36 (February 1986): 6, 9.

[83] Cavanaugh: Cavanaugh et al., "Plague," in Ognibene and O'Neill, *Internal Medicine in Vietnam*, 2: 167–97; Interv, Col Dan C. Cavanaugh, MSC, Ret., with Maj Eric G. Daxon, MSC, Washington, D.C., 17 Apr 85, DASG-MS; Engelman and Joy, *Two Hundred Years of Military Medicine*, p. 40.

[84] Quoted words: Brady, Dorland interv.

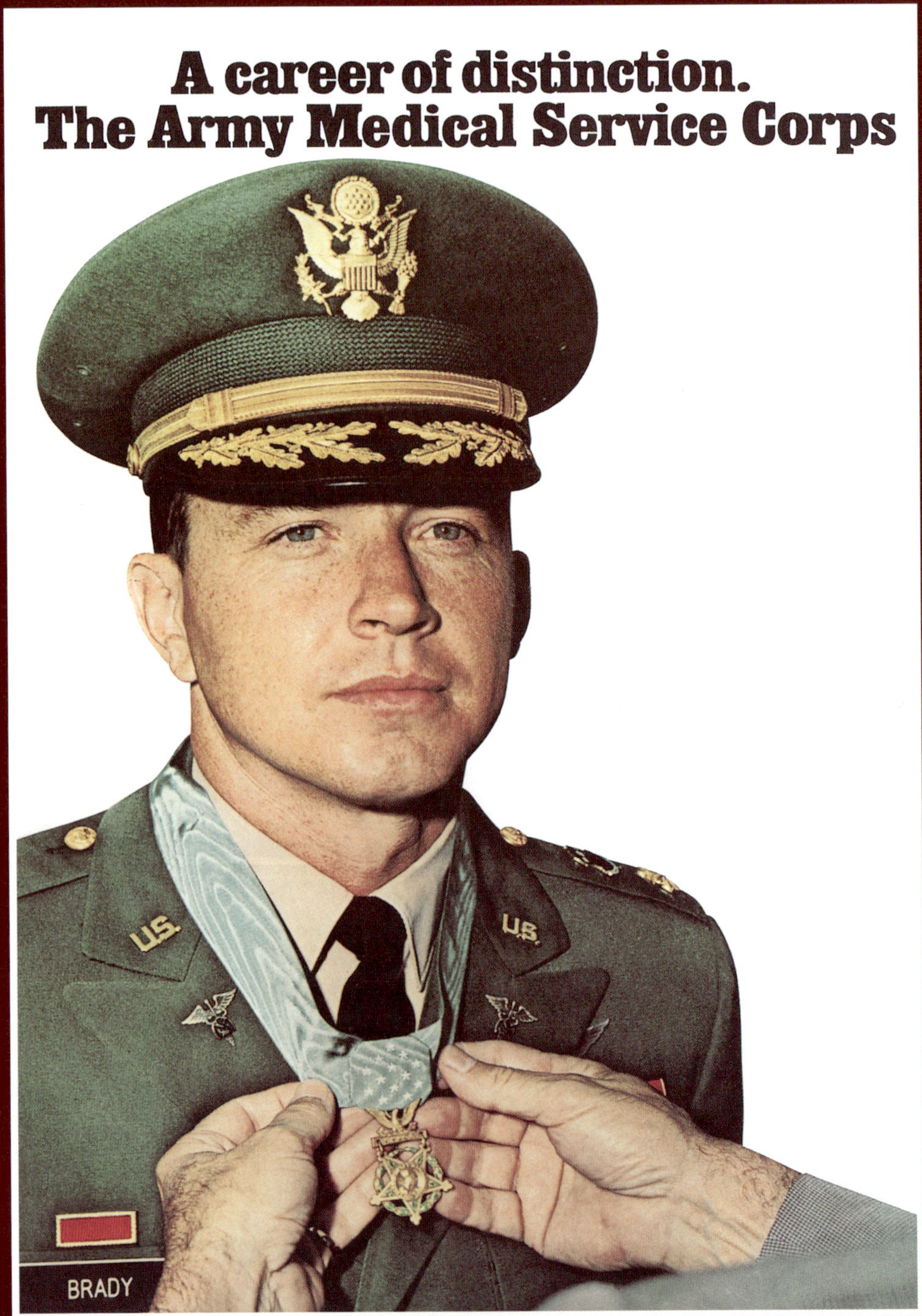

Cover of Medical Service Corps recruiting bulletin, September 1971

11

The Corps During the Vietnam Era

Medical Service Corps officers were important members of the medical team in the Vietnam War from the buildup in 1965 through the peak in 1969 to the final pullout in 1975. But Southeast Asia was not the only place where MSCs found themselves on foreign soil. While the Medical Department's first priority was support of the theater of operations, its attention was also directed to other areas of the world where U.S. national interests were threatened.

A decade of foreign interventions began in 1965 with a sudden deployment of U.S. forces that took some MSCs to the Caribbean. President Lyndon B. Johnson, Kennedy's successor, decided to intervene in the Dominican Republic's civil war between government and leftist rebel forces, a conflict that had its roots in the assassination four years earlier of Raphael Trujillo, the republic's dictator for thirty-one years. The elected government had been overthrown by military revolt in 1963, and rebel activity increased thereafter.[1]

The capital city of Santo Domingo was a battle area when Johnson decided to intervene. In April he ordered the 82d Airborne Division at Fort Bragg, North Carolina, to move a brigade combat team to the Dominican Republic where it would join the 4th Marine Expeditionary Brigade. At the peak of the invasion U.S. forces totaled 23,000. The marines withdrew in June, at which point U.S. military involvement turned to civic action. Withdrawal of U.S. forces was completed in 1966. In all, 14 U.S. military personnel had been killed and 146 wounded in action, of whom 68 required hospitalization.

A clearing company of the 307th Medical Battalion and the medical platoons of two airborne infantry battalions were the first medical units on the island, followed by the rest of the 307th Medical Battalion. As in Korea, command of the medical battalion stayed with the MSC commander, Lt. Col. Charles Anistranski. Similarly, the clearing companies remained under their MSC commanders, including Company D, the first company deployed, commanded by Capt. Robert F. Elliott. Medical additions included the 400-bed 15th Field Hospital from Fort Bragg, the 54th Medical Detachment (Helicopter Ambulance) from Fort Benning, Georgia, and other medical units.

The Medical Department's mission of providing posthostilities support was again evidenced when civic action became the primary mission. By the end of June medical assistance teams had treated nearly forty thousand civilian patients, mostly obstetric, pediatric, and geriatric—a pattern that continued throughout the operation, despite complaints from a few local physicians that the Army was ruining their business. Another lesson relearned was the immediate requirement for optometric support in combat operations. The initial absence of MSC optometrists increased evacuations from the Dominican Republic, since it was necessary to send soldiers to Puerto Rico for the nearest optometric services.

Medical Department Organization

The invasion in the Dominican Republic, the beginning of a large buildup in Vietnam, and the maintenance of a large forward-deployed force in Europe caused the Medical Department to rethink how it was organized to support a world power. In 1967 the Board of Inquiry on the Army Logistics System (the Brown Board) recommended that the Army form a worldwide medical command under the surgeon general. The Medical Department[2] addressed this in 1969 with its Worldwide Organizational Structure for Army Medical Support (WORSAMS) study.[3]

Col. Lewis H. Huggins, MSC, an operations officer, was the study coordinator, and MSC officers headed three of the four study teams. They concluded in 1970 that it was not desirable at that point to extend such an organization to overseas areas. However, they proposed forming a medical command as the single manager for the department's activities in the continental United States, excluding field units. To that end they proposed transfer of the Class I community hospitals to the department's direct control, joining the Class II medical centers. The Army acted upon the recommendation in 1973 when it consolidated the fixed facilities in the continental United States into the U.S. Army Health Services Command (adding the hospitals in Hawaii, Panama, and Alaska the following year). The Medical Field Service School, Fort Sam Houston, Texas, which had moved into a new building in 1972, also joined the new command as the Academy of Health Sciences.[4] Unfortunately, the WORSAMS concept of having the command report directly to the surgeon general was not implemented. Rather, the Health Services Command commander and the surgeon general both reported to the Army chief of staff.

Col. William A. Hamrick, MSC, served as chief of the Medical Service Corps from 1963 to 1969. He was initially "triple-hatted" with the additional duties of executive officer of the Personnel and Training Division and chief of its MSC Branch. Colonel Hamrick was able to persuade Lt. Gen. Leonard B. Heaton, the surgeon general from 1959 to 1969, that the corps needed a full-time chief, and that became his only duty beginning in 1965.[5] Removal of the additional duty of branch chief lessened Hamrick's involvement in the day-to-day business of officer assignments. However, that task continued to require his concurrence, and he was directly involved with key positions.[6] Hamrick was replaced in 1969 by Brig. Gen. Manley G. Morrison, who was followed by Brig. Gen. John E. Haggerty in 1973 (*see Appendix G*). General Morrison had a single duty of corps chief, but Haggerty's concurrent appointment as the surgeon general's director of resources management returned the chief to a "dual-hatted" position. The authority of the MSC chiefs over assignments survived various incursions. For example, the surgeon general rejected an effort in 1966 by the Fourth Army commander to gain assignment control over MSC officers in that command.[7]

Developments in the Corps

In March 1965 the MSC had 4,512 officers on active duty, an increase of 149 in four months as the Vietnam buildup got under way. This number stood at 5,144 in 1972 (*see Appendix K*). MSCs served in forty-two specialties in twenty career fields. This was a reduction from fifty-eight specialties in 1961, but it was still a large number. The corps continued to provide authorizations for medical students, a number that stood at 199 in 1972.[8] When the Army was unable to meet some of its requirements for MSC officers as the Vietnam War accelerated, especially in air ambulance units, Colonel Hamrick took specific actions to increase the availability of MSCs, including calling up graduating ROTC cadets early and drafting optometrists. Nevertheless, by January 1966 the Army was listing commissioned and warrant officer aviators as well as bacteriologists and biochemists as critical shortages.

Colonel Hamrick's greatest concern was pilots. He was upset in 1965 when the department requested ninety flight school slots but received only nine, even though 185 of the available 196 MSC aviators were overseas. By February 1967, 247 aviators were in Vietnam, and some were on their second tour. By November only two had not yet gone. In 1969, 35 percent of the MSC pilots in Vietnam were there for the second time.

By 1969 twenty-one MSC pilots had been killed in Vietnam. Hamrick did not lose sight of the fact that this was the only group of Medical Department officers taking significant losses, and he pressed for more MSC aviators. When challenged as to how they would be used after the war, he responded that it took a year to train a pilot and many were serving multiple dangerous tours in Vietnam. "You fill every requisition you get for training."[9] The problem of providing future career opportunities for MSC aviators was resolved by requiring them to obtain an additional MSC specialty as they advanced through the ranks. This would make them competitive for field grade positions in their secondary specialty and would resolve the dilemma posed by the small number of field grade slots for aviators in medical aviation units.

In 1965 the Medical Department developed a proposal to include a warrant officer aviation specialty in the MSC. That did not materialize, but a plan to use warrant officers as aeromedical pilots did, and the surgeon general identified requirements for 298 of them. The department initially desired a 1:1 ratio of commissioned to warrant officer aviators. It wanted that high percentage of commissioned MSCs because of their familiarity with the Medical Department's entire operations, an expertise they gained through their training and assignments as MSC officers. However, warrant officers came to predominate because the demand for Dustoff aviators exceeded the capacity of the Army to meet all its requirements with commissioned officers.[10]

The corps continued to expand as the war in Vietnam heated up. By May 1966 there were 4,853 officers on active duty. The MSC was more than twice as large as either the Navy or Air Force MSCs and was larger than ten other branches of the Army, including the Quartermaster, Transportation, and Military Police Corps. The number climbed to 5,601 by the end of 1966, peaking at 6,033 in July

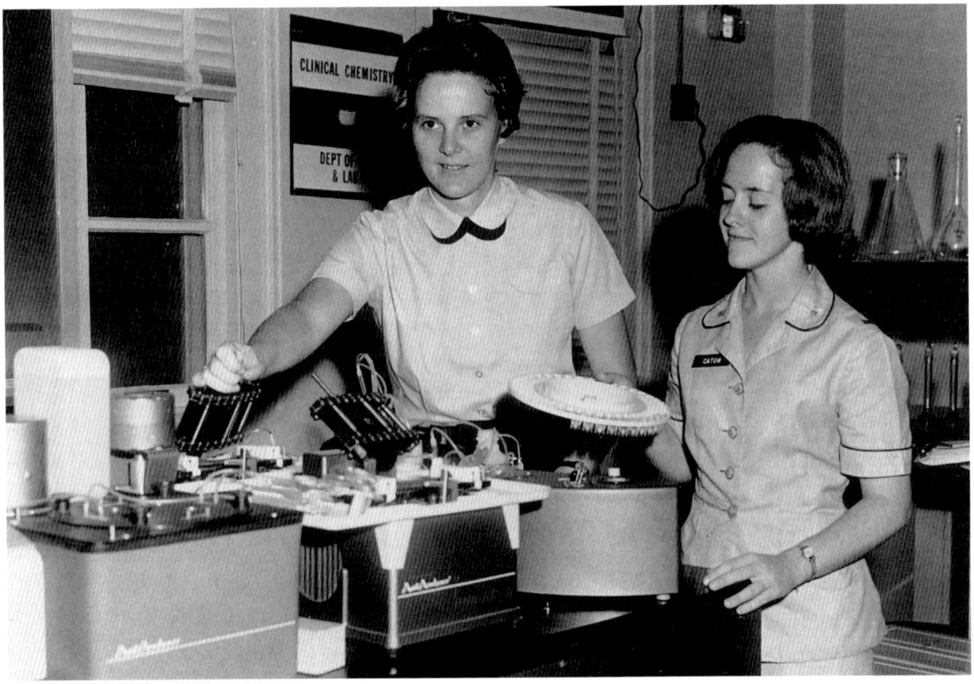

Female officers at the Medical Field Service School, October 1967

1969, when nearly half were serving overseas. The number began dropping as troop reductions began in Vietnam, falling to 4,957 in June 1975. At that point the MSC was the largest of the six Medical Department corps, accounting for 31 percent of its 16,000 officers.[11]

The quality of MSC officers remained an area watched by the chief, and Branch continued sending out "buck-up" letters. There was constant attention to the number and quality of new accessions, and the corps maintained active recruiting programs. There were ten to fifteen applications for every opening during 1967, and in 1968 there were 2,000 applications for 265 spaces. Advertising efforts in 1970 included a new MSC recruitment brochure and pamphlets for the scientific specialties. Brochures in 1971 featured a cover photograph of Maj. Patrick A. Brady, MSC, receiving the Medal of Honor.[12]

The principal sources of officers were ROTC and direct appointments. In addition, West Point graduates were now allowed to select the MSC. The first graduate was appointed in 1965, and by 1968 there were nineteen. OCS also continued as a source of officers, and 100 graduates entered the corps in 1969. Forty of the sixty-two who entered the following year from the Infantry OCS at Fort Benning, Georgia, were in the top third of their class; five were honor graduates. The basic course at the Medical Field Service School bulged with the new accessions, and by July 1966 there were 343 officers in attendance.[13] The number of women in the corps remained low. There were just 7 in 1968: 4 laboratory officers, 2 social workers, and 1 comptroller.

A baccalaureate degree was expected for commissioning in the MSC, and by 1969 nearly 94 percent of the corps had college degrees as opposed to only 70 percent for Army officers as a whole. Hamrick resisted efforts to waive the requirement. "To me, education is simply discipline. I think that anyone can get through school if they are willing to apply themselves sufficiently."[14] The corps also stressed graduate study. In 1969 over one-third of MSC officers had graduate degrees. One of every four Ph.D.s in the Army was an MSC, and there were 960 MSC positions designated as requiring graduate training. Hamrick marveled at the improvement in the quality of MSCs, "the product of an advanced educational experience which confounds the imagination of us old-timers."[15]

The Army-Baylor Hospital Administration Program became the Army-Baylor Health Care Administration Program in 1969, in keeping with the profession's expansion into different health care settings. It remained the only avenue for graduate training in hospital administration open to MSCs. Prior attendance at resident Command and General Staff College or the Armed Forces Staff College was not a bar to selection; conversely, Army-Baylor attendance did not bar an officer's attendance at the staff college. However, it was the rare officer who did both.[16]

Baylor classes averaged fifty-four students; the largest was sixty-two in 1967. The student body included officers from each of the six Medical Department corps, as well as other agencies and countries. A few junior officers were selected for each class; for example, eight officers with less than three years' service were included in the thirty-seven MSCs chosen for the 1968 class.[17]

The department's assignment policies dictated the use of Baylor graduates as hospital executive officers in Vietnam. The commander of the 67th Medical Group took issue with that practice. His complaint was not with the quality of the course but with the lack of field experience of the officers as they continued through their careers. On the other hand, the commander of the 44th Medical Brigade (who was formerly the commander of the 68th Medical Group) thought the Baylor graduates did an outstanding job once in the field.[18]

Baylor continued to apply pressure for higher entrance requirements and tougher courses. It imposed a five-year limit for completion of the degree, a result of continued problems with students who completed the first year of the course but failed to finish their residency-year research project. Of the 536 students from 1964 to 1975, forty failed to graduate from Baylor; most were physicians and international students. Baylor considered establishing its own hospital administration program, which presumably would have absorbed the Army-Baylor Program, but the university concluded that it was not feasible and dropped the idea.[19]

The corps maintained its emphasis on military training. The MSC basic course was eight weeks long in 1966 (as compared to six weeks for the Army Nurse Corps and four and a half weeks for the other Medical Department corps). The MSC advanced course was twenty-one weeks long. The Medical Department's operation of its own school and its provision of different basic courses for the various branches survived a challenge by the Haines Board, a study of Army schools in 1965, and the department went on to lengthen the MSC basic course to sixteen weeks.[20]

MSC boards selected officers for the Regular (resident) Course at the Command and General Staff College at Fort Leavenworth, Kansas. In 1972 Lt. Col. James Van Straten was the first MSC honor graduate, and the following year Maj. Bob Muzio, MSC, convinced the college to include Medical Department officers in the class leadership positions of section and work group leaders. A very small number of MSCs—typically two a year—attended senior service college. The Army created the Army War College Corresponding Studies Course in 1968 to expand war college opportunity to more officers, particularly those in the reserve components. A rigorous two-year program that included two resident summer sessions, it was the only military correspondence course with competitive selection. Col. Larry W. Coker, MSC, was a member of the first graduating class.[21]

There were complaints about the quality of officers assigned to garrisoned field medical units in the later years of the Vietnam period. General Haggerty believed the corps had ignored those assignments. "It bothered me no end when some of our people were being relieved from command."[22] The commander of the lst Corps Support Command at Fort Bragg sounded the alarm in 1973. He complained of a shortage of MSCs in the 55th Medical Group, as well as the lack of depth and experience of those who were assigned. The group operations officer, a captain whose highest military education was the basic MSC course, was filling a major's position that called for a Leavenworth graduate. The commanders of the 5th and 28th Combat Surgical Hospitals were both majors and advanced course graduates when they should have been lieutenant colonels and Army-Baylor graduates. The group executive officer should ideally have been a graduate of both Leavenworth and Army-Baylor, but the incumbent was neither.[23]

Lt. Gen. Melvin Zais, Third Army commander, believed the matter was serious, and he personally asked the surgeon general for remedial action. It was one of the first problems on General Haggerty's desk when he became chief of the corps, and he immediately directed that all graduates of the Regular Course at Fort Leavenworth would go to field unit assignments. "We had two guys . . . who almost passed out because they had thought they were coming right back to The Surgeon General's Office."[24] MSC field medical performance was also helped by the Army's establishment of command selection boards to pick officers for command.

The pressure continued to move MSCs into administrative positions once held only by physicians. It took another turn in 1968 when the Department of Defense (DOD) directed the Medical Department to convert 3 percent of its Medical Corps spaces to MSC. More pressure came in 1973 when Secretary of Defense Elliot Richardson asked the military departments to make better use of their military health care professionals. A legislative proposal for incentive pay for physicians had encountered administration opposition because of the sizable share of the nation's supply of health personnel claimed by the military. The departments were required to remove physicians and dentists from positions "for which they may be best qualified but which can be adequately filled by non-physicians."[25]

In this environment MSC position opportunities continued to improve. MSCs served as chief of staff of the U.S. Army Medical Command (later retitled the 7th Medical Command), headquartered in Heidelberg, Germany, a position

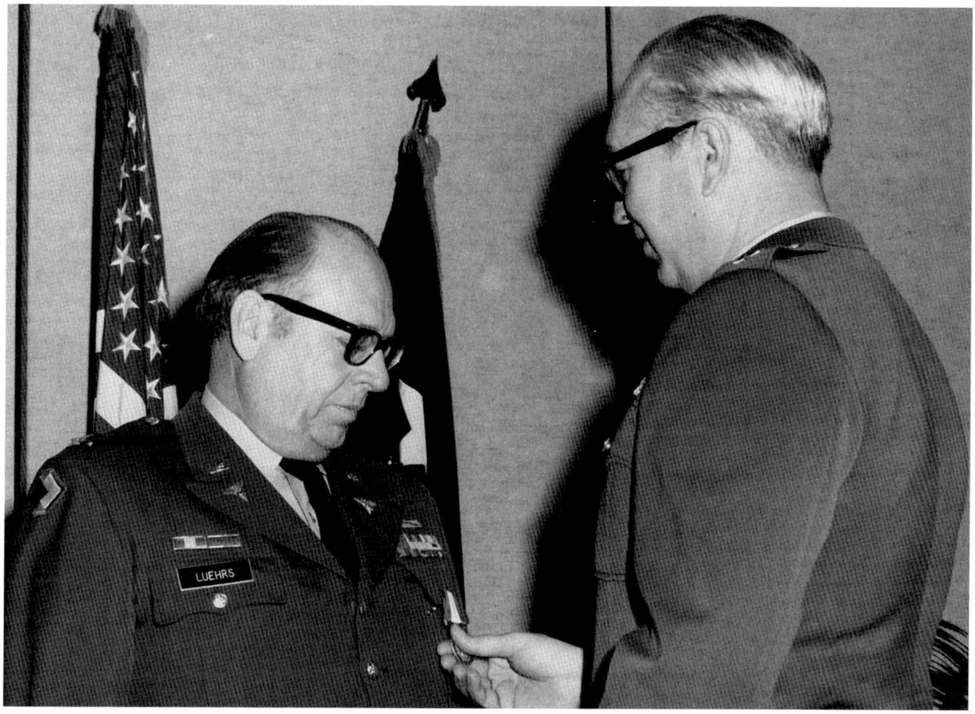

Colonel Luehrs receives the Distinguished Service Medal from General Jennings.

that included the additional duty of executive officer for the chief surgeon, U.S. Army, Europe, and Seventh Army. The hospital executive officer position was firmly established for MSC officers, although Medical Department policy persisted in reserving command of operational medical treatment facilities for physicians. In 1969 Col. William S. Mullins, MSC, replaced a physician as commander of the surgeon general's historical unit, and in 1970 Col. Grover L. Kistler, MSC, became the first nonphysician director of the Civilian Health and Medical Program of the Uniformed Services (CHAMPUS). Col. Charles J. Shively, MSC, was appointed in 1974 as the first commander of the U.S. Army Medical Department Personnel Support Agency.

A major advance occurred in 1969 when Col. William C. Luehrs, MSC, became the executive officer for the surgeon general, a change precipitated by Lt. Gen. Hal B. Jennings, Jr., who replaced Heaton as surgeon general in 1969. Colonel Luehrs' predecessor had argued that it was necessary for the executive officer to be a physician in order to function as a full partner in the department's senior leadership team. Such a policy, he insisted, allowed the surgeon general and his deputy to pursue their duties without "having to be braced for some unexpected cataclysmic event which may have come about innocently" because of the executive officer's lack of medical training. Luehrs was thus initially leery about the job because of such beliefs, but he found that General Jennings gave him unstinting support.[26]

Medical Department doctrine continued to specify that only Medical Corps officers would command units engaged in active patient care, and General Heaton had been outspoken on the subject. However, administrative assignments were no more popular among physicians in the Vietnam War than in other periods. A survey in 1966 showed that fear of a prospective administrative or command assignment was the second most prevalent reason for leaving the Army. Col. William A. Boyson, MC, was surprised by the vehemence of the responses to his survey. He attributed it to the desires of military physicians to maintain clinical proficiency and to the fact that it was "all but impossible to do both clinical medicine and command-administration at the same time."[27]

The Department of Defense intervened in the command issue in May 1973 when the deputy secretary of defense sent a memorandum to the Services directing that "any qualified health professional may command or exercise administrative direction of a military health care facility or serve as executive officer of such a facility without regard to the officer's basic health profession."[28] The memo noted Air Force success with MSC officers as clinic commanders and directed the Army and Navy to submit their implementation plans by 4 June. The Army Medical Department ignored the order.

General Jennings did support a proposal to permanently transfer command of medical battalions to MSCs. The plan, as briefed in 1973, would convert the "dual-hatted" position of division surgeon and medical battalion commander into two separate positions, a Medical Corps division surgeon and a Medical Service Corps battalion commander. That change would enable the division surgeon to concentrate on the division's medical practice, preventive medicine activities, and planning for medical support of operations while permitting the battalion commander to concentrate full time on the administrative functions of command and control. The proposal ran into resistance from the Army Staff, and the chief of staff disapproved it in a decision that retained the "dual-hatted" physician commander. The decision reaffirmed that MSC officers would command garrisoned units but that the MSC commander would step down and become the executive officer when the battalion deployed operationally.[29]

Cohesion initiatives continued. The gold versus silver issue resurfaced when Colonel Hamrick solicited comments on the MSC insignia. He found that younger officers actually preferred a silver insignia because it distinguished them from the other corps of the Medical Department. One observed that the performance of MSCs, not the color of their insignia, would determine their status. This was about the last word on the subject, and the controversy ended. The pride that had developed in the distinctive insignia was evidenced in its use in the Silver Caduceus Society of Korea, a collegial organization formed in 1967 by MSC officers assigned to the U.S. Eighth Army.[30]

There was a renewal of the effort to write the history of the corps. The department reactivated the project in 1965, and Colonel Hamrick chaired a meeting of a reconstituted editorial board. The board reestablished the project as a single-author book with a publication date of 1971. This effort did not succeed either, and by 1975 the MSC volume, while a fully chartered Army project, was in its second decade and again languishing.

TECSTAR

The corps was nearly abolished during the Vietnam era. The reorganization of the Army in 1962[31] led to a follow-up study, the Technical Career Structure of the Army (TECSTAR). By 1964 the Army had abolished five of the branch chief positions, and with the exception of the Corps of Engineers and the "special branches" (Judge Advocate General, Chaplain, and Medical Department), the branch chiefs lost their personnel management functions and had meaningless titles.[32] The reorganization broke the Army's historical branch support pattern, and TECSTAR was an extension of that process.[33]

The TECSTAR plan offered five alternatives, each of which called for the disestablishment of the Medical Service Corps. One alternative retained the MSC for the scientific specialties; the other four called for the abolition of the corps entirely, with varying arrangements for disposing of the officers. Requirements for the administrative and scientific specialties would be met from the general pool of Army officers—for example, medical logistics positions would be filled by Quartermaster, Transportation, or Ordnance Corps officers.

The study infuriated General Heaton. He protested that if allowed to go unchecked it would cause a marked deterioration in medical care. The MSC was an essential part of the Medical Department team, and without it "we could not continue in our presently highly effective fashion—it is that simple." When Heaton could not convince the Army Staff to exclude the MSC from the study, he urged the Medical Department's senior leaders to speak out against it at every opportunity.[34]

Heaton believed that the exceptional quality of MSC officers in branch-immaterial positions in the Pentagon might have whetted the Army Staff's appetite for more. The transfer in 1963 of Col. Leo Benade, MSC, to the Adjutant General Corps was instructive. Benade, called the "indispensable man" by the *Army Times* for his expertise in military compensation, represented the unusually gifted MSC officer, something borne out by his eventual promotion to lieutenant general. Another was Col. Ralph Richards, MSC, a confederate of Benade's in the Surgeon General's Special Projects Office who transferred to the Army Finance Corps and retired as a major general.[35]

Whatever the cause, the threat was real, and Colonel Hamrick saw TECSTAR as a call to arms. "We are in the process of firing a heavy volley of rebuttals, but at this stage cannot predict the outcome." He enlisted Col. Ralph G. LeMoon, MSC, chief of the Special Projects Office, to head a task force. Officers were brought in from the Medical Field Service School to help staff a "War Room" in the Surgeon General's Office, and the battle was joined.[36]

One of the most valuable reinforcements came from the corps' association with the American College of Hospital Administrators (ACHA). Hamrick asked Ray E. Brown, a former ACHA president, to prepare a report on TECSTAR. Brown, the surgeon general's consultant in hospital administration, was director of the Duke University Program in Hospital Administration and a nationally recognized pioneer in the profession, whose energy, writings, and reputation were legendary.[37]

Brown's report said the TECSTAR proposals flew in the face of contemporary hospital administration practice and common sense. "It just doesn't make sense to disrupt the efficient and effective organizational arrangement that you have when it would serve no purpose to do so." It was essential for the department to have its own comptrollers, personnel officers, registrars, and all the other specialties provided by the MSC. "Just as the best pilot on the Mississippi River would be lost on the Amazon, the non-medical specialist cannot appropriately apply and practice his specialty in the medical setting without knowledge of the peculiarities of that setting."[38]

General Heaton laid it on the line. "I must repudiate the TECSTAR detailed plan."[39] The effort that it represented had collapsed, and TECSTAR was rejected to the extent that the chief of staff issued a disclaimer that it was "approved for information only."[40] The Medical Service Corps was saved for another day.

A Star

The absence of general officer opportunity was demoralizing, especially as MSC officers raised their educational levels and moved into positions of increased responsibility. The corps was used as part of the total Army commissioned strength in determining the total number of general officers allowed by Congress, justifying an estimated twenty-three general officers by its officer strength. Yet the MSC was the only male commissioned corps with no opportunity for promotion to general. This was particularly galling since it was larger than ten other Army branches that in the aggregate had thirty-one generals.[41] Awarding one of the existing Medical Department stars to the MSC would have meant taking a star from the Medical, Dental, or Veterinary Corps, an action that no surgeon general was willing to approve. In fact, Col. Vernon McKenzie, MSC, observed that when the department was faced with loss of its Veterinary Corps star, Maj. Gen. Silas B. Hays, the surgeon general at the time, was willing to see it transferred to the Quartermaster Corps rather than put it in the MSC.[42]

Colonel Hamrick counted on Heaton's support, knowing full well that the establishment of a general officer slot would not come to pass without his concurrence. Hamrick's confidence was well placed, for General Heaton declared in writing, "I believe that no other branch or corps within the Army has a greater diversity of scientific, technical, and administrative specialties than the Medical Service Corps."[43]

Another ally was William P. MacCracken, the Washington counsel for the American Optometric Association and the key player in the 1945 legislative attempt to create an optometry corps. MacCracken took up the fight for an MSC star, lobbying in Congress for support of a bill introduced by Congressman Philip J. Philbin of Massachusetts in 1965. The lobbyist made a strong impression on Congressman Durward G. Hall, who told Maj. Gen. James T. McGibony, the deputy surgeon general, that MacCracken frightened him. McGibony assured the congressman that MacCracken was legitimate.[44]

But the Army's position remained unchanged. It did not want general officer authorizations tied to positions, and it opposed the Philbin bill.[45] However, during the course of the debate it also became evident that the Army would support

MSC general officer opportunity as long as it was not tied to a specific position. This new wrinkle came when the Army's judge advocate general, in a reversal of an earlier opinion, ruled that the Army could not promote MSC officers to general officer without a change to the law. General Creighton Abrams, the vice chief of staff, opposed the Philbin bill's tying an MSC star to a position, but he supported removing the statutory bar to MSC general officer promotions.[46]

Hamrick launched a campaign to gain congressional approval, and he and others wrote congressmen "and anybody who would listen." The campaign worked. The bill was placed on the House Armed Services Committee's calendar in spite of Defense Department opposition, the work of Colonel McKenzie through his close association with the committee's senior counsel.[47] Heaton, called to testify in July 1966, was obligated to support the Defense Department's negative position. However, when questioned by members of the committee he made it clear that he personally favored the bill. The same turnabout happened in September when he testified before the Senate Armed Services Committee.[48]

The Philbin bill passed and was signed into law by President Johnson on 24 September. In a compromise designed to satisfy the Department of Defense, it provided for a brigadier general in the Medical Service Corps without specifying that this would have to be the chief. Furthermore, the star did not come from within the Medical Department's allocation. This feat was accomplished by Senator Leverett Saltonstall, chairman of the Senate Armed Services Committee, who "had a sack of stars and he took them out and put them back as he wanted to." On 10 November 1966, Hamrick was promoted to brigadier general.[49]

An MSC general was a matter of pride to the corps. However, the inequity in general officer opportunity when compared to other Army branches remained. In 1972 the MSC had one general for 5,430 officers. However, the Ordnance Corps, with 4,917 officers, had 26 generals. The Quartermaster Corps, with 3,853 officers, had 14; and the Finance Corps, with 1,009 officers, had 4. Transportation Corps officers had twenty-nine times the chance for a star that their MSC counterparts did.[50]

General Morrison attempted to increase general officer opportunity for the MSC. He commissioned a study that identified sixteen Medical Department positions that could be filled by MSC general officers.[51] He gained the support of General Jennings, who asked the Army chief of staff to increase the MSC allocation to three general officers—one major general and two brigadier generals—but the request failed when it ran afoul of a 25 percent cut in Army general officers. Subsequently, Congressman Don Fuqua introduced legislation to change the MSC authorization to five general officers per thousand Regular Army officers. Fuqua's bill would have authorized ten MSC generals, with a major general as chief of the corps and brigadier generals as assistant chiefs. Morrison encouraged senior MSCs to support the legislation on the grounds that establishing those general officer slots by law would create "a strong moral obligation" for the secretary of the Army to allocate stars against the billets. Fuqua's proposal did not succeed, however, and there was no change to the number of MSC generals.[52]

Developments in the Administrative Specialties

In 1961 MSC administrative officers had been serving in thirty-six specialties (*see Appendix H*). A series of actions reduced that by 1972 to twenty-three specialties in nine career fields: comptroller, hospital administration, medical aviation, medical technical intelligence, operations and training, personnel, registrar, supply, and medical equipment repair (*see Appendix K*). These classifications remained dynamic, and a number of changes were made during the Vietnam period. Most officers entered their specialty fields without prior qualification and were not awarded a specialty skill identifier until after completing six to eight years on active duty. Each specialty was represented by a senior officer appointed as a consultant to the chief of the corps.[53]

The registrar specialty numbered 185 officers in 1972. It would change its title to patient administration, a term more in keeping with its expanded functions, which now included quality assurance as well as insurance eligibility under DOD's new Civilian Health and Medical Program of the Uniformed Services (CHAMPUS) for military family members. Some patient administrators, especially Maj. Max Hoyt, MSC, and Col. Boyd E. Cooksley, MSC, were instrumental in adapting the International Patient Diagnostic System to Army systems in 1971, giving the department an automated data base for discharged patients.[54]

There were 149 comptrollers in 1972. Col. Milton C. Devolites, MSC, was the action officer in 1970 for formation of the Surgeon General's Directorate of Resources Management, a consolidation of five separate offices. Devolites became the first deputy director, but Medical Corps general officers served as directors until General Haggerty's dual appointment in 1973. Lt. Col. Donald A. Waller, MSC, in 1970 was appointed the assistant executive to the comptroller of the Army, the first Medical Department officer to serve in that capacity on the Army Staff. An average of three MSCs attended each class of the Army Comptrollership Program at Syracuse University, Syracuse, New York. The program, which had initially focused almost exclusively on financial management, gradually changed to encompass an overall concept of resource management.[55]

The medical supply specialty (433 in 1972) had initial difficulties to overcome in supporting the buildup in Vietnam. Col. Charles C. Pixley, MC, commander of the 68th Medical Group, said that one of his biggest problems was the quality of his medical logisticians.[56] There were not enough experienced officers, a problem attributed to various DOD efficiency drives that had converted depot military positions to civilian. In addition, the transfer of Army medical supply functions to centralized DOD agencies had diminished the department's ability to train officers in medical depot operations. Further, grade authorizations for medical logisticians did not match their levels of responsibility; a medical depot, for example, was authorized a major as the commander. The overall problem of shortages and inexperience was put in a nutshell by a senior MSC logistician. "You give me a lieutenant to run supply and this poor kid has never been in a hospital."[57]

Action was necessary. Training programs were undertaken at the Atlanta Army Depot and the U.S. Army Medical Materiel Agency (USAMMA) at Fort Detrick, Maryland. The department increased the grade of the depot and subdepot commanders as well as the number of officers in the basic medical logistics course at the Medical Field Service School. By 1968 Col. Jesse N. Butler, MSC, the surgeon general's chief of medical supply, concluded that MSC medical logisticians were, on balance, acquitting themselves well in Vietnam. Officers trained in inventory management at USAMMA were well qualified, and the basic course was functioning satisfactorily. Warrant officers served as medical equipment repair specialists, the field that had opened to them in 1961, and in 1972 their number stood at eighty-four. A pioneer, CW4 W. B. "Foxy" King, retired that year, at which time he was assigned to the Surgeon General's Office as the first head of the Medical Department's National Maintenance Point.[58]

MSC aviators (359 in 1972) conducted the Army's portion of the Military Assistance to Safety and Traffic (MAST) program, a project involving the Departments of Defense, Transportation, and Health and Human Services. MAST began in July 1970 at Fort Sam Houston, Texas, as a test of the feasibility of utilizing aeromedical helicopters for evacuating seriously injured highway accident victims. The test was successful, and legislation in 1973 provided a permanent authority for that DOD role. The aeromedical units assigned MAST responsibility provided a 24-hour standby crew of pilot, copilot, crew chief, and medic.[59]

Hospital administration got a boost in 1965 with passage of the Medical Care for the Aged (Medicare) and Medical Care for the Indigent (Medicaid) amendments to the Social Security Act. The federal government's direct financing of medical care uncorked a federal money gusher, but hospitals had to adopt standard business practices to support their claims for reimbursement. Sometimes that meant performing rudimentary business practices, such as preparing budgets, that they had never done before, while learning to adapt to federal regulations and forms. The need for professionally trained managers was more pronounced than ever, and the number of physicians who served as chief executive officers of American hospitals dropped to 813 by 1972.[60]

Federal dollars made the practice of medicine more lucrative, at least initially, further dimming the luster of administrative positions for military physicians, who needed to remain current in the practice of medicine in order to secure clinical appointments when they left active duty. Then, on the heels of Medicare came national concerns over costs and access to care. The federal government translated this into a series of laws unprecedented for their number and the extent of their involvement with health care organizations.[61] The changes were felt by MSC health care administrators, who, like their civilian counterparts, operated within a changing environment and were more and more required to be experts in regulations. Indeed, the growing complexity of federal paperwork was the principal topic at the annual meeting of Army hospital administrators in 1966.[62]

The membership of the American College of Hospital Administrators was now predominately composed of administrators with the professional master's degree in hospital administration. The MSC retained close ties, and in 1966 Hamrick and Col. Ralph G. LeMoon, MSC, advanced to fellowship, the highest level of advancement in the college. Maj. Gen. James T. McGibony, MC, served as the first regent-at-large for military members from 1964 to 1967, and later Hamrick replaced him.[63]

There were concerns with the general health of the operations and training career field, which broadened to include intelligence. The deputy commander of the 44th Medical Brigade maintained that the department's performance in Vietnam was hampered by a shortage of seasoned operations officers. He attributed this to the department's failure to make it an attractive specialty for young officers, who saw less opportunity for graduate education in the specialty, especially the Army-Baylor Program. Generals Hamrick, Morrison, and Haggerty were aware of those perceptions and countered them with efforts to emphasize field assignments and to improve opportunities for operations officers.[64]

Operations officers contributed at all levels of the department. Maj. Roy S. Church, MSC, the S–3 of the 46th Medical Battalion in Heilbronn, Germany, was responsible for the Army's Expert Field Medical Badge, a competitive award earned by medical personnel in the same manner that infantrymen compete for the Expert Infantry Badge. The program was adopted based on a test developed by Church in the 4th Infantry Division. Across the Atlantic, Robert F. Elliott, a major in 1973, was chief of the medical section of the U.S. Army School of the Americas in Panama. His cadre and students regularly conducted civic action missions at a hamlet accessible only by a two-hour trip by motor launch. Some officers were assigned to the Historical Unit of the Surgeon General's Office. One of those, Capt. Robert J. Parks, MSC, completed the training volume of the Medical Department's World War II history, a project begun during the war. Published in 1974, it was one of the last volumes published in that series.[65]

Health facilities planning finally got its own specialty within the Pharmacy, Supply, and Administration Section, and by 1975 there were six officers in the field. Some served as consultants for U.S. allies. Lt. Col. Harold T. Heady, MSC, for example, provided guidance to the Guatemalan Army in 1967 in planning the construction of a 350-bed military hospital. Biomedical information, another emerging specialty, had sixty-one officers by 1975.[66]

A sizable number of MSCs in all specialties, especially operations, served as instructors at the Medical Field Service School. Lt. Col. John E. Persons, MSC, was commander of the officer student battalion during the height of the Vietnam protests, when three Medical Corps officers decided to show their antiwar sentiment by wearing their National Defense Service "Alive in '65" ribbons wrapped in black crepe. They ran into Persons, who introduced himself as their commander. "Oh my goodness. I see my supply sergeant has made a terrible mistake and given you the wrong ribbons," he said as he yanked the decorations from their uniforms. "I'll see that he gets you the right ones."[67]

Developments in the Scientific Specialties

There were 89 pharmacy officers on active duty in 1965, but there were still 161 graduate pharmacists serving as Army enlisted pharmacy technicians. External pressure continued on the department to discontinue using enlisted pharmacists, and the number of officers nearly doubled to 166 by 1972.

The trend toward greater sophistication produced a series of progressive steps over a five-year period beginning in 1966. Fitzsimons Army Medical Center,

Denver, Colorado, and Letterman Army Medical Center, Presidio of San Francisco, California, began additional residency programs in the general practice of pharmacy. Fitzsimons also started the first sterile product and intravenous additive program and the first unit dose program. Walter Reed began a program in oncology pharmacy. Letterman began a nuclear medicine pharmacy service, and Brooke Army Medical Center, Fort Sam Houston, Texas, established an oncology pharmacy for the preparation of antineoplastic agents. The Brooke initiative led to the administering of drugs by pharmacists, an expansion of pharmacy in a way that seemed to reach back to its apothecary roots.[68]

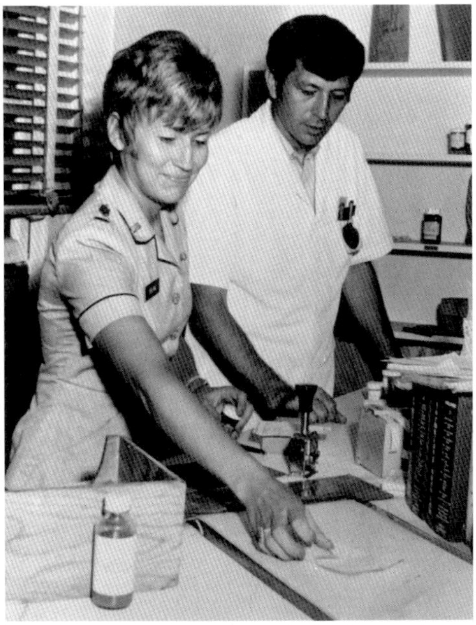

Military and civilian pharmacists at WRAMC, August 1974

The activities of individual pharmacy officers reflected the continued growth. In 1971 the American Pharmaceutical Association selected Capt. Glidden N. Libby, MSC, of the Fort Carson Army Hospital, as the first Army winner of the Military Section Literary Award. The establishment of the Health Services Command at Fort Sam Houston in 1973 included the appointment of Col. Robert B. Tweito, MSC, as the first pharmacy staff officer.[69]

In 1965, 579 officers, or 12.8 percent of the corps, were serving in the Medical Allied Sciences Section in six career fields: psychology, social work, podiatry, entomology, nuclear science, and laboratory science. The last group was the largest, with 213 officers in six specialties: bacteriology, biochemistry, parasitology, immunology, clinical laboratory, and physiology.[70] Regulatory demands, such as those generated by new environmental protection laws, as well as the steady advances in medical technology, added to the number of scientific specialty officers needed by the Army. By 1972 the Medical Allied Sciences Section had increased to 878 officers, or 17.1 percent of the corps. The largest increases occurred in laboratory sciences (from 213 to 286) and social work (from 148 to 260). A program of commissioning dental hygienists as military community oral health managers began in 1969. Six officers held this specialty in 1972, but it was soon abandoned.[71]

The underlying tension between the scientific and the administrative specialties resurfaced in 1972 when a group of nineteen MSC and Army Medical Specialist Corps (AMSC) officers assigned to the 2d General Hospital, Landstuhl, Germany, wrote the surgeon general requesting the transfer of all MSC scientific specialty officers to the AMSC. The Landstuhl group contended that scientific officers were at a disadvantage in a corps predominately com-

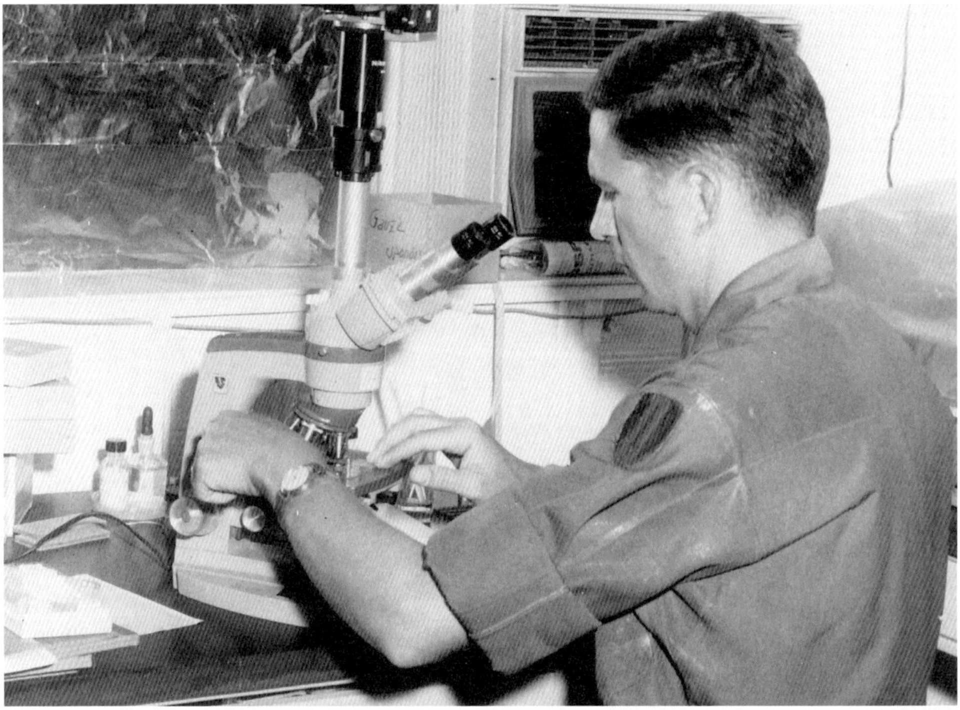

Parasitologist at the 9th Medical Laboratory, Long Binh, Vietnam, 1970

posed of administrative specialists, particularly since they often had administrative officers in their rating chain. Their main complaint was that they were expected to handle additional duties such as inspections, reports of survey, inventories, and other tasks that they believed were demeaning and detracted from their primary responsibilities. All in all, they thought that the AMSC would be a better match.

Col. Donald H. Hunter, MSC, chief of the Medical Allied Sciences Section, offered little comfort. While Hunter agreed that the Army had a responsibility to ensure the appropriate use of its officers, it also had the right to expect them to perform duties inherent in the military calling. Any discipline has an administrative component, and exposure to those duties was an advantage, since they must expect to shoulder managerial responsibilities as they increased in rank. Additionally, Hunter believed that efficiency reports written by administrative officers often helped, rather than hurt, scientific officers.[72]

Scientific specialty officers figured prominently in medical research and development. In 1973, a representative year, eighty-one MSC scientists were serving in research assignments, including seventy-one with doctorates; many conducted "bench work" research. Beginning in 1964, Lt. Col. Dan C. Cavanaugh, MSC, with Lt. Col. John D. Marshall, MSC, carried out landmark plague research at the Walter Reed Army Institute of Research (WRAIR), Washington, D.C. Cavanaugh's work in Vietnam with the WRAIR Medical

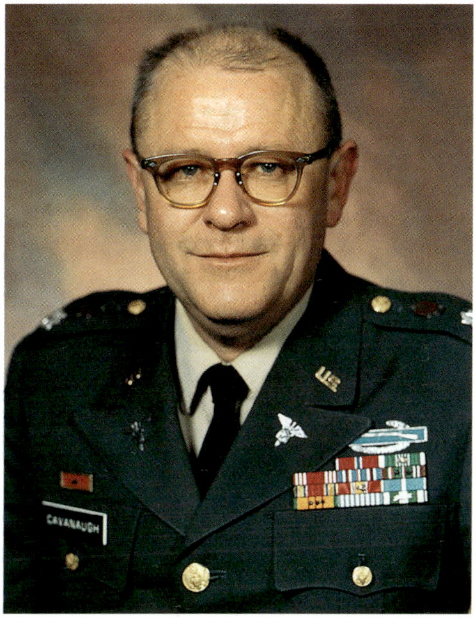

Colonel Cavanaugh

Research Team enabled him to explain the puzzling relationship of plague outbreaks to changes in climate. Cavanaugh was able to demonstrate from his research that hot weather interrupted the process of the disease's transmission via the flea vector, and this phenomenon reduced the incidence of plague during warmer periods.[73] Cavanaugh's international recognition resulted in his election to the Expert Panel for Bacterial Diseases of the World Health Organization. In 1965 Col. Robert B. Lindberg, MSC, a researcher at the U.S. Army Institute of Surgical Research, the Army's burn center at Fort Sam Houston, was credited, along with Arthur D. Mason, M.D., and Col. John A. Moncrief, MC, with developing sulfamylon cream, an antibacterial topical ointment. "Lindberg's butter" was very effective in reducing mortality from severe burns and became the standard treatment. Col. Sidney Gaines, MSC, a bacteriologist assigned to the WRAIR research team in Vietnam from 1965 to 1967, set up the Enteric Bacteriology Laboratory of the Pasteur Institute in Saigon. Other officers contributed to medical research staff work, and in 1970 Lt. Col. John N. Albertson, MSC, a microbiologist, was assigned as the executive officer for the Army's Director of Army Research. Colonel Hunter and Col. Robert J. T. Joy, MC, a research scientist on the staff of the director of defense research and engineering, championed the use of MSC scientists in senior management roles.[74]

MSCs did very well in those roles, but their success fueled criticism from those in the civilian research community who feared that civilian scientists were being denied opportunities for advancement in the Army. This issue became contentious and was finally resolved in 1977 when Lt. Gen. Richard R. Taylor met with some of the Medical Department's critics. Taylor made a distinction between the university-based researchers who were responsible for training teachers and investigators and the military medical researchers whose primary mission was not to teach but to solve military medical problems. That served as the rationale for reserving the senior administrative positions (such as commanders) for uniformed scientists. Civilian scientists were best utilized in science management positions (such as research department chiefs). Further, they had special promotion opportunities based solely on their scientific performance, not their specific position. Taylor's explanation was convincing, and the public criticism ended.[75]

In 1971 Lt. Col. Bruce F. Eldridge, MSC, led a team of Army and Air Force entomologists who studied the mosquito vectors of Venezuelan Equine

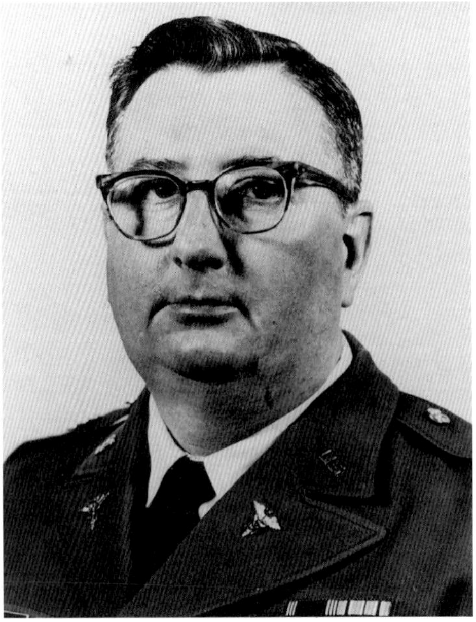

Colonel Camp

Encephalomyelitis (VEE) in several states of the southwest United States where the epidemic had spread from Mexico. VEE, a disease of horses and mules that causes an infection in man similar to influenza, had devastated the horse populations of Latin America and posed a considerable threat to the North American equine population. The work by Eldridge's team enabled the United States to control the spread of VEE using a vaccine developed by Col. Trygve O. Berge, MSC, of the U.S. Army Medical Research Institute of Infectious Diseases, Fort Detrick, Maryland. The risk to laboratory personnel who worked with virulent strains of disease in the institute's research programs had necessitated development of a vaccine for humans. In the early 1960s Berge had been the first test subject inoculated with the TC–50 vaccine for VEE.[76]

MSCs were major contributors to Army blood research. In 1972 Maj. James E. Spiker, MSC, chief of the blood bank at Brooke Army Medical Center, along with the center's medical staff, identified an extremely rare case of Rh negative blood antigen that contributed to the patient's hemolytic disease. In 1973 Maj. John H. Radcliff, MSC, chief of the Walter Reed Army Medical Center blood bank, and Lt. Col. Michael W. Hannagan, MC, developed an automated information storage and retrieval system for blood-banking operations.

Col. Frank R. Camp, MSC, was the Army's giant in blood banking. In 1964 Camp prepared a study with Col. William H. Crosby, MC, that resulted in the development of a fellowship program in blood banking as well as the establishment of the Blood Transfusion Research Division of the U.S. Army Medical Research Laboratory at Fort Knox, Kentucky. He directed the division from its beginning, and at the time of his retirement in 1974 he was the laboratory commander. Author of hundreds of articles, Camp pioneered important developments, including the extension of shelf life through freezing. He was the driving force behind Army blood banking throughout this period, and the Fort Knox blood bank center was named in his honor in 1983.[77]

A shortage of psychologists at the beginning of the period was representative of shortages nationally in various scientific specialties. As an example, in 1964 there were only 519 applicants for 1,750 civilian position vacancies advertised at the American Psychological Association's annual convention. The MSC continued its recruiting efforts, and the number of active duty psychologists increased from 95 in 1965 to 139 in 1972. Col. Charles A. Thomas, Jr., an Army Air Corps enlisted pilot in World War II who had been shot down over occupied France and helped to safety by the French Resistance movement, served as the psychology consultant to the surgeon general for eight years prior to his retirement in 1974, at which time he was also chief of the Medical Allied Sciences Section. Thomas concentrated on expanding the scope of psychologists from narrowly focused diagnostic and therapeutic functions. He recruited psychologists with industrial, educational, and counseling expertise in addition to clinical skills.[78]

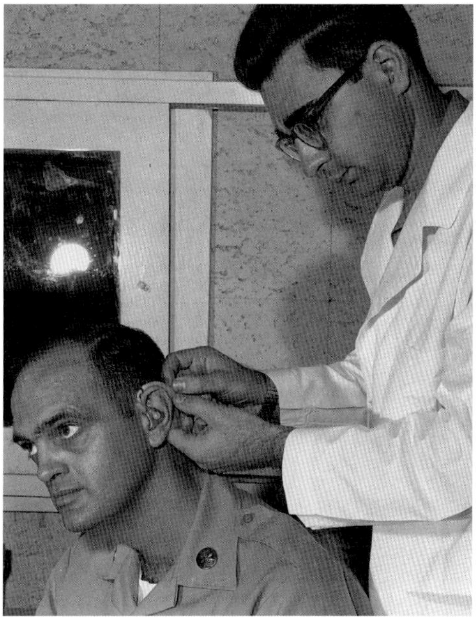

Audiologist at WRAMC fits patient with hearing aid, October 1969.

The graduate psychology student program continued, but was replaced in 1974 by the Health Professions Scholarship Program. Where the earlier program had been specifically set up for psychology students, the newer program was established for training physicians, and the inclusion of other health specialties was not guaranteed. The entry grade for Ph.D. psychologists increased to captain, and training opportunities in the Army improved. Walter Reed Army Medical Center established a counseling psychology internship in 1969 and a child psychology fellowship the following year. Psychologists were added to division medical battalions in 1972.

The first Army Behavioral Science Seminar was held in 1970. This meeting, attended by psychiatrists, psychologists, and social workers, nearly turned into a brawl because of dissension among the different groups. Psychologists were fearful of being tagged as junior psychiatrists, and social workers were fearful of threats to their autonomy. Col. Franklin Del Jones, MC, later the psychiatry consultant to the surgeon general, described the affair as "a good deal of acrimony, a great deal of hurt feelings, and a minimum of useful work." The surprising thing was that the annual meetings continued.[79]

The Army became increasingly sensitive during this period to the problems of hearing loss among soldiers, especially at large training installations. Its attention was concentrated by new Occupational Safety and Health Administration regulations for federal agencies, including the Army. A study in 1962 at Fort Jackson, South Carolina, had revealed severe hearing loss in over half of the weapons instructors. More alarming, a U.S. Army Medical Research and Development Command study in 1975 indicated that over half of combat arms soldiers had a documented hearing loss by their tenth year of service. An article in the *Washington Star* reported that some soldiers used cigarette filters because they were unable to obtain regular ear plugs.[80]

Audiologists emerged as the experts in the prevention and treatment of hearing loss. Commissioning required a master's degree in the specialty, and by 1972 there were twenty-five audiologists on active duty. Two officers were in doctoral programs, and Capt. Don W. Worthington, MSC, served on the Professional Services Board of the American Board of Examiners in Speech Pathology of the American Speech and Hearing Association.

Audiologists' functions were part curative and part preventive as they performed both in clinical care and hearing conservation roles. In their clinical duties they provided hearing aid evaluation, aural rehabilitation, and hearing testing. In their preventive role they were the principal action officers for the Army's hearing conservation program, a function under the supervision of the deputy chief of staff for personnel. In an unusual move, the Army directed in 1974 that 50 percent of audiologists' time would be spent in hearing conservation activities, a step taken to preserve their availability for the preventive function.[81]

In 1965 the American Podiatry Association recognized the Association of Podiatrists in Federal Service, headed by Maj. William A. Potter, MSC, as a component group of the national organization. It presented Potter its Gold Award for his exhibit on fatigue fractures of the foot at the annual meeting. By 1972 there were thirty-nine podiatrists on active duty, a doubling in seven years.

As Medicare expanded, podiatry became a much more lucrative practice because the government funded care for the elderly, a growing market in the aging American population. The change placed military salaries at a disadvantage in podiatry, just as in medicine. Podiatrists sought additional pay, but DOD would not support them because the Army was not experiencing difficulty in recruiting podiatrists as it was with physicians and dentists.[82] Podiatrists also complained about promotion opportunity, and General Hamrick instructed members of promotion boards to give podiatry and optometry officers a "fair shake."[83]

The department depended upon social workers who served as consultants to commanders and clinical staffs in addition to their patient care role, but it experienced a shortage at the beginning of this period. The 148 officers on active duty in 1965 were not sufficient to meet the need, but the Army was competing for social workers at a time when there were an estimated ten thousand openings nationwide, a product of President Johnson's Great Society and other social programs. The social work consultant, Lt. Col. Fergus T. Monahan, MSC, sought assistance from the heads of university programs, and the number on active duty increased to 260 in 1972. Demand continued to increase, and by 1974 his successor, Lt. Col. Paul F. Darnauer, MSC, had identified a requirement for 320 social work officers on active duty.[84]

Requirements for social workers were further increased in 1966 when the Army established the Army Community Service (ACS), a program of family support services at Army installations under the direction of the Army's deputy chief of staff for personnel. It was based on a concept developed by Lt. Col. William S. Rooney, MSC, who saw it as a way to meet the needs created by an Army that was more and more populated by married and single-parent soldiers. By August 1969 there were forty-one MSC social workers assigned to the expanded ACS programs. The ACS positions joined community hospitals, general hospitals, correctional facilities, and an "other" category (instructor, staff officer, and researcher) as practice fields for MSC social workers.[85]

Sanitary Engineering

The Sanitary Engineering Section went from 126 officers in 1965 to 188 in 1972. In 1858 Florence Nightingale had called for creation of "some specially qualified Sanitary Officer, medical or otherwise" to perform environmental science functions for military hospitals.[86] The Army fielded Nightingale's specialist over a century later, when the sanitarian was added to the division surgeon's staff. They joined sanitary engineers, as well as officers from another two specialties, entomology and nuclear medicine, who moved to this section in 1973 from the Medical Allied Sciences Section.[87]

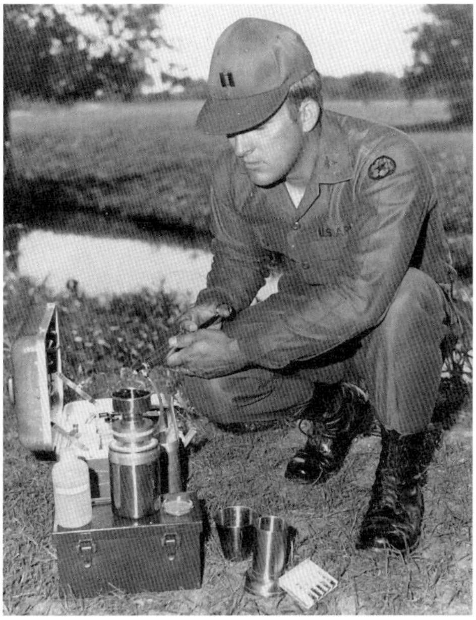

Sanitary engineer tests water at Medical Field Service School, 1970.

The number of entomologists on active duty increased from fifty-six in 1965 to eighty-three in 1972, with about a third of those officers serving overseas. They were active in tri-service coordination of pest control activities, efforts that had been made permanent with DOD's establishment of the Armed Forces Pest Control Board in 1962. Entomologists were essential for the Army's control of insect-borne disease, and the surgeon general emphasized the value of their role as consultants on the staffs of major headquarters in Southeast Asia.[88]

In 1973 sanitarians, by then called environmental science officers (ESO), replaced physicians in preventive medicine and occupational health positions at twenty installations in the United States. There they assumed responsibilities for water quality, food service sanitation, hospital sanitation and infection control, health education, waste disposal and environmental pollution, insect and rodent control, and epidemiological investigations. There were 106 ESOs on active duty by 1975, including the first female, 2d Lt. Karen M. Oxidine, MSC.

In 1971 Col. Bernard L. Goldstein, MSC, the chief of the Sanitary Engineering Section, instituted the Environmental Health Sciences and Engineering Education Program. It was established to commission 100 ESOs over a five-year period by enabling selected enlisted applicants to remain on active duty while they completed their baccalaureate degrees in environmental health. They were commissioned as second lieutenants upon graduation and incurred a four-year active duty obligation. Three classes entered the program either at the University of Texas or at East Tennessee State University beginning in 1972. The program ended in 1976 due to the post-Vietnam reductions. There had been about seven hundred applicants for seventy places. Sixty-nine students graduated, including thirty-two with honors.[89]

In 1972 Col. Hunter G. Taft, Jr., MSC, a sanitary engineer, became the first nonphysician to assume command of the U.S. Army Environmental Hygiene Agency, Aberdeen Proving Ground, Maryland. Twenty-two Sanitary Engineering Section officers were serving with the U.S. Army Medical Research and Development Command by 1973. By 1974 fifteen officers had completed doctoral training.[90] Over 90 percent of sanitary engineers were registered professional engineers, and about a fourth were diplomates of the Environmental Engineering Intersociety Board or certified by related specialty boards.

Colonel Taft, as chief of the section, made several recommendations in 1974 to General Haggerty on the career management of Sanitary Engineering Section officers, especially the use of senior officers. In 1974 there were requirements for two colonels, but because the Medical Department promoted without regard to specialty, six officers held that grade. This had necessitated the assignment of four colonels to staff and command positions typically filled by administrative specialty officers. Hunter observed that as officers in his section became more senior they had fewer demands upon their technical expertise but more requirements for general managerial skills. He suggested that officers who desired to remain in strictly technical positions accept the limitation of a twenty-year career as reservists on active duty. However, those who desired career status in the Regular Army would apply with the understanding that their careers would include generalist—or broadening—assignments. Officers in the latter category would have opportunities for troop duty to prepare them for more varied positions at higher rank. Taft's recommendation was not acted upon.[91]

Optometry

The number of optometrists on active duty increased from 174 in 1965 to 284 in 1972. Their role in Vietnam was important because Army studies reported that about a third of all soldiers needed eyeglasses, a need which also required manufacture of optical inserts for protective masks. Some officers served in roles outside of optometry. In 1965 Lt. Col. Robert W. Bailey, MSC, an optometrist, replaced a physician as the second commander of the U.S. Army Aeromedical Research Laboratory, a position he held until his retirement in 1976. Under Bailey's leadership the laboratory developed the SPH–4 aviator helmet, which provided greatly improved hearing protection for Army helicopter crew members.[92]

Because they were unwilling to volunteer for military service in sufficient numbers, male optometrists joined male physicians, dentists, veterinarians, and nurses as clinical specialties drafted for service in Vietnam.[93] The shortage prompted the surgeon general in August 1965 to ask for a draft of 100 optometrists. DOD did not grant that request, partly because some on the DOD staff feared it would build pressures to appoint optometrists in higher grades and to grant them special pay.[94]

As the surgeon general's staff wrestled with the pros and cons of a draft, Col. Billy C. Greene, MSC, the chief of the Optometry Section, stepped up recruiting efforts at the optometry colleges. However, the shortage worsened. By January

1966, for example, Fitzsimons Army Medical Center reported a half-year wait for routine eye examinations. The draft remained an option, and Hamrick concluded it was the only solution;[95] the Selective Service issued draft calls for optometrists, and four were drafted by mid-July. That precipitated a salute to military optometrists in a special issue of the *JAOA*.[96]

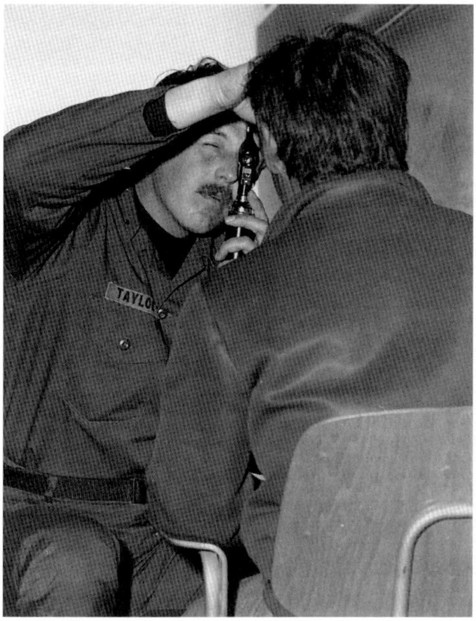

Army optometrist examines the eyes of an Eskimo patient at Chifornak, Togiak, Alaska, July 1973.

The grade of optometrists entering active duty became another point of contention. It was based on a formula in which optometrists received constructive service credit for active duty time based on the years spent in their training. The constructive credit rules helped, at least for a time. On the average, optometrists had six years of training, because the standard curriculum for the Doctor of Optometry degree required a minimum of two years of college plus four years of optometry school. Although some optometrists spent more than that in university training, they were credited with the average time spent by all optometry graduates. The six-year credit equated to two years beyond the standard college degree, and that counted for two years of service when they came into the Army.[97]

That was good enough during the height of the Vietnam War to ensure that optometrists would enter the Army as captains (the same as physicians, dentists, and veterinarians, whose training took longer),[98] because the Vietnam buildup had compressed to twenty-four months the minimum time in the Army necessary for promotion to captain. However, in 1971 the time-in-grade promotion criteria were lengthened, and optometrists reverted to entering active duty as first lieutenants. They viewed this as unfair treatment, pointing out that their peers commissioned in the Public Health Service entered at the equivalent grade of captain rather than first lieutenant, with the expectation of making the equivalent of full colonel much more rapidly than in the Army.

The lower entry grade contributed to a growing unhappiness among optometrists. A $100-per-month specialty pay authorized for optometrists in 1971 failed to improve matters since the pay was still not competitive with private practice.[99] Lt. Col. Budd Appleton, MC, the Surgeon General's ophthalmology consultant, did not help either when he wrote a "dear doctor" letter to his constituents in which he referred to optometrists as "medical assistants," a term which stirred up a small firestorm. Appleton later recanted and told his readers to "disregard the entire content" of the letter, but the damage had been done.[100]

In 1974 Lt. Col. Gene M. Bourland, MSC, chief of the Optometry Section, solicited optometrists for their concerns. He received heated responses. A letter from the former chief of the section, Colonel Greene, summed up the major complaints: lack of upward mobility, restrictions on Medical Department staff assignments, limited education opportunities, lack of control over the optical laboratory program, unrealistic workloads, low promotion rates, lack of properly trained technicians, and inequities in pay and constructive credit.[101]

Colonel Bourland believed morale was the lowest it had been in twenty years. Optometrists complained that their requests for consultations with physicians on the hospital staff were not treated seriously, and there were senior optometrists with "tunnel vision" who refused to deal with the unmet need for care. Optometrists were independent practitioners in private practice, but in the Army they reported to ophthalmologists, who treated them as ancillary personnel.[102]

Many officers complained about prohibitions against an expanded practice. They desired to fit contact lenses, conduct visual training, and perform developmental and low-vision work. They found, instead, that the Army compelled them to provide quantity rather than quality and forced them into "quickie refractions." Fort Bragg optometrists each performed twenty-seven exams a day. At the 196th Station Hospital in Belgium the figure was seventeen to twenty a day; many were complicated examinations for the older staff officers of the Supreme Headquarters, Allied Powers Europe. Officers at Fort Polk, Louisiana, averaged ten to fifteen minutes per patient, even though the professional rule of thumb was thirty.[103]

The level of unhappiness increased to the point that Lt. Gen. Richard R. Taylor, General Jennings' successor in 1974 as surgeon general, asked General Haggerty to personally review the situation. Haggerty flew to Denver, Colorado, where he met with Colonel Bourland and six other optometrists. The Denver group decided upon five basic recommendations: a reorganization of hospitals to make optometry an element separate from ophthalmology; entry grade constructive credit at the same rate as dentists and physicians; authority for the use of diagnostic drugs; enhanced promotion opportunity; and additional staffing for optometry clinics. Surprisingly enough, the group also recommended inclusion of MSC hospital executive officers in the rating chain of optometrists to improve their efficiency reports. Some of the complaints that surfaced in Denver were mundane but still irritating, including the desire for "Doctor" name tags on hospital white coats and parking privileges in the doctors' parking lot. The Ophthalmological Consultation Form was also a source of annoyance, because the title ignored optometry.[104]

The recommendations were on the chief's desk as the period ended. At least there was a truce with the ophthalmology consultant. Appleton wrote Bourland in a positive tone and asked that they work together for those objectives they mutually supported. Bourland responded in kind, expressing his appreciation for Appleton's cooperative attitude.[105]

Summary

The Medical Department's reorganization opened position opportunities for the MSC, principally in new staff jobs, but unanticipated consequences made the chief's job more difficult. The original idea of WORSAMS was to have a central medical organization reporting to the surgeon general, but that was not the reporting channel actually set up in 1973 for the commander of the Health Services Command. The surgeon general ended up in a weaker position than before the reorganization, especially since all the class II hospitals (medical centers) were transferred to the new command, and tensions between the two headquarters were inevitable. There was more discord than before between the surgeon general's statutory responsibility as chief of the Medical Department and his authority to accomplish that mission, a problem shared by the surgeon general's staff, including the MSC chief.

Position opportunities improved in some ways—the opening of the surgeon general's executive officer position was the greatest single advance yet. But the lack of command opportunities for MSC officers remained a source of contention. A fundamental difficulty with the command policy was its departure from contemporary practice in civilian life and the desires of many Army physicians to practice medicine, not administration. The department's objective since World War II had been to create a Medical Corps of competent clinicians. The emphasis on specialty training "on a par with the best in civilian medicine," to use General Heaton's words, had greatly influenced the assignment desires of Army physicians.[106]

Col. William Boyson concluded after he reviewed the results of his survey that an alternative would be for the department to designate administrative positions, including command, for MSC officers, but he believed that senior Medical Corps officers would balk.[107] The issue centered on power, and that went beyond any survey. The deputy secretary of defense memorandum in 1973 ordering the military medical departments to broaden opportunity for command was a major shift in Department of Defense policy regarding operational medical units. DOD did not prohibit the use of physicians in those administrative positions, but stipulated that the military departments closely monitor such assignments. Officers used to the command environment of the Army's divisional units and unschooled in the ways of Washington could not understand how the Medical Department simply ignored the order.

Medical supply operations in Vietnam, Korea, and Europe during this period underscored the primary need to maintain that system under medical control, operated by medical logisticians. The doctrinal point was confirmed in a series of Army and DOD studies after the disastrous experience of consolidating medical supply within the general supply system. The 1966 report of The Administrative Support Theater Army (TASTA) study underscored the point. The following year the Board of Inquiry on the Army Logistics System, the Brown Board, concluded that medical materiel must be managed by the Medical Department as a separate commodity, a recommendation that the Army enacted in 1968 with the establishment of Class VIII supply, a separate category. In 1970 the Besson Board, a DOD study of logistics support in Vietnam, concluded that the Army was the largest user of medical materiel and reasserted that the system had to be responsive to medical direction.[108]

The Besson Board raised an additional point, easily forgotten—the Army, as the nation's ground force, routinely encountered medical logistics requirements that exceeded the customary demands of military units, to include support for refugees, displaced persons, and United States foreign aid programs. The point was demonstrated in the post-hostilities support in the Dominican Republic and throughout the war in Vietnam, as MSCs at all levels supported those requirements as well as medical care for enemy POWs and civilians. The United States depended upon the broad range of MSC administrative and scientific specialties in order to carry out its national objectives in both conflicts.

Redoubling of the star wars in 1965 resulted in the establishment of a brigadier general billet in 1966. This was important for MSC officers, yet its impact extended beyond the Army. Executives of the American College of Hospital Administrators believed it marked a turning point in the recognition of all uniformed Medical Service Corps officers as professional administrators. While the corps had benefited in the past from civil sector advances in professional recognition, this time the roles were, for a moment, reversed.[109]

Notes

[1] Dominican Republic: Study, Capt Daniel G. McPherson, MSC, THU, OTSG, sub: The Role of the Army Medical Service in the Dominican Republic Crisis of 1965, 1968, USACMH; Jay Mallin, *Caribbean Crisis* (New York: Doubleday and Company, 1965), pp. 1–22; Bruce Palmer, Jr., "The Army in the Dominican Republic," *Army* 15 (November 1965): 43–44; Rpt, 82d Abn Div, sub: Medical Service Activities, 1 January–31 December 1965, 28 Feb 66, USACMH.

[2] Department title: Heaton engineered legislation in 1968 that changed the awkward title Army Medical Service back to Army Medical Department. 82 Stat. 170, 4 June 1968; Interv, Col Vernon McKenzie with Ginn, 20 Jun 84.

[3] Brown Board: Chief of Staff Memorandum (CSM) 65–276, sub: Board of Inquiry on the Army Logistics System, 17 Jun 65, and Heaton to Maj Gen Laurence A. Potter, MC, Surg, USAREUR, 12 Oct 66, RG 112, accession 69A–2604, Box 17/38, NARA-WNRC; OTSG, Spread Sheet, Board of Inquiry on the Army Logistics System (Format B), Recommendation V–IV, p. III–35, par. 15.b.(3), sub: Development of Logistics Doctrine, 17 Mar 67, DASG-MS.WORSAMS: Memo, Brig Gen William A. Knowlton, Secretary of the General Staff, OCSA, sub: Study: World-Wide Organizational Structure for Army Medical Support (WORSAMS), CSM 69–75, 28 Feb 69; Office memo, Col. R.P. Campbell, MC, XO, OTSG, sub: Organization of the WORSAMS Study Group, 22 Aug 69; Rpt, OTSG, sub: WORSAMS Final Report, vol. 1, sub: Executive Brief, and vol. 2, sub: Analysis of Alternative Structures, 20 Aug 70, all in JML; SG Conferences, 20 Jan and 17 Mar 67.

[4] HSC: U.S. Army HSC, GO 1, Assumption of Command, and GO 2, Unit Organized, 1 Apr 73, DASG-MS. Academy of Health Sciences: The new building, begun in 1970, had 416,000 square feet of space. Unpublished paper, Eugene A. Venable, sub: A Brief History of the Evolution of the United States Army Academy of Health Sciences from 1920–1980, 21 May 81, DASG-MS, hereafter cited as Venable, AHS History, 1981.

[5] Change: Memo, Heaton for Dir, P&T, sub: Organizational Relationship, 13 Aug 65, MSC-USACMH.

[6] Chief's concurrence: This was described as "jurisdictional cognizance," a nice example of bureaucratic obtuseness.

[7] Key assignments: Office of the Chief, MSC, policy statement 614–6–1, sub: Assignment of Medical Service Corps Officers, 1 Dec 70; Hamrick to Ginn, 22 Aug 88, both in DASG-MS. Control: SG Conference, 25 Mar 66. While the department blocked assignments of MSC officers to positions outside the department (other than selected exceptions), so did it resist encroachment by other branches. See OTSG Form 301, Memo, Lt Col Jon N. Harris, MSC, Spec Proj Off, sub: Detail of Women's Army Corps Officers and Warrant Officers to the AMEDD, 7 Sep 73, approved by Lt Gen Richard R. Taylor, TSG, DASG-MS. See also 10 U.S.C. sec. 3065 (e).

[8] Numbers: Rpt, Manpower Control Div, OTSG, Fiscal Year Reports, Medical Service Corps, FY 1959–67, hereafter cited as MSC Rpts FY 1959–67; Col William A. Hamrick, MSC, Ch, MSC, to Col Othmar Goriup, MSC, Ret., 3 May 66, both in DASG-MS; SG Conferences, 5 Nov 64, 30 Jul 65, 4 Jan and 15 Jul 66, and 11 Aug 67, USACMH; Hamrick, "Entering Second Half-Century of Service," *Medical Bulletin* (May 1968): 165, in JML.The Senior Student Program numbered 100 in 1965. Another thirty-five spaces covered "Excess Leave" for medical students, a program begun in 1960 in which officers were detailed from active duty to medical school. In 1972 Congress established the Health Professions Scholarship Program for graduate students in the health professions at civilian universities. It also funded construction of the Uniformed Services University of the Health Sciences, the DOD medical school in Bethesda, Maryland. The MSC provided spaces for all Army students in those programs.

[9] Aviators: SG Conferences, 25 Jun 65, 3 and 10 Feb 67, 1 Nov and 13 Dec 68, and 17 Jan 69. General Heaton said it was "another shining example of why we do not want our MSC splintered." Quoted words: Interv, Hamrick with Ginn, Washington, D.C., 7 May 83, DASG-MS.

[10] Warrants: DF, Brig Gen Conn L. Milburn, MC, Actg TSG, to DCSPER, sub: Employment of Warrant Officers as Medical Aviators in Air Ambulance Units, 23 Mar 65, RG 112, accession 69A–2603, Box 4/13, NARA-WNRC; Brig Gen Glenn J. Collins, MC, to DCSPER, sub: Army Aviator Requirements Study, 19 Apr 65, and DF CMT 2, TSG to DCSPER, sub: Officer and

Warrant Officer Aviation Requirements, 28 Oct 65, both RG 112, accession 68A–3358, Box 17/33, NARA-WNRC.

[11] Numbers: Lt. Gen. Leonard Heaton, TSG, Statement Before the Committee on Armed Services, United States Senate, 8 September 1966, including backup papers, hereafter cited as Heaton, SASC Statement, plus date; Rpts, Manpower Control Division, OTSG (DASG-RMM), sub: AMEDD Officer Strengths, 29 April 1977, and the MSC From Fiscal Year 1975–Fiscal Year 1981, undated, both in DASG-MS; SG Conferences, 27 Jan 67 and 15 Aug 69; *SG Report* 1970, pp. 77, 104, and 1972, pp. 74, 108. The Navy MSC figure includes warrant officers, physical therapists, occupational therapists, and dietitians—specialties not included in the Army MSC total. 1967 numbers: Engelman, *A Decade of Progress*, p. 96.

[12] Buck-up letters: Chief, MSC, Policy 623-105-2, sub: Buck-Up Letters, 1 Dec 1970, DASG-MS.

Accessions: SG Conferences, 15 July 1966, 27 January 1967, 21 June 1968, and 28 February and 21 March 1969; Hamrick to Goriup, 3 May 1966; MSC Newsletters, 1 May 1968, 1970-73; OTSG, DA, procurement brochures "The Optometry Officer," "Social Work Officers," "Laboratory Sciences Officers," etc., October 1968; Office of the Surgeon General, Department of the Army, full color brochure, "A Career of Distinction, The Medical Service Corps," 1971, all in DASG-MS.

[13] Medical Field Service School: In 1968 the school was operating 70 classrooms and 70 laboratories; had a staff of 225 officers, 250 enlisted personnel, and 15 civilians; and was training 11,500 resident and 15,000 nonresident students. Venable, AHS History, 1981.

[14] Hamrick's support: Hamrick to Lt Col Norman J. Edwards, DC, 15 Nov 65, RG 112, accession 68A–3358, Box 17/33, NARA-WNRC; SG Conference, 18 Jul 69. Education: Ch, MSC, Policy 350–219–2, sub: Long Term Civilian Schooling of Medical Service Corps Officers, Dec 70, DASG-MS. Quoted words: Interv, Hamrick with Ginn, Fort Sam Houston, Tex., 1 Nov 83, DASG-MS.

[15] Education: Hamrick to Goriup, 3 May 66; Heaton, SASC statement, 8 Sep 66; James G. Van Straten, "MSC Educational Legacy," *Medical Bulletin* (October 1970): 26–27; SG Conference, 16 Sep 66; Rpt, Manpower Br, Pers Div, Office of Pers Ops, HQDA, sub: Report on Educational Levels of Army Commissioned Officers, Nov 68, folder 270, box 17/18, MSC-USACMH; MSC Newsletter, 1972. In 1963 slightly over 23 percent of MSCs had master's degrees, 3.5 percent had academic doctoral degrees, and 2.68 percent had professional degrees at the doctoral level. Quoted words: Hamrick, "Entering Second Half-Century of Service," p. 165.

[16] Baylor course: MFR, Lt Col Nathaniel H. Pond, MSC, Pers & Trng Dir, OTSG, sub: DA Board to Review Army School System (Haines Board), 21 Jul 65; Rpt, Lt Col David G. Dougherty, MSC, Adjutant (Adj), BAMC, sub: Proceedings of the DA Board to Review Army Officer Schools, 3 Sep 65, both in RG 112, accession 69A–2606, Box 40/81, NARA-WNRC; MSC Newsletter, 1 May 1968; Memo, Maj C.W. Amidon, Jr., MSC, sub: Ph.D. Time Limit Proposed, 12 Dec 68, DASG-MS; J.V. Williams, Dean, Baylor Graduate School, to Col John P. Valentine, MSC, Dir, Dept of Admin, MFSS, 27 Dec 68, DASG-MS; SG Conferences, 18 May 65 and 15 Aug 69; HCAD, AHS, listing of Army-Baylor students, 1960–1976, undated, DASG-MS; Ch, MSC, Policy 350–219–1, sub: Attendance of MSC Officers at the U.S. Army–Baylor University Program in Health Care Administration, 1 Jul 72, DASG-MS.

[17] Junior officers: MSC Newsletter, 1 May 1970.

[18] Vietnam: Interv, Col W.R. LeBourdais, MC, CO, 67th Med Gp, Da Nang, Vietnam, with Maj Donald A. Lacey, CO, 27th Mil Hist Det, 6 Jun 69; Interv, Col Richard B. Austin, MC, Cdr, 44th Med Bde, with Lacey, Vietnam, 16 Jun 69.

[19] New program: Boone Powell, a Baylor vice president, said it was "too complex a matter." Powell, Baylor Univ, Dallas branch, to Valentine, Nov 67, DASG-MS.

[20] Courses: Rpt, Maj J.J. O'Hara, MSC, Adj, MFSS, sub: Information for DOD Study Group, April 1966, with Incl 4, sub: Officer Education Study; MFSS, Program of Instruction 6–8–C20, sub: Army Medical Department Basic Course (MSC Officers), April 1971, all in DASG-MS; Rpt, OTSG, sub: Professional Education and Training Committee Meeting, Main Navy Bldg, 14 Sep 66, RG 112, accession 69A–2606, Box 40/81, NARA-WNRC. Haines Board: Named for its head, Lt. Gen. Ralph G. Haines, Jr. Rpt, Brig Gen Charles B. Smith, sub: Department of the Army Board to Review Army Officer Schools, 19 Jul 65; MFR, Lt Col Nathaniel H. Pond, MSC, Pers & Trng

Dir, OTSG, same sub: 21 Jul 65; Rpt, Lt Col David G. Dougherty, MSC, Adj, BAMC, sub: Proceedings of the DA Board to Review Army Officer Schools, 3 Sep 65; Rpt, OTSG, sub: Professional Education and Training Committee Meeting, 14 Sep 66, all in RG 112, accession 69A–2606, Box 40/81, NARA-WNRC; Engelman, *A Decade of Progress*, pp. 128–31.

[21] Training: Memo, Maj Thomas H. Korte, MSC, for Col Adams, XO, OTSG, 25 Oct 73; Ch, MSC, Policy 350–10–1, sub: C&GSC/AFSC Selections, 1 Dec 70; Information paper, Maj Leopold, U.S. Army Military Personnel Center (MILPERCEN), sub: U.S. Army War College Corresponding Studies Program, 15 Aug 86, all in DASG-MS; "Medical Service Corps," *Newsletter of the U.S. Army Medical Department* 1 (October 1970): 19, JML. The MSC section of the department's *Newsletter* was used as the corps newsletter throughout its publication.

[22] Quoted words: Interv, Brig Gen John F. Haggerty, MSC, Ret., with Ginn, Washington, D.C., 7 May 83, DASG-MS.

[23] Assignments: Lt Gen Melvin Zais, CG, Third Army, to TSG, 21 May 73; 2d Ind to Lt Gen J. Hay, CG, XVIII Abn Corps, 7 Jun 73; 1st Ind to Col James B. Vought, Cdr, I Corps Support Command, sub: Experience, Quantity and Quality of Medical Service Corps Officers Assigned to the 55th Medical Group, 4 May 73; Haggerty, Ginn interv, 7 May 83, all in DASG-MS.

[24] Quoted words: Haggerty, Ginn interv, 7 May 83, DASG-MS.

[25] 3 percent: SG Conference, 3 May 68. DOD policy: Memo, Elliot L. Richardson, Sec Def, for Secs of the Mil Depts, sub: Strengths of Medical and Dental Officers, 2 May 73, DASG-MS.

[26] Substitution: MSC Newsletter, 1970; Memo, Col Robert P. Campbell, MC, XO, OTSG, for Brig Gen Jennings, DSG, sub: MC vs MSC as Executive to the Surgeon General, 23 Jul 69, DASG-MS, including quoted words; SG Conference, 25 Jul 69. Support: Written interv, Col William C. Luehrs, MSC, Ret., with Ginn, 5 Nov 84, DASG-MS. Luehrs was a pharmacist who served as an infantry officer in World War II and returned to active duty after the war as a Pharmacy Corps officer. He served as a medical battalion commander in Germany from 1961 to 1962 during the Berlin crisis and, an Army-Baylor graduate, as executive officer of three hospitals.

[27] Quoted words: William A. Boyson, "Why Doctors Get Out," *Journal of the Armed Forces* 105 (30 September 1967): 10. Also see Ltr to the editor, Clayton Yeutter, "MSC Officers at Helm of Medical Institutions?" *Journal of the Armed Forces* 105 (November 1967): 3.

[28] Quoted words: Memo, William P. Clements, Dep Sec Def, for Secs of Mil Depts, sub: Staff and Command Assignments of Health Professionals, 1 May 73, DASG-MS.

[29] Battalion command: The plan was briefed to the Surgeon General's Policy Council in February by Col. Knute Tofte-Nielsen, MSC, Ret. See Col Robert E. Adams, MSC, XO, OTSG, sub: Minutes of The Surgeon General's Policy Council Meeting, 20 Feb 73; Briefing Notes, Tofte-Nielsen, Doctrine and International Activities Br, OTSG, MSC, 12 Feb 73; Memo, Maj Gen Ralph L. Foster, SGS, OCSA, for TSG, sub: Combat Division Medical Structure Modification, 27 Jul 73; Msg, DA 271738Z Jul 73, same sub; Tofte-Nielsen, Ginn interv, 23 Oct 84. The final policy was reaffirmed by Brig. Gen. Surindar Bhaskar, DC, Dir Pers, OTSG, in 6th Ind to Ltr, sub: Nomination for the 7th Medical Battalion Commander (19 February 1975), 19 May 75, all in DASG-MS.

[30] Insignia: Ltr, Lt Col John A. Kneepkins, MSC, to Hamrick, 19 Aug 65, RG 112, accession 68A-3358, Box 17/33, NARA-WNRC; Hamrick to Ginn, 22 Aug 88, DASG-MS. Society: Col Richard F. Neitzel, MSC, COS, 8th Med Cmd (Prov), to Ginn, 2 Nov 83, DASG-MS.

[31] 1962: Spurred by Kennedy's Secretary of Defense, Robert S. McNamara.

[32] Branch chiefs: Hewes, *From Root to McNamara*, pp. 364, 406. Loss of power: Maj Gen V.P. Mock, SGS, CSM 64–127, sub: Technical Missions, Structure and Career Development, 31 Mar 64, hereafter cited as CSM 64–127, 31 Mar 64; General Morrison notes that as TSG's representative to the study committee, he was able, with Heaton's support, to preserve the basic organization of OTSG, which would have been transferred from DCSLOG to DCSPER staff supervision. Morrison to Ginn, 18 Aug 88.

[33] TECSTAR: SG Conferences, 10, 15, and 25 Jun 65; General Harold K. Johnson, CSA, "Technical Career Structure of the Army," *Army Information Digest* (November 1964): 5–8; CSM 64–127, 31 Mar 64; DF, Col Walter M. Vann, GS, Dep Chm, TECSTAR Working Group, sub: Project TECSTAR, 19 May 64; Memo, Col Charles H. Moseley, Dir, Pers & Trng, OTSG, for TSG, sub: Project TECSTAR, 11 Jun 65; Memo, Col Ralph G. LeMoon, MSC, Ch, Spec Proj Off,

OTSG, for Dir, Pers and Trng, OTSG, and Ch, MSC, sub: Technical Missions, Structure and Career Development (TECSTAR), 16 Jul 64; DF CMT 2, Heaton to DCSPER, sub: Project TECSTAR Outline Plan, 30 Jul 64; Memo, Col Mahlon E. Gates, GS, DCSPER, for Dir Mil Pers, sub: Formats A&B, TECSTAR, and Memo, Moseley for TSG, sub: Current Status of Project TECSTAR, 30 Sep 64; Memos, LeMoon, sub: TECSTAR, 6, 7 Oct 64; Memo, Lt Col Leigh F. Wheeler, Sr., MSC, Ch, Directives & Pol Br, OTSG, sub: TECSTAR, 7 Oct 64; Memo, Moseley for Heaton, sub: TECSTAR, 22 Oct 64; Memo, Moseley, sub: Status Report on AMEDS [Army Medical Service] Participation in TECSTAR, 23 Nov 64; Ray E. Brown to Heaton, 19 Jul 65; Ltr, Heaton to Maj Gen George M. Powell, MC, CG, BAMC, and twenty-four other addressees, 22 Jul 65, including statement, sub: Position of the Surgeon General on Project TECSTAR; Heaton to Comptroller of the Army (COA) and DCSPER, sub: COA Recommendations on TECSTAR (drafted by LeMoon), 4 Aug 65; Memo, Moseley for TSG, sub: Project TECSTAR, 13 Aug 65; Col Arnold L. Ahnfeldt, MC, Dir, THU, OTSG, to Heaton, 24 Aug 65; Brig Gen Charles A. Corcoran, SGS, CSM 65–576, sub: Project TECSTAR, 22 Nov 65, hereafter cited as CSM 65–576; Hamrick, Ginn interv, 7 May 83; Benade, Ginn interv, 25 Jan 84, all in DASG-MS.

[34] Heaton: SG Conference, 30 Jul 64; DF, Heaton to DCSPER, sub: TECSTAR Detailed Plan, 21 Jun 65 (drafted by Col LeMoon and called "a magnificent paper" by Heaton); Memo, Heaton for COA, sub: COA Recommendations on TECSTAR, 4 Aug 65, both in DASG-MS. Quoted words: DF, Heaton to DCSPER, sub: CSA Recommendations on Project TECSTAR, 30 Jul 64, DASG-MS. Speak out: Heaton to Powell, 22 Jul 65.

[35] Benade: "Indispensable Man," *Army Times*, 12 June 1963. Also see "Col. Cited, Picked for Post in USAREUR," *Stars and Stripes*, 6 June 1966; OTSG News Clip, 10 Jul 62, "Colonel Benade is 'Mr. Big' in Armed Forces Pay Studies," extracted from *Army, Navy, Air Force Journal and Register*, 7 July 1962, DASG-MS. Richards: See Benade, Ginn interv and Morrison, Ginn interv, 7 May 83.

[36] Quoted words: Hamrick to Col Ralph D. Arnold, MSC, XO, HQ Eighth Army, 14 Jun 65, RG 112, accession 68A–3358, Box 17/33, NARA-WNRC.

[37] Ray Brown: DF, Heaton to DCSPER, sub: TECSTAR Detailed Plan, (drafted by Lt Col Lewis Huggins, MSC, Spec Proj Off, OTSG), 21 Jun 65 with 24 incls, including: Rpt, Ray E. Brown, sub: Implications of the Proposal by the TECSTAR Study Group to the Army Medical Care Program, 18 Jun 65; Studies, sub: Codification of MSC Officers' Positions and Trends in Civilian Health Service and Their Relationship to the Army Medical Service; and DA Form 1598, sub: TECSTAR Detailed Plan; Hamrick, Ginn interv, 7 May 83, all in DASG-MS. Brown's active role in support of military hospital administration was later commemorated by the Association of Military Surgeons of the United States, which established the Ray E. Brown Award for "outstanding accomplishments in Federal Health Care Management."

[38] Quoted words: Brown to Heaton, 19 Jul 65; Brown rpt, 18 Jun 65.

[39] Quoted words: Heaton to DCSPER, 21 Jun 65.

[40] Quoted words: CSM 65–576. TECSTAR was not to "be construed as DA policy nor are its conclusions or recommendations to be considered as approved."

[41] TECSTAR and stars: Col Arnold L. Ahnfeldt, MC, Dir, THU, to Heaton, 24 Aug 65, DASG-MS.Ten branches: Quartermaster, Dental, Transportation, Chemical, Adjutant General, Finance, Veterinary, Military Police, Judge Advocate General, and Chaplain Corps. MFR, LeMoon, sub: H.R. 11488, 89th Congress, A Bill "To Authorize the Grade of Brigadier General in the Medical Service Corps of the Regular Army, and for Other Purposes," 6 Dec 65, DASG-MS.

[42] MSC star: SG Conferences, 22 Jul, 12 Aug, and 16 and 30 Sep 66; Benade, Ginn interv, 25 Jan 84; Interv, Hamrick with Dwight D. Oland, 5 Nov 79, USACMH; Hamrick, Ginn interv, 7 May 83; McKenzie, Ginn interv, 20 Jun 84; Summary sheet, Benade, sub: Request for Allocation of One Brig. Gen. Space to the Medical Service Corps, 19 Apr 61; Cyrus R. Vance, Sec Army, to Rep Carl Vinson, Chm, HASC, 4 Sep 62; Rep Durwood G. Hall, Missouri, to TSG (DSG, Maj Gen McGibony), 13 Oct 65; McGibony to Hall, 28 Oct 65; CMT 2, Col David Penson, AGC, Comptroller, TAGO, 25 Oct 65, to DF, Lt Col Louis J. Prost, GS, Ch, Gen Off Br, DCSPER, sub: H.R. 11488. . ., 19 Oct 65; Memo, Heaton for DCSPER, same sub. (includes draft DA rpt), 3 Dec 65; MFR, LeMoon, same sub., 6 Dec 65; DF, Prost, same sub. (includes DA rpt), to TAG, 11 Jan 66, with CMT 2 to Col LeMoon, Spec Proj, OTSG, 12 Jan 66; Summary sheet, Maj Gen J.C. Lambert, TAG, sub., DA Report on H.R. 11488, 89th Cong., 2d sess., 25 Jan 66; Memo, Stanley

R. Resor, Sec Army, for CSA, sub: Statutory Grade Authorizations for Specific Positions, 1 Apr 66; Memo, Gen Creighton W. Abrams, Acting CSA, for Sec Army, same sub, 15 Apr 66; Resor to L. Mendel Rivers, Chm, HASC, 29 Apr 66; Hamrick to Col Othmar F. Goriup, MSC, Ret., 3 May 66; Statement, Heaton before the House Committee on Armed Services, sub: H.R. 11488, 20 Jul 66; Heaton, SASC statement, 8 Sep 66; MFR, LeMoon, sub: House Armed Services Subcommittee no. 1, Hearings on H.R. 420 and H.R. 11488, both 89th Congress, 20 Jul 66, all in DASG-MS; PL 89–603, 24 Sep 66; "Grade of Brigadier General—Medical Service Corps," *Congressional Record, House of Representatives* (15 August 1966): 18453–4, D757–8; Interv, Hamrick with Col Ernest J. Sylvester, MSC, AWC and USAMHI Senior Officers Oral History Program, Feb 84, USAMHI. Hays: McKenzie, Ginn interv notes, 17 May 83, DASG-MS.

[43] Support: Hamrick, Ginn interv, 1 Nov 83. Heaton said the MSC was "a very important cog in our everyday activities." Heaton, McLean interv, 7 Dec 78. Quoted words: Heaton to DCSPER, 3 Dec 65; Heaton, SASC statement, 8 Sep 66.

[44] Frightened: Hall to McGibony, 13 Oct 65. Philbin's bill, H.R. 11488, was identical to H.R. 11727 submitted by Congressman L. Mendel Rivers, South Carolina, chairman of the House Armed Services Committee.

[45] Stars: It was also a zero-sum game: the SASC had a limit of 475 active duty flag officers for all the Services.

[46] Abrams' support: Abrams to Sec Army, 15 Apr 66.

[47] Quoted words: Hamrick, Oland interv, 5 Nov 79.

[48] Testimony: Heaton, when questioned, supported the bill in testimony McGibony called "superb." As Hamrick recalled, "it was very obvious when the congressmen and the senators began to ask him questions that he was in favor of it." Heaton said he justified his request for a star based on the "scope and magnitude" of the chief's position. SG Conference, 16 Sep 66; Hamrick, Oland interv; Heaton, SASC statement, 8 Sep 66.

[49] Star billet: DF, Col Robert P. Campbell, MC, XO, OTSG, to Gen Off Br, DCSPER, sub: General Officer Job Description, 23 Nov 66, RG 112, accession 69A–2604, Box 19/38, NARA-WNRC. Quoted words: Hamrick, Oland interv.

[50] Stars: Morrison to Col John Lada, MSC, 12 Jul 72, including Fact Sheet, sub: U.S. Army Medical Service Corps, 1972, with GO and MSC figures based on OPO STAT REPT–7, 31 Dec 71, folder 40, box 4/18, MSC-USACMH.

[51] Study: Study, Lt Col John W. Bullard, MSC, DASG-MS, sub: Requirements for Medical Service Corps Branch General Officers, 1970, DASG-MS.

[52] Fuqua: H.R. 15201, *Congressional Record, House of Representatives* (30 May 1972), pp. 1284 and 19118; U.S. Congress, House, *Digest of Public General Bills and Resolutions*, 30 May 1972, 92d Cong., 2d sess., Part 11: E–343. Quoted words: Morrison to Lada, 12 Jul 72.

[53] Numbers: CMT 2, Col Griffin, MC, XO, OTSG, to DCSPER, sub: Manpower and Personnel Studies, 30 Sep 65, RG 112, accession 68A–3358, Box 17/33, NARA-WNRC; MSC Rpts FY 1959–67; Rpt, DASG-RM, sub: MSC Requirements, Authorized, Actual, FY 1976–81, both in DASG-MS. A presidentially directed commission required DOD to identify positions it could convert from military to civilian. OTSG reported very little potential in the MSC administrative specialties. Memo, Lyndon Johnson for Robert S. McNamara, Sec Def, 1 Aug 65, included in DCSPER Rpt, sub: Military-Civilian Substitutability Staff Study, 21 Aug 65, and DF, Maj Gen James T. McGibony, Actg TSG, same sub, 1 Nov 65 with Staff Study, OTSG, sub: Feasibility of Converting Medical Service Corps Officer Positions to Civilian Positions, 30 Oct 65, RG 112, accession 69A–2603, Box 4/13, NARA-WNRC; SG Conferences, 29 Mar and 3 May 68.

[54] Automated data systems: SG Conference, 13 Jan 67; OTSG Lessons Learned interv, Maj Max E. Hoyt, MSC, 7 Sep 67, USACMH; Notes of discussion, Col James R. Young, MSC, Cdr, U.S. Army Patient Administration Systems and Biostatistics Activity, with Ginn, 25 Sep 84, DASG-MS.

[55] Comptroller: SG Conference, 8 Sep 67; Unpublished article, Col Milton C. Devolites, MSC, Ret., "The Organization of the Resources Management Directorate, Office of The Surgeon General, Department of the Army," 3 Oct 84; Rpt, Syracuse University, sub: Army Comptrollership Program, 1991; Fact Sheet, Syracuse University, sub: Synopsis of the Army Comptrollership Program (draft), 1990, all in DASG-MS; MSC Newsletter, 1970. The consoli-

dation included Nepthune Fogelberg's Budget Division and Isaac Cogan's Programs Coordination Office.

[56] Inexperience: CMT 2, TSG to ACSFOR, 16 Mar 67, including 32d Medical Depot Opnl Rpt, 10 Nov 66, and TAG Ltr, 2 Feb 67, RG 112, accession 70A–2772, Box 12/43, NARA-WNRC; Interv, Col Charles C. Pixley, MC, Cdr, 68th Med Gp, with McPherson, Vietnam, 23 Jun 67; Wier, McPherson interv, 17 Jun 67; Interv, Col. W.R. LeBourdais, MC, with Lacey, 1969; OTSG Lessons Learned interv, Col Jesse N. Butler, MSC, Ch, Med Supply Div, 14 Nov 68, all in USACMH.

[57] Quoted words: Col Marvin A. Ware, MSC, PS&O, OTSG, in Rand, OTSG interv.

[58] Assessment: Butler, Lessons Learned interv. King: Notes of telephone interv, CW4 W.B. King, Ret., with Ginn, 8 Feb 92, DASG-MS.

[59] MAST: *SG Report*, 1970, p. 121; Information paper, OTSG, sub: MAST, Dec 84, DASG-MS.

[60] Hospital administration: Neuhauser, *Coming of Age*, p. 52.

[61] The laws: PL 89–749, The Comprehensive Health Planning and Public Health Services Amendments of 1966, 80 Stat. 1180, linked hospital construction with regional planning. PL 92–603, The Professional Standards Review Organization Act of 1972, 86 Stat. 1329, set up local agencies to pass on the appropriateness of hospital admissions. PL 92–666, The Health Maintenance Organization Act of 1973, 87 Stat. 914, provided start-up funds for HMOs, insurance plans that provide prepaid benefits to subscribers using providers contracted or owned by the plan.

[62] Changes: See Neuhauser, *Coming of Age*, pp. 66–71; Interv, Richard J. Stull, ACHA President, 1972–78, with Lewis E. Weeks, 9 Apr 80, American Hospital Association, copy in AHA Library, Chicago; Charles V. Letourneau, "Hospital Administration: A True Profession," *Hospital Administration* 13 (Winter 1968): 51–67. Meeting topics: News release, OTSG, sub: Hospital Administrators Plan for the Future, 9 May 66, RG 112, accession 70B–2773, Box 38/55, NARA-WNRC.

[63] ACHA: SG Conference, 16 Sep 66; Stull, Weeks interv; Lt Col Glenn R. Willauer, MSC, USAF, Regent's Newsletter, June 1989, DASG-MS.

[64] Operations officers: Interv, Col Robert D. Pilsbury, MC, with Lacey, 1 May 69. Actions: Hamrick to Lt Col William A. Bost, MSC, 1 Jun 65, and Lt Col John A. Kneepkins, MSC, to Hamrick, 19 Aug 65, RG 112, accession 68A–3358, Box 17/33, NARA-WNRC; Brig. Gen. Manley C. Morrison, "Medical Service Corps," *Newsletter of the U.S. Army Medical Service* 1 (October 1970): 19.

[65] EFMB: Interv, Col Roy S. Church, MSC, Ret., with Ginn, Fort McPherson, Ga., 9–10 Nov 83; Maj Gen T. McGibony, Actg TSG, to DCSPER, sub: Expert Field Medical Badge, 2 Nov 65, RG 112, accession 687A–3358, Box 17/33, NARA-WNRC. Panama: Stanley S. Johnson, "Lab for Living," *Soldiers* 28 (July 1973): 22–25. History: Robert J. Parks, *Medical Training in World War II*, volume in the series Medical Department of the United States Army in World War II (Washington, D.C.: Office of the Surgeon General, Department of the Army, 1974).

[66] Facilities planning: "Army Officer Aids Plans for Guatemalan Hospital," *Southern Command News*, 5 January 1968, DASG-MS.

[67] Ribbon: Called the "Alive in '65" ribbon because it was issued to all military personnel beginning in 1965. Quoted words: Notes of discussion, Lt Col John E. Persons, MSC, Ret., with Ginn, Dustoff Association Meeting, San Antonio, Tex., 1 Mar 86, DASG-MS.

[68] Pharmacy: J.B. Lischke to Sen Vance Hartke, 14 Aug 65, and Col Herschel E. Griffin, MC, XO, OTSG, to Office of the Chief of Legislative Liaison (OCLL), sub: Draft of Reply to Sen. Hartke on Behalf of Mr. J.B. Lischke, 7 Sep 65, RG 112, accession 68A–3558, Box 17/33, NARA-WNRC; MSC Newsletter, 1970–73; Heaton, SASC statement, 8 Sep 66; Lt Col Alfred W. Gill, MSC, Ch, Pharm Br, AHS, Lesson Plan 37–365–320, sub: History and Traditions of Army Pharmacy, 1986, hereafter cited as Gill, Army Pharmacy, both in DASG-MS; SG Conference, 30 Jun 67; Scott C. Martin, "Oncology Pharmacy Residency at Walter Reed Army Medical Center," *Military Medicine* 153 (August 1988): 41.

[69] Libby and Tweito: MSC Newsletter, June 1971; Gill, Army Pharmacy.

[70] MAS numbers: MSC Rpts, FY 1959–67, DASG-MS; *SG Report*, 1972, p. 110.

[71] Oral health: SG Conferences, 31 Jan and 6 Jun 69.

[72] Landstuhl group: Capt David J. Anderson, MSC, et al., 2d Gen Hosp, to TSG, sub: Optimum Utilization of Allied Science Personnel in the Army Medical Department, 27 Sep 72,

with comments to Ch, MSC, including Col Donald H. Hunter, MSC, Ch, MAS, 9 Nov 72, DASG-MS.

[73] Plague: Dan C. Cavanaugh, "Specific Effect of Temperature Upon Transmission of the Plague Bacillus by the Oriental Rat Flea, *Xenopsylla Cleopis*," *American Journal of Tropical Medicine and Hygiene* 20 (March 1971): 264. The WRAIR team served in Vietnam from 1963 to 1971; see Albertson, MSCs in Medical Research and Development.

[74] R&D: MSC Newsletters, 1970–73; Engelman and Joy, *Two Hundred Years of Military Medicine*, pp. 41–48; Rpt, THU, OTSG, sub: Chronology: U.S. Army Contributions to Civilian Medicine, 1971; Ltr, Lt Gen Charles Pixley, TSG, sub: Letter of Instructions to the Nominating Board Considering Officers for Appointment as Assistant Chief, Medical Service Corps, with incls, 6 Oct 80; Curriculum vitae, Col Sidney Gaines, 1969, all in DASG-MS; Joseph Israeloff, "Victories in Army Medicine," *Army Digest* (July 1970): 26. Cavanaugh: Dan C. Cavanaugh et al., "Plague," in Andre J. Ognibene and O'Neill Barrett, Jr., *General Medicine and Infectious Diseases*, volume in the series Internal Medicine in Vietnam (Washington, D.C.: Office of the Surgeon General and U.S. Army Center of Military History, 1982), pp. 167–97; Interv, Cavanaugh with Maj Eric G. Daxon, MSC, Washington, D.C., 17 Apr 85, DASG-MS; Engelman and Joy, *Two Hundred Years of Military Medicine*, p. 40.

[75] Dispute: See account in Albertson, MSCs in Research and Development. The controversy began in 1974. Over eighty letters had been written to Congress at the time of the meeting with General Taylor, and articles were appearing in journals and newspapers. For example, see *American Society for Microbiology News (ASM News)*, March, June, and August 1976, and *U.S. Medicine*, 15 May 1976. A series of actions were interpreted as "the gradual erosion of civilian scientists in positions of authority." "Army Surgeon General Acts Against Civilian Scientists," *ASM News* 42 (March 1976): 133. The Medical Department was said to have a "management philosophy which downgrades the role of civilian scientists." "Civilian Scientists," *ASM News* 42 (June 1976): 350.

[76] VEE: Col Trygve 0. Berge, MSC, draft section, sub: Virology and Immunology, 1958 MSC History Project, p. 17, DASG-MS; MSC Newsletters, 1970–73.

[77] Spiker: Col. James Spiker, MSC, to Ginn, 5 Aug 88, DASG-MS. Camp: Col John P. Canby, MC, Cdr, USAMEDDAC, Fort Knox, to TSG, sub: Naming of the Blood Bank Center, USAMEDDAC, Fort Knox, 2 Aug 83, with CMT 2, Brig Gen France F. Jordan, Ch, MSC, 7 Oct 83, DASG-MS; Engelman and Joy, *Two Hundred Years of Military Medicine*, p. 41.

[78] Psychology: Brochure, OTSG, "Graduate Student Program in Clinical Psychology, Counseling Psychology, Experimental Psychology," Oct 68; Unpublished paper, Harold D. Rosenheim, Ph.D., "A History of the Uniformed Clinical Psychologist in the U.S. Army," presented to the American Psychological Association (APA), Montreal, 2 Sep 80, and Rosenheim to Ginn, 18 Sep 84; Col Robert S. Nichols, Ph.D., MSC, Dir, Human Resource Div, U.S. Army War College, to Haggerty, 12 Aug 74; Col Charles A. Thomas, MSC, Ret., "Contributions of and Challenges Faced by AMEDD Psychology: 1950's–1970's," Proceedings of the 1982 AMEDD Psychology Symposium, 14–19 Nov 82, Fort Gordon, Ga., DASG-MS. Thomas: Lt Col Donald D. Sammis, USAF, Asst Air Attache, U.S. Embassy, Paris, to Thomas, 28 Feb 74; Thomas to Mlle. Adrienne Joffre, 25 Mar 74; OTSG Form 576, Col Charles A. Thomas, MSC, sub: Report on Leave Activities, 13 Jun 74; D. Lucibello, Associacion Republicaine des Anciens Combattants, to Thomas, 26 Mar 1976; Thomas to Ginn, 24 Feb 1988, with enclosures; Notes of fonecon, Ginn with Ms. Diana Brooks, U.S. Embassy, Paris, 19 Apr 88, all in DASG-MS. Thomas was flying as a bomber pilot with the Royal Canadian Air Force. Wounded, he was hidden in Paris by Mlle. Adrienne Joffre, a cousin of Marshal Joseph Joffre, the leader of the French delegation to the United States in 1917 that had requested U.S. help in their war with Germany. In June 1974 the City of Paris invited Thomas to ceremonies honoring the French Resistance on the thirtieth anniversary of the liberation of France. He received the Silver Medal of the City of Paris.

[79] Quoted words: Col. Franklin Del Jones, MC, "Behavioral Sciences in a Changing Army," in Jones, David L. Willard, and Barry N. Blum, "Proceedings of AMEDD Behavioral Sciences Seminar," FAMC, 23 Mar 79, Document ADA 87842, Defense Technical Information Center (DTIC), Defense Logistics Agency, Cameron Station, Va., hereafter cited as Jones, "Proceedings," 1979.

[80] Audiology: Fact sheet, OTSG, sub: Audiologists and the U.S. Army, Jul 71; Briefing, Maj Roy K. Sedge, Ph.D., MSC, TSG Audiology Consultant, for Brig Gen J. Young, Ch, MSC, 8 Feb 86;

Ltr, Maj Gen. Verne L. Bowers, TAG, sub: Establishment and Utilization of Audiologist (MOS 3360) Positions in Hearing Conservation Programs, Feb 72, hereafter cited as TAG Ltr, Hearing Conservation, 1972; Young to Sedge, 29 Apr 79, concerning draft Memo for TSG, sub: Utility of 68Ms (Audiologists) for Hearing Conservation and Clinical Programs, with five incls; MSC Newsletter, 1972, all in DASG-MS; TSG to Rep Paul G. Rogers, 15 Sep 69, response to 21 Aug ltr, RG 112, accession 72A–3501, Box 19/55, NARA-WNRC; AR 40–5, "Health and Environment," 24 Sep 74, PL; Frank Murray, "Soldiers Deafened by Weapons' Roar," *Washington Star*, 21 August 1969.

[81] Hearing conservation: TAG Ltr, Hearing Conservation, 1972; AR 40–5.

[82] Special pay: Seward P. Nyman, D.Sc., Exec Dir, APA, to Heaton, 22 and 23 Sep 65, and Heaton's response, 8 Oct 65, RG 112, accession 68A–3358, Box 17/33, NARA-WNRC; Shirley C. Fisk, M.D., Dep Asst Sec Def (Health and Medical) to Rep Charles S. Grubser, 16 Feb 66, and Heaton to Sen George C. Murphy, 24 Feb 66, both responses to Ltrs, Ronald F. Noble, D.P., Cupertino, Calif., 27 Jan and 8 Feb 66, RG 112, accession 69A–2604, Box 19/38, NARA-WNRC.

[83] Boards: "Look at these people very closely. Give them an opportunity." Hamrick, Sylvester interv.

[84] Social work: Lt Col Anthony C. Mastrolia, MSC, P&T Div, OTSG, to Lt Col Charles L. Franklin, MSC, Office of Surgeon, HQ, Fourth Army, 30 Dec 65, RG 112, accession 68A–3358, Box 17/33, NARA-WNRC; Matthew D. Parrish, "The Changing Field of Army Psychiatry," 1968, in Franklin D. Jones, ed., *M.D. Parrish, M.D.: Collected Papers, 1955–1970* (Washington, D.C.: Office of the Surgeon General, Department of the Army, 1981), Doc ADA–108069, DTIC; SG Conferences, 18 Jun 65 and 22 Jul 66; Rpt, Ross, USMEDCOMV, sub: AMSAR CY 1971, USACMH; Rpt, Academy of Health Sciences (AHS), U.S. Army, sub: Current Trends in Army Social Work, 4–8 Mar 74, Doc ADA–058124, DTIC. Consultants: Brochure, OTSG, "Social Work Officers in the Medical Service Corps," Oct 68, DASG-MS.

[85] ACS: Lt Col Donald A. Myles, MSC, to Ginn, 15 May 83; Myles, The Army Community Services Program, chapter in "A Survey of Community Service Centers: Welfare Problems, Services, Personnel and Resources," Ph.D. dissertation, Catholic University of America, Washington, D.C., 1970; Lt Col William S. Rooney, MSC, Ret., to Ginn, 22 Feb 85, all in DASG-MS.Careers: Samuel G. Duggins, "A Social Work Career," article in Rpt, AHS, sub: Army Social Work Current Trends, 6–11 May 72, pp. 164–69, JML.

[86] 1858: Florence Nightingale, *Notes on Matters Affecting the Health, Efficiency and Hospital Administration of the British Army* (London: Harrison and Sons, 1858), p. 228.

[87] Sanitary engineering: MSC Newsletter, 1972; DF, Col Hunter G. Taft, Jr., MSC, sub: Ph.D. Training for Sanitary Engineering Officers, Sep 74, DASG-MS.

[88] Entomology: OTSG, Annual General Inspection (AGI), Armed Forces Pest Control Board, 4 Jan 65, RG 112, accession 68A–375, Box 10/40, NARA-WNRC; Brochure, OTSG, "Entomologists," Oct 68, DASG-MS; TSG to Rep Paul Findly, RG 112, accession 72A–3501, Box 19/55, NARA-WNRC.

[89] EHSEEP: Rpt, Lt Col James M. Morgan, Jr., MSC, USAR, sub: A Review of the Current Status of Environmental and Sanitary Engineering Officers in the United States Army Reserve, July 1974; Rpt, Morgan, sub: Suggestions for Recruiting Environmental Science and Sanitary Engineering Officers into the Medical Service Corps, April 1978, all in DASG-MS.

[90] Sanitary engineers: Hamrick to Goriup, 3 May 66; Brochure, OTSG, "Sanitary Engineers," Oct 68; Lt Col John F. Erskine, MSC, to Ginn, 11 Aug 83, including news clippings; MSC Newsletter, 1972, all in DASG-MS; OTSG, Annual General Inspection (AGI), U.S. Army Environmental Hygiene Agency, 31 Mar 65, RG 112, accession 68A–375, Box 10/40, NARA-WNRC; SG Conference, 3 Jan 67; DF, Col Ralph J. Walsh, MSC, HQ, USARV, sub: End of Tour Report, 20 Nov 69, USACMH.

[91] Recommendations: Col Hunter G. Taft, Jr., MSC, to Haggerty, 8 Aug 74, with five incls, DASG-MS.

[92] Optometry: CMT 2, Col. Herschel E. Griffin, MC, XO, OTSG, to DCSPER, sub: Manpower and Personnel Studies, 30 Sep 65, RG 112, accession 68A–3358, Box 17/33, NARA-WNRC; Hamrick to Goriup, 3 May 66, DASG-MS; Brochure, OTSG, "The Optometry Officer," Oct 68, DASG-MS; Thomas, USARV Senior Officer Debrief, 12 Nov 70; OTSG, AGI, U.S. Army

Aeromedical Research Unit (USAARU), 15 Jan 65, RG 112, accession 68A–375, Box 10/40, NARA-WNRC; "37% of Soldiers Wear Glasses," *Army Reporter* (U.S. Army, Vietnam) 5 (6 January 1969); Rpt, THU, sub: Chronology: U.S. Army Contributions to Civilian Medicine, 1971, both in DASG-MS.

[93] Draft: Women could not be drafted.

[94] Optometry draft: H.R. 3313, "To Provide Career Incentives for Certain Professionally Trained Officers of the Armed Forces," 89th Cong., lst sess., 2 January 1965; TSG to TAG, sub: Special Call #37 for Physician, Dentist and Veterinarian Registrants, 29 Sep 65; News release 635–65, OASD (Public Affairs), "Selective Service to Provide 1,979 Medical Personnel Beginning in January 1966," 22 Sep 65; Summary sheet, Brig Gen Frederick J. Hughes, Jr., MC, Actg TSG, forwarding Memo to ASD (Manpower), sub: Drafting of Optometrists, including MFR, Hamrick, 22 Oct 65, and Memo, Thomas A. Morris, ASD (Manpower), same sub, to Sec Army, all in RG 112, accession 68A-–358, Box 17/33, NARA-WNRC; SG Conferences, 30 Sep and 1 Oct 65, and 4 Jan and 15 Jul 66; "Military Optometry," *Journal of the American Optometric Association (JAOA)* 37 (April 1966): 331–45. Special Call #37 was for 1,529 physicians, 350 dentists, and 100 veterinarians. Special Call #38 for 900 male nurses (700 Army, 200 Navy) produced 27 warrant and 124 commissioned ANC officers. See Robert V. Piemonte and Cindy Gurney, *Highlights in the History of the Army Nurse Corps*, pamphlet (Washington, D.C.: U.S. Army Center of Military History, 1987), p. 51.

[95] Draft of optometrists: Hamrick said it was his "strong belief" a draft was necessary. Hamrick to Hughes, 22 Oct 65, RG 112, accession 68A–3358, Box 17/33, NARA-WNRC.

[96] Salute: *JAOA* 37, special issue (April 1966): 331–45.

[97] Entry grade: Vernon McKenzie, DASD (HR&P), to Sen Walter D. Huddleston, 13 Dec 73; Brig Gen Surindar N. Bhaskar, Dir Pers, OTSG, to Rep Carl D. Perkins, 15 Jan 74; Maj Gen Robert W. Green, Actg TSG, to William H. McAlister, 1 Apr 74, all in DASG-MS.

[98] Credit: Physicians had on the average nine or more years of training, dentists seven, and veterinarians between six and seven.

[99] Special pay: Memo, Giroux for TSG, sub: Office of the Secretary of Defense (OSD) Legislative Proposal, sub: Armed Forces Medical and Dental Special Pay of 1979, 22 Feb 79; Optometry Newsletter, 1 August 1980, all in DASG-MS. It was opposed by General Morrison because he believed it would be divisive if only one MSC specialty received the pay.

[100] Letter: Ltrs, Lt Col Budd Appleton, MC, WRAMC, to "Dear Doctor," undated (1968), and to "Dear Doctor," 27 Sep 68, DASG-MS.

[101] Complaints: Twenty-seven letters from optometrists to Lt Col Gene M. Bourland, MSC, Ch, Opt Sec, May–Sep 74, DASG-MS, hereafter cited as Letters to Bourland.

[102] Quoted words: Bourland to Haggerty, 27 Aug 74, DASG-MS.

[103] Numbers: Letters to Bourland.

[104] Meeting: Bourland to Haggerty, sub: Recommendations Affecting Army Optometry, with incls, 6 May 74, DASG-MS.

[105] Apologies: Appleton to Bourland, 16 Aug 74; Bourland to Appleton, 3 Sep 74, both in DASG-MS.

[106] Assignments: Heaton, "Medical Support of the Soldier: A Team Effort in Saving Lives," *Army* 19 (October 1969): 86.

[107] Unacceptable: Boyson, "Why Doctors Get Out," p. 10.

[108] TASTA–70: Rpt, HQDA, sub: The Administrative Support Theater Army 1965–1970 (TASTA–70), 8 Jun 66, summarized in CMT 2, OTSG, sub: Review of TASTA, Part I, 23 Feb 68, and MFR to CMT 2, TSG to DCSLOG, sub: Proposal for Development of a Standard Theater Army Support Command (TASCOM) Supply and Maintenance System, 10 Feb 69, RG 112, accession 72A–3501, Box 20/55, NARA-WNRC; Col Campbell, XO, OTSG, to ACSFOR, sub: Operational Report, Lessons Learned, 3 Jan 67, RG 112, accession 70A–2772, Box 12/43, NARA-WNRC; SG Conferences, 15 Apr 66 and 20 and 27 Jan and 17 Mar 67. Brown Board: CSM 65–276, sub: Board of Inquiry on the Army Logistics System, 17 Jun 65, and Heaton to Maj Gen Laurence A. Potter, MC, Surg, USAREUR, 12 Oct 66, RG 112, accession 69A–2604, Box 17/38, NARA-WNRC; Spread Sheet, OTSG, sub: Board of Inquiry on the Army Logistics System (Format B), Recommendation V–IV, p. III–35, par. 15.b.(3), sub: Development of Logistics Doctrine, 17 Mar 67, DASG-MS. Background on the formation of Class VIII (and AR 320–5 def-

inition) in SG Conferences, 17 Mar and 7 Aug 67. Also see DF, Wilbur J. Balderson, Ch, Materiel Coord Br, OTSG, to Ch, Materiel Rqmts Br, OTSG, sub: Establishment of an Army Medical Service Depot Section of a General Depot, 5 Dec 67, DASG-MS. Besson Board: Besson Board, pp. D3–D4.

[109] MSC star: Notes of interv, Richard Kirk Weir, Dir, Developmental Credentialing Programs, ACHA (formerly Director of Membership), with Ginn, Chicago, Ill., 12 Feb 85, DASG-MS.

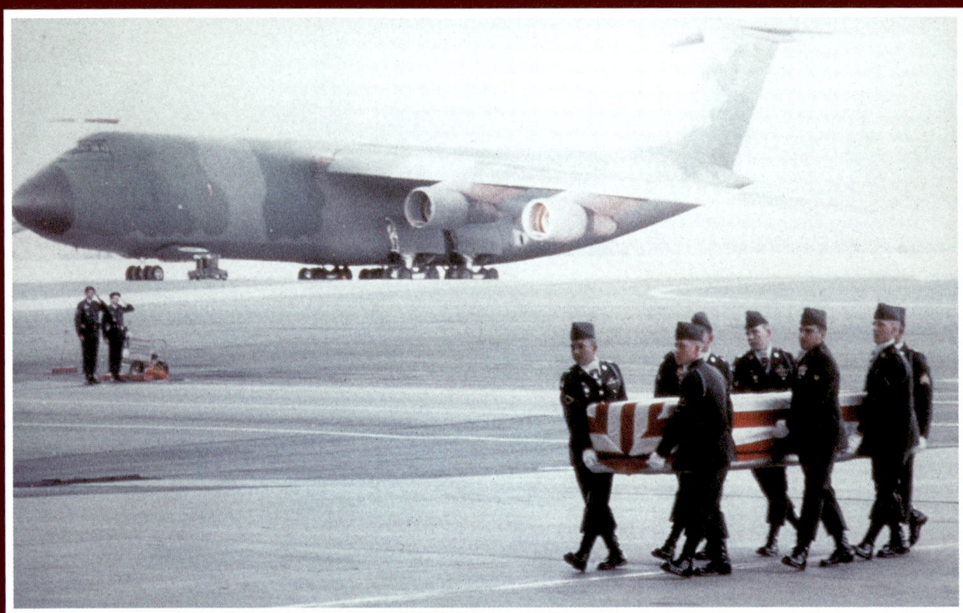

Scene at Dover Air Force Base, Delaware, after military plane crash at Gander, Newfoundland

12

The Post-Vietnam Era

The ending of the physician draft in 1973 coincided with the ending of the Berry Plan, the program that had allowed drafted physicians to defer active duty until completion of specialty training. Lt. Gen. Richard R. Taylor, MC, surgeon general from 1973 to 1977, found his most pressing problem was dealing with the inevitable physician shortage, a condition that only grew worse during his tenure. When his successor, Lt. Gen. Charles C. Pixley, MC, became the surgeon general in September 1977, only 4,056 physicians were on active duty, over 1,200 less than needed. Indeed, the number of serving physicians had dipped to 3,700 earlier that year. Pixley regarded the situation as so bad that he hated to come to work.[1]

To alleviate the shortage, General Pixley expanded physician recruiting efforts, employing over fifty MSCs in forty-three field offices and giving them permission to call him at any time to speak to candidates. Hard work, a rising U.S. medical school enrollment, and a period of peace began to correct the situation, and the number recruited more than tripled from 106 in 1976 to 338 in 1979.[2] The Health Professions Scholarship Program also helped, as did the establishment of new special pay programs for physicians that contributed to a better retention rate of Medical Corps officers beyond their initial tour. As a result of these various factors the recovery from the physician shortage was quicker than expected, dispelling overly pessimistic projections. The number of Army physicians on active duty had increased by nine hundred as Pixley's four-year term as surgeon general ended in 1981. Improvement continued, with the number reaching 5,214 in 1984 and 5,606 in 1991. Nevertheless, the recruitment and retention of physicians in both the active and reserve components remained one of the Medical Department's most vexing problems during the years immediately following the Vietnam War.[3]

Modernization of Field Medical Support

The Army modernized during the post-Vietnam period. A recruiting slogan, "Be All You Can Be," challenged soldiers to meet higher standards, such as a universally applied semiannual physical fitness test and strict weight control rules. Training also became more demanding and realistic; armored brigades, for example, maneuvered against a proficient aggressor force in the Mojave Desert at the National Training Center, Fort Irwin, California. The Army embraced an AirLand Battle doctrine that emphasized flexibility, mobility, and joint Army and Air Force operations.

The Medical Department also took steps to improve its doctrine, force structure, information systems, and equipment. It took a loss, however, when reorganization of combat service support units in 1982 removed the medical battalion from armored and mechanized infantry divisions in a change that established multifunctional forward support battalions (medical, maintenance, and supply and transportation companies) for the maneuver brigades. Conversion of the light divisions followed. This change necessitated forming a medical operations section in the Division Support Command to provide the medical operations staff capability for the division that had existed in the medical battalion. A development called Division 86 restructured division-level doctrine and equipment, converting the battalion surgeon to a warrant officer physician assistant and changing the MSC medical operations assistant in maneuver battalions to the medical platoon leader.[4]

Medical doctrine underwent reexamination, beginning in 1984 with a Medical Systems Program Review at the Academy of Health Sciences, Fort Sam Houston, Texas (which in 1991 became part of the newly organized U.S. Army Medical Department Center and School), a study conducted at the direction of General Maxwell R. Thurman, the vice chief of staff of the Army.[5] The resulting operational concept was termed Health Service Support, AirLand Battle, in 1986 and was further revised in 1991 as Health Services Support for AirLand Operations. Planners focused on building medical units from cellular components and reducing the types of hospitals in the theater of operations. The doctrinal development continued in the early 1990s as Health Service Support (HSS) AirLand Operations. It was intended to improve the evacuation and hospitalization system for future theaters of operations in which combat action would be characterized by speed, lengthened lines of communication, and dispersed units. Automation support for medical command, control, and communications was addressed with the computer-based Theater Army Medical Management Information System (TAMMIS). This automated system had subsystems for patient accounting and reporting, patient regulating, blood management, and medical logistics.[6]

The five echelons of medical support were referred to as levels I through V health service support (*Chart 5*). Medical capability at level I was improved through expanded first aid training for all soldiers (buddy aid) and the creation of a combat lifesaver program that trained selected nonmedical soldiers in the techniques of lifesaving aid, such as administering intravenous fluids to control shock until the medic arrived. The intent was to have a combat lifesaver in every infantry squad or equivalent combat element. At levels III and IV the doctrinal changes were translated into Army organizational changes through Medical Force 2000 (also called MF2K), a force structure proposal based on four types of battlefield hospitals and a medical holding company (a reduction from seven hospitals).[7]

Field medical equipment improvements were highlighted by the Deployable Medical Systems (DEPMEDS), a modernization program for all military field hospital sets. DEPMEDS featured hard-walled expandable shelters for equipment-intensive functions such as surgery, x-ray, and laboratory, as well as special generators and power distribution equipment. DEPMEDS sets were issued to the

CHART 5—POST-VIETNAM ECHELONS OF MEDICAL SUPPORT

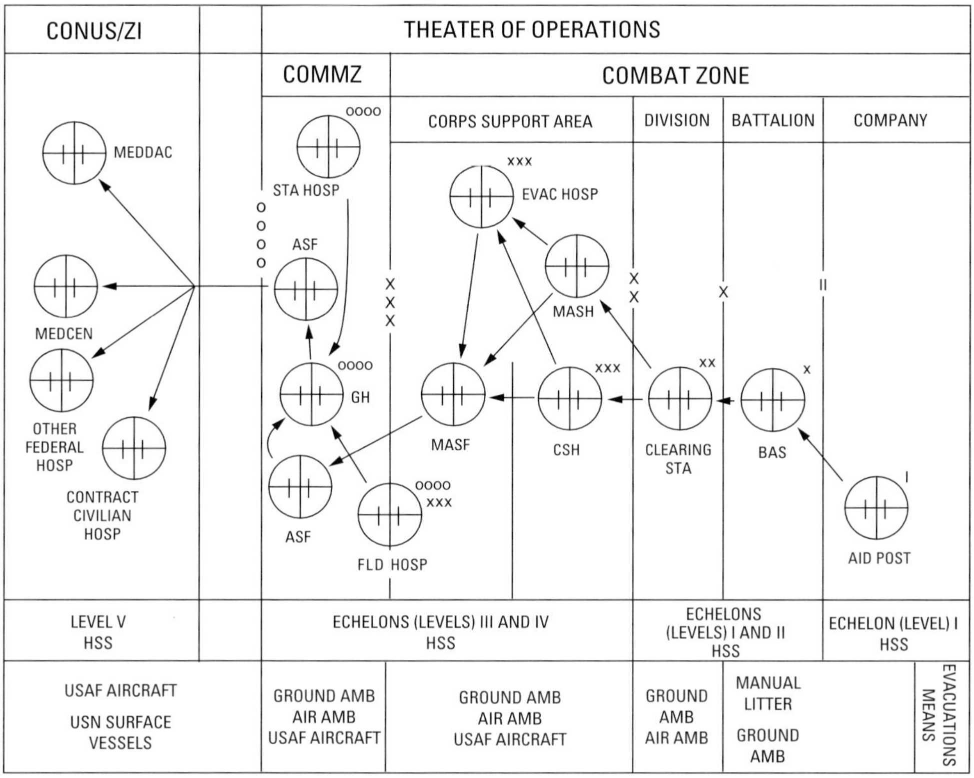

Source: Field Manual 8–10, *Health Service Support in a Theater of Operations*, 1 March 1991, figure 5–1.

forward-deployed numbered hospitals in Europe beginning in 1988 and were pressed into service soon after the sets began arriving.

For example, the 196th Station Hospital, stationed in Casteau, Belgium, conducted the first full surgical inpatient use of DEPMEDS components by an operational Army hospital, using portions of its set for a four-month period beginning in July 1989 when it was forced to close its entire inpatient capability for renovations. Not long thereafter elements of the 5th MASH from Fort Bragg, North Carolina, commanded by Lt. Col. Stephen H. Johnson, MSC, deployed to Europe for the annual Return of Forces to Germany (REFORGER) exercises. It became the first REFORGER medical unit to set up and operate with DEPMEDS. Those experiences demonstrated the advantages of the new equipment.[8]

Developments in the Corps

MSC active duty strength stayed close to five thousand officers throughout this period. In 1982, a representative year, the active component MSC numbered 4,994 officers: 3,563 in the Pharmacy, Supply, and Administration Section; 840 in the Medical Allied Sciences Section; 372 in the Sanitary Engineering Section; and 219 in the Optometry Section (*see Appendix L*). The number of specialties had dropped from forty-two in 1972 to thirty-five. In 1992 the corps numbered 4,920 in the active component, 1,175 in the National Guard, and 8,709 in the reserves, for a total of 14,804 in all components. The MSC also continued to serve as the carrier for various student programs, the graduates of which would be commissioned in other corps of the Medical Department. In 1982 this practice accounted for 205 Army medical students at the Uniformed Services University of the Health Sciences, Bethesda, Maryland (the DOD medical school).[9]

Brig. Gen. James J. Young, MSC, succeeded General Haggerty as corps chief in October 1977. He also replaced Haggerty as the surgeon general's director of resources management, a continuation of the practice of "dual-hatting." Young was followed in October 1981 by Brig. Gen. France F. Jordan, MSC, who continued as the surgeon general's director of personnel and commander of the U.S. Army Medical Department Personnel Support Agency. In March 1984 Jordan was selected as the first MSC to fill the two-star billet of deputy assistant secretary of defense for medical readiness. He was replaced as chief of the Medical Service Corps by Col. Walter F. Johnson III, MSC, the executive officer for the surgeon general. Johnson began his tour with the rank of colonel but was promoted to brigadier general in October 1985, when he also became the first MSC appointed as the surgeon general's director of health care operations. For the first time there were two MSC generals on active duty, a situation that continued until Jordan's retirement in 1987. Brig. Gen. Bruce T. Miketinac replaced General Johnson in November 1988 as corps chief and operations director (*see Appendix G*).

Throughout this period the evolution of the MSC continued. A committee headed by Maj. William E. Lohmiller, MSC, studied the administrative specialties in 1978 and concluded that the corps had emphasized specialization at the expense of more generalized capabilities. His committee recommended managing administrative officers as a group rather than as individual specialties and reducing the number of administrative specialties. All new MSC administrative officers were to have the entry-level skill of field medical assistant (coded as 67B), losing the B suffix when they received their primary and secondary specialties between the seventh and fifteenth years of service.[10]

The important aspect of Lohmiller's recommendations was the concept of administrative officers as a single group with increased flexibility of assignments within that group. The Medical Department was preoccupied with other problems at that time and the recommendations were not acted upon, but the basic principle remained alive. It was incorporated into an MSC management study, organized by General Johnson in 1987, that sought to include the scientific specialties as well. The study was continued by General Miketinac when he became corps chief in 1988.

The new corps structure as it emerged in 1994 from the MSC Management Study reduced from thirty-five to twenty-six the number of Medical Service Corps commissioned and warrant officer specialties, now called areas of concentration (health facilities planning, manpower management, physiology, and psychology associate were eliminated or combined with other specialties). Warrant officers were unchanged, but commissioned officer specialties were arranged into eight groups called medical functional areas (*see Appendix M*). Four of these areas—health services (the administrative specialties), laboratory sciences, preventive medicine, and behavioral sciences—consisted of related specialties. It was believed that this would allow greater flexibility in assigning officers to specialty-immaterial positions in the senior grades. For example, it was estimated that over 90 percent of the colonel positions in the laboratory sciences medical functional area could be filled by officers from any specialty within that grouping. The other four medical functional areas—pharmacy, optometry, podiatry, and aeromedical evacuation—were stand-alone areas of concentration.[11]

Accessions to the corps during the post-Vietnam period were principally through ROTC and direct appointments in the various specialty areas. ROTC accounted for about three hundred new officers each year during much of this period, including graduates from an MSC ROTC program at the University of Pennsylvania. Of that total, the MSC offered about seventy Regular Army commissions to ROTC distinguished military graduates annually. Commissioning of West Point graduates, which had lapsed in the mid-1980s, was reinstituted in 1988 when the Army added the MSC, Adjutant General Corps, and Finance Corps to branches already available to cadets. In 1992 this source accounted for 12 of 435 accessions.[12]

The Army greatly expanded opportunities for women in the early 1980s, the exception being positions with the highest probability of direct combat. A suggestion surfaced in 1983 to commission all female ROTC cadets in the special branches (Chaplain Corps, Judge Advocate General's Corps, and the Medical Department branches). In effect, because of the particular training requirements of the other special branches, this proposal would have meant that most female cadets would be placed in the MSC for duty in the administrative specialties. However, since many MSC junior officer positions were in the category with the highest probability of direct combat, the proposal would have been difficult to implement. In any case, Maj. Gen. H. Norman Schwarzkopf, the director of military personnel management, wanted greater opportunities for women throughout the Army, and he rejected the measure.[13]

Women increasingly sought careers in the MSC. In 1968 there were only 7 women in the corps, but by 1987 the number had risen to 544. Most of the increase had occurred after 1977, and thus their number consisted predominantly of junior officers, with only twenty-six female majors and five lieutenant colonels in the upper echelons. In an attempt to gain insight into the situation of women officers, Capt. Susan R. West, MSC, a management intern in General Johnson's office, surveyed a hundred female MSCs. A common theme of the respondents was their struggle in establishing themselves as Army officers. In general, they indicated satisfaction with their careers, although there were complaints of lingering prejudice. Of those surveyed, 44 percent believed their opportunities were equal to or better than male MSCs, and more than two-thirds regarded the MSC as equal to or better than other Army branches.[14]

As women progressed through the ranks they achieved significant milestones in the active component MSC. In 1991 Donna C. Williamson became the first

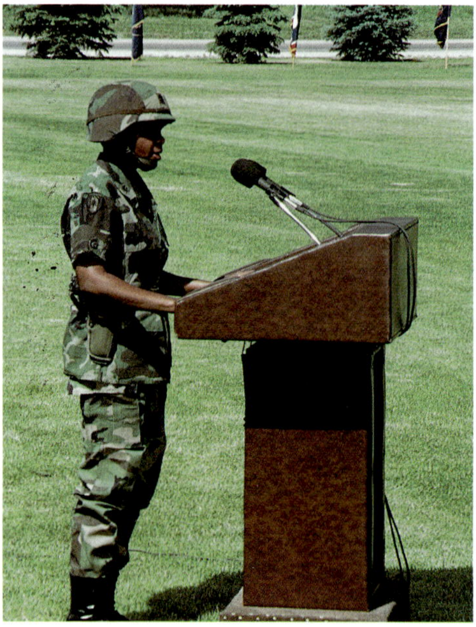

Colonel Alston at her change of command ceremony, June 1994

female promoted to colonel. In 1992 Capt. Katherine H. Moore, MSC, was selected as one of the Ten Outstanding Young Americans by the national Junior Chamber of Commerce. Also in 1992 Lt. Col. Mary Anne Svetlik, MSC, became the first female deputy commander for administration (formerly the hospital executive officer), and in 1994 Lt. Col. Priscilla M. Alston, MSC, became the first female field grade commander. By January 1995 the MSC had 825 female officers, more than any other branch in the Army except the Army Nurse Corps. Nineteen percent of MSCs were women, an increase of 70 percent since 1987 as a percentage of the corps.[15]

Efforts to promote cohesion continued. General Jordan established an MSC medallion to be presented to MSCs retiring from active duty, and the chief's office undertook the manufacture and sale of MSC belt buckles and commemorative coins. An annual directory of all MSCs provided a resource not available to officers in other branches. General Johnson convened a meeting of senior MSCs in 1984 to prepare a strategic plan. They developed thirteen goals grouped into the areas of readiness, management, quality service, professionalism, and cohesion that the chief disseminated as a pocket-size handout.[16]

Generals Johnson and Miketinac both urged senior MSCs to serve as mentors for junior officers, an effort that was particularly needed with the loss of the MSC medical battalion commanders as role models. In Europe, for example, there were nearly two hundred MSCs—mostly lieutenants and captains—assigned to units outside the 7th Medical Command, prompting the command's chief of staff to ask the senior MSCs in each region to work informally with these younger officers as "mentors."[17]

In 1982 General Jordan announced establishment of the MSC Chief's Award of Excellence. It recognized two outstanding junior officers each year, one in the administrative specialties and one in the scientific specialties (*Appendix N*). Duane C. Goodno, a first lieutenant, and Erik A. Henchal, a captain, in 1982 were the first winners. Goodno was recognized for accomplishments as the logistics officer of the 421st Medical Company (Air Ambulance) in Germany; Henchal, a microbiologist at the Walter Reed Army Institute of Research, was honored for his research in dengue. In 1983 General Johnson added an award for a warrant officer. The first winner was CW2 Cornelius L. Reeder, recognized for his duty as a biomedical equipment repair technician at

Dewitt Army Hospital, Fort Belvoir, Virginia. In 1986 Johnson added a fourth category, an officer from the U.S. Army Reserve. Capt. Marisa P. Parker, MSC, 2d Hospital Center, Hamilton Field, California, was selected as the first winner for her contributions during a tour of duty with the Senior Army Reserve Adviser. The Army National Guard joined the lineup in 1990 with the selection of Capt. Mary L. Ivanhoff, MSC, 146th Combat Support Hospital, San Francisco, California.[18]

Another initiative was the establishment of an annual Junior Officer Day with the Chief. The first session in December 1982 was attended by eleven lieutenants and captains who toured the Pentagon, were briefed by MSC staff officers, and lunched with General Jordan and other senior MSCs. By 1987 the event had expanded to a two-day visit by eighteen participants, including commissioned and warrant officers. Yet another innovation began in 1985 when Capt. Eric G. Daxon, MSC, became the first management intern in the chief's office, another program begun by General Johnson.[19]

Some MSCs were recognized in competitive awards of the Association of Military Surgeons of the United States (AMSUS). In 1977 Maj. Richard V. N. Ginn was the first Army MSC awarded the Sir Henry Wellcome Medal and Prize, the oldest award of the association, presented annually for an essay reporting original work in military medicine. General Jordan received the first AMSUS Outstanding Federal Services Health Administrator Award in 1984. Col. Thomas C. Munley, MSC, became the second Army recipient in 1986, and General Johnson was the third in 1988.[20]

The identification of MSCs with field medical service flowered in a special way through the efforts of Lt. Col. Richard J. Berchin, MSC. His single-minded dedication to creating a memorial to the combat medic resulted in the Combat Medic Memorial, which was dedicated in ceremonies at Fort Sam Houston in November 1979. The bronze statue of a medic tending a fallen comrade became a popular icon.[21]

MSCs also figured in an Army initiative to increase unit cohesion by identifying soldiers with the traditions and customs of historic regiments. This led to the establishment of the Army Medical Department Regiment in 1986. All medical officers and enlisted personnel were formally affiliated with the regiment, to include wearing the departmental crest on their uniforms. In 1994 an MSC, Col. James G. Van Straten, Ret., became the second honorary colonel of the regiment, replacing Maj. Gen. Spurgeon Neel, MC, Ret. Primarily a ceremonial position, Van Straten's role was to enhance morale and esprit de corps through the perpetuation of the regiment's traditions and customs. Van Straten, who had retired in 1986, was dean of allied health sciences of the University of Texas Health Science Center in San Antonio.[22]

Opportunity

A continuing theme in military medicine is the ebb and flow of political pressure to reduce the number of physicians in administrative positions. In 1978 DOD representatives testified to the House Committee on Appropriations that

120 Army physicians occupied executive management positions. Congress asked for a 20 percent reduction, and that pressure, as well as the evident capabilities of senior MSCs, continued to open position opportunities. In 1976 Col. Neil J. McDonald became the first MSC appointed as director of personnel for the Surgeon General's Office, and in 1978 Colonel Van Straten became the first MSC assigned as the deputy commandant (later redesignated assistant commandant) of the Academy of Health Sciences. MSCs served as the chiefs of staff of the U.S. Army Medical Command, Europe (renamed the 7th Medical Command in 1978), in Heidelberg, Germany, and the U.S. Army Medical Research and Development Command (USAMRDC), Fort Detrick, Maryland. In 1981 Col. Donald H. Triano became the first MSC chief of staff of the Health Services Command, Fort Sam Houston. Col. Philip Z. Sobocinski became the first MSC deputy commander of the USAMRDC in 1984, and in 1987 Col. Carl E. Pedersen became the first MSC commander of the U.S. Army Medical Materiel Development Agency, a USAMRDC unit also at Fort Detrick.[23]

In 1978 Maj. Gen. Surindar Bhaskar, chief of the Dental Corps, created positions for MSCs as executive officers of U.S. Army Dental Activities (DENTAC). The new organizations, although attached to Army hospitals for support, were independent headquarters; by 1982 there were forty-two MSC administrative positions in grades from captain to lieutenant colonel. General Young believed that these positions were an excellent opportunity for officers who wished to broaden their managerial experience. This and other management changes contributed to a 48 percent increase of productivity by Army dentists from 1978 to 1983.[24]

Despite these advances, a promotion slowdown became a serious morale problem during this period. The reductions of the Army after the Vietnam War had not cut enough MSCs. That was due principally to the physician shortage that left the department with vacant Medical Corps authorizations each year. The Surgeon General's Office, fearing the loss of those spaces (the rule of "use or lose"), converted some to MSC so that it could keep the authorizations filled. Unfortunately, in so doing it retained more MSCs in low- to mid-level grades than could be accommodated by the corps' normally pyramidal rank structure. Thus promotions became more competitive for Vietnam-era officers, because selections were based on the year of an officer's entry on active duty. Vietnam-era year groups bulged, a problem compounded when the department was able to resolve the physician shortage and took back the authorizations it had temporarily placed with the MSC. The ensuing reductions in the overstrength year groups forced many promising officers out of the service or into other branches.[25]

The Defense Officer Personnel Management Act of 1981 (DOPMA) increased the size of the Regular Army, and the Army elected to have a career force (major and higher) of all Regular officers. The act allowed field grade reserve officers on active duty to apply for Regular Army integration, and many reserve MSCs applied. But the practice only added to the year group problem, because those reserve officers who would have retired when they reached their twentieth year of service tended to stay on active duty. Furthermore, DOPMA's ideal selection rates—80 percent for major, 70 percent for lieutenant colonel, and 50 percent

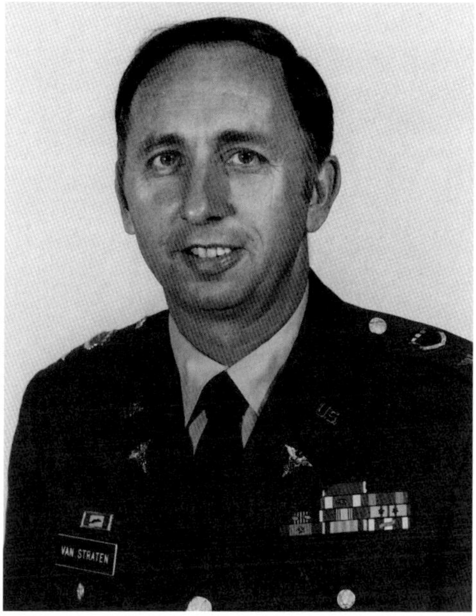

Colonel Van Straten

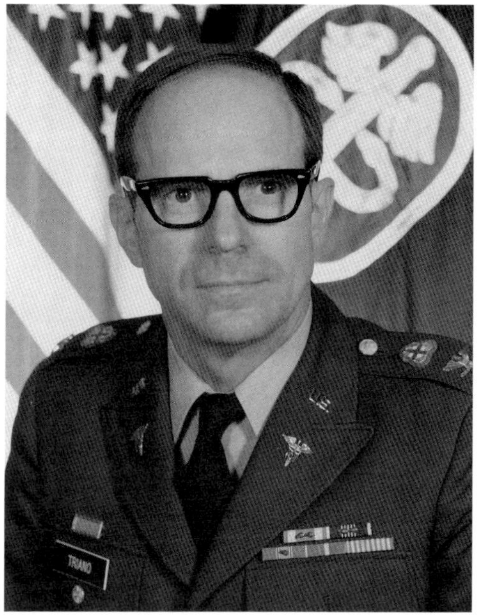

Colonel Triano

for colonel—were initially used by MSC promotion boards and added to the overstrength problem in certain year groups.

By 1983 MSCs were falling behind in promotions when compared to their peers in other Army branches. Predictions were that by 1989 they would be over three years behind the rest of the Army for promotion to major and four years behind for lieutenant colonel. General Johnson was able to gain the assistance of Delbert L. Spurlock, Jr., assistant secretary of the Army for manpower and reserve affairs, who told the Army chief of staff that the promotion problem was distressing.[26] Some officers in other branches who worked for MSCs were promoted so rapidly that they ended up supervising their previous bosses. In a typical example, Captain Daxon, the chief's first management intern, was one year behind his West Point classmates when he was promoted to major in June 1985.

The problem was resolved through a combination of actions. The Army provided some relief through additional field grade promotion authority in 1986. The Medical Department tightened its management of year groups: it retired or separated officers in the overstrength year groups and approved their requests for transfers to other branches. In 1987 the MSC underwent the Army's first selective early retirement board, a process that picked officers for involuntary retirement.[27] In addition, the Army used promotion rates generally lower than the goals of DOPMA. For example, the 1987 Medical Department colonel promotion board, which considered officers who came into the Army during the Vietnam War, had a 35 percent selection rate for those considered for the first time, a contrast to earlier boards that had used higher rates (such as the 1979 board that had used a 52 percent first-time selection rate). By using lower selection rates, the Army was able to avoid stagnation of promotion timing. In other words, it promoted fewer officers, but those who advanced did so at an accelerated rate.

Stars

The corps continued to have the lowest percentage of general officers of any branch in the Army except the Army Medical Specialist Corps (AMSC). In 1982 the corps had one brigadier general for 4,901 officers. All other Medical Department corps (except the AMSC) fared better, and if the MSC were compared to the branches most frequently mentioned as possible substitutes—Adjutant General, Ordnance, Quartermaster, Chemical, Signal, and Transportation—it had an elevenfold disadvantage at best. For example, Ordnance Corps officers had a thirty-two times better chance for stars than MSCs. The MSC continued to lose promising officers because of the lack of opportunity beyond the rank of colonel.[28]

DOPMA also changed the basis for calculating the number of general officers and theoretically gave MSCs the same opportunity as other Army officers. However, that was subject to the constraints imposed by the number of generals that Congress appropriated for the Army and that the Army in turn allocated to the Medical Department, a number that totaled twenty-two in the post-Vietnam era and fell to sixteen by 1994.[29] Lt. Gen. Bernhard T. Mittemeyer, surgeon general from 1981 to 1985, supported the appointment of a second MSC general officer, but that did not materialize.[30]

The promotion of General Johnson while General Jordan was still on active duty had been accomplished through the use of a Medical Corps star. Whether that situation would last depended on the desire of the surgeon general who would be serving when Jordan retired. When he did retire in 1988 the corps reverted to only one general officer on active duty. The pressure within the department for the star was such that Lt. Gen. Quinn H. Becker, Mittemeyer's replacement as surgeon general from 1985 to 1988, was unwilling to leave it in the MSC.[31]

Education and Training

Despite problems with rank, MSC educational levels remained high. In 1981 41 percent of the corps had master's degrees (as compared to 24 percent for all Army officers) and 7.4 percent had doctoral degrees (versus 1 percent for the Army). The corps provided two avenues for university training: baccalaureate degree completion for warrant officers and graduate programs for commissioned officers. The corps chief approved training starts based on validated requirements by specialty area, and officers could apply for graduate training between their fifth and eighth year of service. From 1980 to 1985 MSCs obtained 83 doctoral and 100 master's degrees at civilian universities. There was also opportunity for a master's of science in logistics at Army Logistics Management Center, Fort Lee, Virginia, and a master of military art and science for students in the resident course of the Command and General Staff College, Fort Leavenworth, Kansas. Fully funded university graduate school opportunities in 1988 included doctoral training in ten disciplines and master's in twenty-one. A new opportunity appeared in 1995 when the Army provided the Medical Department with four openings in the Training with Industry (TWI) program. Officers selected for this graduate (but non–degree producing) training would be stationed with a private sector company for one year to obtain firsthand experience in management skills and business practices which they would then apply in a subsequent utilization assignment.[32]

By 1981 the Army-Baylor Program had awarded 991 master's degrees since its affiliation with Baylor in 1951, and by 1989 it was second of all U.S. graduate programs in the total number of degrees awarded each year.[33] In 1976 the course changed from a semester to a trimester schedule of 42 graduate credit hours; class size was reduced to thirty-four students (including twenty-one Army MSCs); and most undergraduate-level work was removed. Later the course lengthened to a full twelve months with four semesters totaling sixty graduate hours. Class size averaged in the mid-thirties. For example, the class that entered in 1987 had thirty-two students, including eighteen Army MSCs. Baylor officials viewed the course as difficult, and students said all they did was "eat, sleep and study."[34]

The program maintained a one-year residency requirement in spite of a move away from residencies by many civilian programs, a trend that was challenged in the early 1990s as the profession found that students and faculty had lost touch with practical experience.[35] Residencies were performed at Army hospitals. However, the class that entered in 1976 participated in three experimental residencies outside the Medical Department with the Department of Health, Education, and Welfare; the Veterans Administration; and the Office of the Secretary of Defense (OSD). The initiative was not supported by the surgeon general, and there were no others until 1990 when an OSD residency resumed.

A survey in 1981 by the Accrediting Commission on Graduate Education for Health Services Administration accelerated some changes. The report cited the program's strength in student motivation, but it faulted the faculty for conducting little research and publishing less, for its high turnover, and for credential weaknesses.[36] Furthermore, the commission believed that admissions were more an Army administrative process than a genuine review of academic capability. General Jordan took corrective actions, stabilizing faculty tours, increasing opportunity for doctoral training for potential faculty members, encouraging research, and requiring completion of the advanced course as a prerequisite for attendance. Baylor tightened its admission requirements and made it clear that it would not waive a minimum Graduate Record Examination score of 1,000 and a 2.7 grade point average (or 3.0 for the last sixty undergraduate hours). The actions were effective, and the program tied with Duke University as thirteenth of the sixty U.S. graduate programs in a survey of program directors conducted in 1990. In 1993 the program received accreditation by the commission through the year 2001.[37]

The Medical Service Corps strongly emphasized the importance of military training throughout the post-Vietnam era, and MSCs were prominent figures in the Academy of Health Sciences (later reorganized into the Medical Department Center and School) at Fort Sam Houston, Texas, both as students and members of the staff and faculty. By 1979 the school was training 25,000 resident students a year.[38] In 1982 its MSC Officer Basic Course increased from eight weeks to a variable twelve- to sixteen-week length, depending upon individual background and specialty. There continued to be changes to the course, and by 1993 it had been reduced in length to nine weeks conducted in two phases. The first portion, attended by officers of all AMEDD corps, consisted of a core of instruction required by the U.S. Army Training and Doctrine Command in soldier skills and knowledge, leadership, and organization of the Army. The second phase was designed with courses pertinent to each corps.[39]

The Officer Advanced Course (OAC), also conducted at Fort Sam Houston, was twenty-two weeks long in 1982. It decreased to twenty weeks and remained a requirement for all MSCs, who attended between their third and fifth year of service. MSC aviators continued to attend the Aviation Branch advanced course at Fort Rucker, Alabama, but the follow-on portion at Fort Sam Houston was terminated. In 1992 the surgeon general directed the Center and School to establish a single OAC for all of the Medical Department's corps and to significantly shorten the course. A series of reviews ensued, a shortened course opened for the Medical Corps, and a single ten-week OAC for all corps was scheduled to begin in January 1997. Another OAC option for MSCs was the Combined Arms Logistics Advanced Course (CLOAC) conducted at Fort Lee, Virginia. The formation of multifunctional forward support battalions (FSBs) had led in 1992 to the development of a multifunctional logistics specialty, also known as functional area 90 (FA 90), and CLOAC was designed to support that concept. General Miketinac believed that MSCs would not be eligible for FSB command without attending CLOAC, and six MSCs were in the first class in 1992. Capt. Mary R. Martin was an honor graduate; Capt. Noel J. Cardenas was on the Commandant's List; and Capt. Raymond S. Dingle won the Ironman Award for physical fitness. The goal was to send between eighteen and twenty-four MSCs a year.[40]

In 1981 MSCs also began attending a new Army course, the Combined Arms and Services Staff School (CAS^3 or popularly "CAS Cubed"). Structured to prepare captains for duty as staff officers, the course was conducted in two phases: a correspondence portion and a nine-week resident phase at Fort Leavenworth, Kansas. By 1986 CAS^3 was mandatory for MSCs, and officers were scheduled for attendance at the second phase prior to their entering into the promotion zone for major. Some MSCs also attended the Combat Casualty Care Course (C–4), initially a one-week and later a two-week course conducted at Fort Sam Houston beginning in 1980 that taught medical officers field medicine. Another opportunity opened in 1983 when Col. Robert J. T. Joy, MC, USA, Ret., chairman of medical history at the Uniformed Services University of the Health Sciences, collaborated with Col. Thomas C. Munley, MSC, chief of the Military Sciences Division of the Academy of Health Sciences, in establishing at the university a ten-month fellowship in military medical history to prepare officers to serve as instructors in the subject at the Academy of Health Sciences. Capt. William H. Thresher, MSC, was the first officer selected. A few MSCs attended the Program Manager Course, a joint course taught at the Defense Systems Management College, Fort Belvoir, Virginia, that prepared officer and civilian executives of the three Services for DOD materiel development and acquisition positions. Capt. Lawrence K. Lightner, the first MSC to attend, completed the course in 1986.[41]

Selection for attendance at the resident course of the Command and General Staff College at Fort Leavenworth or (until 1990) the Armed Forces Staff College at Norfolk, Virginia, remained extremely competitive, averaging between fifteen and twenty MSCs a year (nineteen in 1994). General Miketinac noted that while the number of resident seats was small (35 for the Medical Department in 1994), it could be argued that this was offset by the much greater opportunity for MSCs to attend graduate school. The Army placed great emphasis on completion of staff college, as did the Medical Service Corps, and it became essential for promotion to lieutenant colonel. Most Army officers completed it through nonresident programs; in 1980, 366 MSCs were enrolled in this way.[42]

The Goldwater-Nichols DOD Reorganization Act of 1986 (named for Senator Barry Goldwater and Congressman Bill Nichols) further tightened the unification provisions of the National Security Act of 1949 by forcing the three Services into "jointness," i.e., joint operations. The Norfolk command and staff course ended in 1990 as the Armed Forces Staff College assumed the mission of training officers of all the Services for joint assignments. Its centerpiece was a twelve-week intermediate Joint and Combined Staff Officer School that officers attended following completion of their Service staff college to prepare them for joint staff assignments. No MSCs attended the first classes.[43]

There continued to be fierce competition for the very small number of slots each year for the resident and nonresident courses of the Army War College at Carlisle Barracks, Pennsylvania, and of the Industrial College of the Armed Forces (ICAF) at Fort McNair, Washington, D.C. The nonresident course continued as a two-year program universally considered more difficult than the resident program, and in 1985 the Army combined the resident and nonresident selection boards into one board to establish a single order-of-merit list. In 1987, a representative year, eleven MSCs were among twenty-seven Medical Department officers selected for senior service college; six were enrolled in the resident and five in the nonresident courses.

New options for resident senior service college opened with the establishment of Army fellowships that awarded senior service college credit under the auspices of the Army War College. Lt. Col. Douglas A. Braendel, MSC, was the first Medical Department officer to enroll in this program when he was selected for an Army intragovernmental fellowship at the Department of Health and Human Services in 1988. Similarly, Col. Steven J. Stone, MSC, in 1994 was the first officer selected for an environmental policy fellowship at the Army Environmental Policy Institute at the Georgia Institute of Technology in Atlanta, Georgia. This fellowship was developed by Col. Robert J. Fitz, MSC, the chief of the Sanitary Engineering Section. Lt. Col. Scott S. Beaty, MSC, in 1994 was the first officer to enroll in a health policy fellowship at George Washington University in Washington, D.C., an opportunity created by Col. Timothy Jackman, MSC. In 1994 MSCs accounted for twelve of the twenty-nine Medical Department senior service college students with five resident and four nonresident Army War College seats, one ICAF seat, and two fellowship seats. Yet in spite of these changes the overall opportunity for Medical Department officers to attend resident senior service college continued to trail all other branches of the Army.[44]

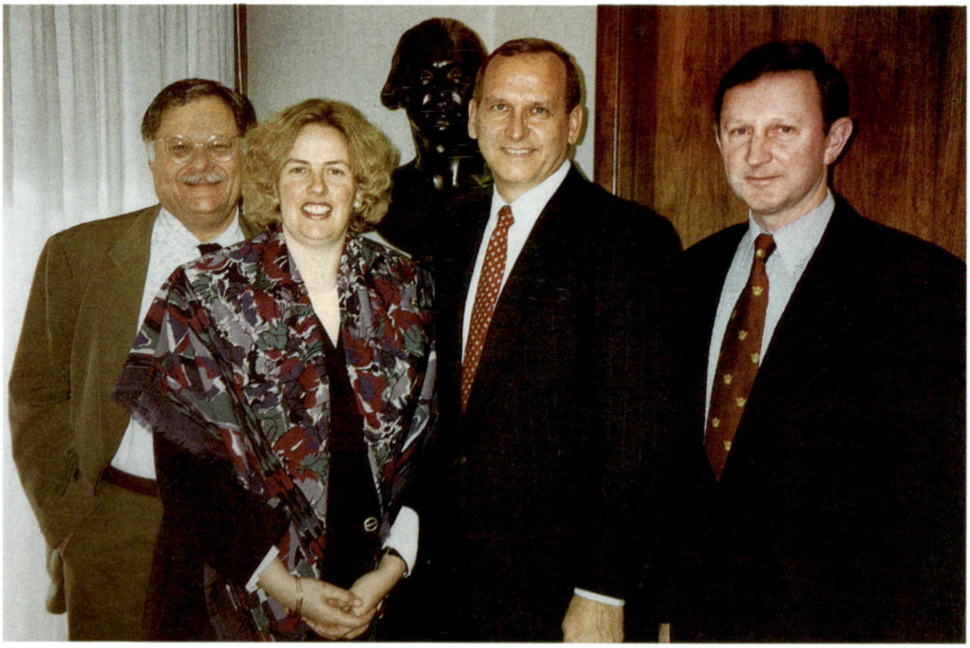

*Colonel Beaty (*second from right*) at George Washington University*

MSCs competed for other advanced training programs. A special opportunity opened in 1986 when Lt. Col. William H. Bell, Jr., began a year's tour as a fellow at the Arroyo Center of the Rand Corporation in Santa Monica, California. One MSC enrolled each year through 1994 in this program, established to develop a stable of officers trained in health policy analysis. Some MSCs attended the Interagency Institute for Federal Health Care Executives, the well-established forum conducted in two two-week sessions each year. In 1985 the institute moved from St. Louis, Missouri, and sponsorship by the Washington University, to Washington, D.C., where it was conducted by the George Washington University. Ten MSCs each year were among a total of 110 health care executives selected annually by the Army, Navy, Air Force, Public Health Service, and Department of Veterans Affairs to attend the institute because of their potential for senior management positions. Lt. Col. Frederick R. McLain, MSC, and William H. Bell, Jr., now a colonel, served as president of the institute's alumni association from 1987 to 1988 and from 1990 to 1991, respectively. A new opportunity opened in 1995 for Medical Department officers to obtain skills in industrial procedures and practices by participating in the Army's Training with Industry Program. Officers selected for this program would spend a year with health care firms in the private sector as preparation for specific departmental positions. Eight MSCs were enrolled by the end of 1995.[45]

Command

The issue of hospital command remained controversial. A 1978 War College paper by a Medical Corps officer argued that "the pendulum is swinging back, rapidly, in civilian medicine to place the physician in firm, formal control of civilian hospitals," implying that the Services should follow that supposed trend.[46] In 1980 the Strategic Air Command surgeon wrote a notorious letter objecting to the assignment of MSCs as hospital commanders by drawing an analogy to the rule that an aircraft commander must always be a pilot. "In the pecking order of the Military Health Care System, the physician is the biggest pecker. Let's keep it that way."[47]

Others disagreed. In 1987 Lt. Gen. Kenneth B. Cooper, the deputy commander in chief of the U.S. Army in Europe and Seventh Army, told the annual MSC meeting in Germany that he believed MSC health care administrators should be used as hospital commanders. Cooper repeated that recommendation in a letter to Robert N. Smith, M.D., the assistant secretary of defense for health affairs. He said he had discussed the matter with Maj. Gen. Marshall E. McCabe, MC, commander of the 7th Medical Command, and had concluded that progress would come only from pressure external to the Army and in Washington. Dr. Smith acknowledged that there was evolutionary development in hospital management, but he did not believe the time was right for his intervention.[48]

However, the issue continued to resurface. The shortage of physicians forced a succession of assistant secretaries of defense—John H. Moxley, John F. Beary, and William E. Mayer—to pressure the Army to reduce the number of physicians in administrative positions. Moxley noted that Navy and Air Force MSCs were commanding seven hospitals and twenty-five clinics in 1980. Beary criticized the Army for failing to implement the 1973 memorandum from Deputy Secretary of Defense William P. Clements that had directed the opening of command positions. Mayer reaffirmed the Clements mandate and argued that physicians should not receive the incentive pay bonus if they were not practicing their primary specialty.[49]

The Medical Department wavered in 1978 when a Department of the Army Inspector General report concluded that changing medical unit commanders upon the outbreak of hostilities constituted a threat to unit combat effectiveness. The surgeon general, required to take corrective action, responded that the best qualified officer would command medical units in peace and war "without regard to specific AMEDD corps."[50] In fact, no action was taken to change the policy. Later, as the Army surgeon general was testifying to Congress that physicians must command hospitals, the Navy surgeon general was testifying to the contrary, and the Marine Corps, which had Navy MSCs commanding its medical battalions, made it plain that it rejected the Army's position.[51]

Although the opportunity to command operational medical treatment facilities was denied MSCs, a wide variety of other opportunities was opened. The Army established command selection boards to select lieutenant colonel and colonel commanders. As a rule, administrative specialty officers in the field medical service "track"—as exemplified by completion of the resident Command and General Staff College course—were selected to command garrisoned medical battalions. Officers in the health care administration track—characterized by completion of the Army-Baylor Program—were selected for command of garrisoned field hospitals. In addition, General Mittemeyer opened the command of medical groups and nondivisional medical battalions in both peace and war to MSCs.

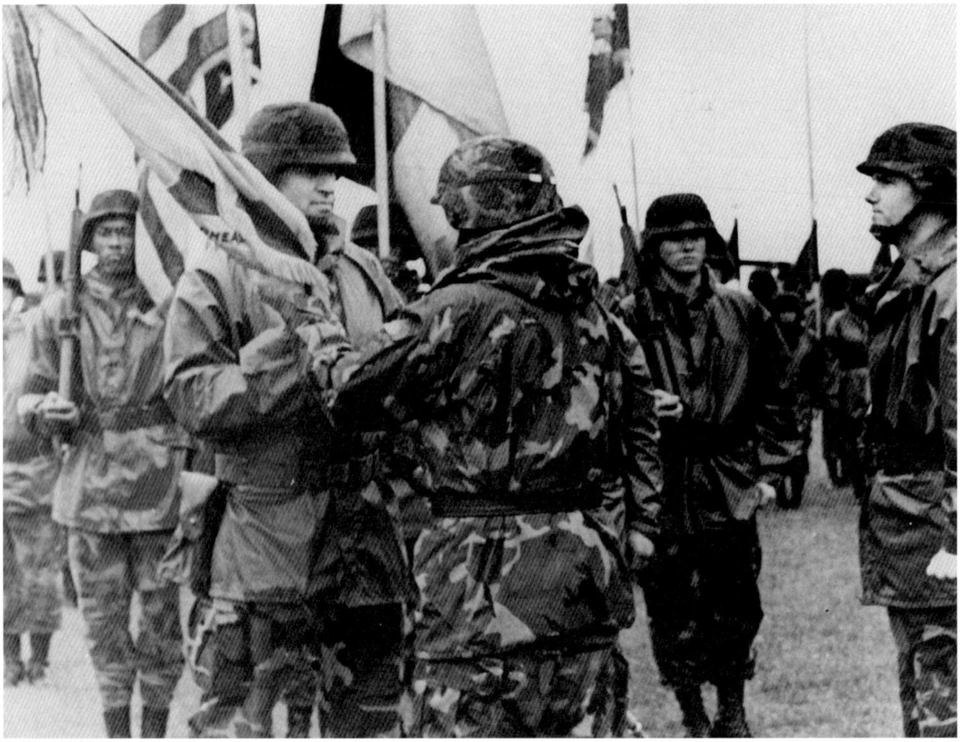

*Colonel Bradshaw (*left*) assumes command.*

Beginning in 1981 scientific specialty officers were also eligible to command field medical units, and additional billets, including scientific specialty units, were added to the initial Command Designated Position List, which had been restricted to field medical unit commands. For example, a 1982 change added the U.S. Army Medical Materiel Agency; the U.S. Army Environmental Hygiene Agency, Pacific; the U.S. Army Garrison, Fort Detrick; and the troop commands of two stateside medical centers.[52]

The loss of medical battalions in the heavy (armored and mechanized) divisions removed the opportunity for command of those units in garrison, but that was replaced with an opportunity for command (in both peace and war) of the forward support battalions, the maneuver brigade support units that absorbed the medical battalions, as well as the main support battalion (MSB) that provided divisionwide and area support. Presumably MSCs would command a third of the forward support battalions, since a medical company was one of the three support companies in each. In April 1982 Lt. Col. Jerry L. Fields, MSC, assumed command of the 3d FSB in the 9th Infantry Division at Fort Lewis, Washington, the first FSB organized in the Army. The opportunity for command of FSBs and MSBs also opened the way for MSCs to compete for Division Support Commands (DISCOMs), the next level of command. Col. Edward G. Bradshaw became the first MSC to achieve this distinction when he assumed command of the 1st Armored Division DISCOM, Frankfurt, Germany, in 1988.[53]

Unfortunately, the Medical Service Corps fared poorly in the ensuing selections for FSB and MSB commanders, averaging just three officers each year from 1983 to 1989. It was argued that the principal reason for the poor selection rate was a failure to ensure that MSCs received experience as operations officers and executive officers of the battalions, the types of assignments that, in addition to company command, were necessary to be competitive for battalion command. General Miketinac set a goal of having at least five MSCs in each FSB and MSB, both for the leadership development of the officers to ensure that they could ultimately compete for battalion command and for their utility in advising the commanders on the employment of medical assets. Branch took measures to implement that guidance, and the average number of MSCs selected for FSB command increased to five per year from 1989 to 1992, although it dropped to zero in 1993. Most MSCs who actually assumed command of these units were selected from alternate lists, as the Army named a total of only two MSCs among ninety officers as primary selections for FSB command from 1989 to 1993. Only one MSC was among twenty-four officers on primary lists for command of MSBs during the same period.[54]

In 1994 MSCs had the opportunity within the Medical Department for 200 company commands as well as 24 lieutenant colonel commands and 13 colonel commands that were listed in the official Army Command Designated Position List (*see Table 4*). The overall story was mixed. The opportunity for command of operational treatment units remained blocked as the Medical Department continued to ignore the 1973 Clements memorandum. Opportunities that had previously existed for command of divisional medical battalions had diminished with the FSB and MSB experience. Further, there was a portent of things to come. In 1983, in a throwback to the period before World War II, General Mittemeyer began placing physicians back in command of some medical companies and battalions. The idea, soon abandoned, was to have physicians commanding sixteen medical companies and four medical battalions. The policy reappeared in 1991, when some TOE hospitals and the 44th Medical Brigade at Fort Bragg, North Carolina, were designated for Medical Corps commanders.[55]

Developments in the Administrative Specialties

In 1982 the Pharmacy, Supply, and Administration Section accounted for 3,563 officers (71.3 percent of the corps) in pharmacy and eleven administrative specialties (*see Appendix L*). Administrative specialties numbered 3,348 officers (67 percent of the corps). The largest specialty, with 1,677 officers, was field medical assistant, the entry-level designation for newly commissioned officers who had not further specialized.

The special requirements placed on patient administration officers were demonstrated in 1985 when a battalion of the 101st Airborne Division (Air Assault) returning from peacekeeping duty in the Sinai crashed in Gander, Canada. With 256 victims, it was the greatest disaster in military aviation histo-

TABLE 4—MSC COMMAND OPPORTUNITY, 1994*

200 Company Commands
109 Table of Organization and Equipment (TOE) [Field Units]
91 Table of Distribution and Allowances (TDA)

24 Lieutenant Colonel Commands
11 Battalions and TOE Hospitals
5 Evacuation Battalions
4 Logistics Battalions
4 Scientific/Technical Commands

13 Colonel Commands
7 Brigades/Troop Commands/Groups
3 Logistics
3 Scientific/Technical
1 Installation

*Army Command Designated Position List (CDPL) commands only

Source: MSC Newsletter, March 1994, DASG-MS.

ry. Identifying the victims became enormously complicated because the soldiers had their medical and dental records on the plane, and in many cases records recovered from the crash had been severely damaged by fire, water, and fuel. Lt. Col. Michael A. Shannon, MSC, led a team at the Pentagon's Army Operations Center that worked around the clock to coordinate efforts to reconstruct the records and provide the information to pathologists at the mortuary at Dover Air Force Base in Delaware. In some cases Shannon's team used dental records from hometown civilian dentists who had treated the soldiers and learned of the identification problems from news broadcasts.[56]

The capability of MSCs in a new specialty, biomedical information systems, was put to good use in the identification effort. On 18 December Lt. Col. Gary L. Swallow, MSC, and 1st Lt. Beverly J. Rice, MSC, reported to Dover with seven microcomputers. They automated preparation of the autopsy protocols and death certificates and led the processing effort that operated on eighteen-hour days through the rest of the month.

Officers in the personnel specialty (271 in 1982) provided the department's military personnel management support as a distinctive component of the Army's personnel system. Lt. Col. Thomas B. Pozniak, MSC, of the Surgeon General's Personnel Policy Division, organized the Army's Exceptional Family Member Program in 1982, a major undertaking that brought the Army into compliance with the statutory requirement for the Department of Defense Dependent Schools to provide services for handicapped children. Also in 1982, the Army established a system of personnel proponency, an initiative by General Edward C. Meyer, the chief of staff, to involve the functional proponents in the policy decisions affecting their specialties (for example, the commanding general of the Infantry School for infantry

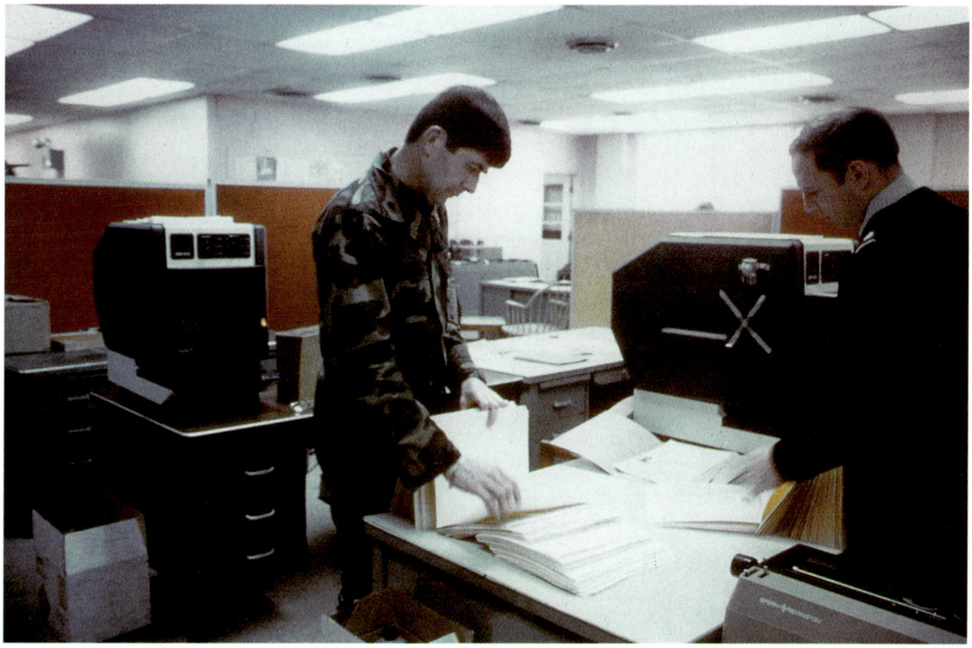

*Colonel Shannon (*right*) and Maj.Donald Fornier peruse records after Gander crash.*

soldiers). The Medical Department established an Enlisted Proponency Office in the Surgeon General's Office that was later expanded into the Personnel Proponency Directorate, organized at the Army Medical Department Center and School with Col. William J. Leary, Jr., as its head. It became the analytical arm of the Medical Department for all officer, enlisted, and civilian specialties.[57]

MSC personnel officers had to adjust their operating practices as the Army more fully integrated the management of Medical Department officers into its centralized personnel systems during the 1980s. In 1985, acting upon a study commissioned in 1982 by then Lt. Gen. Maxwell R. Thurman, the deputy chief of staff for personnel, the Army abolished the U.S. Army Medical Department Personnel Support Agency and transferred its personnel management functions to a newly formed Health Services Division (headed by an MSC) of the Officer Personnel Management Directorate (OPMD), a component of the U.S. Army Military Personnel Center, later renamed the U.S. Total Army Personnel Command (PERSCOM). While the surgeon general remained the proponent for military medical specialties, officer personnel management was centralized in PERSCOM, much as enlisted management had been earlier, and all Medical Department officers became "OPMD-managed." In 1988 the Health Services Division relocated from offices in Buzzard Point, Washington, D.C., to join the rest of OPMD in the Hoffman Center, Alexandria, Virginia.[58]

In 1982 there were 101 MSC comptrollers to handle the planning, programming, budgeting, and execution of the Army's medical programs as unit and DA and DOD staff officers. Graduate training was available through the Army

Comptrollership Program, a fourteen-month Syracuse University master of business administration program. Two MSCs were recognized during this period for being the top students in their classes: Capt. Fred Goeringer in 1979 and Capt. Kenneth L. Quaglio in 1991. A shortage of MSC comptrollers led the corps to establish a one-year master's degree program in public administration at Harvard University and to increase attendance at Syracuse from three to four MSCs in each class.[59]

There were 117 operations officers in 1982 (the Health Services Plans, Operations, Intelligence, and Training specialty). Opportunity for a master's in strategic intelligence at the Defense Intelligence School, Washington, D.C., began in 1980. A special event occurred in 1989 when the annual operations meeting at the Fitzsimons Army Medical Center, Denver, Colorado, was named in honor of Col. John R. Sperandio, USA, Ret., "a great soldier and dedicated Medical Service Corps officer" who had died the year before.[60]

New position opportunities opened on the staffs of the major medical commands, the Office of the Surgeon General, the Organization of the Joint Chiefs of Staff, and the Office of the Secretary of Defense. Some officers were assigned to the U.S. Army Center of Military History during the early part of this period, and 1st Lt. Gaines M. Foster, MSC, completed *The Demands of Humanity: Army Medical Disaster Relief*, published by the center. Some operations officers found challenge in military assistance assignments on advisory teams in Saudi Arabia and Central Africa. In May 1983 President Ronald Reagan ordered the deployment of a medical training team to El Salvador. Robert F. Elliott, now a colonel, was deputy chief of the team that trained 400 enlisted medics in six months and designed a medical infrastructure for the military forces. In 1987 the U.S. Army Medical Intelligence and Information Agency, Fort Detrick, became the Armed Forces Medical Intelligence Center, a tri-service activity under the command of Lt. Col. Jimmy Walker, MSC. Operations officer functions included operations security (OPSEC). An Army-wide program to recognize significant contributions to OPSEC resulted in the selection of Capt. William B. Miller, MSC, of Headquarters, Health Services Command, as the winner of the Individual Achievement Award for 1992.[61]

The perception that the operations specialty was overshadowed by others was largely reversed during this period. The 1977 annual meeting in Denver produced a report that listed fifty proposals to improve the specialty, including establishment of an operations course, incorporation of the manpower specialty, emphasis on a diversity of assignments, and increased recognition for officers who served in command positions.[62]

In 1979 a study group made nineteen further recommendations. Although many were routine changes to existing policies, others sought to improve the organizational climate, such as a recommendation to handle command assignments on a more personal basis. Some were adopted in part or not at all. Examples were the recommendation for the transfer of the manpower specialty—partially adopted in 1983 with the transfer of that division within the Surgeon General's Office to the director of health care operations—and the proposal for an operations course, which was dropped.[63]

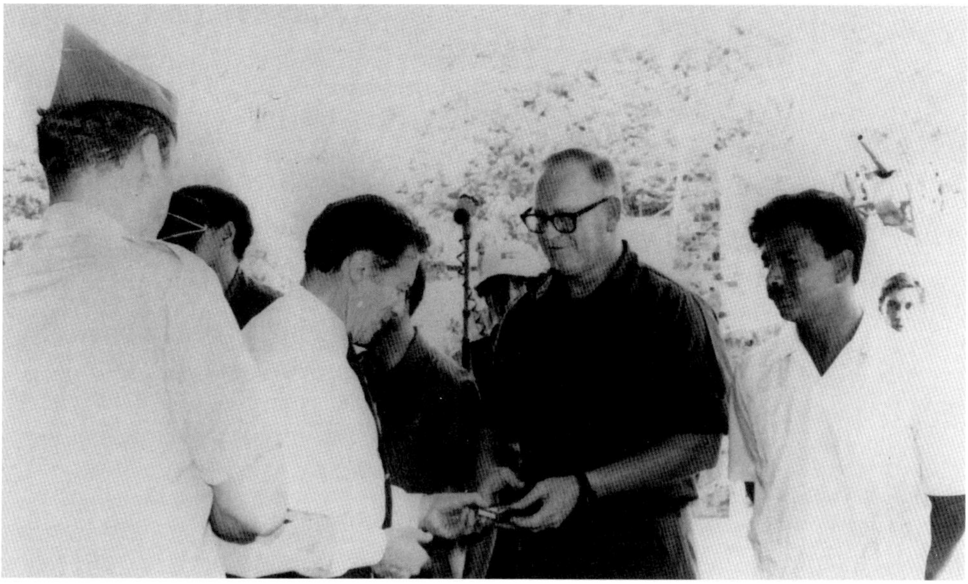

Colonel Elliott in El Salvador

In 1991 Col. Timothy Jackman, MSC, the specialty's consultant, published a handbook for operations officers that was a comprehensive guide to all aspects of a career in this specialty. In an article the following year he described operations officers as "keepers of the readiness flame" for the Medical Department. Training opportunities had expanded and now included a "track" in the Army-Baylor Program for operations officers. General Miketinac had agreed that they would retain their 67H operations identifier after completing the course rather than being reclassified as 67A, the specialty code for health care administration. He argued that 67 "Hotels" needed operational hospital experience, especially to prepare them for duties in medical center and regional strategic planning. The Baylor course was a step in that direction.[64]

MSC medical logisticians (343 in 1982) occupied key medical logistics positions, including chief of the Surgeon General's Logistics Division and commanders of medical depots; the U.S. Army Medical Materiel Agency (USAMMA), Fort Detrick; and the U.S. Army Medical Equipment and Optical School (USAMEOS), Denver, Colorado. In addition, some were assigned to various DOD logistics agencies and to the Army Combined Arms Support Center, Fort Lee.

They rested their case for medical control of medical supply on two principal points: the need for experts knowledgeable in its intricacies, and the need for a higher standard of performance than that required by the general supply system.[65] While the arguments were clear to experienced medics, they were not so evident to logisticians outside the department, who continued to challenge the department's position. MSCs assumed a continuing responsibility in communicating those arguments to the general logistics community through such devices as articles in *Army Logistician*, an Army publication. The explanations began at the ground level, as seen in an article published in 1995 by 1st Lt. Christine M. Nelson-Chung, MSC, the division medical supply officer for the 25th Infantry Division, Hawaii. Chung's article, "Medical Supply 101," was a primer for unit commanders.[66]

Medical depots of the theater of operations were organized into medical supply, optical, and maintenance (MEDSOM) units (later redesignated as medical logistics battalions), also under the command of MSC officers. MSCs commanded the depot in Pirmasens, Germany, a consolidation of three MEDSOMs into the U.S. Army Medical Materiel Center, Europe (USAMMCE), which the Secretary of Defense designated as the single manager for medical materiel in Europe. It provided medical logistics and optical fabrication support to Army, Navy, Air Force, and State Department activities in Europe, Africa, and the Middle East. Its staff of 641 processed 27,000 orders a month, maintaining an inventory of 16,000 different items in 800,000 square feet of warehouses on a 93-acre installation. USAMMCE shrink-wrapped stacked medical supplies in clear plastic, a technique introduced to the depot by Col. E. Kistler, MSC, to facilitate loading, shipping, and identification.[67]

Medical logistics officers completed the entry-level Medical Logistics Management Course at the Academy of Health Sciences. Advanced training was offered through two USAMMA courses: a six-month Medical Materiel Management Course and the Procurement Officer Program, a one-year course. In October 1982 Capts. Lawrence M. Foltz, MSC, and Warren F. Heinemann, MSC, were the first graduates of the Biomedical Equipment Maintenance Orientation Course, a four-month program at the U.S. Army Medical Equipment and Optical School (USAMEOS), Aurora, Colorado, that trained them in medical equipment installation, calibration, and repair. Some officers completed the Logistics Executive Development Course, a ten-month program leading to a master's degree in logistics management from the Florida Institute of Technology in Melbourne, Florida.[68]

The department appointed about ten warrant officers each year as health services maintenance technicians (there were a total of ninety-three in 1982). Candidates selected from enlisted applicants attended a fifteen-week course at USAMEOS, served in field positions, and returned for advanced training. MSC warrant officers also replaced Corps of Engineers warrant officers in field hospitals equipped with the new DEPMEDS sets.[69]

Health facilities planning became part of the logistics field during this period. Officers in this specialty (twenty-two in 1982) had opportunities for a master's degree and Ph.D. in architecture. Their principal assignments were as project officers at various construction sites. In 1975 the Army approved the formation of the U.S. Army Health Facilities Planning Agency (HFPA), an activity collocated with the Surgeon General's Office under the direction of Col. Charles E. Christ, MSC, its first commander. The agency (with a staff of thirty-two by 1995) provided a single point of control and continuity for all Army health facilities projects and oversaw an ambitious construction program of nearly $2 billion from 1975 to 1994. However, the trend of ever-increasing funding for construction projects was reversed in 1994 when the Office of the Secretary of Defense cut the Army, Navy, and Air Force program for fiscal years 1996 to 2001 by a billion dollars.[70]

MSC health care administrators belonged to an established profession. In the Army, the rules for awarding the specialty favored graduates of the Army-Baylor Program, but the corps did not close the door to other sources. Outside the military, the emergence of large hospital corporations and a host of smaller firms helped to turn health care administrators into hospital chief executive officers and the number of American hospitals with physicians as CEOs dropped to 202 by 1983. There was a return of women to the profession, and in 1981, 51 percent of the students in graduate programs were female.

The American College of Hospital Administrators numbered over nineteen thousand affiliates in 1985 when it changed its name to the American College of Healthcare Executives (ACHE), but only 200 of 1,200 military affiliates were Army officers, a reflection of the lack of emphasis by the MSC. Fourteen of the sixty-five military fellows (the highest rank in the ACHE) were Army MSCs, an improvement from eight in 1982, but still a small number. At the initiative of General Johnson, the corps sponsored the first "Army Day" at the 1986 meeting, and this added emphasis by the corps leadership resulted in increasing enrollment. Col. Douglas A. Barton, MSC, selected as the Army regent in 1992, spearheaded an effort to get the number over 500 so as to get a second regent for the Army. By August 1994 there were 517 Army affiliates, and his goal was assured. The number of Army fellows had increased to thirty-three, another indication of the improved record.[71]

General Johnson, with the support of Col. Gerald D. Allgood, MSC, the Health Services Command chief of staff, engineered a change in 1985 of the position title for the senior MSC in Army hospitals from executive officer to deputy commander for administration (DCA). This occurred as the title of the senior physician changed from chief of professional services to deputy commander for clinical services (DCCS). Johnson's intention was to equalize the authority between those two positions and to prevent a situation in which the executive officer would report to the DCCS rather than directly to the commander, although the department continued to prohibit the DCA from assuming command in the absence of the commander or the DCCS. The Health Services Command chief of staff position was given the additional duty of DCA for the same reason. Allgood believed that step could also help to restore the star his position had when the command was formed, thereby opening a new MSC opportunity. General Johnson planned to establish boards for selecting DCAs beginning in fiscal year 1986, but that plan was dropped and selections for those positions remained the province of the corps chief and the MSC Branch chief (the title reverted from Career Activities Office in 1985).[72]

Some MSCs gained regional and national recognition in health care administration. Col. Robert I. Jetland, MSC, retired from active duty in 1969, becoming the administrator of Harborview Medical Center in Seattle, Washington. He was named emeritus by that institution in 1985 and was honored as an outstanding retired alumnus by the Army-Baylor Alumni Club in 1990. Other MSCs were recognized with AMSUS awards. The Ray E. Brown Award, named for the pioneer in health care administration, was presented to General Haggerty in 1978 and to Col. James B. Stubblefield, Jr., in 1985. In 1981 Maj.

Richard V.N. Ginn was the first winner of the Young Federal Health Care Administrator Award. In 1987 Maj. Paul B. Mouritsen became the second Army officer to receive that award, and Maj. David A. Patillo was the third in 1991. Col. Philip L. Dorsey received the American Hospital Association's Federal Health Care Executive Award of Excellence in 1991, and Lt. Col. George V. Massi received the association's Federal Health Care Executive Special Achievement Award in 1993.[73]

MSC aviators (332 in 1982) played important roles in development of the Army's Utility Tactical Transport Aircraft System (UTTAS), a general-purpose helicopter that replaced the workhorse Bell UH–1 Huey models. Lt. Col. John W. Hammett, MSC, who worked with UTTAS from 1966 to 1970, found his biggest challenge was getting the Army to accept a requirement for a helicopter large enough to accommodate litters across the fuselage rather than longitudinally, as in the Huey. The resulting UH–60 Black Hawk, built by Sikorsky Corporation, was larger, more powerful, and faster than the Huey and met the desired medical requirements. It utilized a four-litter patient "carousel" that was inserted into the cabin. While a sophisticated device, it took up a lot of room and limited the patient capacity. Prototypes of an improved Black Hawk, the UH–60Q, as exhibited in 1993, abandoned the carousel for a specialized patient suite. The Q model incorporated twenty-three features that combined to make it a "Cadillac" of air ambulances. However, its cost was prohibitive, making it unlikely that the Army could procure it in its full array.[74]

In February 1979 1st Lt. Karen D. Anderson became the first female MSC aviator. There were thirty spaces for MSCs in flight school in 1980, a typical year, and 332 aeromedical evacuation officers in 1982. The Dustoff tradition continued, its camaraderie facilitated by the formation of the Dustoff Association, which held its first convention in 1980. In 1992 the association published a compilation assembled by Capt. Randall G. Anderson, MSC, of the unit histories of all sixty-nine active and reserve component air ambulance units.[75]

Nevertheless, the threat to the integrated Medical Department evacuation capability continued. In 1983 the Army formed the Aviation Branch, resurrecting the old Army Air Corps branch insignia. Immediately there were intense pressures to place MSC aviators in the new branch, and only concerted effort by the surgeon general's staff in actions coordinated by Lt. Col. Thomas C. Scofield, MSC, forestalled a takeover. Once again, a surgeon general laid it on the line: Mittemeyer protested that the Army's proposal would "result in death and suffering to our soldiers by changing a critical portion of total patient care which has already been tested and proven in combat." General Schwarzkopf, the acting deputy chief of staff for personnel, and General John A. Wickham, Jr., the vice chief of staff, weighed in with support, and Mittemeyer's argument was sustained. But Col. Douglas E. Moore, MSC, the surgeon general's executive officer, cautioned that the MSC could lose the next time. Paper bullets of the Pentagon could hurt worse than real ones.[76]

In 1985 the 52d Medical Battalion was activated in Korea under the command of Lt. Col. Jack R. Roden, Jr., MSC. It was the first evacuation battalion since Vietnam. Pilots of its 377th Air Ambulance Company were required to be fully familiar with the entire 153-mile width of the demilitarized zone, and all operations stressed night flying. MSC aviators continued performing Military Assistance to Safety and Traffic (MAST) operations. By 1984 the thirty-one participating units (twenty-four of which were Army) had evacuated nearly 33,000 emergency civilian patients. MAST units had flown 30,500 missions, often at night, in marginal weather, and/or from unimproved landing sites.[77]

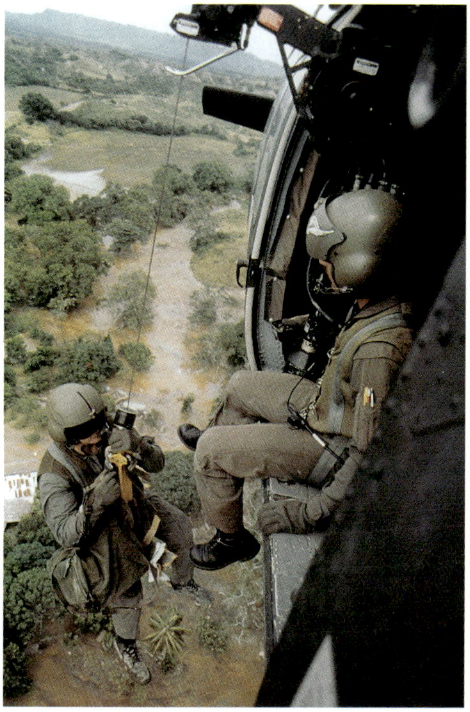

A medical technician is lowered from a U.S. Army UH–60A Black Hawk helicopter to look for survivors following the eruption of a volcano in Colombia, November 1985.

Dustoff crews were subject to immediate deployment. In 1985 two eruptions of a Colombian volcano unleashed avalanches of mud and water that crested at a depth of fifty feet, engulfing fourteen towns and villages. The disaster killed 23,000 people and left 22,000 homeless. The 214th Medical Detachment, stationed in Panama under the command of Maj. Robert E. Whiting, MSC, deployed two Black Hawks for the ensuing relief operations. The crews found that volcanic ash and rains had inundated areas with a sea of mud so deep that a nine-foot pole would not touch bottom. They subsequently conducted hoist missions to rescue survivors and used water trucks to hose off the victims, who were caked with crystallized mud.[78] Elsewhere the 421st Medical Company, now stationed in Germany, was reorganized in 1987 into the 421st Evacuation Battalion. It participated in Operation DISPLAY DETERMINATION, an exercise in which three Black Hawks deployed to Turkey for training planned and executed by the 2d Platoon commander, Capt. Analou R. Eisner, MSC.[79]

Military training was affected by the formation of the Aviation Branch. The Army stipulated that MSC aviators attend the Aviation Branch advanced course at the U.S. Army Aviation Center, Fort Rucker, Alabama. That was followed by a special six-week MSC advanced course at the Academy of Health Sciences where the officers were "re-marooned" (the Army's heraldic color for medical branches is maroon). However, such matters are never completely settled, and in 1986 the center proposed that the Aviation Branch absorb the aeromedical mission into general aviation with "beans and bullets forward, bodies and blood to the rear." The measure was again rejected, but it promised to be a continuing concern. While this move died down, the practice of sending the aviators to the follow-on course at Fort Sam Houston after Fort Rucker ceased.[80]

Developments in the Scientific Specialties

A Defense Audit Service survey in 1982 of commissioned pharmacists, optometrists, clinical psychologists, and physician assistants in the military revealed a commonly held perception that opportunities for promotion in these areas were less than in the administrative MSC fields. But several analyses of the matter by the Surgeon General's Office failed to substantiate that perception. For example, the promotion opportunity from 1986 to 1991 for major, lieutenant colonel, and colonel was similar among the two groups; sometimes the scientific specialty officers fared even better. There were several reasons for this relative equity. The success of each specialty was closely monitored by the various consultants whose feedback to the personnel system was continuous and direct. The presence of scientific specialty officers on promotion boards also ensured promotion parity. The letter of instructions provided to each board was another. It typically mentioned the special requirements of officers in the scientific fields, and beginning in 1991 it also included "floors" (or mandatory minimum promotion quotas) for individual specialties as another guarantee of promotion equity.[81]

The issue of compensation for certain scientific specialties took a new turn in 1994. While the 1982 survey did not expose a morale problem associated with pay, the perception persisted over the years that military pay was a source of dissatisfaction for officers in certain specialties involved in direct patient care, especially psychology, which continued to have difficulty in retaining officers. In a move that surprised the Army, in 1994 the assistant secretary of defense for health affairs directed the military services to implement a special pay program ranging from $2,000 to $5,000 annually for a number of nonphysician health care providers. What had started out as a special pay program to reward psychologists who had achieved diplomate status was expanded to other categories of Medical Department officers who achieved board-certified status. In the case of the MSC this applied to audiologists, optometrists, pharmacists, podiatrists, and social workers.[82]

Pharmacy officers added capabilities in clinical treatment programs, the preparation of customized sterile intravenous fluid therapies, and inpatient unit dose systems of prepackaged medications for each patient issued daily to hospital wards (to reduce the potential for medication errors). The 215 pharmacy officers in 1982 was a slight increase from an average of 200 officers in the late 1960s. Most pharmacists were commissioned from ROTC, and in 1988 the newly formed U.S. Army Cadet Command was holding ten to fifteen spaces a year as delayed entry spaces for those ROTC students desiring to complete pharmacy training prior to entry on active duty. Pharmacy officers also had opportunities for graduate training leading to a master's of science, doctor of pharmacy, or Ph.D. in pharmacology.[83]

A nuclear pharmacy program at Letterman Army Medical Center, San Francisco, California, trained five Army officers who were among the first sixty-three nuclear pharmacists certified by national examinations of the Board of Pharmaceutical Specialties in 1983. That same year Capt. Michael S. Edwards, MSC, became the first resident in an oncology pharmacy practice program begun at Walter Reed Army Medical Center under Lt. Col. John J. Pelosi, MSC, one of two programs in the United States accredited by the American Society of Hospital Pharmacists. By 1988 there were oncology pharmacy training programs at the Army medical centers in the United States; the residents administered chemotherapy and participated in all phases of clinical drug trials.

In 1974 Capt. Terry V. Guilbert, MSC, established the U.S. Army Allergen Extract Laboratory at Walter Reed Army Medical Center, which by 1988 provided diagnostic and immunotherapy stocks to a number of federal hospitals and maintained 20,000 patient profiles. Some pharmacy officers received national recognition. The AMSUS Andrew Craigie Award, recognizing advancement of pharmacy in the federal government, was presented to Col. George A. Sommers, MSC, in 1980; Col. A. Gordon Moore, MSC, in 1981; Col. Douglas J. Silvernale, MSC, in 1984; and Col. David L. Schroder, MSC, in 1991. In 1987 Lt. Col. Gerald L. Wannarka, MSC, shared the Secretary of the Army's Award for Outstanding Achievement in Materiel Acquisition for managing the Army's development of a cyanide antidote for chemical weapon defense. It combined a longer shelf life with a smaller size that made it easier for soldiers to use, while saving about $10 million a year.[84]

In 1982 the 840 officers of the Medical Allied Sciences Section represented 16.8 percent of the corps (*see Appendix L*). There were 253 social work officers, 163 psychologists, 70 audiologists, and 52 podiatrists. Laboratory sciences was the largest group, numbering 302 officers, with 56 microbiologists, 81 biochemists, 18 parasitologists, 30 immunologists, 92 clinical laboratory officers, and 25 physiologists. A byproduct of the MSC Management Study was a better understanding that requirements for those specialties were derived from military necessity. General Miketinac stressed that there was no need for scientific officers to believe they had to have administrative assignments along the way in order to be competitive for promotion; their duty was to perform in their designated specialty.[85]

Educational opportunities continued to be an attraction for military service. Offerings included doctoral programs in audiology, biochemistry, immunology, microbiology, psychology, and toxicology. Other programs included a master's in toxicology, a two-year advanced social work program in family studies, a one-year postgraduate residency program in podiatry, and a one-year medical technology program for clinical laboratory officers.

Some scientific specialty officers received national recognition. Lt. Col. Robert T. Usry, MSC, as president and in other leadership roles from 1979 to 1982, oversaw the growth of the Society of Armed Forces Medical Laboratory Scientists to over 750 members. In 1983 the director of the Army Aeromechanics Laboratory of the Ames Research Center at Moffet Field, California, presented the Director's Award for Technological Achievement to Capt. James W. Voorhees, MSC, an engineering research psychologist. Voorhees, the first military officer so recognized, was honored for developing visual and speech symbols for a prototype "friend or foe" radar warning indicator. In 1984 the National Aeronautics and Space Administration (NASA) selected a reserve officer, Capt. Millie Hughes-Fulford, MSC, an associate professor of biochemistry at the University of California, as the only female scientist selected for the Spacelab program from outside NASA. In June 1991 Hughes-Fulford, then a Veterans Affairs researcher in San Francisco, conducted blood studies as a payload specialist on the shuttle *Columbia*. Maj. Daryl J. Kelly, MSC, a microbiologist at the Walter Reed Army Institute of Research, received the Army Research and Development Award in 1987 for developing a portable test kit for field diagnosis of typhus. Award of the "A prefix" designator to scientific specialty officers that began in 1961 continued as a distinctive recognition for selected officers.[86]

In 1978 there were fifty-three audiologists on active duty (forty-three at the master's level and ten at the Ph.D.); by 1982 there were seventy. The establishment of the Exceptional Family Member Program, an effort which included provisions for children with hearing impairment, added to the requirements for audiologists. But hearing conservation remained the primary reason for having military audiologists. In 1984 the Veterans Administration paid over $161 million to veterans with service-connected hearing losses, and DOD civilian employees collected over $25 million in claims.[87]

The Army continued to mandate that audiologists devote one-half of their time to hearing conservation, but the emphasis proved difficult to maintain at posts with heavy clinical demands. Consequently, Maj. Roy K. Sedge, MSC, the consultant, disapproved a proposal that all hospitals conduct hearing aid evaluation and aural rehabilitation. Sedge insisted on reserving those functions for the medical centers so as to ensure that smaller facilities would be able to perform their hearing conservation mission. The Army Audiology and Speech Center at Walter Reed Army Medical Center was the center of activity, ranking sixth of two hundred such centers nationally in 1979. Its developments included the use of biofeedback with hypertensive voice-disordered soldiers, brain-stem evoked response audiometry, and an inpatient aural rehabilitation program. Elsewhere, new initiatives included a mobile van developed by Capt. Michael J. Mouel, MSC, at Fort Carson, Colorado, that was able to test six soldiers simultaneously. In 1993 Col. Rodney M. Atack, MSC, the specialty consultant, said that Army audiology was one of the "great success stories" of military medicine for its development of new technologies in hearing conservation, training of hearing conservationists, and audiology research.[88]

The number of podiatrists on active duty increased to fifty-two in 1982. Capt. Peter C. Smith, MSC, a podiatrist assigned to Bassett Army Community Hospital, Fort Wainwright, Alaska, was recognized in 1993 with the William Kershisnik Award of the Society of Armed Forces Podiatrists, as was Capt. Katherine A. Ward, MSC, of Walter Reed Army Medical Center, in 1994. The shortage of physicians prompted their expanded use, and nine podiatrists were assigned to assist orthopedic surgeons during the worst period. The Medical Department also identified procedures that podiatrists could perform in emergency situations: they could serve as skilled surgical assistants, debride major wounds and second degree burns, and reduce fractures of the ankle and tibia. A move in 1984 to place podiatrists in the Medical Corps, where they presumably would have greater opportunities, was opposed by the American Medical Association on the grounds that reassignment would make them eligible for command of hospitals, "dilute the integrity" of the Medical Corps, and make it more difficult to attract physicians to Army service. The proposal died.[89]

A boom in personal fitness added to the demand for podiatric services and made it harder for the Army to compete for podiatrists. In 1980, 75 percent of MSC podiatrists had less than four years of active duty, a reflection of the specialty's expansion and the difficulty in retaining these specialists. It was necessary to offer educational opportunities to overcome inexperience and stimulate retention. A residency program began at Brooke Army Medical Center in 1981, and by 1988, 65 percent of its graduates went on to postgraduate residency training programs. The department also established a program of postgraduate residencies at accredited civilian institutions. Maj. Douglas R. Beirne, MSC, attended the University of Texas in 1980 as the Army's first resident selected in this program.[90]

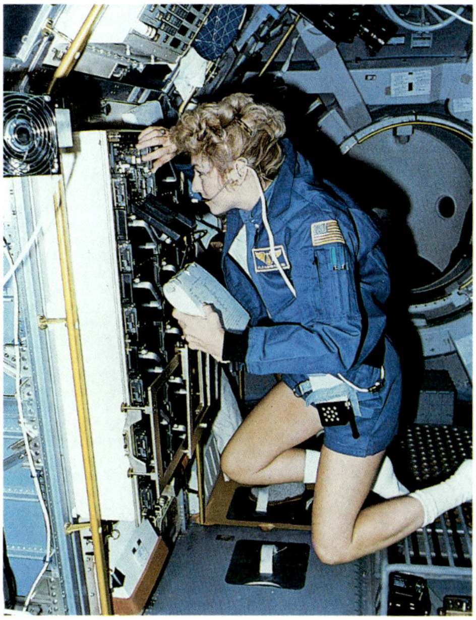

Captain Hughes-Fulford kneeling in front of an animal cage on the Shuttle Columbia, *June 1991*

There were 163 MSC psychologists in 1982, including 87 clinical psychologists, 45 research psychologists, and 31 psychology associates. The Health Professsions Scholarship Program (HPSP) was the prime source for psychologists, accounting for 42 percent of accessions from 1979 to 1981. Plans to increase accessions by quadrupling the number of scholarships were dashed when DOD restricted HPSP in 1981 to entering medical students. HPSP was reinstituted for psychology in 1990 with three spaces each year. The Ph.D. was the standard for Army practice and was the preferred prerequisite for commissioning in that specialty, although some psychologists were commissioned at the master's level pending completion of their doctoral requirements. Those officers who had completed all their Ph.D. requirements except the dissertation received the title of psychology associate (formerly behavioral science associate).[91]

Military requirements spanned the field's diversity. Maj. Larry H. Ingraham, MSC, told the 1975 meeting of the American Psychological Association that the Medical Department had to maintain a mix of skills to be able to respond immediately to changing needs. He cited the drug control program as an example of a mission that had required an immediate response. Hospital privileges of Army clinical psychologists now routinely incorporated patient assessment and treatment functions; some performed 24-hour on-call duty for psychiatric emergencies. Others were engaged in the Army's alcohol and drug treatment programs, an effort estimated to return to duty about 15,000 soldiers each year, the equivalent of a division. Psychologists assigned to divisions provided mental hygiene consultation services at the grass roots level.

Capt. Lawrence E. Klusman, MSC, stationed in Germany with the 1st Armored Division, surveyed his fellow Seventh Army psychologists and found their greatest success rate with problem soldiers came from early intervention. Their expertise was especially valuable in advising Army leaders in a time when over 56 percent of soldiers were married. Maj. Frederick N. Garland, MSC, and Lt. Col. Franklin R. Brooks, MSC, described this capability in an article they published in 1992 in *Military Review*, the journal of the Army Command and General Staff College. Their article, aimed at a line officer audience, discussed the special problems of military families who were potential targets of terrorist attacks, particularly those stationed overseas.[92]

In 1980 the clinical psychology consultant, Col. Cecil B. Harris, MSC, reported that 70 percent of all MSC psychologists would leave active duty by their eighth year of service. An Academy of Health Sciences survey of 130 psychologists on active duty and 69 who had left the Army indicated that these officers were satisfied with the work environment, supervisors, and coworkers, but dissatisfied with pay and promotions.[93] A DOD request that the Army grant psychologists departmental autonomy was rejected by the surgeon general.[94] Dissatisfaction with pay and promotions was offset to a degree by educational opportunities. In 1981 Madigan Army Medical Center, Fort Lewis, Washington, began postdoctoral fellowships in child psychology and neuropsychology. The latter was started by Capt. Raymond A. Parker, MSC, as training that linked behavioral change to neurological problems and was especially useful in treating brain-injured patients.[95]

Some psychologists filled assignments outside the specialty. In 1981 Colonel Harris left his post as assistant professor of medicine at the Uniformed Services University of the Health Sciences to become the executive officer of the 5th General Hospital, Bad Cannstatt, Germany. In 1984 Lt. Col. Frank J. Sodetz, Jr., became the first MSC to command the South East Asia Treaty Organization (SEATO) Laboratory in Bangkok, Thailand, a U.S. Army Medical Research and Development Command (USAMRDC) activity.

Research was another attraction, and Sodetz' appointment as the first research psychology consultant in 1979 marked the establishment of that field as a separate specialty. Major Ingraham and Maj. Frederick J. Manning, MSC, reilluminated the old problem of combat exhaustion, a problem that they called combat stress reaction. Manning also caught the eye of Army leaders with research on sleep deprivation. His team from the U.S. Army Medical Research Unit–Europe, a USAMRDC activity, observed the members of an artillery battalion during exercises in Germany. They found that sleep deprivation was risky for those in positions requiring mental alertness. Their report cut across ingrained beliefs that chronic fatigue was a mark of dedicated leadership. To the contrary, their findings demonstrated that sleep for leaders was an important factor in a unit's effectiveness.[96]

In 1979 there were 269 social work officers, 169 of whom were assigned to the Health Services Command where chiefs of social work reported directly to the hospital deputy commanders for clinical services. A 1982 study found that Army social workers were generally satisfied with their military careers. Some were assigned to duties outside their primary specialty. For example, Col. Paul F. Darnauer, MSC, was appointed the inspector general of the 7th Medical

Command in 1980, and at the time of his retirement in 1986 he was the USAMRDC chief of staff. However, hospital-based social work remained a principal area of concentration, and in 1982 the social work consultant, Col. David P. Jentsch, MSC, coauthored *Social Work in Hospitals*, a practical guide for students and beginning social workers.[97]

The postdraft All-Volunteer Army with its higher percentage of family members increased the Army's attention to family support, and some officers completed the two-year Advanced Social Work Program in Child and Family Studies at Walter Reed Army Medical Center. The new emphasis was reflected in the activities of social work officers in family therapy and marital counseling in which they addressed such problems as family violence, terminally ill patients, rape victims, handicapped children, single parents, and pregnant unmarried soldiers and their dependents. Accordingly, social workers were assigned to family advocacy and community service programs and alcohol and drug abuse clinics. As Col. Robert A. Mays, Jr., MSC, the social work consultant in 1993, noted: "Commanders frequently use social workers to handle situations which require tact, diplomacy, sensitivity, and soldier skills."[98]

Sanitary Engineering

There were 372 officers in the Sanitary Engineering Section in 1982 (7.5 percent of the corps), including 94 sanitary engineers, 143 environmental science officers, 54 nuclear medical science officers, and 81 entomologists (*see Appendix L*). Accessions depended upon ROTC and direct commissions, and assignments included the U.S. Army Environmental Hygiene Agency (AEHA) at Aberdeen Proving Ground, Maryland, an agency commanded by MSCs. Some officers were assigned to the Army Corps of Engineers for duty with the Army Pollution Abatement Program. The USAMRDC provided other opportunities, and Col. John F. Erskine, MSC, a sanitary engineer, became the command's chief of staff in 1986.[99]

Demand for environmental science officers (ESOs) accelerated as the department assigned them to field units and converted positions for preventive medicine and occupational health physicians at twenty installations to ESOs. Capt. John Y. Young, MSC, Fort Ord, California, prepared a handbook for soldiers taking part in 7th Infantry Division maneuvers in 1985 on the Caribbean island of St. Lucia. Young, commander of an environmental sanitation unit, the 172d Medical Detachment (LB), provided guidance on topics ranging from water to insects. He warned soldiers to "be prepared or prepare to be miserable," but also related that snakes were almost nonexistent due to a large mongoose population which "seems to be taking care of the chickens as well."[100]

Nuclear medical science officers enabled the department to meet the strict requirements of federal regulatory agencies for the use of radioisotopes, x-ray equipment, and other electronic devices; there were fifty-four officers in 1982. The majority came directly from civilian life, but their retention was adversely affected by perceptions of inequities in promotion opportunity and pay. In 1978 the Medical Department estimated that a pay gap of twenty-five to thirty thousand dollars per year existed between the military and civilian sectors of their field and, as in other specialties, attempted to improve retention through educational and position opportunities. In 1982, for example, Col. Bobby Adcock, MSC, became the first nonphysician director of the Armed Forces Radiobiological Research Institute in Bethesda, Maryland.[101]

Optometry

The Optometry Section accounted for 219 officers in 1982, or 4.4 percent of the corps (*see Appendix L*). Retention was a problem for this specialty. A 1979 study showed that 36 percent of all optometrists left the Army by the end of their third year on active duty, and 84 percent were gone by the end of the tenth. A difference in earnings between military and civilian careers, estimated at more than $278,000 over a 28-year period, made Army careers a hard sell. That had not been helped in 1975 when special pay for optometrists was halted. It was reinstated in 1979 at the original $100 monthly rate even though the Army had argued for much more. The number of optometrists on active duty dropped to 179 in 1985, and the department let hospitals in the United States go short in order to keep positions filled overseas, resulting in appointment backlogs of up to six months. Although the situation improved as the number rose to 219 in 1982, the gains proved temporary. By 1988 the number dropped to 150, of which 110 were committed overseas, again necessitating shortchanging stateside hospitals as the cycle repeated itself.[102]

Recruiting was hampered by an incident at the Academy of Health Sciences in 1976 when a group of optometrists in the basic officers course, already sensitive to perceptions of second-class status, were denied administrative absences to take their state licensure board examinations after being told, "You're not doctors, you're Medical Service Corps officers." With a generous dash of salt in an old wound, tempers flared. The flap went public in the *Journal of the American Optometric Association*. One optometrist solicited his colleagues for support in separating from the MSC; he received twenty-nine letters of support. The AOA president and three other officials met with General Pixley and his staff in the Pentagon. Their meeting resolved the contretemps, and a subsequent editorial encouraged graduates to consider the Army as a career.[103]

Recruiting was hurt by the ending of the HPSP scholarships for optometry students in 1980. It had provided about twenty accessions per year for the Army, almost the sum total of new officers annually. The optometry profession again cried foul, and Congressman Bill Nichols of the House Armed Services Committee asked the Department of Defense to lift the restriction. That was to no avail, and by 1987 there was again a shortage of optometrists. HPSP was finally reinstituted for optometry in 1988 with twenty-five openings per year, and by 1993 the program was accepting over fifty students a year.[104]

Col. Arthur R. Giroux, MSC, was appointed chief of the Optometry Section in 1975. He served as an effective spokesman until his retirement in 1983, spearheading a variety of initiatives. Those included recruiting trips to schools of optometry, increasing HPSP scholarships (until the program ended), and an advertising campaign that proclaimed that Army optometry "Deserves a Closer

Look."[105] Position opportunities included head of the Optical Directorate of the U.S. Army Medical Materiel Center, Europe, an activity that fabricated 15,000 pairs of spectacles a month.[106]

Giroux established nineteen clinical clerkships for optometry students at Army hospitals, a good recruiting tool. He also began an annual three-day Optometric Management Course and designed a master's program in clinical optometric management at the Pacific University College of Optometry, Portland, Oregon. Giroux maintained close ties with the AOA, whose Council on Clinical Optometric Care began accrediting Army optometry clinics; that also added to the attractiveness of Army programs. The council surveyed eight hospitals in 1979 and nine in 1980.[107]

Optometrists were also unhappy over their inability to enter the service as captains, and Colonel Giroux was the catalyst in resolving that problem in 1980 with the "50-75 rule," a marvel of Byzantine language in DOPMA. Under this rule, a graduate of a professional school was eligible for constructive credit for all the time spent in the school—four years in the case of optometry—if it could be established that 50 percent or more of the professional schools for that specialty required three or more years of undergraduate studies and if 75 percent or more of the students in the entering classes of those schools exceeded that requirement by one or more years. The result was that physicians, dentists, veterinarians, optometrists, podiatrists, and clinical psychologists all entered active duty as captains.[108]

The efforts to improve recruitment and retention worked. Twenty-four optometrists were recruited in 1981 and twenty-one in 1982, as compared to five per year from 1977 to 1979. Retention of officers beyond their initial obligation, a dismal 5 percent in fiscal years 1975 to 1976, improved to 41 percent in 1979 and reached 55 percent by 1981. The recruiting efforts attracted optometrists who later received special recognition that attested to their contributions to military medicine. In 1990 and 1993 the Armed Forces Optometric Society elected Capt. Francis L. McVeigh and Maj. George L. Adams III, respectively, as the Military Optometrist of the Year. In 1991 the Society of U.S. Army Flight Surgeons presented its Outstanding Achievement Award to Maj. Morris R. Lattimore, Jr., MSC, a research optometrist of the U.S. Army Aeromedical Research Laboratory, Fort Rucker, Alabama, for contributions to Army aviation through his work in contact lens wear by aviators. Lattimore was also recognized by the Medical Department's Award of Excellence in 1992 for this project.[109]

Scope of practice continued to be a sensitive matter. Although the Army permitted optometrists to use topical anesthetics and cycloplegic drugs for refractions, it required the immediate availability of a physician for adverse reactions. The AOA protested that civilian optometrists had never been under the supervision of physicians, and Maj. Gen. William C. Augerson, the deputy assistant secretary of defense for health affairs, formed a tri-service working group of optometrists and ophthalmologists to resolve the conflict. DOD pressure and Colonel Giroux's prodding produced results. In 1981 the surgeon general submitted a change to Army regulations authorizing optometrists to use diagnostic drugs and to prescribe "glasses, contact lenses and other therapy as appropriate."[110]

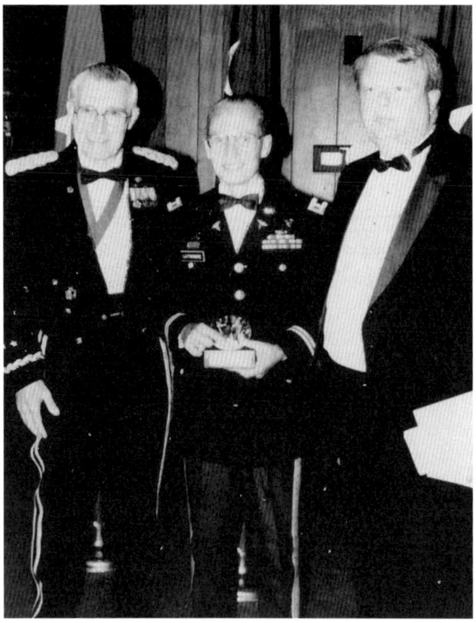

Major Lattimore (center) *receives the AMEDD Award of Excellence in Allied Health Care.*

Summary

General Haggerty had criticized the department for continuing to block MSCs from its top positions at the beginning of the post-Vietnam period. MSCs, he maintained, were the logical candidates for a variety of key posts such as Chief of Staff, Health Services Command; Commander, U.S. Army Medical Research and Development Command; Commandant and Deputy Commandant, Academy of Health Sciences; and Deputy Commander, 7th Medical Command. Two of his recommendations came to fruition.[111] Col. Vernon McKenzie, a retired MSC and the principal deputy assistant secretary of defense for health affairs, said in 1984 that he would advise a young person contemplating a career in the MSC to consider it very carefully because of the barriers to reaching the top in the Army Medical Department. Those perceptions were not uncommon. However, such misgivings should not obscure the improvements that occurred in the growing opportunities for positions of increased responsibility, a point made by those who counseled that MSCs were "too good to be ignored." Yet McKenzie's caution remained valid, for the top jobs continued to be blocked.[112]

Promotion lags during this period were offset somewhat by educational opportunities. Recruitment and retention problems continued in certain specialties such as psychology; in some fields, such as optometry, the swings in the number on active duty were exaggerated, resulting in periods in which the department was unable to meet its mission requirements. Overall, there was increased professionalism through training, advancements in position opportunity, and the recognition of officers by professional guilds. The external associations continued to play a role in the internal developments of the corps, and their awards—for example, those by the Association of Military Surgeons—were evidence of the validation of MSC specialty groups and officers according to national standards.

Ironically, there was an obverse side to the expansion of position opportunity. The newly opened jobs were among the department's most demanding. Their pressures were very great and often required family relocations to areas that, if not undesirable, were more costly or at the least constituted one more move among many in a career. Yet the normal incentives of progression to the top jobs and further promotions were not present. Indeed, some MSC colonels moved into positions vacated by generals, Col. Neil McDonald being an example. In other words, the department expected MSCs to take its most responsible positions without adequate opportunities for rewards, to shoulder "unusual challenges without hope of unusual recognition."[113] The situation served to emphasize anew both the corps' steady progress and its continuing status as a less than equal partner in the Medical Department.

Notes

[1] Shortage: Rpt, Manpower Mgmt Div, OTSG (DASG-RMM), DCSPER–46, pt. 1, sub: AMEDD Officer Strength, FY 64–82, 4 Jan 83, DASG-MS; Paul Smith, "Army Physician Shortage Finally Easing," *Army Times* (31 August 1981): 12. Pixley: "Improving Manpower: Pixley's Early Days," *U.S. Medicine* (15 September 1981): 19. Also see "Military Doesn't Attract Young MDs," *U.S. Medicine* (1 November 1978): 1.

[2] Physician recruitment: Neil Roland, "General Pixley Credited With Turning the Tide," *Army Times*, 22 November 1982. Also see Maj. Charles M. Lott, MSC, "USAMEDDPERSA History," *'Persanality'*, USAMEDDPERSA Newsletter, 31 October 1985 (final issue); Pixley, "Army Physicians: Medics on the Mend," incl to DF, Col Guy D. Plunkett, MC, Ch, Professional Svcs, BAMC, sub: Communication from Pixley, 1980; Pixley said they did a "magnificent job." Interv, Pixley with Ginn, Bethesda, Md., 1 Nov 84, all in DASG-MS.

[3] Pessimism: The variable incentive pay (VIP) program was structured in such a way as to encourage retention. It proved to be an effective initiative, and projections after its first full year of operation in 1976 that the overall DOD physician shortage would not resolve until 1981 were soon revised downward to 1979. Briefing, Capt Larry Kobe, Ofc of the Asst Sec Def for Health Affairs (ASD [HA]), sub: Variable Incentive Pay, 19 Aug 77, author's notes, DASG-MS. MC numbers: Information (info) papers, Maj Thomas C. Clegg, MSC, USAMEDDPERSA, sub: Medical Corps End Strength, and Medical Corps Specialty Shortages, 15 April 82; Lt. Rpt, Col Thomas E. Broyles, MSC, Manpower Div, OTSG (DASG-RM), sub: Medical Corps Strength (Actual), End Fiscal Years 1973 to 1991, 18 Dec 94, all in DASG-MS.

[4] Loss of medical battalion: DF, Deputy Chief of Staff for Operations (DCSOPS), to TSG, sub: Read Ahead for 5 Mar 82 CSA Decision Brief, 24 Feb 82, and CMT 2, TSG, 25 Feb 82, Health Care Doctrine Div (DASG-HCD); Info paper, Lt Col Joseph F. Yohman, MSC, DASG-HCD, sub: Division 86 Relook, 24 Feb 82, DASG-HCD; MSC Newsletter, 15 February 1985, all in DASG-MS. The loss of the medical battalion was a fundamental reordering of field medical support. The author agrees with critics who argue "We took a great step backward." Ltr to the editor, Maj. Neal Trent, MSC, "AMEDD and Readiness," *Army* 44 (December 1989): 5.

[5] Medical Systems Program Review (MSPR): The study reflected the personal involvement of the academy commandant, Maj. Gen. William P. Winkler, MC. Briefing slides, Winkler, sub: MSPR, 31 May 84, DASG-MS.

[6] Doctrine: Discussion based on U.S. Army Training and Doctrine Command (TRADOC) Pamphlet 525–5, *AirLand Operations*, 1 Aug 91; Field Manual 8–10, *Health Service Support in a Theater of Operations*, 1 Mar 91; TRADOC Pam 525–10, *U.S. Army Operational Concept for Health Service Support, AirLand Battle*, 11 Apr 86; Briefing slides, Ofc of Asst Ch of Staff, Opns (ACSOPS), 7th Medical Command (MEDCOM), sub: Health Service Support, AirLand Battle (HSSALB), 25 Feb 87, DASG-MS; Info paper, Maj Phillip T. Martinez, MSC, ACSOPS, 7th MEDCOM, sub: HSSALB, 19 Feb 87, and Briefing, 25 Feb 87, Neckargmuend, Federal Republic of Germany (FRG), author's notes, DASG-MS; Rpt, Academy of Health Sciences, U.S. Army (AHS), sub: Health Service Support AirLand Operations, in AMEDD Stockholders Rpt, 27 Jul 91, pp. 1, 24; Memo, Col James J. Truscott, MSC, Asst Cmdt, Force Integration, AMEDD Center and School, sub: Health Service Support, 17 Jan 91, all in DASG-MS. FM 8–10 is described as "the keystone manual for the Army Medical Department" (p. iii). Experiments: One discarded concept was a "TOE carved out of TDA" in the stateside hospitals that would have identified field hospital units within the organization of the fixed facilities—with the field unit component deploying for contingencies. Health Services Support AirLand Battle (HSSALB): HSSALB was suspended in 1986 at the request of the commander in chief of the U.S. Army, Europe, and Seventh Army, who said it would clutter the corps area with recuperating patients and hospital units. The Seventh Army surgeon estimated it would increase the requirement for patient beds in the corps area from 15,000 to 33,000, an unacceptably large logistical "tail." Msg, CINCUSAREUR to DCSOPS, DA, (DAMO-FD), 171700Z Oct 86, sub: Programming of HSSALB, DASG-MS. Implications of changes: See Chapter 2 of this book and Karl D. Bzik and Ronald F. Bellamy, "A Note on Combat Casualty Statistics," *Military Medicine* 149 (April 1984): 229–31; Eran Dolev and Craig H. Llewellyn, "The Chain of Medical Responsibility in Battlefield Medicine," *Military Medicine* 150

(September 1985): 471–75; Ronald F. Bellamy, "Contrasts in Combat Casualty Care," *Military Medicine* 150 (August 1985): 409–10, and Ltr to the editor, *Military Medicine* 151 (January 1986): 63–64.

[7] Four hospitals: Medical Force 2000 hospitalization was provided by four hospital units: mobile Army surgical hospital, combat support hospital, field hospital, and a general hospital plus a medical holding company. FM 8–10, *Health Service Support in a Theater of Operations*, app. J, 1 Mar 91, PL.

[8] Deployable Medical Systems (DEPMEDS): Info paper, Capt John H. Brown, MSC, HQ, 7th MEDCOM, sub: DEPMEDS, 20 Feb 87; Msg, Sec Def (ASD-HA), 142227Z Apr 86, sub: FY87 DEPMEDS Budget; Presentation, Capt David Stanley, MSC, sub: DEPMEDS, at the MSC annual meeting, Garmisch, Federal Republic of Germany (FRG), 11 May 88 (author's notes), all in DASG-MS. Operational use: Brett D. Walker and Richard V.N. Ginn, "Continued Operations with DEPMEDS During Hospital Closure," *AMEDD Journal*, (August/September 1991): 13–20 (until 1987 the central house organ is cited as *Medical Bulletin*; thereafter it is cited as *AMEDD Journal*, plus the date, as the *Medical Bulletin of the U.S. Army, Europe*, was renamed in 1987 the *Medical Bulletin of the U.S. Army Medical Department*, and shortly thereafter, the *Journal of the U.S. Army Medical Department*); Briefing, Lt Col Stephen H. Johnson, MSC, Cdr, 5th MASH, sub: REFORGER After Action Report, HQ, 7th MEDCOM, Heidelberg, FRG, 12 Feb 90, notes by Lt Col David Forshey, MSC, DASG-MS.

[9] MSC numbers: MSC Newsletter, 30 September 1981; Rpt, Personnel Distribution Div, OTSG (DASG-PTH), 1 Sep 82; Briefing slide, DASG-PTH, sub: MSC Strength, 1 Sep 84; Rpt, Ch, MSC, sub: Directory of MSC Officers, 15 Jan 87; Rpt, Personnel Directorate, OTSG (DASG-PTZ), RQTDEC91, 11 Feb 92, all in DASG-MS; Bernhard T. Mittemeyer, "Facing Challenges, Army Goals Endure," *U.S. Medicine* 18 (15 January 1982): 42. There were 4,957 MSCs in 1975; 4,834 in 1980; 4,901 in 1982; 5,025 in 1984; 4,981 in 1987; and 5,005 in 1991.

[10] Lohmiller: Memo, Maj William Lohmiller, MSC, for Dir Pers, OTSG, sub: MSC Officer Classification and Utilization System, 26 Sep 78, DASG-MS.

[11] MSC study: Presentation, Lt Col William J. Leary, Jr., MSC, AHS, sub: MSC Management Study, MSC Meeting, Garmisch, FRG, 14 May 90, author's notes; Info paper, Lt Col Peter Leventis, MSC, AHS, sub: MSC Management Study Implementation Update, undated; Info paper, Col Timothy Jackman, MSC, sub: MSC Management Study, 17 Oct 89; MSC Newsletter, 15 December 1987 and 29 March 1991, all in DASG-MS; AR 611–101, Commissioned Officer Classification System, change 5, 1 Jul 94.

[12] ROTC: Rpt, Col James M. Morgan, MSC, USAR, sub: Suggestions for Recruiting, Apr 78, DASG-MS. Of the 400 officers commissioned in 1981, 125 were direct appointments from 800 applicants. USMA: Bernard J. Adelsberger, "980 Academy Cadets Choose Branches," *Army Times* (18 April 1988): 10. 1992 accessions: 271 ROTC, 27 Health Professions Scholarship Program (HPSP), 60 USUHS (medical students), 32 direct commissions, 13 clinical psychology interns, 12 USMA, 16 other—total 435. This compares to 442 MC and 482 ANC accessions the same year. Info paper, Mil Pers Mgmt Div, OTSG (DASG-PTM), sub: AMEDD Officer Personnel Strength Management, 1 Feb 93, DASG-MS.

[13] Women in the Army (WITA): Policy statement, DCSPER, sub: Speaking With One Voice: Interim Position Regarding Women in the Army, 2 Sep 81, DASG-MS; Memo, Ginn for TSG, sub: Women in the Army In-Process Review, 13 Apr 83 (follow-up to DCSPER WITA Rpt, 12 Nov 82), DASG-MS.

[14] Women: MSC Newsletter, May 1968; Ch, MSC, MSC Directory, 1987, both in DASG-MS. Numbers and survey: On 15 January 1987, there were 544 women among 4,981 active duty MSCs (11 percent): 5 lieutenant colonels, 26 majors, 327 captains, 102 first lieutenants, and 84 second lieutenants. Rpt, Capt Susan R. West, MSC, DASG-MS, sub: Questionnaire, 30 Nov 87, DASG-MS.

[15] Numbers in 1995: On 15 January 1995, there were 825 women among 4,432 active duty MSCs (19 percent): 2 colonels, 28 lieutenant colonels, 151 majors, 323 captains, and 321 lieutenants. By comparison, the percentage of females in the other Medical Department corps was: Medical Corps, 16 percent; Army Nurse Corps, 71 percent; Dental Corps, 9 percent; Army Medical Specialist Corps, 36 percent; and Veterinary Corps, 24 percent. By January 1995 there were two deputy commanders for administration and two commanders. Rpt, Health Svcs Div, Officer Pers Mgmt Dir (TAPC-

OPH), U.S. Total Army Personnel Cmd (PERSCOM), Alexandria, Va., sub: AMEDD Gender Statistics, 9 Jan 95, DASG-MS; Jim Tice, "Minorities, Women Gain in Downsizing Active Force," *Army Times* (21 November 1994). Williamson: Msg, 7th MEDCOM, 051159Z Aug 91, DASG-MS. Moore: A. J. White, TAPC-PDA, info paper, 17 Jun 93, DASG-MS.

[16] Goals: Rpt, DASG-MS, sub: MSC Strategic Planning Conference, 30 October–2 November 1984; Handout, Ch, MSC, sub: MSC Goals and Objectives, 1985, both in DASG-MS.

[17] Mentors: Info paper, Maj Richard B. Parry, Jr., MSC, HQ, 7th MEDCOM, sub: MSC Officer Mentorship, 29 Jan 88, DASG-MS.

[18] Award: MSC Newsletter, 9 April 1982; OTSG Reg 15–31, The Chief, Medical Service Corps Award of Excellence, 22 Aug 83, DASG-MS. Winners: MSC Newsletters, 1984–90.

[19] Intern: MSC Newsletters, 8 October 1984 and 14 August 1987.

[20] AMSUS awards: Insert, "Annual Awards Program," *Military Medicine* 153 (January 1988); Richard V.N. Ginn, "Of Purple Suits and Other Things: An Army Officer Looks at Unification of the Department of Defense Medical Services," *Military Medicine* 143 (January 1978): 15–24; MSC Newsletter, 15 December 1987.

[21] Statue: AMEDD Medical Museum, Fort Sam Houston, Tex., insert included with prints of the statue, 1990, DASG-MS. In addition to Berchin, the Combat Medic Memorial Fund Committee included Col. Robert E. Mathias, MSC; Maj. Michael D. Cordy, MSC; Maj. Jerry P. Devine, MSC; CSM George J. Pierce; and CSM (Ret.) Edward O'Boyle.

[22] Honorary colonel: "AMEDD Regiment Gets New Honorary Colonel," *Mercury* (U.S. Army Health Services Command newspaper, March 1994), DASG-MS.

[23] Number: U.S. Congress, House, Department of Defense Appropriations Bill, 1980, 95th Cong., 2d sess., 1978, p. 43. Positions: MSC Newsletters, 2 August 1982, 5 December 1983, and 25 July 1984; Lott, "USAMEDDPERSA History"; Biographical summaries, unit directories, and MSC Newsletters, 1978–88, DASG-MS.

[24] Dental Activities (DENTACs): L. Robert Woods, "A New Managerial Approach: Army Dentistry and the Medical Service Corps Officer," *Military Medicine* 146 (December 1986): 886–88; MSC Newsletters, 1 December 1978, 4 January 1980, and 22 October 1982; U.S. Congress, House, *Hearings Before the Subcommittee on the Department of Defense of the Committee on Appropriations*, 98th Cong., 2d sess., 1984, pt. 3, p. 117, hereafter cited as HAC, *DOD Appropriations for 1985*. Productivity was measured by daily procedures per dentist.

[25] Promotions: Memo, Col Eugene Lail, MSC, Ch, MSC Career Activities Office, sub: MSCs Personnel Turbulence, 8 May 78; MSC Newsletters, 20 August 1978, 30 March 1979, 30 September 1981, and 15 December 1987; Col James D. Van Straten, CofS, 7th MEDCOM, to Jordan, 6 Sep 83; Info paper, Lt Col Jack O. Harrington, MSC, Pers Policy Div, OTSG (DASG-PTB), sub: Defense Officer Personnel Amendments Act 1982, 31 Mar 82; OCSA, Dir Program Analysis and Evaluation (PA&E), Major Commanders Conference 1984; Interv, Pixley with Ginn, Pentagon, 1 Nov 84, DASG-MS; Johnson to Van Straten, sub: MSC Washington Update, 11 Oct 84; Memo, Gen Maxwell R. Thurman, VCSA, Memo for TSG, sub: AMEDD Promotion Opportunity, 18 Jan 85; MFR, Col James G. Vermillion, MSC, Dep Dir Pers, OTSG, 18 Jan 85; Memo, Delbert Spurlock, Jr., Asst Sec Army (M&RA), for CSA, sub: Army Medical Department Promotions, 1 Oct 85; Memo, Spurlock for Principal Dep ASD (HA), sub: Army Medical Promotions, 17 Dec 85; Info paper, Lt Col Peter Tremblay, MSC, DASG-PTM, sub: AMEDD Force Management Process, 30 Dec 87; Info paper, Lt Col Ray Elizondo, MSC, DASG-PTM, sub: AMEDD (less MC/DC) Promotions, 28 Dec 87; Briefing slides, Col Thomas B. Pozniak, MSC, ACSPER, 7th MEDCOM, sub: OACSPER Issues, DCA Conf, Heidelberg, Germany, 25 Feb 88; Info paper, DASG-PTM, sub: Evolution of AMEDD Promotions, 12 Apr 91, all in DASG-MS.

[26] Promotion problem: Spurlock to CSA, 1 Oct 85.

[27] Retirement: Officers selected had to retire within six months of the secretary of the Army's approval of the board's recommendations.

[28] Stars: CMT 2, Col Fred L. Walter, MSC, 7 May 80 to DF, Maj Peter M. McLaughlin, MSC, Asst to Ch, MSC, sub: MSC Action Plan, 2 Apr 80; Johnson to Van Straten, sub: MSC Washington Update, 11 Oct 84; Rpt, DASG-PTB, sub: General Officer Distribution, 23 Jan 85; MSC Newsletters, 27 April 1984 and 30 October 1985; all in DASG-MS; HAC, *DOD Appropriations for 1985*, 3: 768. Loss of officers: An example of officers who sought their fortunes

elsewhere was Col. William H. Wunder, MSC, who transferred as a colonel to the Adjutant General Corps in 1975. Wunder retired in 1982 to follow a career in education that included the position of president of Marymount College in Kansas. In 1995 he was elected president of the International Association of Lions Clubs. U.S. Army War College Newsletter, Fall 1995, DASG-MS.

[29] AMEDD stars: 22 in 1985: 1 lieutenant general, 8 major generals, and 13 brigadier generals; 16 in 1994: 1 lieutenant general, 6 major generals, and 9 brigadier generals. The number by corps:

	MC	*DC*	*VC*	*MSC*	*ANC*	*AMSC*	*Total*
1985	16	3	1	1	1	0	22
1994	12	3	0	1	1	0	16

Source: HAC, *DOD Appropriations for 1985*, 3: 768; Rpt, Army Medical Department Center and School (AMEDDC&S), sub: AMEDD Immaterial Command Leader Development Action Plan, 7 Sep 94, DASG-MS.

[30] Support: Jordan to Brig Gen Manley Morrison, MSC, Ret., 22 Feb 84.

[31] MC star: SG Staff Conference, 15 Feb 85, as related to the author, author's notes, 15 Feb 85, DASG-MS. General Mittemeyer announced that a board would convene in May 1985 to select an MSC brigadier general, using a star taken from the Medical Corps. The ultimate disposition of that star would be at the call of General Becker, his replacement as surgeon general.

[32] Education: MSC Newsletters, 19 October 1979, 12 November 1980, and 30 October 1985; Rpt, MSC Career Activities Office (CAO), U.S. Army Medical Department Personnel Support Agency (USAMEDDPERSA), (SGPS-MS), sub: Active Duty Officers Who Failed to Complete LTCT, 30 Jan 80; Msg, Education and Training Div, USAMEDDPERSA (SGPS-EDA), 181900Z Feb 88, sub: MSC Long Term Civilian Training (LTCT) Selection Board, all in DASG-MS. Training with Industry: AR 621–108, sub: Military Personnel Requirements for Civilian Education, 3 Mar 92, PL; Info paper, Lt Col James E. Sutton, MSC, DASG-PT, sub: Medical Readiness Brief—AMEDD, 10 January 1994, DASG-MS.

[33] Army-Baylor: MSC Newsletters, 12 November and 30 December 1980; U.S. Army–Baylor University Alumni Club Newsletter, May 1987; MFR, Col George R. Krueger, Ch, MSC CAO, sub: Selection Board, U.S. Army–Baylor University Program in Health Care Administration FY 75, Jan 74; Rpt, Col Melvin E. Modderman, MSC, Dir, Army-Baylor Program, sub: A Report to Alumni and Friends, 1987; Memo, Young for President, U.S. Army–Baylor University Program in Health Care Administration Selection Board, sub: Corps Chief's Policy Guidance, 1979; Darryl E. Crompton, J.D., ACEHSA Fellow, to Lt Col Thomas Janke, MSC, Dir, Army-Baylor Program, 2 Aug 81; Office notes, Maj Peter M. McLaughlin, MSC, Office of Ch, MSC, 7 Nov 80, all in DASG-MS; Jay Green, "Graduate Programs Get Back to Basics," *Modern Health Care* (27 August 1990): 28–37, 52, hereafter cited as Green, "Graduate Programs." Flexible residencies: HEW: Maj. Franklin J. Goriup, MSC; VA: Maj. Eric H. Myrland, MSC; OSD: Maj. Richard V.N. Ginn, MSC.

[34] Quoted words: Nancy Barcus, "Fort Sam's Unique Students," *Baylor* (June–July 1984): 27.

[35] Residencies: See Green, "Graduate Programs," pp. 28–30.

[36] Report: Rpt, Darryl E. Crompton, J.D., ACEHSA Fellow, sub: Report of Visiting Committee Site Visit to Lt Col Thomas Janke, Dir, Army-Baylor Program, 12 Aug 81, DASG-MS.

[37] Ranking: Green, "Graduate Programs," p. 52. Accreditation: MSC Newsletter, August 1993.

[38] School: Venable, AHS History, 1981.

[39] Basic course: MFSS, Program of Instruction (POI) no. 6–8–C2O, sub: Army Medical Department Basic Course (MSC Officers), Apr 71; Briefing slide, AMEDDC&S, MSC Basic and Advanced Courses, undated (1993); MSC Newsletters, 2 August 1982 and 30 October 1985, all in DASG-MS.

[40] Advanced course: AHS, POI no. 6–8–C22, sub: AMEDD Officer Advanced Course, Jun 78, as revised 23 Aug 78; Briefing slide, AMEDDC&S, MSC Basic and Advanced Courses, undated (1993); Briefing slides, Lt Col James E. Sutton, MSC, OTSG, sub: Military Education Update, 18 Aug 94, hereafter cited as Sutton, Military Education Update; MSC Newsletters, 2 August 1982 and 30 October 1985, all in DASG-MS. CLOAC: MSC Newsletter, 15 January 1993. Functional Area 90: Memo, Col Boyd C. Bryant, General Staff (GS), Ch, Combat Svc Spt Div, Officer Pers Mgmt Dir (OPMD), PERSCOM, sub: Notification of Functional Area 90 Designation Board, 15 Dec 92, DASG-MS. Training policy: Memo, MSC Br, HSD, OPMD, PERSCOM, sub: Statement of Policy 93–1, undated (March 1993), DASG-MS.

[41]CAS^3: Info paper, Maj Mary Anne Svetlik, MSC, SGPS-ED, sub: CAS^3, 26 Mar 82; Info paper, Maj H. Berriman, GS, ODCSPER, sub: CAS^3, 2 Sep 86, both in DASG-MS. C–4: Jay P. Sanford, "USUHS 'Innovative' in Teaching Design," *U.S. Medicine* (January 1988): 29. General Young said the MSCs who attended as role models for physicians in a field environment "performed magnificently." MSC Newsletter, 31 July 1980.

[42] CGSC: MSC Newsletters, 1 December 1978, 19 October 1979, and 30 September 1981; Speech, Young, sub: State of the Corps, 29 Feb 80; Info paper, Berriman, sub: To Provide Information Concerning the Nonresident Command and General Staff College, 2 Sep 86, all in DASG-MS; Sutton, Military Education Update, 18 Aug 94; Interv, Brig Gen Bruce T. Miketinac with Ingeborg Sosa, in *AMEDD Journal* (May/June 1993).

[43] Act of 1986: Department of Defense Reorganization Act of 1986, 100 Stat. 922, 1 October 1986. The bill was commonly referred to as the Goldwater-Nichols Act, after its sponsors, Senator Barry Goldwater and Congressman Bill Nichols.

[44] SSC: MSC Newsletters, 30 December 1980 and September 1994; Info papers, Maj Mark Leopold, ODCSPER, sub: SSC Selection Board Procedures and U.S. Army War College Corresponding Studies Program, 15 Aug 86; Memo, John O. Marsh, Jr., Sec Army, sub: Instructions to the 1987 Army Competitive Category Senior Service College (SSC) and Academic Year 1988–90 Army War College Corresponding Studies Course (AWCCSC) Selection Board, 21 Jul 1987; Sutton, Military Education Update, 18 Aug 94, all in DASG-MS. Difficulty: Jim Tice, "Senior Service College Board Meets July 6," *Army Times* (11 April 1988): 3. Fellowships: Maj Gen John C. Ellerson, Dir of Strategy, Plans and Policy, ODCSOPS, to Col Robert Fitz, MSC, 14 Oct 93; Ellerson to Col Timothy Jackman, MSC, 14 Oct 93, DASG-MS. Opportunity: The number of officers selected in 1994 for resident SSC compared to the number eligible reveals the following:

Category	*Selected/Eligible*	*Percentage*
Basic Branches	346/4,523	7.6
Chaplain Corps	4/142	2.8
Judge Advocate General's Corps	5/189	2.6
Army Medical Department	18/1,457	1.2

Source: Memo, Col Michael L. Leahy III, Ch, Functional Area Mgmt and Development Div, OPMD, PERSCOM, sub: FY 1994 Senior Service College Selection Board, 7 Sep 94, DASG-MS.

[45] Advanced training: MSC Newsletter, 30 October 1985; OTSG Reg 5–6, Army Medical Department Programs at Arroyo Center, 6 Apr 90, DASG-MS; Sutton, Military Education Update, 18 Aug 94.

[46] Quoted words: Unpublished paper, Col Kenneth A. Cass, MC, sub: The Requirement for Medical Corps Officers (Physicians) To Be Medical Facility Commanders and Major Medical Staff Officers in NATO and HSC, 12 May 78, USAMHI.

[47] Quoted words: Brig Gen William H. Greendyke, MC, USAF, Strategic Air Command Surgeon, to Lt Gen Paul W. Myers, AFSG, 1 Mar 80, DASG-MS.

[48] Cooper letter: Lt Gen Kenneth B. Cooper, DCINC, USAREUR, to Robert N. Smith, M.D., ASD(HA), 16 Jun 77, and Smith to Cooper, 24 Aug 77, DASG-MS. Smith's response was drafted by Capt. Peter A. Flynn, MC, USN, who added: "There is no arguing that some physician commanding officers are absolute dolts—but then so are some senior MSCs—physicians have no corner on the market for stupidity." Flynn to Smith, 22 Jul 77, DASG-MS.

[49] Clements: Memo, William P. Clements, Dep Sec Def, for Secs of the Mil Depts, sub: Staff and Command Assignments of Health Professionals, 1 May 73, DASG-MS. Moxley: Memo, John H. Moxley III, M.D., for ASA-M&RA, sub: Physicians in Executive Management Positions, 16 Jul 80, DASG-MS. "I know of no substantive reason why the Army should not be moving in the same direction as the Air Force and Navy." Beary: The policy "is herewith restated." John F. Beary III, M.D., to Sen Daniel K. Inouye, 8 Mar 73, DASG-MS. The Army said it was "not mandated": Army response, 10 Aug 83, to Draft DOD IG Report, sub: Defense IG/Audit Service Report on Utilization of MC, DC, MSC, 10 Jun 83; Memo, Col Melvin E. Modderman, MSC, Dep Dir Pers, OTSG, to DSG, same sub, 12 May 83, all in DASG-MS. 1984: William E. Mayer, M.D., in HAC, *DOD Appropriations for 1985*, 3: 760–61.

[50] Field command: DAIG, inspection of 3d Armored Div, USAREUR, finding 140, sub: Medical Unit Commanders, May 78, with response, Col Charles A. Mateer, MSC, XO, OTSG, 13 Dec 78; Draft rpt, DOD IG, 10 Jun 83, all in DASG-MS; AR 600–20, Army Command Policy and Procedures, 15 Oct 80, PL.

[51] Army: General Mittemeyer testified that the physician "is the most qualified officer of the healthcare team to supervise direct hands-on care." HAC, *DOD Appropriations for 1985*, 3: 767. The Navy and Air Force surgeons general testified that seven hospitals and twenty-three clinics were commanded by USN or USAF MSCs. U.S. Marine Corps (USMC): Memo, Commandant, USMC, for DOD IG, sub: Review of the Utilization of Medical Service Corps Officers in Executive Management Positions (Project 21J–141), 21 Mar 83; Draft rpt, DOD IG, 10 Jun 83, all in DASG-MS.

[52] Command selection: MSC Newsletters, 31 July 1980, 30 September 1981, 26 February and 22 October 1982, and 28 June 1984.

[53] Fields: Lt Col Jerry L. Fields, MSC, to Maj Gen Robert M. Elton, CG, 9th Inf Div, sub: Award of Alternate Skill Identifier 92, 11 Jan 83, with 1st Ind, Col William J. Buchanan, Jr., Cdr, 9th Div Spt Cmd (DISCOM), 24 Jan 83; 2d Ind, Elton, CG, 9th Inf Div, 2 Mar 1983; and 3d Ind, Jordan, Ch, MSC, 5 Apr 83. Also see Ltr, Lt Gen Richard H. Thompson, DCSLOG, to Mittemeyer, 28 Jun 83, and Mittemeyer to Thompson, 26 Jul 83, DASG-MS. Forward Support Battalions (FSBs): Memo, Mittemeyer, DASG-PTB, for DCSPER, sub: Command Selection Procedures for FSB and DISCOM Command, 25 Oct 83; Jordan to Ginn, 2 Oct 1988. DISCOMs: Johnson to Van Straten, 11 Oct 84. DISCOM Commanders: A second MSC, Lt. Col. (P) Randy P. Maschek, MSC, was slated in 1995 for the 4th Infantry Division DISCOM at Fort Carson, Colorado, but was deferred from command when that unit was announced for inactivation. In 1987 Fields, then a colonel, had assumed command of the 6th Infantry Division DISCOM at Fort Richardson, Alaska, but not as an MSC since he had transferred to the Quartermaster Branch prior to assuming command. Fields was subsequently relieved of command.

[54] Command of FSBs: Rpt, DASG-PTM, sub: Battalion Commander Selections, 22 Oct 91; Rpt, Col John A. Sierra, Jr., MSC, Dep Dir Pers, OTSG, sub: Number of MSC FSB Cdrs, 1983–1992, 14 Feb 92; Memo, Brig Gen Gary L. Brown, OPMD, sub: Selection List for FY93 Lieutenant Colonel Level Command, 24 Jun 92, all in DASG-MS; Timothy Jackman, "Army Medical Department Plans, Operations, Training, Security and Intelligence Officers: Then, Now and Next," *AMEDD Journal* (May/June 1992): 6–10, hereafter cited as Jackman, "Operations Officers."

[55] MSC commanders: HAC, *DOD Appropriations for 1985*, 3: 766; MSC Newsletters, 22 October 1982, 28 June 1984, and March 1994; MSC Directory, 1991, all in DASG-MS. MC commanders: MSC Newsletter, 25 March 1983; *Army Times* 28 (March 1983): 2.

[56] Gander crash: Notes of interv, 1st Lt Beverly J. Rice, MSC, with Ginn, Pentagon, 16 Jan 86; Rpt, Lt Col Gary L. Swallow, MS, Automation Mgmt Ofc, OTSG (DASG-AMO), sub: Gander Crash After Action Report, 18 Jan 86; Rpt, Lt Col Michael A. Shannon, MSC, Professional Services Directorate, OTSG (DASG-PS), sub: Medical Records Construction, 26 Feb 86, all in DASG-MS. Also see David Fulghum, "Identification 'Tremendous Emotional Experience,'" *Army Times* (2 June 1980): 8, 46.

[57] Personnel: Memo, Col Richard C. Harder, MSC, Ch, Education and Tng Div, for Cdr, USAMEDDPERSA, sub: Organization of a Health Services Personnel Manager Task Force, 7 Jun 77; Draft ltr, Col Neil J. McDonald, MSC, Cdr, USAMEDDPERSA, to AMEDD Pers Mgmt Conf, sub: Summary of Findings of the Health Services Personnel Managers Task Force (HSPM/TF), 17 Apr 79. Also see Col Marion Johnson, MSC, XO, BAMC, to Young, 12 Sep 80; all in DASG-MS. Proponency: Briefing slides, Maj Richard V.N. Ginn, DASG-PTB, sub: AMEDD Specialty Proponency, Apr 82; Mittemeyer, TSG, to Maj Gen Raymond R. Bishop, Jr., CG, HSC, 17 Jan 83; Info paper, Lt Col R. Ginn, sub: AMEDD Enlisted Proponency, 4 Apr 83, all in DASG-MS. Exceptional Family Member Program: Info paper, Lt Col Thomas R. Pozniak, MSC, DASG-PTB, sub: Provision of Health Related Services to Handicapped Dependents, 1 Apr 82, DASG-MS.

[58] Personnel Command: USAMEDDPERSA Newsletter, 31 October 1985 (final issue); Info paper, TAPC-OPH, sub: History of the Health Services Division, OPMD, 1974–1994, 30 Jan 94;

Memo, Col Charles A. Henning, GS, Ch, Officer Div, ODCSPER, sub: Draft FY96 Officer Distribution Plan (ODP) Policy Guidance, 8 Dec 94, all in DASG-MS.

[59] Comptroller: MSC Newsletter, 29 September 1986; Msg, DA, sub: MSC LTC Selection Board, DASG-MS. Syracuse: Ms. Anne P. Twist, DAC, Student, Army Comptrollership Program (ACP), Syracuse Univ, to Ginn, 5 Sep 91; Rpt, ACP, sub: ACP 1952–1991, Syracuse Univ, 1991, all in DASG-MS.

[60] Quoted words: Ch, MSC, plaque presented at the Sperandio Conference, 11 Sep 89.

[61] Operations: DA Msg, 18 Feb 88; MSC Newsletters, 9 January and 30 December 1980 and August 1993; Information booklet, U.S. Army Health Services Command (HSC), sub: Fort Detrick, undated, 1988, DASG-MS. Foster: Brig Gen James L. Collins, Jr., Cdr, USACMH, to Cdr, USAR Components and Admin Ctr, sub: Active Duty Training—1LT Gaines M. Foster, 21 Jan 76, box 19/18, MSC-USACMH; Foster, *The Demands of Humanity: Army Medical Disaster Relief* (Washington, D.C.: U.S. Army Center of Military History, 1983). El Salvador: Msg, DA, 191923Z Jul 83; Memo, Col Robert F. Elliott, MSC, for Sec Def, sub: Medical MTT Objectives and MEDEVAC Requirements, 7 Sep 83, and Rpt, sub: Humanitarian Medical MTT, 20 Jan 84, all in DASG-MS. Col. Herman Morales, MC, was team chief.

[62] Role of operations specialty: Col Charles R. Angel, Ch, MAS Sec, to Young, sub: Visit to Fort Campbell, Kentucky, 23 Feb 76, DASG-MS. Proposals: Rpt, Col Charles A. Mateer, MSC, Course Dir, sub: Meeting, Current Problems in Medical Plans and Operations, June 1978, to Young, 8 Sep 78; Mateer to Young, 18 Oct 78, with DF, Young to DASG-RM, sub: Review and Evaluation of Current Problems and Trends in Medical Plans and Operations, 20 Oct 78, all in DASG-MS.

[63] Operations study: Young to Jordan, sub: Organization of a Health Services Plans, Operations, Intelligence and Training Task Force, 20 Jul 79; MSC Newsletter, 9 January 1980; Rpt, Jordan, Chm, 67H Study Gp, sub: A Review of Plans, Operations, Intelligence and Training, Jan 81; Staff notes, McLaughlin, Asst to Ch, MSC, 19 Jan, 24 Feb, and 2 Jun 81; Jordan to Ginn, 2 Oct 88, all in DASG-MS.

[64] Guide: Rpt, Directorate of Health Care Opns, OTSG (DASG-HCZ), sub: Health Services Plans, Operations, Training, Security, and Intelligence Officer Professional Development Handbook, Sep 91, DASG-MS. Quoted words: Jackman, "Operations Officers," p. 10.

[65] Logistics: MSC Newsletters, 9 January 1980, 19 April 1985 (issue devoted to medical logistics), and 15 December 1987. An MSPR session, 17–18 December 1984, chaired by General Maxwell Thurman at the Academy of Health Sciences, challenged this premise. Notes of discussion, Lt Col William D. Finical, MSC, DASG-RMM, with Ginn, 19 Dec 84. Other challenges are in Jordan, 3d Ind to Ltr, Lt Col Jerry L. Fields, MSC, sub: Award of Alternate Skill Identifier 92, 5 Apr 83; Lt Gen Richard H. Thompson, DCSLOG, to Mittemeyer, 28 Jun 83; Mittemeyer to Thompson, 26 Jul 83, all in DASG-MS.

[66] Articles: Thomas E. Kistler, "A Case for the Separate Medical Logistics System," *AMEDD Journal* (December 1985): 5; Richard V.N. Ginn, "Medical Logistics: A Lesson From Vietnam," *Army Logistician* (November/December 1993): 36–38; Philip E. Livermore and Angel Cintron, "Medical Logistics: Pillar of Health Care Delivery," *Army Logistician* (March/April 1994): 9–11. MSC logisticians were closely attuned to Army field programs. For example, see George E. Shultz, "NBC Protection—A Personal Matter," *Army Logistician* (May–June 1985): 22–24.

[67] USAMMCE: Irene Weber, "Medical Materiel: The Army's Best Kept Secret," *MEDCOM Examiner* (7th MEDCOM newspaper, March 1988): 1, 8–9; Weber, "Kistler: A Man for All Reasons," ibid., p. 9, DASG-MS.

[68] Training: Col George L. Brown, MSC, Cdr, U.S. Army Medical Equipment and Optical School, to Maj Peter Tancredi, MSC, Asst to Ch, MSC, 2 Nov 82; MSC Newsletters, 9 January and 12 November 1980, 23 January 1984, and 15 December 1987; DA Msg, 18 Feb 88, all in DASG-MS.

[69] Warrant officers: MSC Newsletters, 1 December 1978 and 31 July 1980; Info paper, Maj Phil Dorsey, MSC, Asst to Ch, MSC, sub: Biomedical Equipment Repair Technician, MOS 202A, 13 Feb 78; Rpt, Hlth Svcs Div, OPMD, MILPERCEN, sub: AMEDD Officer Active Duty Strength Report as of 30 November 85, Jan 86; Info paper, Lt Col Roy A. Bryan, MSC, DASG-PTM, sub: Warrant Officer Issues, 30 Dec 87, all in DASG-MS; "Management Transition Stalls for WOs," *Army Times* (19 October 1987): 7. The specialty code changed in 1987 from 202A to 670A.

[70] Health facilities: Memo, Lt Gen Richard R. Taylor, TSG, for Asst Sec Army (Installations and Logistics), sub: Program Manager for Medical Facility Construction, 10 Jul 75; MSC Newsletter, 30 December 1980; DA Msg 18 Feb 88; Rpt, U.S. Army Health Facilities Planning Agency (USAHFPA), sub: Funding Trend for Army Health Facilities, 15 Aug 91; Rpt, Dedi Graham, USAHFPA, sub: Medical Appropriations, FY80 Thru FY93, 3 Aug 94. Program reductions: The five-year program was reduced from $2.273 to $1.232 billion. The cut included deletion of $223 million for a new Fitzsimons Army Medical Center. Briefing slides, Col Edward P. Phillips, Jr., Cdr, USAHFPA, sub: USAHFPA, 10 Feb 95, all in DASG-MS.

[71] Health care administration: MSC Newsletters, 30 March 1979, 26 February 1982, 15 February 1985, and 22 January 1986; Office notes, McLaughlin, 16 Sep 80; Van Straten to 7th MEDCOM XOs, 17 Oct and 24 Dec 84; DASG-MS, "The AMEDD in an Era of Transformation," Army Day Program, ACHE, 10 Feb 86; Col Douglas A. Barton, MSC, ACHE Army Regent's Newsletter, September 1994; Memo, Barton for Ginn, sub: ACHE Stats, 11 Oct 94, all in DASG-MS. Applicants for the health care administration specialty (67A) were required to have a master's in a field approved by the ACEHSA or in administration (MA, MPA, MS, or MBA) from an accredited university. In 1980 General Young unsuccessfully attempted to restrict degrees to those accredited by the ACEHSA in order to prevent the recognition of weak programs. Health care changes: Neuhauser, *Coming of Age*, pp. 2, 52–54, 69–71; Rpt, Korn/Ferry International and Association of University Programs in Health Administration, sub: Health Administration Employment, 1979–83, 1983, DASG-MS.

[72] DCA: Notes of telephone conversation, Col Gerald D. Allgood, MSC, Ret., with Ginn, 31 Aug 91; Notes of telephone conversation, Brig Gen Walter F. Johnson III, USA, Ret., with Ginn, 10 Feb 92, both in DASG-MS; AR 611–101, Commissioned Officer Classification System, 30 Oct 85, PL.

[73] Awards: MSC Newsletters, 9 April 1982, 22 January 1986, 15 December 1987, 17 December 1991, and August 1993; "Annual Awards Program," *Military Medicine* 153 (January 1988), insert; Rpt, Lt Col Glenn R. Willauer, USAF, MSC, ACHE Regent at Large, sub: Regent's Report, Jan 1986 and Jan and Jun 1988; *The Bear Facts: U.S. Army–Baylor University Alumni Club Newsletter*, Winter 1990, all in DASG-MS.

[74] UH–60: Interv, Lt Col John W. Hammett, MSC, Ret., with Capt Peter G. Dorland, MSC, THU, OTSG, Oct 75, USACMH. UH–60Q: Rpt, Lt Col Richard R. Beauchemin, MSC, Aviation Consultant, OTSG, sub: Aviation Update, in Memo, Col Timothy Jackman, MSC, sub: Health Services Plans, Operations, Training, Security and Intelligence Newsletter, 15 Jun 93, DASG-MS, hereafter cited as Jackman, Operations Newsletter.

[75] Aviation: MSC Newsletters, 30 March 1979, 9 January and 3 July 1980, and 21 December 1984 (issue devoted to medical aviation); *SG Report*, 1970, p. 121; Meeting program and author's notes, Dustoff Assn Seventh Annual Mtg, San Antonio, Tex, 28 Feb–2 Mar 86; Author's notes of presentation, Lt Col Jack Roden, MSC, "The First Evacuation Battalion," Dustoff mtg, 1 Mar 86, all in DASG-MS; Reginald G. Moore, Jr., Peter P. Smith, and Mark W. Yow, "Twofold Challenge," *Military Medicine* (October 1987): 495–96. Unit histories: Rpt, Capt Randall G. Anderson, MSC, sub: The Dustoff Report, printed by the Dustoff Assn, undated (Nov 92), DASG-MS. Anderson's report listed 27 active component, 17 reserve, and 25 Army National Guard aeromedical detachments and companies.

[76] Threat: MSC Newsletter, 21 December 1984; Memo, Maj Gen H. Norman Schwarzkopf, ADCSPER, for CSA, sub: Aviation Branch Composition, 13 Apr 83, as annotated by the Director of the Army Staff, Vice CSA, and CSA; Memo, Mittemeyer for DCSPER with tabs A–E, sub: HQDA Aviation Implementation Plan, 5 Apr 83; Jordan to Ginn, 2 Oct 88, all in DASG-MS. TSG arguments also included the danger of losing protected status for Dustoff crews under the Geneva Conventions. Quoted words: Memo, Mittemeyer for DCSPER, sub: HQDA Aviation Implementation Plan, 5 Apr 83. Also see notes of telephone interv, Lt Col Thomas C. Scofield, MSC, with Maj Gen Spurgeon Neel, MC, Ret., Mar 83, all in DASG-MS. Moore: Speech, Col Douglas Moore, MSC, XO, OTSG, sub: DUSTOFFer, Dustoff meeting, 1 Mar 86, author's notes, DASG-MS.

[77] MAST: Info paper, OTSG, sub: Military Assistance to Safety and Traffic (MAST), Dec 84, DASG-MS. MAST had increasing competition from civilian programs. Editorial, Howard F.

Champion, "Helicopters in Emergency Trauma Care," *Journal of the American Medical Association* 249 (10 June 1983): 3074.

[78] Colombia: Presentation, Maj Robert G. Whiting, MSC, sub: Disaster Operations in Colombia, Dustoff mtg, Mar 86, author's notes, DASG-MS. This was the Nevado del Ruiz volcano.

[79] 421st: Presentations, Lt Col William T. Stahl, MSC, sub: DUSTOFF Europe, and Maj Reuben G. Pinkson, MSC, sub: Pacific Deployment Training, Dustoff mtg, Mar 86, author's notes, DASG-MS.

[80] Quoted words: In notes of interv, CW4 Mike Novosell, Jr., U.S. Army Aviation Center, Fort Rucker, Ala., with Ginn, Dustoff mtg, San Antonio, Tex., 2 Mar 86, DASG-MS.

[81] Promotions: Memo, Merle Meling, Assoc Dir, Finance and Manpower Audits, Defense Audit Service, Arlington, Va., for ASD (HA), sub: Survey of Non-Physician Health Care Providers, 5 Aug 82 (the survey canvassed 9 percent of 2,472 officers); Memo, Sec Army for President, Colonel, Medical Service Corps, Army Nurse Corps, Army Medical Specialist Corps, and Veterinary Corps Promotion Selection Board, sub: Selection Board Procedures, 31 May 91; Info paper, DASG-PTM, sub: Evolution of AMEDD Promotions, 12 Apr 91, all in DASG-MS.

[82] Special pay: Memo, Stephen C. Joseph, ASD(HA), for Asst Sec Army (Manpower and Reserve Affairs), sub: Diplomate Pay for Psychologists and Board Certified Pay for Non-physician Health Care Providers, 22 Sep 94, DASG-MS.

[83] Pharmacy: Lt Col Alfred W. Gill, MSC, Pharm Br, AHS, Lesson Plan 31–365–320, sub: History and Traditions of Army Pharmacy, 1986, DASG-MS; Bernard J. Adelsberger, "Retention," *Army Times* (8 February 1988): 276; Scott C. Martin, "Oncology Pharmacy Residency at Walter Reed Army Medical Center," *Military Medicine* 153 (August 1988): 414, 416; Frank A. Cammarata et al., "Pharmacy Practice in the United States Army," *American Journal of Hospital Pharmacy* 44 (April 1987): 756–59; Msg, DA, 181900Z Feb 88, sub: MSC LTC Selection Board, hereafter cited as DA Msg 18 Feb 88, all in DASG-MS.

[84] Allergen laboratory: Cammarata, "Pharmacy Practice in the Army"; Notes of discussion, Ginn with Capt Ralph R. Watson, MSC, Ch, Allergen Extract Lab, WRAMC, 1985–88, at 196th Station Hospital, Casteau, Belgium, 6 Oct 88. Awards: MSC Newsletters, 20 September 1981, 15 December 1987, and 17 December 1991; "Annual Awards Program," *Military Medicine* 153 (January 1988): insert.

[85] Medical Allied Sciences Section: Rpt, DASG-PTH, 1 Sep 82; DA Msg 18 Feb 88, both in DASG-MS. Consultants: Col Dan C. Cavanaugh, MSC, Ch, MAS, to Young, sub: Staffing Responsibility of Laboratory Sciences Consultant, 10 Sep 80; Brig Gen Garrison Rapmund, ASG (R&D), to Consultants Div, OTSG (DASG-PC), sub: Consultant Roster Update, 16 Jul 81; Rapmund to Young, 21 Jul 81, and CMT 2, Lt Col William J. Shaffer, MSC, Asst to Ch, MSC, to Rapmund, 26 Aug 81; Ltr, Maj Gen Enrique Mendez, Jr., DSG, sub: Military Consultants to The Surgeon General, Department of the Army, FY 1981, 18 Sep 80, all in DASG-MS. Policies: Miketinac, remarks to senior MSCs at MSC mtg, Garmisch, FRG, 16 May 90, author's notes, DASG-MS.

[86] National recognition: MSC Newsletters, 22 August 1983, 3 December 1984, and 15 December 1987; Capt James W. Voorhees, MSC, to Jordan, 18 Dec 83, DASG-MS; "Reservist Picked for Astronaut Program," *CAR* [Chief Army Reserve] *Notes* (March–April 1984): 2, DASG-MS; Terry Jemison, "VA Astronaut Will Stick to Lab on Earth," *U.S. Medicine* 27 (September 1991): 1, 43. "A" prefix: An OTSG board selected twenty-three MSCs for this honor in 1992, a typical year. MSC Newsletter, December 1992.

[87] Audiology: MSC Newsletters, 1 December 1978 and 4 January and 30 December 1980; Audiology Consultant, audiology newsletter, 1 September 1980; DF, Maj Roy K. Sedge, MSC, to Ch, Otolaryngology Service, WRAMC, sub: Transfer of 68M Consultantship to MSC 68M Audiologist, 14 Apr 77; Briefing, Sedge for Brig Gen Young, sub: The Army Audiology Program, 8 Feb 78; Maj Donald R. Ciliax, MSC, Ch, Audiology Sec, Dwight David Eisenhower Army Medical Center (DDEAMC), to Sedge, sub: Formulating Policies for HAE's and AR's for the SE Medical Region, 21 Feb 79, with 1st Ind, Sedge, 2 Mar 79; DF, Sedge to TSG, sub: Assignment of 68Ms, 20 Jul 79; Sedge to TSG, sub: Consultant Visit to Federal Republic of Germany, 25 Apr 1980; Maj Gen Spencer B. Reid, MC, Cdr, 7th MEDCOM, to Sedge, 5 May 80, all in DASG-MS; Bernhard T. Mittemeyer, "Facing Challenges, Army Goals Endure," *U.S. Medicine* 18 (15

January 1982): 42, 51; J. Monique Bebout, "Audiology in the Armed Forces," *Hearing Journal* (September 1985): 7–14.

[88] Walter Reed: The ranking was by the American Speech and Hearing Association in 1979. MSC Newsletter, 4 January 1980. Quoted words: Rodney M. Atack, "Army Audiology: Yesterday to Today," *AMEDD Journal* (November/December 1993): 49.

[89] Podiatry: MSC Newsletters, 1 December 1978, 31 July 1980, 30 September 1981, and August 1993; Hamrick, Sylvester interv, 21 Feb 84; Rpt, Manpower Control Div, OTSG, sub: FY Reports, MSC, FY 59–67, 27 Jan 67, hereafter cited as OTSG, MSC FY 59–67; Rpt, DASG-PTH, 1 Sep 82; DA Msg 18 Feb 88, all in DASG-MS; *SG Report*, 1972, p. 110; Mittemeyer, "Facing Challenges," p. 42; Terry D. Weaver et al., "The Role of the Podiatrist in a Wartime Scenario," *Military Medicine* 153 (August 1988): 391-93. Quoted words: Rpt, James H. Sammons, M.D., Pres, AMA, to Senate Conferees on S. 2723, "1985 Department of Defense Authorization," p. A14, PL.

[90] Podiatry residency: MSC Newsletter, 31 July 1980.

[91] Psychology: MSC Newsletters, 30 March and 14 October 1979, 4 January 1980, and 30 September 1981; Memo, Col Franklin Del Jones, MC, Psychiatry and Neurology Consultant, for TSG, sub: Army Psychologists, 1978, including speech, Maj Larry H. Ingraham, MSC, sub: New Directions in the Procurement of Army Uniformed Psychologists, American Psychological Association Convention, Chicago, 30 Aug 75; Rpt, Maj Thaddeus A. Krupka, MSC, DASG-PTH, sub: Psychology, 13 Aug 78; Memo, Jones for TSG, sub: Army Psychologists, 1980; Col Robert S. Nichols, MSC, to Young, 4 May 79; Unpublished paper, Harold Rosenheim, sub: History of the Uniformed Clinical Psychologist in the U.S. Army, 2 Sep 80; Info paper, Col Cecil Harris, sub: Issues of Concern—Army Clinical Psychology, 1 Dec 80; DASG-PTB, DA Form 2028, Changes to AR 611–101, Dec 81, all in DASG-MS; Jones, "Proceedings," 1979. Health Professions Scholarship Program (HPSP): Fact sheet, Capt Frank E. Blakely II, MSC, DASG-PTH, sub: HPSP Scholarship Reductions, 31 Mar 82; Louis Marangoni, Ch, Mil Pers Div, HQ, U.S. Army Medical Research and Development Command (USAMRDC), to Ginn, 16 Sep 91, DASG-MS.

[92] Utilization: Presentation, Lt Col James L. Maury, MSC, sub: Alcohol and Drug Program, MSC mtg, Garmisch, FRG, 10 May 88 (author's notes); Memo, Capt Lawrence E. Klusman, MSC, 120th Med Det, 1st Armored Div, sub: USAREUR Psychologists' View of Problem Soldiers, 9 Aug 79, all in DASG-MS; Frederick N. Garland and Franklin R. Brooks, "Military Families: Strategic Targets in a Subtle War," *Military Review* 72 (April 1992): 55–56.

[93] Survey: Study, David A. Mangelsdorf, Ph.D., AHS, sub: Psychologist Retention Factors, Jan 78, Doc ADA 059374, DTIC; also see Meling, Defense Audit Service Survey, 5 Aug 82, both in DASG-MS.

[94] Autonomy: Vernon McKenzie, PDASD(HA), memo to ASA(M&RA), sub: Utilization of Psychologists in the Military Health Care System, 2 Aug 1978, and response, Pixley to ASD(HA), (drafted by Lt. Col. James Rumbaugh, MC), 11 Sep 1978, DASG-MS.

[95] Education: MSC Newsletter, 30 September 1981; DF, Capt Raymond A. Parker, MSC, Asst Ch, Psy Svc, Madigan Army Medical Ctr, sub: Request for Approval to Offer a Post-Doctoral Fellowship in Clinical Neuropsychology, 27 Mar 79; Memo, Col Ben F. Dobson, MSC, for Ch, MSC, sub: Establishment of a Post-Graduate Fellowship in Neuropsychology, 18 Apr 80; Memo, Col France F. Jordan, MSC, Dir of Pers, for TSG Policy Council, sub: Postgraduate Fellowship in Neuropsychology, 9 Jul 81.

[96] Combat exhaustion: Larry H. Ingraham and Frederick J. Manning, "Psychiatric Battle Casualties: The Missing Column in a War Without Replacements," *Military Review* 60 (August 1980): 20, 29. Sleep: Manning to Lt Col Richard E. Hartzell, MSC, TSG Psychology Consultant, 28 Nov 78; Rpt, Manning, sub: Human Factors in Sustaining High Rates of Artillery Fire (Final Report), 1979, both in DASG-MS; Manning, "Continuous Operations in Europe: Feasibility and the Effect of Leadership and Training," *Parameters* 9 (June 1979): 8–16. Ingraham also got attention with an article that attacked the Army's new officer efficiency report that was fielded in 1979. He charged that reports were inflated and were leading to an officer corps of "sequestered vegetables." He predicted its collapse by 1987. Ingraham, "The OER Cudgel: Radical Surgery Needed," *Army* 35 (November 1985): 54–56.

[97] Social work: Lt Gen Taylor, TSG, to Gen Frederick J. Kroesen, CINC, USAFORSCOM, and Gen William E. Dupuy, CG, USATRADOC, 24 Mar 77; Memo, Col David P. Jentsch, MSC, sub:

Army Social Work Program Up-Date, 4 Jul 80, all in DASG-MS; Col Jones, "Behavioral Sciences in a Changing Army," in Jones, "Proceedings," 1979; Bascom W. Ratliff, Elizabeth M. Timberlake, and David P. Jentsch, *Social Work in Hospitals* (Springfield, Ill.: Charles C. Thomas, 1982). Study: Rpt, Maj Edward R. Hamlin III, MSC, Elizabeth M. Timberlake, Col David P. Jentsch, MSC, and Maj Edwin W. VanVrankin, MSC, sub: U.S. Army Social Work in the 1980's, WRAMC, Washington, D.C., 5 May 82, JML. The researchers received 130 questionnaires from 259 social workers surveyed, a 50 percent return rate.

[98] Quoted words: Col. Robert A. Mays, Jr., MSC, in MSC Newsletter, August 1993.

[99] Sanitary engineering: MSC Newsletter, 4 January 1980; OTSG, MSC FY 59–67; Rpt, DASG-PTH, 1 Sep 82; Rpt, Lt Col James M. Morgan, Jr., MSC, USAR, sub: A Review of the Current Status of Environmental Science and Sanitary Engineering Officers in the United States Army Reserve, Jul 74; Rpt, Morgan, sub: Suggestions for Recruiting, Apr 78, all in DASG-MS.

[100] Quoted words: Pamphlet, Capt John Y. Young, MSC, sub: Preventive Medicine Considerations: Exotic Palm, 1985, DASG-MS.

[101] Nuclear science: OTSG, MSC FY 59–67; Rpt, DASG-PTH, 1 Sep 82; DF, Col Robert T. Wangemann, MSC, Nucl Med Sci Consultant, OTSG, to Ch, MSC, sub: Recruitment and Retention of Nuclear Medical Science Officers (NMSO), 29 Dec 78; MFR, Herndon, sub: Report of the Second Sanitary Engineering Section Senior Officer Meeting, 4 Jun 82, all in DASG-MS; Mittemeyer, "Facing Challenges," p. 42.

[102] Optometry: Rpt, DASG-PTH, 1 Sep 82; Info paper, Col Arthur R. Giroux, MSC, Ch, Opt Sec, sub: Army Optometry, 25 Sep 77; Memo, Giroux for TSG, sub: OSD Legislative Proposal, "Armed Forces Medical and Dental Special Pay of 1979," 22 Feb 79; Memo, Giroux, for Ch, MSC, sub: Retention Rates, 21 Nov 79; Optometry Newsletter, 1 August 1980, all in DASG-MS; Bernard J. Adelsberger, "Retention Troubles Plague Medical Corps," *Army Times* (8 February 1988): 26–27. It was called a "critical shortage" in 1980 (MSC Newsletter, 9 January 1980).

[103] Flap: Editorial, Milton J. Eger, in *Journal of the American Optometric Association* (JAOA) 48 (March 1977): 275–76. Gmelin: Lt Col Robert T. Gmelin, MSC, to attendees at FAMC Optometry Conference, 27–31 August 1984, DASG-MS. Meeting: DASG-MS file, sub: AOA Meeting, assembled for Brig Gen Young, including a variety of documents; Pixley to Eger, 16 Jan 78; Notes of address, Young to Military Optometry Short Course, FAMC, 18 Sep 78; Eger to Pixley, 15 May 78; Eger to Giroux, 3 Aug 78; Maj Jerry D. Davis, MSC, Optometry Instructor, AHS, to Giroux, 1 Oct 79, all in DASG-MS; Eger editorials in *JAOA*, March 1977 and June 1978. Editorial: Eger editorial, June 1978; Eger to Giroux, 3 Aug 78, DASG-MS.

[104] HPSP: MSC Newsletter, 30 September 1981; Survey, Meling, 5 Aug 82; Info paper, Giroux, sub: Manpower Status, Optometry Officers, 6 Nov 79; Lee W. Smith, Exec Dir, Assn of Schools and Colleges of Optometry, to Moxley, 20 Aug 80; Info paper, Giroux, sub: Issues of Concern—Army Optometry, 10 Nov 80; Rep Bill Nichols to Moxley, 20 Nov 80; DF, Beck, sub: SG Reports, 1976–1980; Col John Leddy, MSC, Ch, Opt Sec, to Ginn, 4 Sep 88; Lou Marangoni, Ch, Mil Pers Div, HQ USAMRDC, to Ginn, 16 Sep 91; Briefing slide, Officer Procurement Div, OTSG, sub: Recruiting Initiatives, 15 Mar 93, all in DASG-MS.

[105] Recruiting: MSC Newsletters, 30 July 1980 and 30 September 1981; Memo, Giroux for TSG, sub: Interim Report—Visits to Optometry Schools and Colleges, 14 Feb 79 and 18 Apr 80; Optometry newsletter, Giroux, sub: Army Optometry Information Letter, 1 Aug 80, DASG-MS. Quoted words: *JAOA*, 1977, in Young, AOA mtg folder, 28 Apr 78, DASG-MS.

[106] Positions: Irene Weber, "Medical Materiel: The Army's Best Kept Secret," *MEDCOM Examiner* (March 1988): 1, 8–9; DASG-MS.

[107] Course: MSC Newsletter, 31 July 1980. Accreditation: Optometry Newsletter, 1 December 1979.

[108] Constructive credit: Young, AOA mtg folder, 20 Apr 78; Alvin Levin, O.D., Pres, AOA, to Giroux, 23 Aug 79; Memo, John H. Moxley, M.D., ASD (HA), for Mil Depts, sub: Revised Constructive Service Credit for Optometrists and Podiatrists, 26 Oct 79; DF, Giroux to Ch, MSC, sub: DA Procurement Circular 601–1, 27 Feb 80; Giroux to 1980 optometry school graduates entering active duty, sub: Date of Entry on Active Duty and Entry Grade Determination, 7 May 80; Memo, Moxley, sub: Revised Constructive Service Credit, 14 Apr 81; Memo, Jordan, Dir Pers, OTSG, for Ch, MSC, same sub, 29 Apr 81; Optometry Newsletter, 1 December 1979, all in DASG-MS.

[109] Retention: MSC Newsletters, 31 July 1980, 30 September 1981, 22 August 1983, and 17 December 1991; Fact sheet, Consultants Div, OTSG, sub: Optometry, 1980; DF, Alfred M. Beck, USACMH, to Health Care Opns Dir, OTSG, sub: Surgeon General's Report, 1976–1980, 10 Feb 1984; Young, address to Military Optometry Short Course, FAMC, 18 Sep 78; Memo, Giroux for TSG, sub: After Action Report—USAREUR Optometry Conference, 19–23 May 1980, Jun 80; Optometry Newsletters, 1 December 1979 and 15 December 1980, all in DASG-MS. Awards: MSC Newsletter, August 1993; USAMRDC Newsletter, November 1991; Notes of telephone conversation, Col Jerry D. Davis, Ch, Optometry Sec, MSC, with Col Richard V.N. Ginn, 12 Oct 94, all in DASG-MS.

[110] Scope: Charles W. McQuarrie, Pres, AOA, to John C. Stennis, Chm, SASC, Nov 77, and to Melvin Price, Chm, HASC, same sub and date; Memo, Maj Gen William S. Augerson, MC, USA, Dep Asst SecDef for Health Affairs, for SGs, sub: Scope of Optometric Services in Military Health Care Facilities, 27 Sep 79; Augerson to SGs, sub: Eye Care Services in the Direct Care System, 16 Nov 79; Memo, Pixley for ASD(HA), sub: Policy Regarding the Utilization of Optometry Officers, 3 Dec 79, including DF, Col Frederick C. Biehusen, MC, Ch, Consultants Div, OTSG, sub: Optometry Policy Statement Update, approved by Lt Gen Taylor, TSG, 4 Apr 77; Pixley to ASD(HA), sub: Eye Care Services in the Direct Care System, 6 Dec 79; Memo, McLaughlin for Young, 17 Dec 79; McKenzie, PDASD(HA), to Mil Depts, sub: Eye Care Review, 22 Apr 80; Rpt, Giroux, sub: After Action Report—USAREUR Visit, 16 Jun 80; DASG-PTB, DA Form 2028, sub: Publication Changes, change to AR 611–101, Dec 81; Optometry Newsletter, 1 December 1979, all in DASG-MS; Amy Goldstein and Susan Schmidt, "In Annapolis," *Washington Post*, 6 March 1988.

[111] Haggerty: Haggerty, Israeloff interv, 6 Jul 76, folder 130, box 9/18, MSC-USACMH.

[112] Frustrations: Vernon McKenzie, Ginn interv, 20 Jun 84. Quoted words: Jordan, remarks to staff luncheon, Washington, D.C., 5 Sep 84, author's notes, DASG-MS.

[113] Quoted words: CMT 2, Col Fred L. Walter, MSC, 7 May 80, to DF, Ch, MSC, 2 Apr 80, DASG-MS.

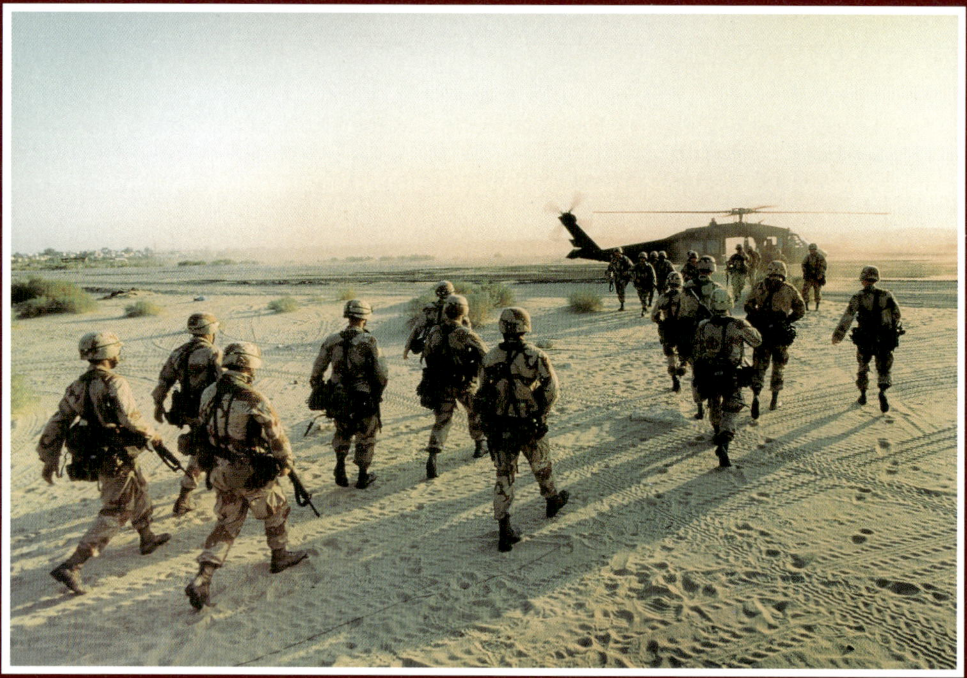

Soldiers move to and from a UH–60 Black Hawk helicopter during Operation DESERT SHIELD, *January 1991.*

13

Beyond the Cold War

The Army's efforts to raise the standards expected of medical soldiers and to update doctrine, equipment, and systems were tested in a series of deployments in the post-Vietnam era. One of the first followed Israel's withdrawal of its occupation forces from the Sinai in 1982, when the United States agreed to maintain one infantry battalion there as part of a United Nations peacekeeping force. MSCs were part of that effort, and 2d Lt. John B. Witmer, MSC, medical platoon leader in the 101st Airborne Division (Air Assault), died in December 1985 along with 255 other members of his battalion when their plane, returning from the Sinai, crashed in Gander, Canada—the greatest disaster in military aviation history.[1]

The first sizable American combat operation after Vietnam was the invasion of Grenada. In 1983 the Caribbean "isle of spice" seemed well on its way to becoming a satellite of Communist Cuba, as Cuban military advisers and workers moved in and began to construct a 12,000-foot airstrip, apparently intended for use by Soviet military aircraft. The situation deteriorated in October when Grenada's prime minister was executed by leftist rivals. Nearly eight hundred American medical students attending school on the island made an attractive target for hostage-taking. The prospects were especially alarming to President Ronald Reagan's administration, which had moved into the White House in 1981 on the heels of President Jimmy Carter's bitter experience with Americans taken hostage by Iran.[2]

Under presidential orders, the invasion began in the early morning of 25 October with a combat jump of two Army Ranger battalions and an assault by helicopter-borne marines. By the next evening the Ranger and airborne battalions of the 82d Airborne Division, Fort Bragg, North Carolina, had evacuated the medical students. The United States reported 19 killed and 115 wounded; it estimated that 70 hostile Cubans and Grenadians had been killed in action and 394 wounded.

Lt. Col. Edward B. Wilson, MSC, remained in command of the 82d Airborne's 307th Medical Battalion. Other medical units included elements of the 5th Combat Support Hospital, which deployed to Grenada from Fort Bragg on 2 November under the command of Lt. Col. Joseph J. Costanzo, MSC. Aeromedical evacuation was provided by the 57th Medical Detachment, commanded by Maj. Arthur W. Hapner, MSC. Lt. Col. Joseph P. Jackson, MC, headed the advance party of the 307th, and his medical team received casualties through 2 November when hostilities ended. The team's experience highlighted a basic lesson in medical logistics as their operations were initially jeopardized because the detach-

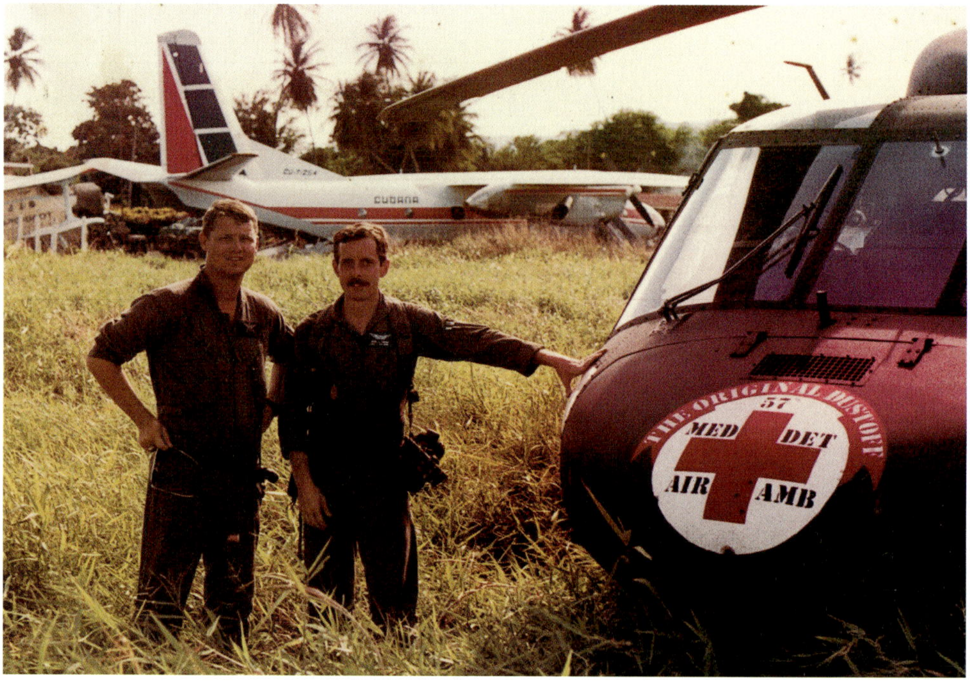

*Major Hapner (*left*) in Grenada, October 1983*

ment's materiel had at the last minute been bumped from its place in the air transport queue at Pope Air Force Base, Florida, when the division ordered in more combat soldiers than originally scheduled. Also relearned was the requirement for medical support of refugees and enemy prisoners of war, and Col. James Rumbaugh, MC, the XVIII Airborne Corps surgeon, organized a medical civic action program before the hostilities ended.

Lt. Col. Hugh M. McAlear, MSC, and Capt. William B. Andrews, MSC, both sanitary engineers, along with Capt. John B. Czachowski, MSC, were members of the preventive medicine team that assembled on the island. Czachowski, an environmental science officer from Womack Army Hospital at Fort Bragg, came under sniper fire while inspecting water points. His arrival was a welcome event for Lt. Col. N. Joe Thompson, MC, the first preventive medicine officer on the island, who was "never so happy in his life as when Czachowski showed up." McAlear, assigned to the U.S. Army Environmental Hygiene Agency, Aberdeen Proving Ground, Maryland, left for Grenada on a 24-hour notice. Riots and a garbage strike prior to the arrival of the American forces, coupled with a water shortage caused by a loss of electricity for pumping, combined with the island's heat to create sanitation challenges. The lackadaisical attitude of some soldiers toward sanitation required command intervention to compel them to adhere to basic field sanitation principles.[3]

MSCs at all levels of the intervention in Grenada quickly shifted from support of combat operations to support of the transition to peace. As in previous

U.S. military engagements, their actions were especially valuable in restoring sanitation and providing health care to POWs and the civilian population. They were active participants in the Army's role in civil-military operations, the creation of a democratic government, and the departure of U.S. forces.

Panama

Disorder in Latin America was not ended, however. Increasing troubles in Panama caused by the regime of dictator Manuel Noriega subjected Panamanians to brutal oppression and threatened U.S. citizens and interests in the Canal Zone. The crisis began in mid-1987 as Noriega, faced with an outpouring of dissent, moved toward armed repression, turning his army against both Panamanians and Americans. Violence escalated and the situation became increasingly chaotic and untenable. The United States increased its troop presence in 1988 as the situation deteriorated and Noriega continued his anti-American tirades. In 1989 Noriega nullified national elections held in May, and he survived a coup attempt in October. In December his forces killed an American Marine lieutenant at a roadblock and later abused a Navy lieutenant and his wife. Thereupon President George Bush ordered an invasion with the purpose of securing the Panama Canal, restoring the Panamanian government to its elected officials, protecting U.S. personnel, and turning Noriega over to U.S. officials to stand trial on a drug-trafficking indictment.

In the early morning hours of 20 December a joint force of about twenty-six thousand U.S. military personnel under the command of General Maxwell R. Thurman, the U.S. Southern Command commander, began a complex operation against targets in twenty-six locations. In short order the American forces captured Noriega, secured the Panama Canal, disarmed the Panamanian military, and restored Panama's government to the country's elected leaders. The intervention was over in a matter of days. The United States had 23 combat deaths; Noriega's forces lost 314, and the Catholic Church estimated the civilian death toll at 655.[4]

A joint force of 7,000 military including elements of the 82d Airborne Division and the 16th Military Police Brigade from Fort Bragg, North Carolina; the 75th Ranger Regiment from Fort Stewart, Georgia; and the 7th Infantry Division from Fort Ord, California, flew from the United States for the attack. In Panama they joined the 193d Infantry Brigade, based in Panama, which had been joined previously by elements of the 5th Infantry Division, Fort Polk, Louisiana; the 7th Infantry Division; and additional support forces. Corps-level medical support was provided by units led by Col. Jerome V. Foust, MSC, commander of the 44th Medical Brigade, Fort Bragg. The 142d Medical Battalion, under the command of Lt. Col. David W. Foxworth, MSC, moved 233 patients by ground ambulances. The 5th Mobile Army Surgical Hospital (MASH), under the command of Lt. Col. Stephen H. Johnson, MSC, and the 56th Medical Battalion, commanded by Lt. Col. Ira F. Walton III, MSC, set up two forward surgical teams that established a 22-bed facility on the airfield of Howard Air Force Base in the Canal Zone. The establishment of a mobile surgical capability forward in

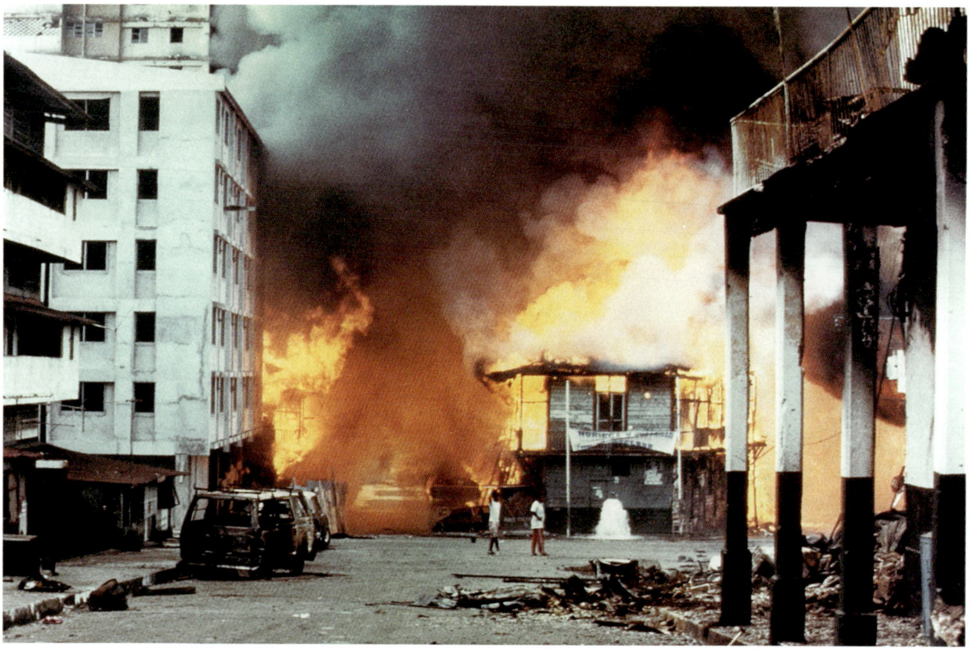

Flames engulf a building following the outbreak of hostilities between the Panamanian Defense Force and U.S. forces during Operation JUST CAUSE, October 1990.

the combat zone was reminiscent of the 25-bed World War II portable surgical hospital that augmented clearing stations of task forces or divisions, especially in jungle or amphibious operations.[5]

Unit-level medical service was provided by the medical platoons of the maneuver battalions under the direction of their MSC platoon leaders. The medical platoon leader of the 5th Infantry Division's battalion task force, 1st Lt. David W. Roberts, MSC, set up his platoon's aid station in Balboa High School. There they treated 140 casualties, receiving their first patients fifteen minutes after the shooting started. Division-level medical support was provided by the medical clearing companies of the 7th Division, the 82d Airborne Division, and the 193d Infantry Brigade. MSCs in special operations, air evacuation, and preventive medicine, as well as those assigned to Gorgas Army Hospital in the Canal Zone and to other units, contributed to the medical support of the combat operations.[6]

The Panama invasion taught several medical lessons—fundamentally the necessity of employing the complete military medical team in support of combat operations. The absence of MSC medical logisticians from the operational planning caused deficiencies in medical supply. In part because the deployed treatment unit included no MSC patient administration officers, the casualty reporting system was unable to meet the demands made upon it, and some wounded soldiers called home before their families were officially notified. Ground ambulance support was inadequate, and the planners were handicapped by the Army's deficiencies in doctrine for conflict resolution—especially the necessity of planning for early transition to humanitarian relief missions. For example, most of the casualties treated by Lieutenant Roberts' aid station were civilians, and within a short while after the fighting ceased his platoon was deluged with 5,000 refugees who had fled to the security of the American soldiers. The medics handed out blankets, medical supplies, and food and delivered two babies.[7]

The Persian Gulf

Despite the instability in Latin America, the most dangerous spot in the contemporary world continued to be the Middle East. Grenada and Panama were eclipsed when on 2 August 1990 Iraq's President Saddam Hussein seized his neighbor, the tiny monarchy of Kuwait. On 7 August President Bush, in response to a request from Saudi Arabia, ordered United States military forces into neighboring Saudi Arabia to head off the danger of an invasion by Iraq, which might have given the dictator control of 40 percent of the world's oil supply. Within thirty days the United States had deployed 41,000 troops to an area located 7,000 air miles and 12,000 sea miles from the continental United States. The 82d Airborne Division and the 1st and 2d Marine Expeditionary Forces, the first combat forces into the region, established an immediate defensive capability for Saudi Arabia. They were followed by the 101st Airborne Division (Airmobile), with its Apache helicopter tank killers and airmobile infantry, and the heavier forces of the 24th Infantry Division (Mechanized), the 1st Cavalry Division, and the 197th Infantry Brigade (Mechanized). MSCs in unit- and division-level medical organizations were part of that rapid deployment. A medical platoon leader in the 24th Infantry Division, 2d Lt. Christopher A. Hutchinson, MSC, was one. He found himself "caught up in an adventure not quite my own, preserving a brittle peace on the front lines of a distant desert."[8]

By 15 August thirteen nations had aligned against Iraq under a United Nations mandate, and the multinational force assembled in Saudi Arabia included 110,000 troops. The United States began calling up reserve and National Guard units and deployed the 2d Armored Division and the 3d Armored Cavalry Regiment. By 13 October the United States had 200,000 troops in place. Those forces were insufficient to provide the allies an offensive capability, and on 8 November the Pentagon announced the deployment of the VII Corps and elements of the V Corps from Germany, adding to the growing array the heavy forces of the 1st and 3d Armored Divisions, the 1st Infantry Division (Mechanized), and the 2d Armored Cavalry Regiment. Equipment, materiel, and personnel continued to pour into the Persian Gulf; by the end of the year about 300,000 United States troops were in Saudi Arabia awaiting the call to action. In January 1991 Congress voted Bush the authority to use armed force to expel Iraq from Kuwait. At mid-month a coalition force of 680,000 troops from twenty-four nations were preparing for war. The United States was the dominant presence in the coalition, and American troops numbered over 415,000, with 4,200 tanks, 2,800 infantry fighting vehicles, and 3,100 artillery pieces. They faced 540,000 Iraqi soldiers armed with 7,000 tanks and armored vehicles and 3,000 artillery pieces.

Operation DESERT SHIELD became DESERT STORM on 17 January 1991 as the United States unleashed an unremitting air campaign aimed at disrupting Saddam's command and control apparatus and eliminating key targets, especially antiaircraft radar and missile sites and nuclear, biological, and chemical weapon production facilities.[9] The 1,000-hour air war ended on 24 February when the allies launched a ground assault. Over the twelve-day period leading up to the attack, General H. Norman Schwarzkopf, commander in chief of the U.S. Central Command (CENTCOM), had shifted two corps with a combined strength of over 200,000 troops to the west at distances of up to 300 miles. In a celebrated maneuver, the coalition forces outflanked and routed the Iraqi Army in 100 hours. The United States had deployed 541,000 military, but suffered only 145 killed and 357 wounded.[10] Iraqi casualties were estimated in the tens of thousands, and Schwarzkopf's forces were swamped with enemy prisoners of war. Lieutenant Hutchinson's medical platoon saved the lives of many Iraqi soldiers who were brought to his aid station.[11]

MSCs at all levels of the military establishment were important contributors to Operation DESERT STORM, and over 1,350 active component officers deployed to the theater of operations. The full range of administrative and clinical specialties was essential, from handling "paperwork" (which increasingly meant the flow of electrons) to serving as essential members of the preventive medicine team that controlled and prevented the spread of disease.[12]

MSCs figured prominently in the command structure of units at corps level and echelons above corps (*Table 5*). Colonel Foust remained in command of the 44th Medical Brigade as it deployed from Fort Bragg to Saudi Arabia to support the XVIII Airborne Corps. Eight medical groups deployed to the theater of operations, six of which were commanded by MSCs.[13]

Col. Benjamin M. Knisely, MSC, CENTCOM's deputy surgeon and the senior MSC on the CENTCOM staff, deployed with that headquarters from MacDill Air Force Base, Tampa, Florida. He made national news in November when he appeared on the ABC program *Nightline*. An earlier broadcast had alleged that CENTCOM was not prepared to support combat operations, principally because of inadequate medical equipment and a lack of medical preparedness. Knisely assured the viewing audience that conversion of the hospital units to Deployable Medical Systems (DEPMEDS) sets was proceeding well and that CENTCOM was assembling a fully capable medical support apparatus.[14]

Anticipating heavy casualties, the United States sent a robust medical force of sixty-five hospitals to the Middle East. The Army deployed 198 medical units, which included the organic support units of 8 divisions and 44 hospital units (16 from the active components and 28 reserve) with 13,580 beds.[15] General Schwarzkopf praised the Medical Department for performance during the buildup that "was nothing short of spectacular."[16]

Preparing for War

The U.S. Army Health Services Command (HSC) undertook the challenge of multiple missions in support of the deployment. First, it designated its six stateside medical centers as primary casualty receiving hospitals and made over ten

TABLE 5—PERSIAN GULF MEDICAL COMMAND AND CONTROL

Echelons Above Corps	
3d Medical Command (AC)—Col. Demetrious Tsoulos, MC	
173d Medical Group (USAR), Chicopee, Massachusetts	Col. Douglas A. Stephens, MSC
202d Medical Group (ARNG), Jacksonville, Florida	Col. Spessard Boatright, SC
244th Medical Group (ARNG), Brooklyn, New York	Col. Thomas P. Meany, MSC
VII Corps	
332d Medical Brigade (USAR)—Brig. Gen. Michael D. Strong, MC	
30th Medical Group (AC), Ludwigsburg, Germany	Col. Jesse K. Fulfer, MSC
127th Medical Group (ARNG), Ashland, Alabama	Col. Dalton E. Diamond, MC
341st Medical Group (USAR), Mesquite, Texas	Col. Robert G. Smith, MSC
XVIII Airborne Corps	
44th Medical Brigade (AC)—Col. Jerome V. Foust, MSC	
1st Medical Group (AC), Fort Hood, Texas	Col. Eldon H. Ideus, MSC
2d Medical Group (AC), Fort Lewis, Washington	Col. William E. Ethington, MSC

Source: John R. Brinkerhoff, Ted Silva, and John Seitz, Office of the Chief, Army Reserve, Rpt, sub: U.S. Army Reserve in Operation Desert Storm: Reservists of the Army Medical Department, 23 Sep 1993, p. 50, PL.

thousand beds available for that purpose. Second, it provided clinical officers, principally physicians and nurses, for the U.S. Forces Command units deploying to the Gulf. This was achieved with the Professional Filler System (PROFIS), a program established in 1979 when mobilization exercises had demonstrated that the peacetime personnel requisition system was not fast enough to meet the needs for rapid deployments or mobilization. PROFIS was designed to provide officers to the gaining units within seventy-two hours of notification (forty-eight hours in certain cases). Over twelve hundred officers in HSC units were deployed to units in the Persian Gulf through this mechanism.[17]

However, a third mission had been unanticipated. The command's task became vastly more complicated when the Army chief of staff ordered that HSC would not curtail its care for family members, retirees, and other beneficiaries during the mobilization. Lt. Col. Ralph E. Bradford, MSC, chief of HSC's Personnel Management Division, handled the intense coordination effort as PROFIS underwent a severe test. Bradford, who had signed into HSC on the day before it was alerted to the Persian Gulf requirements, found himself on a roller coaster of frenzied activity, working 22-hour days. "I was astounded at what humans can do when the adrenalin starts flowing." Mobilization planning had assumed the sus-

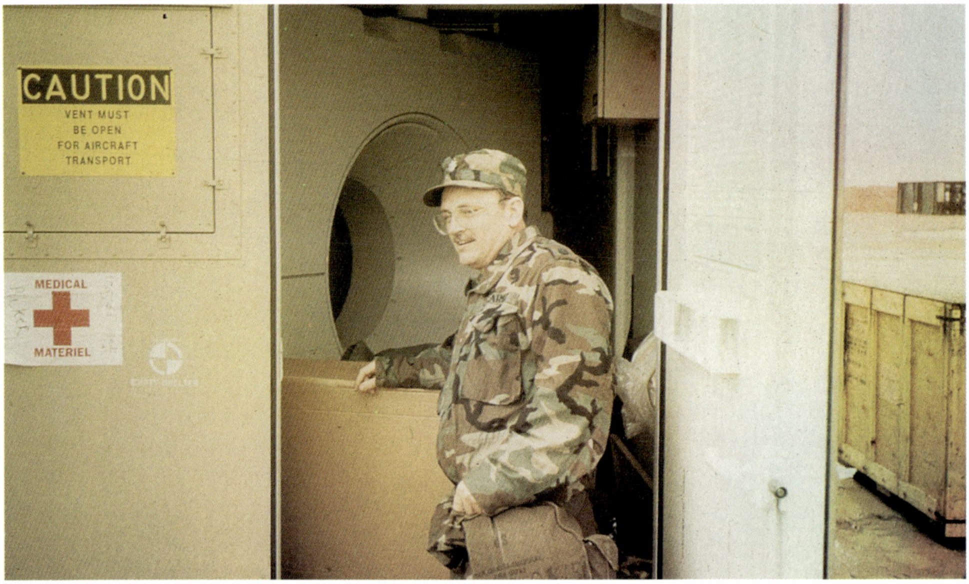
CAUTION
VENT MUST
BE OPEN
FOR AIRCRAFT
TRANSPORT
MEDICAL
MATERIEL

Fielding mobile CT scan to 86th Evacuation Hospital at King Khalid Military City, Saudi Arabia, January 1991

pension of care for other than active duty military, and the chief of staff's order meant that Colonel Bradford and his team would have to find replacements for the officers deployed to the Gulf under PROFIS. It was made even more difficult when HSC had to come up with eighty-seven clinical officers to backfill units deploying from Germany.[18]

Their first source for replacing the PROFIS officers was the pool of officers remaining in HSC. Other sources included the units of the reserves and individual reservists who volunteered for temporary active duty tours. PROFIS worked "amazingly well" according to one report, but the unforeseen requirement to keep HSC hospitals running at full capability for all beneficiaries caused an enormous amount of work for MSC personnel officers.[19] The deployment brought into focus the need to make major improvements, including intensive management of the supporting automated data base and the establishment of a means for the automatic replacement of PROFIS officers through the individual mobilization augmentee program of the reserves. For Bradford, though, it was the experience of a lifetime. "Everyone should have the chance to do what I did."[20]

The deployment placed large demands on Army medical facilities in the United States and Europe. For example, MSC optometrists assigned to eye clinics and optical fabrication laboratories were hard pressed to meet the demand for the more than 112,000 deploying soldiers who did not have the appropriate spectacles or protective mask inserts.[21] As another example, family support efforts received strong command emphasis as senior leaders demanded the establishment of support networks for the families of soldiers sent to the Persian Gulf. This was even more important for families in Europe who were already isolated

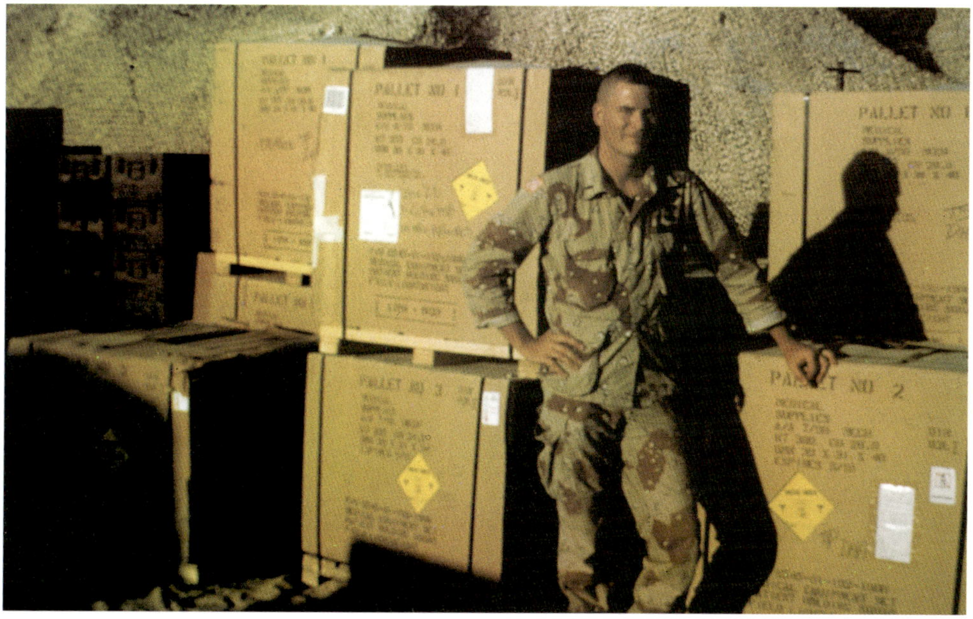

24th Infantry Division medical supply officer in Saudia Arabia, November 1990

by being overseas. MSC psychologists were valued contributors to those programs, including planning for the special needs of children. Nearly every student and teacher in schools on military installations had family members or close friends deployed for war. Psychologists who assisted the schools in responding to the deployment dealt with the possibility that up to twenty children in any one classroom might lose a parent.[22]

The 7th Medical Command in Germany sent 12 units, 1,300 soldiers, and 17 DEPMEDS hospital assemblages while supporting the deployment of 70,000 soldiers from Europe.[23] It tripled its operating capacity and designated its three largest hospitals as primary receiving facilities, setting aside 1,820 beds for combat casualties. The 7th MEDCOM was replenished by Army Reserve and National Guard units called to active duty. The 3,000 soldiers from those units who backfilled 7th MEDCOM units prevented the collapse of the Army's health care system in Europe, which continued to support the force remaining in Europe and the family members of the soldiers deployed to DESERT STORM. The reserve component soldiers were a welcome addition to the medical force in Europe. For example, an Army National Guard unit from Maine, the 112th Medical Company (Air Ambulance), received special commendation by General Crosbie E. Saint, the USAREUR commander, who said it "established an outstanding reputation providing medevac support to the theater."[24]

One of 7th MEDCOM's Dustoff units, the 45th Medical Company (Air Ambulance), commanded by Maj. Richard S. Ellenberger, MSC, flew twelve Black Hawk helicopters 3,500 miles from Darmstadt, Germany, to Dhahran, Saudi Arabia, in late August. The trip, which was spread over five days, took the crews south from Germany, through Italy, Greece, Cyprus, and Egypt, and into Saudi Arabia—the longest self-deployment of the Black Hawk ever attempted. It challenged their resourcefulness. One crew repaired a rotor blade skin separation by drilling holes in the blade with a hand drill and injecting glue using syringes from their medical supply kit.[25]

Once in the Persian Gulf the crews dealt with the ever-present elements of heat, sand, desert navigation, and flying with night-vision goggles. Capt. Randall G. Anderson, MSC, a pilot with the 57th Medical Detachment of the XVIII Airborne Corps, said his crew of four found that the Black Hawk helicopter was a multipurpose vehicle in addition to being an ambulance. The constant requirement for mobility necessitated keeping all their personal effects with them at all times, and they used every nook and cranny of the aircraft for storage. They found that the four-litter carousel support device in the cabin afforded the crew an excellent place to sleep. The helicopter's main rotor blade served as a hanger for a shower bucket and, despite the fact that bathers were covered by blowing sand by the time they dried off, the shower made them feel (and smell) clean. So equipped, Anderson's crew evacuated four thousand patients during the operation, including over a thousand enemy prisoners of war.[26]

MSC commanders took their hospital units to Saudi Arabia and then stepped down from command to serve as executive officers, in accordance with a standing Medical Department doctrine that would be strongly criticized after the war. Lt. Col. Scott Beaty, MSC, commander of the 47th Field Hospital, deployed his unit in August from Fort Sill, Oklahoma, sixteen days after he was first alerted. The 47th set up in a former British compound in the far northeast corner of the tiny island country of Bahrain. The temperature soared to 130 degrees during the day, making the use of air-conditioned shelters essential. Once the unit was operational, Beaty was replaced as commander by a physician in accordance with the existing Army doctrine. Reverting to duties as the 47th's executive officer, Beaty coordinated the unit's use of a hospital set that had been pre-positioned in that region some twenty years earlier. Much of the stored equipment was obsolete and some had deteriorated—a World War II lesson relearned. The experience taught Beaty that going to war "is never going to be the way you thought it was going to be."[27]

Maj. Tommy R. Hancock, MSC, deployed as the executive officer of the 159th Mobile Army Surgical Hospital, a Louisiana Army National Guard unit. The 159th crossed the Iraqi border on 25 February and was operational for a little over two weeks, during which time it received 300 patients, a third of whom were enemy prisoners of war. Lt. Col. Joseph H. Cohen, MSC, was executive officer of the 403d Combat Support Hospital, a reserve unit in Phoenix, Arizona. His unit, which was activated the day before Thanksgiving, had just completed training with DEPMEDS equipment at Camp Pendleton, California. It was good preparation for what they faced in Desert Storm.

The medical logistics effort was a noteworthy performance. The 32d Medical Supply, Optical, and Maintenance (MEDSOM) Battalion, commanded by Lt. Col. Ray G. Brueland, MSC, arrived in Saudi Arabia on 8 August. Col. Philip E. Livermore, MSC, arrived at the end of the month as the senior medical logistician for the Army component of CENTCOM (ARCENT). The 32d MEDSOM was joined by the 47th MEDSOM in September; they were combined into a single organization and designated the U.S. Army Medical Materiel Center, Saudi Arabia, under the direction of Lt. Col. Richard L. Ursone, MSC, commander of the 47th. It functioned as the joint medical logistics organization for the theater. The 980th MEDSOM, a reserve unit from California commanded by Lt. Col. Jeffrey Gidley, MSC, replaced the 32d, which then relocated to support the XVIII Airborne Corps. The newly formed materiel center processed over 200,000 customer requests for over $200 million in supplies and equipment—an average of sixty-five air line of communication (ALOC) pallets daily.[28]

Two more MEDSOMs arrived in December: the 428th, commanded by Lt. Col. Clarence R. Wills, MSC, deployed from Germany with the VII Corps, and the 145th, a reserve unit commanded by Lt. Col. Gene Johnson, MSC, deployed from Texas to the western region of the theater. The 7th MEDCOM's U.S. Army Medical Materiel Center, Europe, located in Pirmasens, Germany, under the command of Joseph J. Costanzo, now a colonel, provided the communications zone medical supply support for DESERT STORM. Its workload skyrocketed; it shipped to the theater 5.6 million pounds of medical supplies valued at $56 million, and at one point had 1,606 ALOC[29] pallets awaiting unloading for further distribution throughout Europe and Saudi Arabia. It sent seventeen DEPMEDS hospital sets, and its optical section filled nearly 71,000 orders for spectacles and protective mask inserts.

Deployed hospitals were retrofitted with DEPMEDS equipment, an enormous undertaking that converted twenty-eight units in Saudi Arabia and upgraded equipment in all the Army hospitals. The work was accomplished by a modernization team of twenty personnel headed by Maj. John T. Harris, MSC, supported by a staging facility at the port of Ad Dammam headed by Capt. Jettaka V. M. McGregor, MSC. The teams delivered over two thousand military vans (MILVANS) and international shipping overseas (ISO) containers of medical equipment to the field units in the largest medical force modernization ever conducted. Capt. James A. Signaigo, MSC, had the task of expediting transportation of the equipment from the port to the field sites. By January the heavily trafficked two-lane Tapline road, which headed northeast 500 kilometers to Hofar al Batin near King Khalid Military City, became essentially impassable for Captain Signaigo's trucks. He arranged for the use of a flatcar railroad train and put together an 800-kilometer combination train and truck route to the same destination. Signaigo's train ran daily, and he had to fend off efforts to steal or borrow it for other purposes.[30]

In the Gulf War American forces faced their first serious chemical threat since World War I. The genuine potential for Iraqi use of chemical agents sent the military scrambling. Scientific specialty MSCs of the U.S. Army Medical Research and Development Command (USAMRDC) were again revealed as a national resource, in this case for their expertise in chemical agent protection. One of the command's tasks was to provide training to the medical clinicians who would handle any chemical casualties. That mission was executed by the U.S. Army Medical Research Institute of Chemical Defense (USAMRICD), whose deputy commander, Lt. Col. George C. Southworth, MSC, coordinated the logistical support for the effort and served as the institute's acting commander throughout this period as its teams provided the Medical Management of Chemical Casualties Course for 6,600 health care providers, principally physicians and nurses, in the United States, Germany, and Saudi Arabia.[31]

The threat of chemical weapons necessitated the protection of aircrews who were issued an aviator version of a new protective mask. Unfortunately, the mask could not accommodate spectacles, so the surgeon general approved aircrew wear of contact lenses on a voluntary basis, expanding an earlier program for Apache and special operations crews. Lt. Col. Morris R. Lattimore, Jr., MSC, of the U.S. Army Aeromedical Research Laboratory at Fort Rucker, Alabama, directed a protocol that outfitted 349 aviators, using a team of eleven optometrists in the United States and Germany who did the contact lens workups. The project established aviator wear of contact lenses as a viable alternative to spectacles and determined that fears of eye injury from desert sand conditions were unfounded.[32]

Of perhaps even greater concern was the potential for Iraqi use of biological weapons. A United Nations inspection team after the war confirmed that Iraq had the capability of producing, at its biological research facility in Salman Pak, fifty gallons weekly of anthrax, *Clostridium perfringens*, and botulinum toxin, amounts sufficient to kill thousands of people.[33] Defense against those agents also fell to the USAMRDC, whose MSC researchers and administrators were part of the team that constituted a defense against this lethal threat. One of the potential agents, botulism, was the most potent bacterial toxin known, and USAMRDC accelerated the fielding of a highly purified equine antitoxin. Lt. Col. Michael A. Balady, MSC, a U.S. Army Medical Materiel Development Activity immunologist, coordinated with the manufacturer and provided oversight for testing schedules, and, with Lt. Col. Gregory P. Berezuk, MSC, the command's human use review officer, secured its approval by the Food and Drug Administration (FDA) for use as an investigational new drug. Maj. William R. Cline, MSC, of the U.S. Army Medical Research Institute of Infectious Diseases, handled its distribution. Other MSC researchers contributed to gaining similar FDA approval for use of pyridostigmine, a nerve gas pretreatment.[34] In addition, the U.S. Army Medical Research Acquisition Activity, commanded by Lt. Col. John L. Chaffee, MSC, executed an emergency procurement of centoxin, required for treatment of septic shock, and ciprofloxacin, a broad-spectrum antibiotic necessary for defense against biological agents. Chaffee's organization awarded the $45 million contract for the drug within forty-eight hours of being notified of the requirement.

On the Ground

Women were a sizable presence in the United States military force deployed for Operation DESERT STORM. Maj. Carolyn A. Albanese, MSC, executive officer of the 350th Evacuation Hospital, deployed with her 400-bed reserve unit from Ohio to King Khalid Military City. Albanese, an associate professor at the University of Akron, believed her gender had no effect on her ability to carry out her duties. "I have the position because I earned the position, and I have the respect of my staff for that particular reason."[35] Lt. Col. William C. Long, MSC, executive officer of the 86th Evacuation Hospital (and the hospital's commander when in garrison at Fort Lewis, Washington), found no difference in the performance of male and female soldiers in his unit. A patient administration officer with the 173d Medical Group, 2d Lt. Melissa A. Gagnon, MSC, was representative of many female MSCs at all levels of the command. Lieutenant Gagnon was on duty in the group's tactical operations center 25 February 1991 when a Scud attack on Dharhan killed twenty-eight soldiers and wounded ninety-eight. She coordinated the evacuation of casualties from the incident, which accounted for one-third of all American deaths in the war.[36]

MSCs were challenged and tested by the deployment, and there were lessons for medical operational planners. There was common agreement that medical supply was more responsive than the other classes of supply; some essential commodities (such as Class IX, spare parts) never functioned at the required level of performance. An enormous logistical problem for the hospital units was the lack of sufficient organic transport, which made moving an arduous task. "Over here there ain't no trains, there ain't no boats," said one captain. Priority of transportation assets went to movement of tactical units and, as MSCs found out, "if you weren't a fighter or if it wasn't bullets or food, you just didn't get trucks."[37] United States forces were heavily dependent upon Saudi vehicles; Colonel Foust went to war in a Toyota.

The DEPMEDS sets received praise, but the deployment made plain the immobility of DEPMEDS-equipped hospitals and the deleterious effect of fielding the sets to the hospitals in Europe without all their equipment (a problem when those sets were pressed into service). Foust believed DEPMEDS was outstanding, but much too heavy.[38] He reduced his combat support hospitals and MASHs to a size that could be moved by their organic vehicles so that they could keep up with the combat units. General Strong agreed. He said that DEPMEDS was "a wonderful system for providing medical care, but a terrible system to try to move."[39]

As in Vietnam, the hospitals were not authorized any fuel trucks. Capt. Steven R. Gilreath, MSC, S–4 of the 86th Evacuation Hospital, had a 36,000-gallon fuel storage capability, but "had I not been able to bootleg a 5,000-gallon civilian tanker we'd never have been able to support ourselves. Once the battle was under way there was no way we could get tanker support from anyone."[40] The 47th Combat Support Hospital deployed with MUST equipment and converted to DEPMEDS in Saudi Arabia. Capt. David O. Hill, MSC, the hospital's logistics officer, estimated the daily fuel requirement for its MUST set at 7,000 gallons, an unsupportable rate under combat conditions, especially without its own fuel truck.[41]

There were other problems in medical support. Col. James A. Martin, MSC, head of the Walter Reed Army Institute's research psychology team in Germany, did an assessment of corps and division mental health support in the Gulf before, during, and after the ground war. He found that mental health teams, with some exceptions, were not sufficiently prepared to handle their combat missions, and he concluded that this would have led to unnecessary evacuations from the theater if the conflict had produced heavy casualties or had been prolonged. He was particularly critical of a general unpreparedness for handling combat stress casualties,

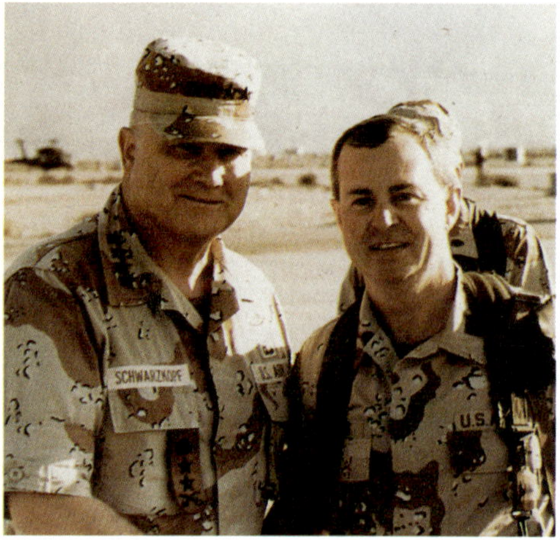

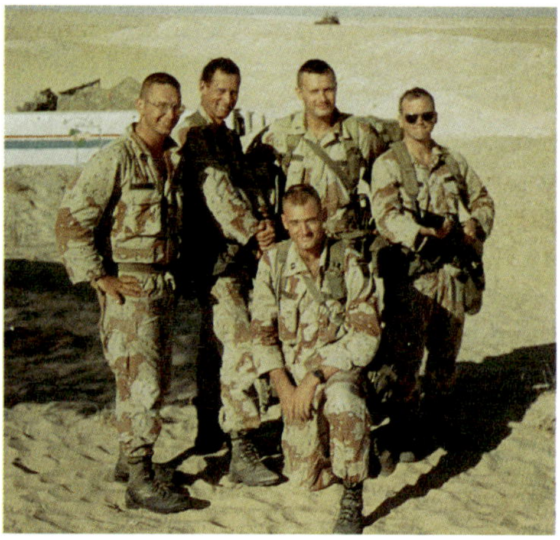

Scenes from the Gulf War

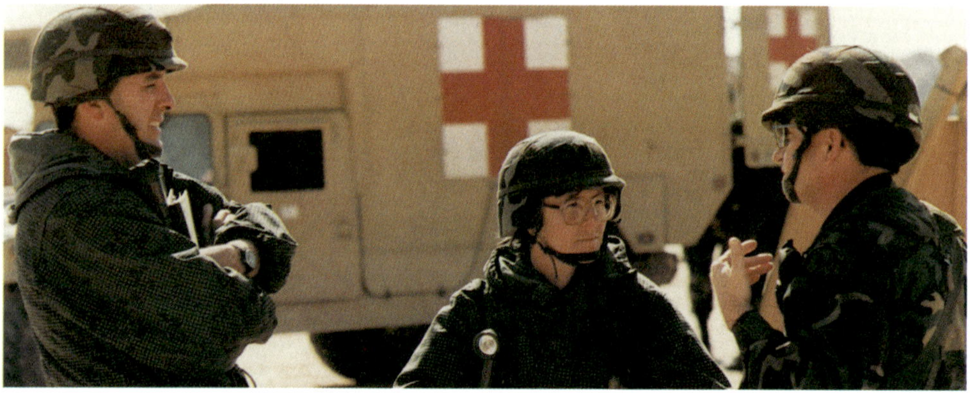

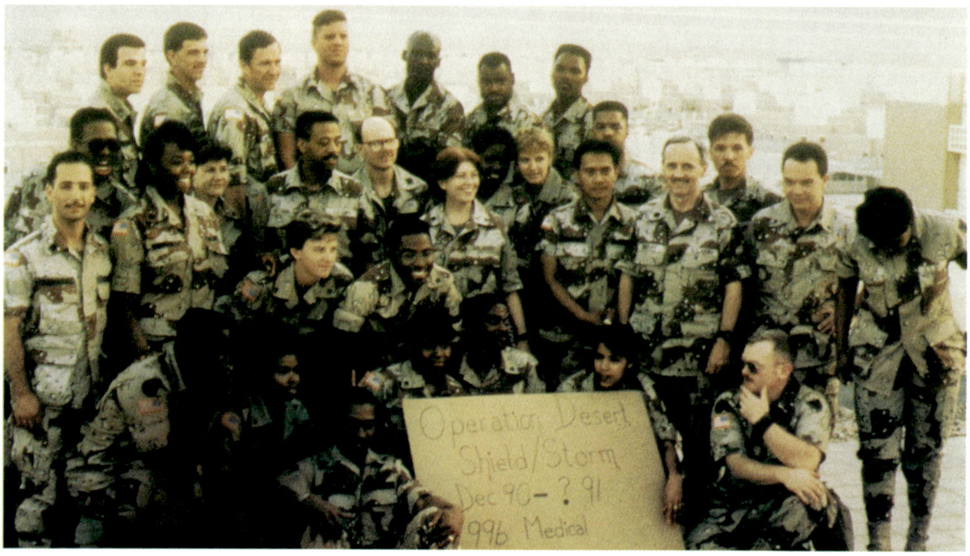

and he emphasized the need to implement lessons that had been painfully learned and relearned since the Civil War. As Colonel Martin put it, "One of the most important roles for any mental health officer in the combat theater is to curb the tendency of line and medical leaders to evacuate [stress] casualties out of the theater of operations as quickly as possible."[42]

MSC patient administration officers had other challenges and headaches. The chief of patient administration for the 47th Combat Support Hospital, 1st Lt. Damon T. Mathis, MSC, said the evacuation system was effective once the ground war started, but prior to that had been "a gnarly mess."[43] In Panama and DESERT STORM, war was covered by live television for the first time, and patient administration officers were faced with the overwhelming expectations of families and commanders that medical information should be superior in timeliness and accuracy to that provided by the omnipresent news media. The Surgeon General's Office received over sixty thousand phone calls a day on a hotline it set up for families to call. None of the DOD systems was able to meet the insatiable desire for information. Patient data were contained within four different computer systems that operated independently of each other. Col. Fred R. McClain, Jr., MSC, commander of HSC's Patient Administration Systems and Biostatistics Agency, recommended formation of a joint patient tracking and information system as a solution for this difficult problem.[44]

The Gulf War, like the operations in Grenada and Panama, demonstrated the need for MSC administrative and scientific specialty officers as part of the military medical team in the posthostilities medical care of enemy prisoners of war (POWs) and refugees. The extent of those requirements tended to catch planners off guard, and their resolution required a variety of MSC skills to handle. As an example, hospital units of Col. Douglas Stephens' 173d Medical Group admitted 6,225 patients during its deployment from December 1990 to April 1991. Over a third were POWs and refugees and, as in previous wars, hospital personnel cared for tired and hungry patients who were infested with lice. Support provided by the 173d to United States POW camps was inspected by a team of the International Committee of the Red Cross who communicated with their home office in Geneva with a microwave transmitter, an example of the increasing electronic sophistication of the twentieth century battlefield.[45]

And as in other times and places, soldiering in the Persian Gulf had a uniquely human dimension as the GIs accommodated to foreign places and customs. Lt. Col. Philip K. Schenck, MSC, the executive officer of the 173d Medical Group, reported that his staff took advantage of the local laundry in the Dharhan area until their own washers and dryers arrived. They quickly discovered that the laundry's one-hour service sometimes took two weeks, that buttons disappeared, and that clothes shrank two sizes in the first washing. After about a month in tents, they moved into a large housing complex. There they found that because Saudis did not use toilet paper, the building drain pipes were of a smaller diameter than those in the United States. This necessitated placing diaper pails in each bathroom for disposing of the used paper. Schenck and his comrades at arms lived with the incongruity of plastic pails gaily decorated with teddy bears and little cherubs.[46]

As MSCs had been challenged by the deployment, so were they put to the test in the redeployment once hostilities ceased and the Army turned to getting soldiers and materiel shipped home. National Guard and reserve soldiers returning to civilian life were required by law to have a physical examination, principally in order to assess future disability claims against the government. A hearing test was part of the examination, but the field medical facilities were not equipped for that procedure. In response to this need an audiologist, Lt. Col. Richard W. Danielson, MSC, led a group of 11 MSC audiologists, 1 noncommissioned officer, and 39 enlisted technicians to Saudi Arabia where they located with the 47th MEDSOM. They brought with them ten 32-foot trailers that were specially equipped for hearing testing. Danielson broke his group into teams of one officer and two soldiers who then fanned out to the evacuation hospitals. They tested over twenty-nine thousand soldiers, and in so doing speeded up the return of the soldiers to the United States. A different sort of homecoming was handled by MSC social work officers at Walter Reed Army Medical Center who served as case managers for five American prisoners of war repatriated by the Iraqis after the conflict. These were the first POWs since Vietnam.[47]

Soldiers learn in basic training that they have to clean and put away their equipment when they come in from the field. For the medics this required rebuilding thirty-five DEPMEDS-equipped hospital sets so that the equipment could be returned to their home stations in a condition that was redeployable. MSC medical logisticians managed the project for both reserve component and active component units, and by August 1993 they had rebuilt the equipment in 610 ISOs and MILVANs. Some 426,000 items had been returned to inventory for reissue, and 4,600 pieces of equipment had been repaired. MSCs also helped Kuwait put itself back together. Maj. John T. Watts, MSC, a health facilities planner, went to Kuwait in 1992 to assess the damage to the country's medical facilities and to identify rebuilding requirements.[48]

Overall, United States military leaders were pleased that the doctrine, equipment, and staffing changes of the post-Vietnam period had worked. General Thurman, one of the architects of the modernized Army, believed DESERT STORM proved that high-quality people with good quality equipment, training, and leadership could do almost anything. The United States had moved half a million military personnel halfway around the world in six months, the fastest deployment for a force of that size in America's history. In Europe, an entire forward-deployed corps had redeployed 77,000 military personnel and all their equipment in forty-five days, leaving their family members overseas—an unprecedented action.[49] Lt. Gen. Frank F. Ledford, Jr., General Becker's successor as surgeon general in 1988, said the Medical Department had "performed superbly" in a deployment that had tested the department's preparedness "to its limits." Once on the ground in the Gulf medical personnel had handled over 20,000 hospital admissions and over 200,000 outpatient visits.[50]

A lot of things had been done right in Panama and Iraq. The effects of the Goldwater-Nichols Act of 1986 were evident. The Services had worked together, and General Colin Powell, the chairman of the Joint Chiefs of Staff, was the undisputed senior military leader.[51] President Bush had clearly stated the objectives in both operations and had effectively marshaled the support of the American people. The United States employed overwhelming combat power, gave authority to the military command structure, and made the care of family members a matter of constant attention at all levels of command.[52]

A Time of Change

The Army Medical Service Corps remained an important national asset in United States military planning for the twenty-first century. MSCs were essential leaders in the Army's health care system, which at the beginning of the last decade of the twentieth century numbered over 200,000 officer, enlisted, and civilian personnel in all the components of the Army, including 91,000 in the active component. MSCs provided administrative and scientific expertise for a medical enterprise that was funded at over $3 billion annually and operated 50 hospitals and 544 health and dental clinics for nearly four million beneficiaries. The fixed plant, complemented by a large field medical apparatus, constituted most of the United States military capacity for meeting medical contingencies. The Academy of Health Sciences (which in 1991 became part of the newly organized U.S. Army Medical Department Center and School) was training more than 35,000 officer and enlisted students per year in the largest military medical training institution in the world. The U.S. Army Medical Research and Development Command was also the largest organization of its kind. But with the end of the Cold War, the most momentous world events since World War II began to influence the Army's medical establishment. As the Soviet Union neared collapse, the challenge would be to preserve the specialties of the MSC as part of the military medical team of the future.[53]

Elements of the 5th MASH arrived in Europe in November 1989 from Fort Bragg for the annual Return of Forces to Germany (REFORGER) exercises while ecstatic Berliners danced on the Berlin Wall to celebrate startling changes on the Continent. Eastern Europeans were pulling the Iron Curtain open, and thousands of little smoke-belching Trabant and Wartburg automobiles were pouring through the openings to clog the autobahns of West Germany.

Those pitiful cars on western European roads were happy evidence of the change. Soviet President Mikhail Gorbachev's policies of *glasnost* (openness) and *peristroika* (restructuring) had unleashed the exuberance of freedom. The phenomenal changes under way in the Soviet Union came to a brief halt with an abortive Communist coup in August 1991, but resumed with renewed vigor shortly afterward. The Soviet empire and its ruling party were nearing collapse and by the end of the year had ceased to exist. The events of 1990 and 1991 made it plain that the course of international events could confound the wisest pundits. The West had won the Cold War.

Exhilaration over the defeat of the Soviet Union was soon followed by the sobering reality that great instability continued to trouble the world and that universal peace was not assured. Yet United States military doctrine had enshrined containment of communism as its centerpiece; suddenly it was swept away, and no one was certain what would take its place. United States military actions on the heels of the Persian Gulf war in deployments to Turkey, Croatia, Somalia,

Rwanda, and Haiti illustrated the changing nature of the nation's role in the post–Cold War era. A measure of the Army's response to diverse and continual deployments was its awarding of over seven hundred Purple Hearts in the period from the collapse of the Soviet Union to the beginning of 1993. A major revision in 1993 of the Army's fundamental war-fighting doctrine, Field Manual 100-5, *Operations*, recognized those changing realities to the extent of including a new chapter on operations other than war.[54]

Some argued that one of those missions, humanitarian and disaster assistance relief, should move to the forefront of the Army's planning. Saddam Hussein provided an opportunity to demonstrate the U.S. military's capability for humanitarian assistance immediately after the Persian Gulf war when his persecution of the rebellious Kurdish minority in Iraq resulted in the flight of over 1.4 million refugees to neighboring Turkey. A European Command combined task force of 21,000 personnel from twelve nations under the command of Lt. Gen. John M. Shalikashvili provided humanitarian assistance in Operation PROVIDE COMFORT. The U.S. involvement that began in April included about one hundred soldiers of the 7th Medical Command who deployed principally for the preventive medicine effort as the command's U.S. Army Medical Materiel Center, Europe (USAMMCE), shipped emergency lifesaving supplies. Lt. Col. Stuart A. Mervis, USAMMCE's head of materiel management, described those shipments as the largest humanitarian assistance effort in the unit's history.[55]

Shortly afterward Mother Nature provided an opportunity for the military to demonstrate its capability for disaster relief at home. In August 1992 Hurricane Andrew, one of the worst storms of the century, struck near Miami, Florida, with 140-mile-an-hour winds, leaving hundreds of thousands of people without shelter, water, and power and causing damage that was still being repaired two years later. The Florida governor's request for federal assistance brought in 17,000 active component soldiers, principally elements of the XVIII Airborne Corps, headquartered at Fort Bragg, North Carolina, and 7,000 soldiers of the Army Reserve and Army National Guard. MSCs in various specialties were part of the effort. Maj. Dale R. Brown, MSC, a health facilities planner, went to the hardest-hit area, Homestead, Florida, where the wind gauge at Homestead Air Force Base had broken at 216 miles per hour. Brown assessed the damage to civilian hospitals as part of the effort to restore essential services. He found that while the buildings were structurally intact, unprotected windows had broken and inadequate roofing had torn apart. This enabled the storm's wind and water to ravage the interior of the facilities. Roof-mounted components, such as air-conditioning equipment and vents, tore off in the high winds, and Major Brown warned that those items should either not be reinstalled on roofs or should be adequately protected.[56]

First Lt. Timothy G. Bosetti, MSC, a sanitary engineer, also went to Homestead where he had firsthand experience with reestablishing a public water system after a natural disaster. He encountered the frustrating complexity of dealing with local, state, and federal officials who had conflicting roles in the matter. Bosetti had to deal with the political ramifications attendant to the restoration of basic public services, especially the pressure to remove an order to boil drinking

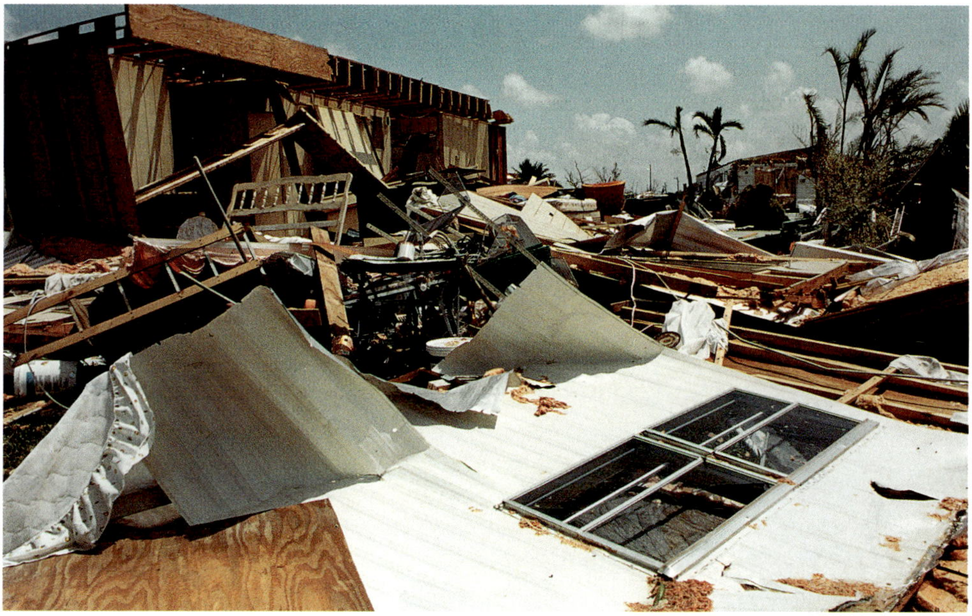

Destroyed buildings at Homestead Air Force Base, Florida, in the aftermath of Hurricane Andrew, September 1992

water that had been imposed in the several jurisdictions throughout the area hit by the hurricane. Elected officials, who desired to stay in office, were feeling the heat from their constituents to restore normal service, no matter what the consequences. They released areas from the boil-water notice in spite of Bosetti's objections that this was premature in some cases due to positive coliform tests in samples taken by the Army at different points in the distribution system.[57]

The next crisis again directed America's attention overseas. The breakup of Eastern European communism unleashed ancient animosities in regions previously dominated by the Soviet Union. A bloody civil war erupted in the former Yugoslavia, and the United Nations dispatched a peacekeeping force to the area in an attempt to moderate the hostilities. In October 1992 Col. Charles G. Stevens, MSC, commander of the 68th Medical Group in Wiesbaden, Germany, was appointed commander of Joint Task Force PROVIDE PROMISE and placed in command of all European Command elements in Croatia. Stevens deployed elements of his command, principally the 212th MASH, to Croatia as the first six-month rotation of a series of Army, Navy, and Air Force field hospitals supporting the 22,000-member U.N. protective force. The 212th set up on an airfield in Zagreb. Much of the surrounding area had been mined by the Yugoslavian National Army before its withdrawal from the separatist province. The hospital's dental clinic became the busiest section, as word of the availability of modern American dentistry quickly spread among the U.N. troops, especially the Eastern Europeans.[58]

Humanitarian assistance soon included aid to Russia as well. In 1992 Lt. Col. Edward P. Phillips, Jr., MSC, took a team to Soviet Georgia to set up a 1,000-bed contingency hospital in the capital city of Tbilisi. The following year MSC medical logisticians transferred $28 million worth of medical equipment from two 1,000-bed hospitals that had been in storage during the Cold War to eight hospitals and a dental clinic in Moscow.[59]

At the end of 1992 the threat of starvation in Somalia as the result of a bitter civil war among competing warlords prompted President Bush, in the last days of his administration, to dispatch his final humanitarian relief effort. Col. Ian L. ("Red") Natkin, MSC, commander of the 67th Medical Group, Fort Lewis, Washington, moved elements of his command to Somalia where he was also appointed the joint task force surgeon. The United States involvement ended in March 1994 when Bush's successor, President Bill Clinton, pulled out all United States troops after the relief operation turned into combat operations that produced two posthumous medals of honor.[60]

Among those in Natkin's command was entomologist Capt. Steve Horosko III, MSC, commander of the 485th Medical Detachment that deployed to Somalia in January 1993 to assume the vector control mission of the preventive medicine team. Horosko reported that the human side of war had not changed. The availability of one five-minute phone call each week for his soldiers after the unit had been in Somalia for six weeks proved to be an enormously important morale booster for soldiers feeling very far from home.[61]

Lieutenant Bosetti, on the heels of his experience in Florida, had another opportunity for a preventive medicine mission as the executive officer of the 485th Medical Detachment, an entomology team that deployed to Somalia in January 1993. His team's primary mission was pest control, with additional capabilities for water testing, mess inspections, and sanitation services. They used several pieces of equipment for the pesticide dispersal operations that made them a welcome presence for the marines operating in Bardera, an area threatened by malaria and dengue fever, and for the soldiers of the 10th Mountain Division in Jalib, a malarious area. Bosetti said the insects were so bad in Bardera that when they sprayed "the sky would rain dead bugs." Bosetti's water-testing mission took him throughout the country to certify potential water sources for quartermaster water production companies, the final product of which he found was superior in quality to most of the imported bottled water. One of his more eerie moments occurred when he had to test the water in a 50 by 100 by 200 foot above-ground tank. He climbed down inside armed only with his 9-mm. pistol, a flashlight, and two sample containers. "It was so humid in there it was actually raining."[62]

Other military deployments to Third World countries benefited from the talents of MSCs. In July 1994 civil war erupted in Rwanda, resulting in an estimated 500,000 deaths in the largest mass murder since the Khmer Rouge pogrom in Cambodia in 1975. The slaughter was of such ferocity that in a matter of days over two million Rwandans fled westward into neighboring Zaire, creating a dreadful refugee situation that was unprecedented for its size and speed. The refugees principally concentrated in the cities of Goma and Bukava, described by *Newsweek* magazine as a "bleak landscape teeming to the horizon with a solid carpet of refugees," where they were subjected to a deadly cocktail of crowding, contaminated water, starvation, and filth.[63] The United Nations responded with humani-

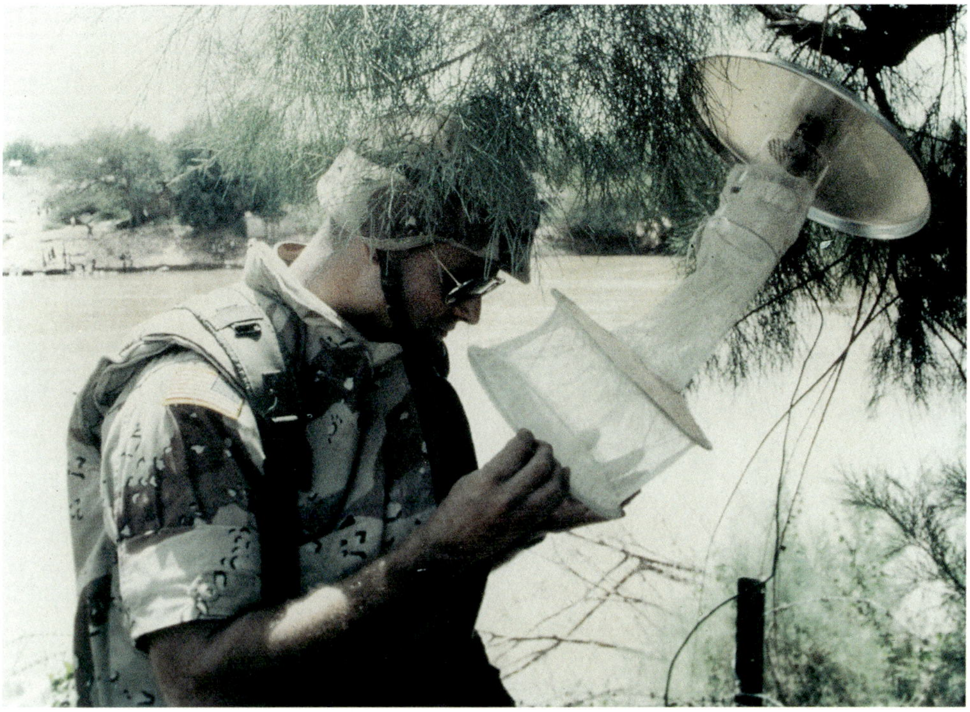

Captain Horosko inspects a mosquito light trap on the banks of the Juba River, Bardera, Somalia, February 1993.

tarian aid to ward off an explosive disease situation that included outbreaks of cholera, typhoid, and dysentery. With thousands of people dying, President Clinton ordered the European Command to provide a joint task force to conduct a humanitarian relief mission in Rwanda resembling the earlier mission to aid Kurdish refugees in northern Iraq. About 2,300 Americans were dispatched to Rwanda. MSCs were in the first deployments as members of the 71st Medical Detachment (Sanitation) and a forward distribution team detachment of the 37th Medical Logistics Battalion.[64]

Similarly, MSCs were valued members of the 20,000-member U.S. joint task force (including 17,500 soldiers) sent to Haiti, a desperately impoverished country, in September 1994 to intervene in a chaotic, violent situation that had intensified with a military coup in 1991 against Haiti's elected president, Jean-Bertrand Aristide. An estimated three thousand people, mostly Aristide supporters, had been killed in the intervening period, principally by government forces. The U.S. military oversaw the removal of the military regime and the return of Aristide to power. Soldiers patrolled the outlying areas, restored the country's infrastructure, and disarmed hostile elements. Medical personnel included medical assessment teams that assisted civilian hospitals and relief agencies. Maj. Arthur P. Lee, MSC, a sanitary engineer, was a member of the preventive medicine team charged with establishing the prevention measures that would keep soldiers healthy in a

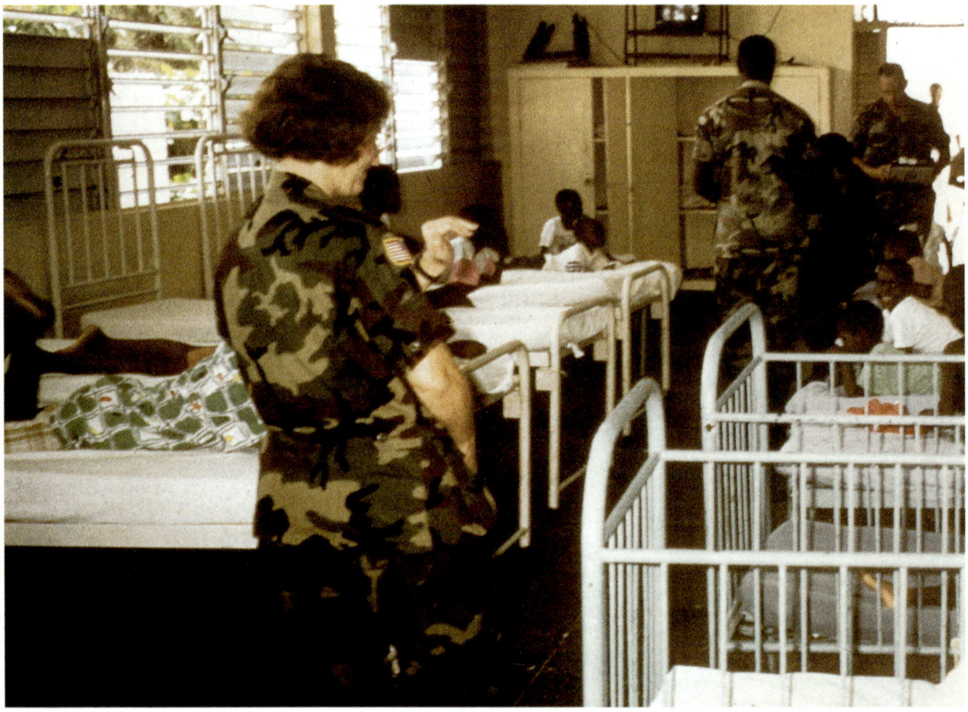

Children's ward at a hospital in Haiti

country with widespread conditions that spread infectious disease. Lee conducted environmental assessments of Haitian hospitals, including one in which chickens were walking around one of the wards. Dale Brown, now a lieutenant colonel, headed a health facility assessment team that completed reports on ten hospitals and clinics. They also provided designs to expand two hospitals and a plan to convert a hotel to a hospital. Brown's team found that in spite of many deficiencies, mostly due to the lack of resources, the rudiments of a system were present. For example, he noted after his visit to St. Catherine's Hospital in the Port-au-Prince area that "for where it is located and what it does it is not in bad shape." In one of the more unusual assignments for a Medical Department officer, Capt. Berthony Ladouceur, MSC, a native French and Creole speaker, served as the personal interpreter for the U.S. joint task force commander, Lt. Gen. Henry H. Shelton.[65]

In such a rapidly changing world, the future of the United States military was uncertain. The planned pullout of U.S. forces from Europe and the overall reductions in strength were both temporarily halted by the war with Iraq. But both resumed in 1991 as the Army began the drawdown of its active duty force from eighteen to ten divisions, complemented by six National Guard divisions. The active duty strength of the Army in 1989 was 780,000; it peaked at 863,000 in 1991 with the call-up of Army Reserve and Army National Guard soldiers for the Persian Gulf war. By the summer of 1993 the active duty number had dropped to 575,000 as the Army drew down in earnest; in a twelve-month period it had moved 400,000 soldiers and released 177,000 (many of whom were veterans of Panama and Iraq) from active duty. The Army was the smallest it had been in forty-four years, since the year before war broke out in Korea. By July 1993 there were more soldiers on the retired rolls than on active duty for the first time in the history of the Army. The number on active duty fell to 540,000 at the end of fiscal year 1994 and was projected to drop to 495,000 in 1996. The United States brought home its overseas cold warriors in droves. It deactivated VII Corps in Germany in order to cut the number of soldiers stationed in Europe from 183,000 in 1990 to 100,000 by 1995, and from 1990 through 1994 closed over nine hundred overseas military installations. Further reductions were planned.[66]

In the aftermath of the Cold War, the Medical Service Corps braced itself anew for the inevitable cuts. The Medical Department was a sizable portion of the Army, and it accounted for 20 percent of all Army officers. This was a prominent target as reductions got under way on a trajectory that would decrease the department's total active component numbers 37 percent through 1997. The number of officers was programmed to drop from 18,478 in 1991 to 14,793 in 1998, a reduction of 20 percent. MSC strength, which had remained relatively constant at 5,000 officers during the post-Vietnam period and numbered 5,080 in 1991, was at 4,571 (*see Appendix M*) in 1994 and was projected to fall to 4,041 in 1998, an overall reduction of 20.5 percent.[67]

Various programs were used to reduce the Army through voluntary and involuntary means that had not been available for the military during previous drawdown periods. These eliminated the need to conduct a reduction in force (RIF) in the MSC, as after the Korean and Vietnam Wars. Younger officers who were not eligible for retirement were offered a variety of attractive bonuses as incentives for separating from active duty. For example, a captain with six years' service could collect a onetime bonus of $32,350, or elect to receive annual payments of $5,390 for twelve years.[68]

The most painful of the drawdown programs were selective early retirement boards (SERBs), which forced officers into involuntary retirement and contributed to an atmosphere termed by the *Army Times* as "the blue mood of the officer ranks." SERBs of MSCs in 1987, 1990, and 1992 through 1995 forced out 250 officers. The odds of being selected were high—23 to 28 percent of eligible colonels were selected each year; in effect, retirement-eligible field grade MSCs were serving on year-to-year contracts. Believed to be an essential mechanism for drawing down the Army while maintaining promotion opportunity, SERB was an agonizing process for those involved in its management. The Medical Department SERB became such a malignant undertaking that by 1995, 95 percent of the MSC colonels selected for forced retirement were rated by the Personnel Command in the top two categories of officers, the result of the unrelenting winnowing of that group each year. Further, although the entire Medical Department was drawing down, by 1995 the MSC by itself accounted for nearly 47 percent of all of the department's officers hit by the SERB since it began. The effect on morale was predictable. While selected officers left active duty with full retirement benefits, their unceremonious departure in this way made for a bitter ending to the careers of a group that included many Vietnam veterans who had gone through two Army drawdowns, had demonstrated superb talent, and had contributed to the dramatic rebuilding of the Army after Vietnam. Army officers remaining on active duty no longer believed that promotion to colonel was a reasonable aspiration. Captains believed their horizons had diminished and now viewed a successful career within the limits of promotion to lieutenant colonel and retirement after twenty years of active duty.[69]

The shape of the MSC for the future was a subject of intense debate. Efforts in 1991 and 1992 to decide how to apply the cuts that were necessary to achieve the drawdown targets produced a draft plan that entailed a drastic reduction of selected MSC specialties. This was particularly true with the more technically complex fields and especially the scientific specialties. Some would have been entirely eliminated, including health facilities planning, research psychology, podiatry, physiology, and biochemistry. Others, such as comptroller, information systems, audiology, and immunology, would have been nearly eliminated. Relief eventually came at the end of 1992, when the MSC figures were adjusted upward and some specialties previously slated for elimination were retained (*see Appendix J*). However, there were no guarantees for the future. Brig. Gen. Jerome V. Foust, promoted and appointed chief of the corps in September 1992, predicted "some tough years ahead of us in regards to the downsizing." To assist him in planning for the future of the corps, Foust formed a board of directors comprising the assistant corps chiefs and eight senior MSCs in a variety of key positions, selected to widen his sources of advice.[70]

As in previous postwar reductions, the future of uniformed scientists in the Army was especially cloudy. The same pressures that had appeared in previous drawdowns predictably reappeared in the post–Cold War period, and questions again were raised as to the viability of the MSC scientific specialties. Indeed, those statements of concern could have been taken verbatim from the transcript of the 1948 meeting on the medical allied scientists. MSC scientists such as Lt. Col. Wilbur K. Milhous, MSC, a microbiologist, worried out loud that the Army could end by losing a valuable asset—the uniformed scientist—who brought to the research mission rapid deployability, focus on military relevance, and individual talent and experience. Often, Milhous argued, medical problems that were of great importance to the military were of no interest to the civil sector. For example, he warned that infectious diseases such as malaria and leishmaniasis remained a worldwide threat to U.S. military operations. However, without the military's support and sponsorship there would be no development of the drugs and vaccines necessary to defend soldiers against those disease threats. His concerns for the future were echoed by the Army's scientific community at large, prompting pledges of support for "green-suit" scientists by Army senior leaders.[71]

There were other concerns. Some senior officers worried over the best way to ensure the proper development of MSCs for the varied settings and challenges they would face in their careers. The MSC Management Study, completed in 1990, attempted to mold a leader development pattern to qualify senior officers for specialty-immaterial assignments. Another aspect was the old issue of alley cats and house cats, the challenge of developing officers with experience in both the wartime and peacetime components of the health care system. Over the years efforts had been made to reward officers who pursued field assignments, and yet some specialties still tended to shield their officers from a mix of assignments between garrisoned and operational medical units. In 1993 Col. Timothy Jackman, MSC, argued that difficulties arose when garrisoned field units deployed to the Persian Gulf, where they were joined by their full complement of clinicians. MSCs in leadership positions whose careers had not included assignments to operational medical units were disadvantaged at that point by a lack of understanding of the clinical mission and of the clinicians themselves. Jackman said this caused organizational stresses at different interpersonal, cultural, and management levels. He noted that his observation would be controversial to some, "especially those who have prided themselves on never having been assigned to a hospital." His solution was to require officers who desired those leadership opportunities to have assignments to operating medical units, such as hospitals, as part of their leader development pattern.[72]

During the early nineties, the Army Medical Museum at Fort Sam Houston, Texas, sold maroon T-shirts emblazoned with the MSC silver caduceus and the motto, "So Others May Live." The MSC would take that credo and the lessons from its history into the next century. Time and again, the United States had found in wartime that it needed medical administrative and scientific specialties. The evolution of the MSC from its precursors into a permanent corps was evidence of that need. After World War I the Medical Department had attempted to capitalize on its experience with the U.S. Army Ambulance Service and the Sanitary Corps, but World War II was needed to show once and for all that the military could not afford to dispense with the contributions of the Medical Administrative Corps and Sanitary Corps. A permanent Medical Service Corps emerged in 1947, and the new corps proved itself in Korea, where it was a source of strength. It demonstrated impressive maturity and cohesion with its own internal leadership during the difficult drawdown period after Korea. Its lifesaving work was in evidence throughout Vietnam. MSCs again showed their courage and expertise in the Persian Gulf, only to face once again the challenges of a postwar drawdown.

The Future

An estimated $898 billion bill for U.S. health care in 1993, accounting for 14.3 percent of the gross national product, and an unsuccessful yet high-priority attempt at health care reform by the Clinton administration kept the cost of health care in the news. DOD's annual cost of over $15 billion also attracted attention.[73] Rising concern by Congress over costs pressured the Department of Defense into further consolidation along the lines of a "purple suit," or amalgamation of the Army, Navy, and Air Force health care organizations.[74] The changes at the top of the military health care system would affect the structure of the Army Medical Department and the form its Medical Service Corps would take in the future. Army MSCs would be instrumental in designing that formulation as well as key players in its operation, but the department would most certainly have to resist more attacks on the MSC. Since the American Revolution, the periods of greatest growth of the MSC and its precursors came during wartime; regression occurred as funds dried up and the appreciation for the full dimension of medical support for combat operations was forgotten. Such periods had been characterized by direct assaults on individual MSC specialties as well as on the continued existence of the corps itself, and these attacks could be expected to reoccur under similar circumstances.

The process was evident in 1990 when the Army undertook Project VANGUARD, a study intended to find ways to cut the Army. Brig. Gen. Bruce T. Miketinac, the chief of the corps, believed it was the department's task to convince the Army Staff and others of the Army's need for MSCs in the various specialties. For example, in the case of resource managers the Medical Department had to communicate its requirement "to train MSC officers to be comptrollers, not comptrollers to be MSCs." The Medical Department resembled other specialized organizations that required their own unitary structure of people, units, equipment, and doctrine to execute their missions. In a similar vein, another effort to move medical logistics away from medical control was put to rest in 1993. The technical complexity of medical logistics, its time sensitivity for the user, and its pivotal role in the delivery of health care had not changed.[75]

Expertise remained a key to the corps' future. The MSC and its precursors had contributed to modernizing military medicine, principally by giving the Medical Department access to new technologies. The inclusion of experts in varied technical fields changed doctrine, equipment, and clinical practice, and the presence of scientific expertise—such as that embodied by Colonels Cavanaugh and Angel during the Vietnam War—was genuinely a national resource. Modernization extended to the administrative specialties as well. Improvements to the evacuation system were pioneered by administrative specialty officers skilled in the pioneering automotive technology of the World War I era, a time also marked by the first American attempts at developing a system of aeromedical evacuation.

The need for modernization was evident in the post–Gulf War period as well. As General Thurman insisted, the United States had to begin preparing immediately for the next war because every element of its military force had been exposed to the view of all countries, friendly and unfriendly.[76] Military medicine had to modernize as part of that process. Accordingly, the Academy of Health Sciences undertook a series of lessons-learned sessions. Problems that had surfaced in Panama and Iraq had to be identified and solved, and much more had to be done to improve joint operations. The Medical Service Corps would be a source of innovators who would develop the new technologies, doctrine, training, and equipment necessary to position military medicine for future challenges.

An example moved to the forefront in 1991. Lt. Col. Fred Goeringer, MSC, had over a several-year period personally shepherded the Medical Department's development of filmless radiology from its early days as a project of the U.S. Army Medical Research and Development Command. Goeringer, a medical logistics officer and institutional entrepreneur, organized an imaging system that combined computer applications with advanced phosphorous plate technology. His project promised to revolutionize military medicine with computer technology that had the potential of billions of dollars in applications in both military and nonmilitary settings. Goeringer oversaw a spinoff of that technology in a successful test of teleradiology in the Gulf War in which scans from a computed tomography (CT) scanner were transmitted via satellite and telephone links to Brooke Army Medical Center in San Antonio, Texas. Goeringer's effort expanded into a network of computer-based systems, called the Medical Diagnostic Imaging Support System (MDIS), that tied together a variety of systems such as CT, ultrasound, magnetic resonance imaging (MRI), and computer radiology. In 1991 the Army awarded a $209 million contract to Loral Corporation for the MDIS project. In 1992 Goeringer was recognized with a Federal 100 Award by an industry journal, the *Federal Computer Weekly*.[77]

Goeringer's efforts formed the Medical Department's core of visionary technology called telemedicine that was strongly championed by Lt. Gen. Alcide M. LaNoue, appointed as surgeon general in 1992, and was demonstrated in 1994 at the Advanced Warfighter Experiment at the National Training Center, Fort Irwin, California. In September 1994 telemedicine became a tri-service effort with the Army as its executive agent under the auspices of the assistant secretary of defense for health affairs. Goeringer, by then a colonel, said that the joint effort was an opportunity "to redesign the process of diagnostic imaging in the military."[78] LaNoue said it provided "the ability to virtually project the skill mix and clinical capabilities found in our medical centers, totally independent of real time and distance limitations."[79]

Another example of a pioneering advance led by MSCs was found in Col. Henry C. Beumler's work as the Health Services Command's (HSC) chief of coordinated care during the period in which the Army's direct health care system evolved into a system called Gateway to Care. This was an expansion of a demonstration project mandated by Congress called Catchment Area Management that began in the Army at the Fort Carson, Colorado, and Fort Riley, Kansas, hospitals in 1989. It represented a major shift in the demands placed upon hospital commanders, who were now required to account for the management of all military health care within the catchment area of their hospitals, including expenditures by the Civilian Health and Medical Program of the Uniformed Services (CHAMPUS), the military's health insurance program for family members. Primary care providers for beneficiaries enrolled in the program would arrange and approve all care for patients as a means of ensuring quality and controlling costs. As implemented in eleven hospitals in 1992, Beumler's Gateway to Care enabled HSC to demonstrate savings in its health care delivery. In 1994 it was subsumed in a DOD regionally controlled program called TRICARE.[80]

A principal theme of the MSC history is opportunity, the lifeblood of a vibrant corps. Opportunity for education, positions, and promotions has everything to do with the Army's ability to retain its best and brightest officers, because it defines the horizons of their aspirations, goals, and ambitions—in a word, their hopes. While the story of MSC opportunity is an evolutionary one, it is also the story of adversity. Nothing that MSCs enjoyed in the late twentieth century was achieved without the vision and struggle of officers who had gone before. Often, visionary Medical Corps officers had provided the leadership for that progress.

Educational opportunity advanced after World War II with graduate education programs and the establishment of the Army-Baylor Program in Healthcare Administration. Military training also opened up, with opportunities for staff college, senior service school, and other military courses that prepared MSCs for greater responsibilities. Position opportunities expanded with MSC replacement of and substitution for physicians and others in such senior positions as commanders, hospital executive officers, and command chiefs of staff. Promotions improved with the repeal of the 2 percent cap on colonels. MSCs could look forward to promotion opportunities through that rank and, beginning in 1966, a chance for brigadier general.

There continued to be good opportunities for Army MSCs in the post–Cold War era. Educational opportunities remained excellent; in fact, two programs were added in 1994. A study directed by the Army chief of staff of branch-immaterial command in medical units held the promise of new position opportunities. And throughout the drawdown the MSC maintained its promotion opportunity close to the goals of DOPMA and sometimes better than that afforded officers of other Army branches.[81]

While young MSCs in the 1990s benefited from the legacy of those who had gone before them, this did not end the evolution of their corps. The talent, skill, and ambitions of MSCs continued to outstrip the Medical Department's willingness to fully accommodate their aspirations. For that reason, some talented officers continued to transfer to other branches or left the Army for better opportunities elsewhere. MSCs could certainly go farther in the 1990s than before, but hope for the future comes from a conviction that tomorrow will be better than today. The challenge to the department's leaders was to provide that hope to officers who had served it faithfully. The removal of obstacles to opportunities for education and training, promotions, and assignments to positions of increased responsibility had strengthened the Medical Department over the years. The imperative was to eliminate the remaining elements of institutional discrimination that continued to block the department from using the full potential of MSCs and officers of other branches and accepting them as full members of the military medical team.

The Army Medical Department began the last decade of the century with the process of transformation incomplete and with some barriers to opportunity still in place. A fundamental theme of the MSC history is the repeated demonstration of a need for a corps of officers who specialized in administrative skills—beginning with control of "paper work"—that surfaced repeatedly in the Revolution, Civil War, Spanish American War, World War I, and World War II. The need for specific medical management skills—for example, medical logistics—was a lesson often relearned. By the time of the Korean War the benefit of a permanent MSC was accepted.

The handmaiden to the evolution of the MSC was pressure from sources outside the Medical Department, such as the War Department and political groups in World War II, who forced modernization and the adoption of modern business practices upon the management of military medicine. Individual MSC specialties had been greatly affected by the demands of professional guilds, especially for professional recognition. Pharmacy from the period after World War I through the formation of the MSC in 1947 was an example. Optometry, sanitary engineering, laboratory sciences, and health care administration were other specialties whose outside practitioners affected the military role.

The pressure to use MSCs to substitute for physicians in administrative positions could be expected to ease in the early 1990s, as American medical schools produced a surfeit of physicians. The federal coffers for the financing of health care opened in 1965 with the advent of Medicare and Medicaid, and the number of physicians expanded to meet the federally funded demand. Some states built new medical schools, existing schools added capacity, and the federal government got in the act with the construction of its own school, the Uniformed Services University of the Health Sciences. The number of graduates from American medical schools more than doubled from 1965 to 1980, peaking at over 16,000 in 1984 (declining slightly after that to 15,499 in 1991). The number of physicians per 100,000 population increased 59 percent over the same period, going from 139 in 1965 to 237 in 1990. The greatly increased physician supply had lessened the department's problems in recruiting physicians, improved the quality of those on active duty, and increased the department's willingness to use them in administrative positions rather than for clinical duties. Political pressure to capitalize on the clinical training of physicians, while perhaps muted for the moment, would undoubtedly return in the future as the supply of physicians changed, as national pressure increased to reduce costs in health care, or if the United States again drafted physicians for military service.[82]

The command issue remained unsettled and unsettling, and there were still those who argued against using MSCs as commanders.[83] Yet bright spots existed. The U.S. Army Medical Research and Development Command (renamed the U.S. Army Medical Research and Materiel Command in 1994) continued to be an exception to the department's policy, routinely appointing officers based on their individual qualifications, and MSCs commanded USAMRDC laboratories, activities, and field research units. Further, at least one surgeon general did not object to MSCs commanding hospitals. General Pixley, in a 1984 interview, said that he believed MSCs could command the smaller community hospitals (although he did have reservations about their commanding operational field medical treatment units).[84]

In 1991 the Senate Appropriations Committee continued to challenge the Army to follow the lead of its sister Services in appointing nonphysician commanders of medical facilities.[85] By 1992 MSCs commanded 18 of 109 Air Force treatment facilities and 21 of 44 Navy hospitals and clinics.[86] In Grenada and Panama—as in Korea and the Dominican Republic—MSCs had remained in command of operational medical treatment units and medical battalions in spite of the rule that called for the relinquishment of command to a physician. In the Gulf War, MSCs remained in command of a medical brigade and all the medical groups they commanded in garrison. However, Medical Department policy dictated the designation of PROFIS commanders for operational treatment units, and MSCs were required to turn over the command of those units as they deployed, often to officers with little if any training and experience to prepare them for that duty. The commanding general of the Medical Department's Center and School believed there was "an inherent fallacy" in this policy.[87] The question to be answered in the 1990s was how the department would act in light of its experiences in recent crises. Would it take the initiative to unharness the talents of MSCs in a new system of free competition? Or would it remain chained to its past?

By 1994 it appeared that the Army was prepared to open up command of medical units to officers of any Medical Department corps. General LaNoue launched a series of revolutionary changes upon his appointment as surgeon general, including the formation of a three-star U.S. Army Medical Command that replaced the Health Services Command and merged a number of organizations under his command (with Henry Tuell, now a colonel, as its first chief of staff). Subordinate units included eight regional health service support areas commanded by the medical center commander in each region. LaNoue sought to appoint Brig. Gen. Nancy R. Adams, the chief of the Army Nurse Corps, as one of those commanders.[88]

Coincidentally, the failure of the PROFIS command policy in the Gulf War, continued congressional pressure to reduce the number of clinicians in administrative roles, and political pressure by the Defense Advisory Commission on Women in the Service forced a review of the Medical Department's command policy. The issue catalyzed when the 212th MASH deployed to Zagreb in December 1992 and underwent a PROFIS change of command from MSC to MC. This resurfaced the complaints about last-minute changes of command that had been voiced by line officers during the Gulf War, and in January 1993 the assistant secretary of the Army for manpower and reserve affairs directed the surgeon general to review the Medical Department's command policy. In June, LaNoue wrote the Army chief of staff, General Gordon R. Sullivan, of his intent to implement Medical Department branch-immaterial slating of medical unit commanders. General Sullivan concluded that the Medical Department's leader development program was not sufficiently developed to support this change, and he suspended action on General LaNoue's request until the department developed a program that would enable any of its officers to prepare for command. Sullivan directed the formation of a formal study that would report its recommendations to him. That effort was under way as this book went to press. The indications were that the Army would approve some form of branch-immaterial command of selected medical units.[89]

Such a change would be a major advance in the opportunities open to MSC officers. Throughout their history MSCs had petitioned the department's leaders for an opportunity for fair and open competition for the largest challenges.[90] It was their hope that, when records were thrown on the table to select officers for the highest positions in the Medical Department, the records of MSCs would be on that table as well, so that their capability, training, and experience would be fairly considered. The hope was that if the Confederate hospital commander, Capt. Sally Louisa Tompkins, were alive in 1995, she would have a fair shot at the job she had performed so well 133 years before.

Notes

[1] Gander: Rice, a first lieutenant commissioned directly from civilian life, processed the death records of Lieutenant Witmer, who as a fellow student in the officer basic course at Fort Sam Houston had taught Rice how to polish her boots just a few months before. Notes of interv, 1st Lt Beverly J. Rice, MSC, with Lt Col Richard V.N. Ginn, Pentagon, 16 Jan 86, DASG-MS.

[2] Grenada: After action rpt, Lt Col Jack R. Roden, MSC (ACSOPS, 44th Med Bde), sub: 44th Medical Brigade, Operation URGENT FURY, 15 Mar 85, hereafter cited as Rodin, Grenada rpt; Roden to Ginn, 28 Mar and 28 Apr 86; Press release, sub: Award of Combat Medical Badge to Maj. Arthur W. Hapner, MSC, and Capt. Kevin J. Swenie, MSC, 44th Med Bde, XVIII Abn Corps, 18 Jan 84; Notes of informal intervs, Ginn with Lt Col Jack Crabtree, Inf, (S–4, 82d Abn Div in Grenada), Brussels, Belgium, 10 Feb 88, and with Lt Col Edward B. Wilson, MSC, OTSG, 25 Apr 86; Notes of discussion, Col Joseph E. Herndon, MSC, Ch, San Eng Sec, MSC, with Ginn, 23 Apr 86, hereafter cited as Herndon notes, all in DASG-MS; Lt Col Joseph P. Jackson, MC, to Cdr, USACMH, 23 May 85, USACMH; Richard Gabriel, *Military Incompetence: Why the American Military Doesn't Win* (New York: Hill and Wang, 1985).

[3] Sanitation: Roden to Ginn, 28 Mar 86, and Roden, Grenada rpt; Herndon notes. Quoted words: N. Joe Thompson and John B. Czachowski, "Preventive Medicine in the Grenada Intervention: Detained Personnel and Civilian Populations," *AMEDD Journal* (November/December 1991): 5.

[4] Panama: Rpt, WRAMC, sub: Casualty Data Analysis, Operation JUST CAUSE, 11 Jan 90; Briefing, Col Jerome V. Foust, MSC, Cdr, 44th Med Bde, sub: Operation JUST CAUSE, presented at MSC mtg, Garmisch, FRG, 14 May 90, author's notes, hereafter cited as Foust, Operation JUST CAUSE; Briefing, Maj Jay Harmon, MSC, sub: Operation JUST CAUSE, 7th MEDCOM Ambulatory Patient Care Conference, Garmisch, FRG, 15 Oct 90, author's notes, all in DASG-MS; Donna Miles, "Operation JUST CAUSE," *Soldiers* (February 1990): 20–24; Kenneth J. Jones, *The Enemy Within: Casting Out Panama's Demon* (Panama: Focus Publications, 1990), p. 145; Lawrence A. Yates, "Joint Task Force Panama: JUST CAUSE—Before and After," *Military Review* 71 (October 1991): 59, 70. United States deaths were twenty-one killed in action plus two who died of wounds later. About 54 percent of the 150 casualties air evacuated on 20 December were jump injuries from the very low (500 feet) combat jumps. Civilian casualty estimates were disputed. They were principally in the Chorillo slum district surrounding the Comandancia, Noriega's headquarters.

[5] Medical operations: Foust, Operation JUST CAUSE; Info paper, Maj Paul E. Bluteau, MSC, sub: Medical Support for Operation JUST CAUSE, 1 Mar 90; Briefing slides, Lt Col Susan McCall, ANC, Chief Nurse, 5th MASH, sub: JUST CAUSE Medical Operations, presented to HQ, 7th MEDCOM, Heidelberg, FRG, 30 Jan 90, all in DASG-MS. Lessons learned are in after-action reports assembled by the 44th Medical Brigade, in Memo, Lt Col Gerald A. Palmer, MSC, COS, 44th Med Bde, for Cdr, 1st COSCOM, 10 Jan 90, including: Maj Ted A. Martinez, Dep ACOSLOG, 44th Med Bde, undated; Lt Col Robert C. Leeds, DC, Cdr, 257th Med Det (DS), 9 Jan 90; Capt Talford V. Mindingall, MSC, Cdr, HQ and HQ Co, 44th Med Bde, 8 Jan 90; Capt Robert J. Yates, ANC, 8 Jan 90; Maj Priscilla M. Alston, MSC, Acting Cdr, 28th Combat Spt Hospital (CSH), 9 Jan 90; Lt Col Elwood L. Stephens, Cdr, 32d MEDSOM, undated; Lt Col Ira F. Walton III, MSC, Cdr, 56th Med Bn, 9 Jan 90; Maj Lee A. Porisch, ANC, 7 Jan 90; Maj David E. Rivera, MC, 1st FST, undated; and Lt Col Muench, MC, FST, 30 Dec 89, all in DASG-MS. Forward surgical team (FST): The FST handled 129 casualties and performed 73 operations, 22 of which required general anesthesia. The portable surgical hospital, which it resembled, was developed in the Pacific and adopted by the Army as T/O 8–572S "to furnish definitive surgical care in areas where it is impractical to use larger, more specialized units." *Military Medical Manual*, rev. October 1944 (Harrisburg, Pa.: Military Service Publishing Company, 6th ed., 1945), pp. 643–44.

[6] Roberts: Tom McNiff, "Remembering Days of War," *Palatka [Florida] Daily News*, 24 March 1990.

[7] Logistics: Foust said the problem was "unbelievable." Foust, Operation JUST CAUSE. Refugees: McNiff, "Remembering Days of War"; Notes of discussion, Capt David W. Rogers, MSC, with Ginn, Alexandria, Va., 11 Jul 94, DASG-MS. Only 34 of the 140 casualties treated by the aid station were American soldiers.

[8] Control of oil: Robert Woodward, *The Commanders* (New York: Pocket Star Books, 1991), p. 206. Woodward cited Nicholas Brady, Bush's secretary of the treasury. Iraq had 20 percent of the world's supply, as did Saudi Arabia. DESERT SHIELD: "'A Line in the Sand'—A Chronology," *Stars and Stripes* (*S&S*), 31 December 1991; "Our Deployment into the Persian Gulf," essays by Generals Glenn K. Otis, Frederick J. Kroesen, and Louis C. Wagner, *Army* 40 (November 1990): 14, 16. Quoted words: Christopher A. Hutchinson, "Dispatches From a Distant Desert," *Duke* 77 (February–March 1991): 10.

[9] Buildup: *S&S*, 10 January 1991; United Press International (UPI), "More Than a Million Troops with Vast Arsenals Face Off," and Associated Press (AP), "Congress Vote Gives Bush Power To Wage War in Gulf," *S&S*, 13 January 1991; "Chronology," in special issue, "The Gulf War," *Military Review* 71 (September 1991): 65–78. The vote in Congress was 52 to 47, Senate, and 250 to 183, House. Forces: AP, "Pentagon Braces for Word To Go," *S&S*, 16 January 1991; "Operation DESERT STORM," *S&S*, 28 January 1991; John Barry and Evan Thomas, "A Textbook Victory," *Newsweek* 121 (11 March 1991): 38. Operations: Association of the United States Army (AUSA), "Special Report: The U.S. Army in DESERT STORM" (Arlington, Va.: AUSA, June 1991), DASG-MS.

[10] Ground assault: Schwarzkopf said, "We're going to go around, over, through, on top, underneath and any other way it takes." Ron Jensen, "Land War Launched To Liberate Kuwait," *S&S* (25 February 1991). Casualties: "Medicine in the Gulf War," *U.S. Medicine* 27 (August 1991): 6, hereafter cited as "Gulf War," *U.S. Medicine*. General Ledford testified to the Senate Armed Services Committee that CENTCOM had predicted thirty to forty thousand casualties, including fifteen thousand KIA. "Army Anticipated 15,000 Gulf Deaths," *U.S. Medicine* 27 (June 1991): 1.

[11] Iraqi casualties: Barry and Evans, "Textbook Victory," p. 38; Ltr to the editor, Hutchinson, *Duke* 77 (June–July 1991): 33. "I was surprised at my own lack of feeling as we rolled over the charred remains of bodies and half-bodies recently killed."

[12] Medical support: Discussion of the medical support for Operations DESERT SHIELD and DESERT STORM is based principally on the following documents: USACMH intervs in the Persian Gulf, Capt Donald E. Hall, MSC, with Lt Col Joseph H. Cohen, MSC, USAR, XO, 403d CSH, 19 Mar 91; Col Jerome V. Foust, MSC, Cdr, 44th Med Bde, 29 Mar 91; Col Harold C. Schade, MSC, XO, 114th Evac Hosp, 7 Mar 91; Brig Gen Michael D. Strong, CG, 332d Med Bde, 21 Mar 91. USACMH intervs in the Persian Gulf (interviewer not identified) with Capt Steven R. Gilreath, S–4, 86th Evac Hosp, 12 Mar 91; Maj Tommy R. Hancock, MSC, Capt Randall L. Gaines, MSC, and Capt Paul Arbour, MSC (all Louisiana Army National Guard), 159th MASH, 8 Mar 91; Lt Col William C. Long, MSC, Cdr (XO during operational status), 86th Evac Hosp, 12 Mar 91. USACMH intervs in the Persian Gulf, Col Richard A. Bowman with Maj Carolyn A. Albanese, MSC, USAR, XO, 350th Evac Hosp, 6 Mar 91; Lt Col Scott Beaty, MSC, XO, 47th Fld Hosp, 23 Feb 91; 1st Lt Damon T. Mathis, MSC, Maj Robert J. Meyers, MSC, and Capt David O. Hill, MSC, 47th CSH, 8 Mar 91. XVIII Airborne Corps interv, Maj Robert B. Honec III, and SSgt LaDona S. Kirkland with Lt Col Roger R. Sexton, MSC, XO, 62d Med Gp, 26 Feb 91, all in USACMH; Intervs, Cols Robert P. Belihar, MC, USAF, and Benjamin M. Knisely, MSC, USA, in "Gulf War," *U.S. Medicine*, pp. 45–56; Interv, Ingeborg Sosa with Maj Gen Michael J. Scotti, Jr., Cdr, 7th MEDCOM, in *AMEDD Journal* (January/February 1992); Interv, Sosa with Lt Gen Frank F. Ledford, Jr., TSG, in *AMEDD Journal* (March/April 1992). Also see Memo, Maj Gen William L. Moore, Jr., Cmdt, AHS, for Dir, Special Proj Study Gp, U.S. Army Combined Arms Center, Fort Leavenworth, Kans., sub: DESERT STORM Lessons Learned Final After Action Review, 21 Jun 91, hereafter cited as Moore, Lessons Learned; Rpt, Col Philip E. Livermore, MSC, Ch, Log Div, OTSG, sub: Medical Logistics, Mar 91, hereafter cited as Livermore, Medical Logistics, all in DASG-MS; Frank F. Ledford, "Army Overcomes Combat Challenge," *U.S. Medicine* 28 (January 1992): 30–31; Robert M. O'Brien and Alexander M. Sloan, "Medical Support to DESERT SHIELD/STORM: The USEUCOM Surgeon's Perspective," *AMEDD Journal* (March/April 1992): 3–9. An especially valuable document is Rpt, John R. Brinkerhoff, Ted Silva, and John Seitz, Ofc, Ch, Army Reserve, sub: U.S. Army Reserve in Operation DESERT STORM: Reservists of the Army Medical Department, 23 Sep 93, PL, hereafter cited as Brinkerhoff, AMEDD Reservists.

[13] Medical groups: George A. Fisher, Howard A. McClelland, and Robert F. Griffin, "Preparing and Organizing Medical Support to VII Corps: Operation DESERT SHIELD and STORM," *AMEDD*

Journal (March/April 1992): 16–19; Edward K. Jeffer and Shirley L. Jones, "The Medical Units of the Army National Guard (ARNG) and Operation DESERT SHIELD/DESERT STORM," *AMEDD Journal* (March/April 1992): 20–22, hereafter cited as Jeffer and Jones, "ARNG Medical Units in DESERT STORM." 332d Medical Brigade: The 341st and 127th Medical Groups, both reserve units, remained operational. General Strong chose to organize all his hospitalization assets into three "vertical bands" because the distances were so great that command and control would otherwise be compromised. Rather than sticking with the doctrinal arrangement of assigning medical units behind a division to one medical group, Strong clumped his hospitals into three groups. The first level (or band), closest to the divisions, was composed of the MASH hospitals and constituted the 127th Medical Group. The 341st Medical Group commanded the second band, which had all combat support hospitals. The evacuation hospitals, which were farthest from the divisions, formed the third band and were grouped into a provisional "Task Force Evacuation."

[14] Knisely: "Gulf Update," *Nightline* (ABC News), 6 December 1990. The panel included Senator John Glenn and John Moxley, M.D., former ASD (HA). The earlier show's thesis had been that "the medical machine was struggling to catch up with the war machine." James Walker and Nancy Synderman, M.D., reporters; Peter Collis, M.D., Prin Dep ASD (HA); and John Beary, M.D., former ASD (HA), panelists, author's notes, *Nightline*, 20 November 1990, DASG-MS.

[15] Numbers: "Gulf War," *U.S. Medicine*, p. 6.

[16] Quoted words: Ltr, General H. Norman Schwarzkopf, USA, Ret., to "Members of the U.S. Army Medical Department," reprinted in *AMEDD Journal* (May/June 1993).

[17] PROFIS: Rpt, Maj Michael E. Dunn, Inf, Pers Opns Br (HSPE-MO), HQ, Health Services Command (HSC), sub: Staff Study, PROFIS, 25 Apr 91, hereafter cited as Dunn, PROFIS Study; Memo, Maj Gen Frederick N. Bussey, Dep Surg Gen, sub: Government Accounting Office Draft Report, "Operation DESERT STORM: Full Army Medical Capability Not Achieved," dated March 31, 1992 (GAO Code 393500), 16 Apr 92, hereafter cited as GAO Rpt, Operation DESERT STORM, 1992; Notes of telephone interv, Lt Col Ralph Bradford, Ch, Mil Pers Div, HQ, HSC, (HSPE-M), with Col Richard V.N. Ginn, 25 Jul 94, all in DASG-MS; "U.S. Hospitals Scramble to Backfill," *U.S. Medicine* (August 1991). Quoted words: Dunn, PROFIS Study.

[18] Quoted words: Bradford, Ginn telephone interv.

[19] Quoted words. Dunn, PROFIS Study. The personnel officers made it work, but at a cost. "Previous mobilization exercises, such as PROUD EAGLE 90, had wished away all the mundane, routine work associated with transporting fillers to their TO&E [Table of Organization and Equipment—i.e., field] units and moving backfill health care providers to the MTFs [medical treatment facilities] in need." Ibid.

[20] Quoted words: Bradford, Ginn telephone interv.

[21] Optometry: Memo, Maj David J. Walsh, MSC, Pgm Mgr, Developmental Eyewear, U.S. Army Medical Materiel Development Activity, sub: Trip Report, Natick Research, Development, and Evaluation Command, Natick, Massachusetts, 7 Oct 91, DASG-MS. The number represented 44 percent of those who wore glasses.

[22] Psychology: Roger Lehman, Jefferey E. Hansen, and Harry L. Musinger, "Crisis Management of Children During DESERT STORM," *AMEDD Journal* (January/February 1992): 39–41. Planning extended to establishing death notification procedures.

[23] 7th MEDCOM: Crosbie E. Saint, "War Adds New Dimensions to Europe's Role," *Army* 41 (October 1991): 91. The 7th MEDCOM provided the U.S. Army, Europe, portion of the U.S. European Command requirement to provide 5,500 contingency beds. O'Brien and Sloan, "Medical Support to DESERT STORM," p. 3.

[24] Quoted words: Jeffer and Jones, "ARNG Medical Units in DESERT STORM," p. 22.

[25] Dustoff: Rpt, 45th Med Co (AA), sub: Darmstadt to Dhahran: Self-Deployment to DESERT SHIELD, 25 Dec 91, DASG-MS; Rosemary Sawyer, "Chopper Ride to Gulf Gives Medical Unit Some Hot Times," *S&S*, 6 September 1990.

[26] Anderson: Randall G. Anderson, "Forward Aeromedical Evacuation," in *Perspectives on the Gulf War* (Arlington, Va.: Association of the United States Army Institute for Land Warfare, August 1993), pp. 49–52, PL.

[27] Criticism of command policy: See Brinkerhoff, AMEDD Reservists, p. 53; Moore, Lessons Learned.Quoted words: Beaty, Bowman interv.

[28] Logistics: Livermore, Medical Logistics; Rpt, AHS, sub: AMEDD Stockholders Report, 27 Jul 91, pp. 4–5, DASG-MS; O'Brien and Sloan, "Medical Support to DESERT STORM." General Scotti, 7th MEDCOM commander, said the medical logisticians "deserve great respect for having accomplished this monumental task." Scotti, Sosa interv.

[29] Pallets: These were model no. 463A air line of communication (ALOC) pallets.

[30] Train: "Gulf War," *U.S. Medicine*, p. 44.

[31] USAMRICD: Frederick R. Sidell, "The Medical Management of Chemical Casualty Course in CONUS and Europe During DESERT SHIELD," *AMEDD Journal* (March/April 1992): 10–12. Sidell was pleased with the outcome. "I believe that at the onset of DESERT STORM, the U.S. military medical personnel were as well prepared to deal with chemical agent casualties as any military medical personnel have ever been." Ibid., p. 12.

[32] Contact lenses: Morris Lattimore et al., "Contact Lens Use by U.S. Army Aircrews on Operations DESERT SHIELD/STORM," *AMEDD Journal* (November/December 1993): 13–17. Maj. Francis L. McVeigh, MSC, in unpublished paper, U.S. Army Command and General Staff College, sub: The History of Army Optometry: The Battles, Triumphs, and Future Challenges, June 1993, DASG-MS. Aviator use of Forward Looking Infrared Night Vision Goggles also dictated the issue of contact lenses. Optometrists also issued selected soldiers Ballistic-Laser Protective Spectacles.

[33] U.N. team: Bernie Ankney, "Iraq Possessed Large Biological Research Program, U.N. Team Says," *U.S. Medicine* (February 1992).

[34] BW/CW defense: *USAMRDC News* (monthly newsletter), August 1990–July 1991, DASG-MS; "Gulf War," *U.S. Medicine*, pp. 13–14; Notes of conversation, Walter E. Brandt, Ph.D., Dir, Biological Systems, U.S. Army Medical Materiel Development Agency, with Col Richard V.N. Ginn, Fort Detrick, Md., 22 Oct 91, DASG-MS.

[35] Quoted words: Albanese, Bowman interv.

[36] Scud attack: Rpt, Lt Col Philip K. Schenck, MSC, XO, 173d Med Gp, sub: The 173d Medical Group and the Gulf War, 12 May 91,DASG-MS, hereafter cited as Schenck, After Action Report.

[37] Quoted words: Bowman intervs with Mathis, Meyers, and Hill.

[38] DEPMEDS weight: Foust, Hall interv. Also see "Army Identifies 'Lessons Learned' from DESERT STORM" (interview with Brig. Gen. Ronald Blanck), *U.S. Medicine* (February 1992): 3.

[39] Quoted words: Strong, Hall interv.

[40] Quoted words: Gilreath, USACMH interv.

[41] Fuel requirement: Bowman interv with Mathis, Meyers, and Hill.

[42] Quoted words: James S. Martin, "Combat Psychiatry: Lessons from the War in Southwest Asia," *AMEDD Journal* (January/February 1992): 44.

[43] Quoted words: Bowman interv with Mathis, Meyers, and Hill.

[44] Patient administration: Col Fred McClain, Jr., Cdr, Patient Administration Systems and Biostatistics Agency, Ft. Sam Houston, Tex., in AHS, AMEDD Stockholders Rpt, pp. 5–10. The four systems were the Automated Quality Care Evaluation Support System (AQCESS), Comprehensive Health Care System (CHCS), Theater Army Medical Management Information System (TAMMIS), and Defense Medical Regulating Information System (DMRIS)

Phone calls: Maj. Gen. Ronald R. Blanck, Director of Professional Services, OTSG, in *U.S. Medicine* (February 1992).

[45] Enemy prisoners: Schenck, After Action Rpt; Notes of telephone conversation, Schenck with Col Richard V.N. Ginn, 14 Jun 94, DASG-MS. Of the 6,225, 4,136 were American patients, 1,138 were enemy POWs, and 951 were in other categories. The Red Cross representatives were pleased with the quality of the American medical support for the enemy POWs.

[46] Diaper pails: Schenck, After Action Rpt.

[47] Audiology: Richard W. Danielson, "Deployment of Audiologists: Forward to the Troops," *AMEDD Journal* (November/December 1993): 50–52. Repatriated POWs: Robert H. Gemmil and Calvin Neptune III, "Social Work Service to Army Repatriated Prisoners of War at Walter Reed Army Medical Center," *AMEDD Journal* (January/February 1992): 45–48.

[48] DEPMEDS rebuild: Richard I. Donahue, "Rebuilding Deployable Hospital Readiness," *AMEDD Journal* (November/December 1993): 9–12. Kuwait: MSC Newsletter, December 1992, DASG-MS.

[49] Satisfaction: Speech, Gen Maxwell R. Thurman, USA, Ret., to the Annual Meeting of the Army and Air Force Mutual Aid Association, Fort Myer, Va., 9 Apr 91, DASG-MS, hereafter cited as Thurman Speech.

[50] Quoted words: Lt. Gen. Frank F. Ledford, Jr., "Army Overcomes Combat Challenge," *U.S. Medicine* 28 (January 1992): 30. Numbers: GAO Rpt, Operation DESERT STORM, 1992.

[51] Changes: Editorial, John G. Roos and Glenn W. Goodman, Jr., in *Armed Forces Journal* (April 1991): 5.

[52] Lessons learned: Thurman Speech.

[53] Numbers: Rpt, DASG-PTZ, RQTDEC91, 11 Feb 92, DASG-MS. The active component numbered 18,171 officers, 37,550 enlisted, and 35,171 civilians. Scope: Msg, Lt Gen Quinn H. Becker, 261330Z Mar 85, sub: Early Appraisal—Becker Sends no. 1; Becker, statement before the House Subcommittee on Defense, Committee on Appropriations, House, 99th Cong., 1st sess., 16 Apr 85, both in DASG-MS. There were also 275 health clinics and 269 dental clinics.

[54] New doctrine: Department of the Army, FM 100–5, *Operations*, June 1993. Chapter 13, "Operations Other Than War," includes thirteen missions, including noncombatant evacuation operations, humanitarian and disaster assistance relief, nation assistance, and peacekeeping operations. For background on this revision see James R. McDonough, "Building the New FM 100–5: Process and Product," *Military Review* 71 (October 1991): 12. Purple Hearts: General Gordon R. Sullivan, CSA, statement to the House National Security Committee, DCSPER electronic mail msg, 24 Feb 94, DASG-MS.

[55] Operation PROVIDE COMFORT: "EUCOM Plays Supporting Role: PROVIDE COMFORT," *U.S. Medicine* (August 1991): 87–88; "A Record of Misery," *Newsweek* 124 (1 August 1994): 37.

[56] Facilities: Frank Sabatino, "Hurricane Andrew," *Hospitals* 66 (20 December 1992): 26–30.

[57] Water supply: MSC Newsletter, December 1992; Info paper, 1st Lt Timothy G. Bosetti, MSC, sub: Disaster Relief—Water System Reconstruction, 3 Nov 93; and Memo, Bosetti, sub: Sanitary Engineering Support of Operation Andrew and Hurricane Disaster Relief, 15 Sep 92, all in DASG-MS.

[58] Croatia: Steve Vogel, "First U.S. Army Unit Arrives in War-Torn Yugoslavia," *Army Times*, 23 May 1992; Vogel, "MASH Provides Aid to U.N. Troops," *Army Times*, 10 May 1993; Harry Noyes, "U.S. Medics Serve U.N. in Croatia," U.S. Army Health Services Command newspaper *Mercury*, August 1993; Presentation, Col Gregg S. Stephens, MSC, to Health Svcs Div, OPMD (TAPC-OPH), PERSCOM, Alexandria, Va., 7 Oct 93, author's notes, DASG-MS.

[59] Aid to Russia: MSC Newsletter, December 1992, DASG-MS; "U.S. Hospital Supplies Sent to Moscow," *Washington Times*, 11 July 1993.

[60] Somalia: Jack Lancaster, "Combat in Mogadishu," *Washington Post*, 20 October 1993.

[61] Entomology: Rpt, Capt Steven Horosko III, sub: After Action Report, Operation RESTORE HOPE, 10 Apr 93, DASG-MS.

[62] Quoted words: Rpt, Capt Timothy G. Bosetti, MSC, sub: Preventive Medicine in Somalia: 485th Medical Detachment, 28 Jun 94, DASG-MS.

[63] Quoted words: "A Race with Death," *Newsweek* 124 (1 August 1994): 26. Dr. Florence Parent, a relief worker, said: "We can't do anything, I'm afraid. They just die and die and die, and they keep coming and coming and coming." "1994 Perspectives," *Newsweek* 124 (26 December 1994): 70.

[64] Rwanda: Briefing slides, Health Care Opns Div (DASG-HCO), OTSG, sub: Rwanda Refugees, 22 Jul 94; Briefing, Col Rick Erdtmann, MC, and Maj David S. Heintz, MSC, sub: Rwanda, 22 Jul 94, author's notes; Msg, DASG-HCO, sub: DASG SITREP no. 3 Rwanda Relief Operations (Operation SUPPORT HOPE), 28 Jul 94, all in DASG-MS; Thomas W. Lippman and Rebecca Fowler, "U.S. and U.N. Rush Relief to Rwandans," *Washington Post*, 22 July 1994; Thomas W. Lippman, "U.S. Sends 4,000 Troops to Help Relief Efforts," *Washington Post*, 23 July 1994; "Army Units Help Ease Tragedy in Rwanda Refugee Camps," *Mercury* (September 1994), DASG-MS; Thomas W. Lippman, "U.S. Troop Withdrawal Ends Frustrating Mission to Save Rwandan Lives," *Washington Post*, 3 October 1994; Steve Harding, "Hope Comes to Rwanda," *Soldiers* 49 (October 1994): 13.

[65] Haiti: Memo, Togo D. West, Jr., Sec Army, for Sec Def, sub: The Weekly Report, 4 Oct 94, DASG-MS; Douglas Farah, "Haitian Police Attack Crowd; U.S. Troops Watch," *Washington Post*, 21 September 1994; Evan Thomas et al., "Here We Go Again," *Newsweek* 124 (26 September

1994): 20–24; Don Kirkman, "GIs Get Warning on AIDS in Haiti," *Washington Times*, 1 October 1994. Assistance efforts: Rpt, Lt Col Dale R. Brown, MSC, Ch, Health Facility Assessment Team, 44th Med Bde, sub: Final Report Assessment and Design Concept, extracts in DASG-MS; "Haiti's Bugs Defy Health Care," *Army Times*, 17 October 1994. Quoted words: Soraya S. Nelson, "U.S. Medics Pitch in at Haitian Hospital," *Army Times*, 10 October 1994.

[66] Army reductions: "U.S. Army Details Major Withdrawal," *Jane's Defence Weekly* 16 (24 August 1991): 300; Memo, Maj Gen Gerald A. Putman, Cdr, PERSCOM, sub: Chain Teaching Program: The Army in Transition—Update 3, 30 Jun 93, DASG-MS; *Army Times*, 15 March 1993 and 27 June 1994; Memo, OCSA, sub: CSA Weekly Summary, 6 May 94, PL. Number retired: On 31 July 1993, the number of retirees was 582,530 and the number on active duty was 579,224. Press release, Retirement Svcs Div, U.S. Army Community and Family Spt Ctr, Alexandria, Va., Nov 93, DASG-MS.

[67] Numbers: Briefing slide, Manpower Div, OTSG, sub: Revised Five Year AMEDD Capability Plan, 12 Oct 94; Briefing slides, AMEDD Personnel Proponency Dir, AMEDDC&S, sub: FY 96 AMEDD Corps Breakout, 4 Oct 94, both in DASG-MS. The total authorized numbers by fiscal year end strength were as follows:

1991	1994	1995	1996	1997
18,478	16,628	15,842	15,377	14,862

[68] Drawdown programs: Voluntary early release and retirement program (VERRP), voluntary separation incentive program (VSIP), lieutenant retention boards, early retirement program, and selective early retirement boards (SERB). MSC Newsletter, December 1992; Rpt, Personnel Svcs Br (PSB), TAPC-OPH, sub: Drawdown Plan, 22 Nov 94, both in DASG-MS. Bonuses: VSIP bonuses came in two forms. As a special separation benefit (SSB) the bonus was a lump-sum payment based on a formula that incorporated base pay and the number of years of active federal service. A captain with fourteen years' service (i.e., with prior enlisted service) could collect nearly $90,000. The alternative was extended payments available under an option called the voluntary separation incentive (VSI), which, as in the case of SSB, was computed with a formula that incorporated base pay and years of service. Using the VSI option, a captain with fourteen' years service would collect about $15,000 a year for twenty-eight years, for a total of nearly $420,000. Rpt, TAPC-OPH-PSB, sub: Voluntary Separation Incentive Program, 27 Dec 94, DASG-MS.

[69] Quoted words: Bernard Adelsberger, "As Officer Cuts End, Uncertainty Begins," *Army Times*, 26 December 1994. SERB: Briefing slide, DASG-PTM, sub: SERB History, undated (1994); Memo, DASG-PTM for DCSPER, sub: AMEDD FY95 SERB, 16 Sep 94; Rpt, TAPC-OPH, sub: AMEDD SERB Background, 15 Dec 94, all in DASG-MS. The 250 total included 109 colonels, 120 lieutenant colonels, and 21 majors.

Year	Col.	Lt. Col.	Maj.	Total
1987	22	17		39
1990	10	10		20
1992	20	20		40
1993	18	26	21	65
1994	20	28		48
1995	19	19		38
Total	109	120	21	250

During this period the Army SERBed a total of 538 Medical Department officers. In addition to 250 Medical Service Corps officers, there were 113 Army Nurse Corps, 99 Medical Corps, 68 Dental Corps, and 8 Veterinary Corps officers. No Army Medical Specialist Corps officers were SERBed. Quality of officers: PERSCOM used four rankings to evaluate officer efficiency reports based on a comparison of each officer's overall file with those of his or her peers: A for above center of mass; P for center of mass, top half (plus); M for center of mass, bottom half (minus); and B for below center of mass. The schema is depicted in Adelsberger, "As Officer Cuts End, Uncertainty Begins." Ninety-five percent of the MSC colonels were rated A or P. This was in contrast to the Medical Corps colonels selected by the same board, 96 percent of whom had M or B files. Rpt, TAPC-OPH, sub: FY95 AMEDD SERB, 30 Nov 94, DASG-MS. Captains: Briefing, Lt Col Ernest R. Morgan III, sub: Army Leadership Study, 20 Sep 94, PERSCOM, Alexandria, Va., author's notes. The study team interviewed 1,625 captains worldwide (including 80 Medical Department officers).

[70] MSC reductions: Briefing slides, APPD, AMEDDC&S, sub: MSC Downsizing FY94 and FY96, undated (Dec 92); Memo, Col Frederick J. Manning, MSC, Research Psychology Consultant, for Research Psychologists, sub: Rumors of Your Demise, undated (Dec 92), both in DASG-MS. Quoted words: MSC Newsletter, August 1993, DASG-MS.Board of directors: The membership included the chief of the MSC; assistant chief of the MSC; chiefs of the four MSC sections; chiefs of staff of the Health Services Command, U.S. Army Medical Research and Development Command, 7th Medical Command, 18th Medical Command, and AMEDD Center and School; director of health care operations, OTSG; chief of the MSC Branch, Health Services Division, OPMD, PERSCOM; and a representative of the Surgeon, U.S. Forces Command. Memo, Lt Col Michael D. Wheeler, MSC, Asst to Chief, MSC, sub: MSC Strategic Planning Conference, 4 Nov 92, DASG-MS.

[71] Concerns for scientists: Memo, Lt Col Wilbur K. Milhous, MSC, for Lt Col George C. Southworth, OTSG, sub: The MSC Soldier/Scientist, 22 Apr 92, DASG-MS; Ralph E. Hay, "The Uniformed Scientist—An Uncertain Future," *Army Research, Development, and Acquisition Bulletin* (July/August 1989): 17–19. Support: Lt. Gen. William G.T. Tuttle, Jr., CG, U.S. Army Logistics Center, Fort Lee, to Editor, *Army Research, Development, and Acquisition Bulletin* (July/August 1989): 45.

[72] MSC Study: Briefing slides, William J. Leary, Jr., MSC, sub: Medical Service Corps; Building for the Future, undated (Mar 90); Memo, Gary L. Tonniges, Ch, AMEDD Pers Proponent Div, AHS, sub: Recommended Changes to Military Occupational Classification Structure, 29 Jan 90, both in DASG-MS. Quoted words: Jackman, Operations Newsletter.

[73] U.S. costs: "A Checkup for Health Care," *U.S. News and World Report* (13 June 1994): 63. DOD costs: Speech, Katherine Ladd Railey, Ofc of the Asst Sec Def for Health Affairs, sub: Internal Accountability, presented at the Federal Day of the annual meeting of the American College of Healthcare Executives, Chicago, Ill., 2 Mar 92, author's notes, DASG-MS. Costs included military personnel and construction.

[74] Pressure: Andy Pastor, "Military Medical System, Beset by Budgeting Ills and Riddled with Waste, Needs Some Doctoring," *Wall Street Journal*, 26 August 1991.

[75] Project Vanguard: MSC Newsletter, 20 November 1990; Rpt, Col Richard V.N. Ginn, MSC, IG, 7th MEDCOM, to Ch, MSC, sub: Historical Perspectives on Project Vanguard with Special Emphasis on Two Administrative Specialties: Aeromedical Evacuation Officer and Health Services Comptroller, 26 Sep 90, both in DASG-MS. Medical logistics: Memo, Gene A. Markel, U.S. Army Logistics Evaluation Agency, New Cumberland, Pa., for DCSLOG, sub: Medical Logistics Policy Proponency Study—Decision Briefing, 1 Oct 93, DASG-MS; Philip E. Livermore and Angel Cintron, "Medical Logistics: Pillar of Health Care Delivery," *Army Logistician* (March–April 1994): 9–11.

[76] Thurman: "If your weapons, doctrine or tactics went to war, you can assume it has been [sic] compromised." Thurman Speech.

[77] Teleradiology: Michael A. Cawthon, Fred Goeringer, et al., "Preliminary Assessment of Computed Tomography and Satellite Teleradiology from Operation DESERT STORM," *Investigative Radiology* 26 (October 1991): 856. MDIS: Larry D. Cade et al., "Project Management in Military Medicine: The Medical Diagnostic Imaging Support System (MDIS) Project," *AMEDD Journal* (November/December 1993): 18–20. Goeringer headed a team that included seven MSCs with a variety of specialties.Award: *Federal Computer Weekly* 6 (March 1992).

[78] Telemedicine: Nancy Tomich, "Telemedicine: 'Off-the-Shelf' Phenomenon," *U.S. Medicine* (July 1994); Donna Miles, "Medicine by Monitor," *Soldiers* 49 (October 1994): 32–34. Quoted words: Nancy Tomich, "MDIS Will Proceed 'Tri-Service,'" *U.S. Medicine* (October 1994).

[79] Quoted words: Memo, Lt Gen Alcide LaNoue, TSG, sub: Telemedicine, 1 Nov 1994, DASG-MS.

[80] Gateway to Care: Rpt, Rand Corporation, Santa Monica, Calif., sub: Evaluating the Catchment Area Management Demonstration, Jun 90; Rpt, Ann L. Price, Manpower Div, OTSG, sub: Army Management Initiatives, Demonstrations, and Alternative Health Care Delivery Systems, 20 Apr 93; Harry Noyes, "Gateway to Care Shows Medical Future" and "Local Control Is Key Part of Gateway Program," in flyer, sub: Gateway to Care...the Army's Coordinated Care Program, undated (1992), extracted from *Mercury*; Harry Noyes, "DOD Orders Active-Duty TRI-

CARE Enrollment," *Mercury* (September 1994), all in DASG-MS; "Catchment Area Management Found Effective in Reducing Health Costs," *U.S. Medicine* (October 1991); Frank F. Ledford, "Army Overcomes Combat Challenge," *U.S. Medicine* 28 (January 1992): 31; Harry Noyes, "TRI-CARE: The Parable of the Genie and the Guru," *Mercury* (August 1994), DASG-MS.

[81]76. Opportunity in the 1990s: Interv, Brig. Gen. Jerome V. Foust with Ingeborg Sosa, in *AMEDD Journal* (November/December 1993). The new offerings were master's programs in marketing and health care economics. Promotions: Briefing slides, Mil Pers Mgmt Div, OTSG, sub: Promotions and Loss Management, 4 Dec 92, DASG-MS. The DOPMA goals consisted of selection opportunity rates of 50 percent for colonel, 70 percent for lieutenant colonel, and 80 percent for major. The opportunity rate was calculated based on the entire population eligible for selection, i.e., officers considered for the first time, plus those previously considered and not selected, plus those selected from below the zone (early promotions).

[82] Numbers: American Medical Association, *Physician Characteristics and Distribution in the U.S.* (Chicago: AMA, 1991); annual education issues of the *Journal of the American Medical Association*, 1965–1991; Karen Sandrick, "U.S. MD Glut Limits Demand for Foreign Medical Graduate Physicians," *Hospitals* 62 (5 February 1988): 67.

[83] Opposition to MSCs: Edward K. Jeffer, "Medical Units: Who Should Command?" *Military Medicine* 155 (September 1990): 413–17. Actually, Jeffer's apparent purpose was to defend the use of physicians as commanders. This is an entirely valid position in the author's view, but not at the expense of denying the opportunity to everyone else. The problem comes in denying the validity of utilizing officers with other specialty backgrounds as commanders no matter what their individual capability. That denial was the underpinning of Jeffer's analogy of the physician as the only conceivable "quarterback" of the health care team.

[84] Pixley's view: Pixley, Ginn interv, 1 Nov 84. In an earlier interview he stated that "the most qualified member of the health team should assume command." "Improving Manpower: Pixley's Early Days," interv in *U.S. Medicine* 17 (15 September 1981).

[85] SAC: Draft rpt, Senate, Appropriations Committee, *Department of Defense Appropriations Bill, 1992*, 102d Cong., 1st sess., September 1991.

[86] Navy command: Memos, Lt Col Larry K. Hammerbacher, AMEDD Ctr and School, sub: Command of Navy Medical Treatment Facilities, and Command of Air Force Treatment Facilities, 19 Oct 94, both in DASG-MS.

[87] Quoted words: Moore, Lessons Learned. Colonel Foust thought it a significant problem. "We had some very bad experiences with physicians taking command." Foust, Hall interv.

[88] Medical command: HQDA GO 20, sub: Organization of the United States Army Medical Command (MEDCOM), 10 Aug 94, PL. The order redesignated HSC as the MEDCOM and assigned to it the U.S. Army Medical Department Center and School, U.S. Army Medical Research and Materiel Command, U.S. Army Environmental Hygiene Agency (AEHA), U.S. Army Dental Command, U.S. Army Veterinary Command, U.S. Army Health Service Support Areas, all medical centers and medical activities, and the medical installations at Walter Reed Army Medical Center, Fitzsimons Army Medical Center, and Fort Detrick, Maryland. AEHA was soon thereafter redesignated the U.S. Army Center for Health Promotion and Preventive Medicine and placed under the command of General Adams. Adams: General Adams was an outspoken advocate of changing the command policy in order to provide members of her corps with the opportunity to command. "Army nurses are qualified and ready to be commanders." Ltr to the editor, Brig. Gen. Nancy R. Adams, "Nurses Ready to Lead," *Army Times,* 14 November 1994.

[89] Command opportunity: Lt Gen Alcide M. Lanoue, TSG, to Gen Gordon R. Sullivan, CSA, 23 Jun 93; Memo, Lt Gen John H. Tilelli, Jr., DCSOPS, sub: Leader Development Decision Network (LDDN) to Study Implementation of Branch Immaterial Army Medical Department (AMEDD) Command Opportunities, 2 Feb 94; Memo, Lt Col Larry K. Hammerbacher, MSC, Ch, Officer Pers Proponent Div, AMEDD Pers Proponent Directorate (APPD), AMEDDC&S, sub: AMEDD Immaterial Command LDDN Council of Colonels, 7 Sep 94, including Rpt, sub: AMEDD Command Leader Development Action Plan; Council of Colonels, AMEDDC&S, Fort Sam Houston, Tex., 18–19 Oct 94, author's notes, all in DASG-MS. The Tilelli memo established a requirement for quarterly briefs by TSG to the CSA and review of the three "pillars" of leader development: institutional training, operational assignments, and self-development.

[90] Petition: Michael J. Tolk, "Who Should Command Medical Units," *Army* (December 1993): 12–13.

Appendixes

Appendix A

Milestones in the Evolution of the Medical Service Corps 1775–1994

30 April 1775: Provincial Congress of Massachusetts Bay establishes the Apothecary General.

14 May 1818: Permanent Medical Department established including Apothecary General and two assistants.

22 May 1862: War Department General Orders 55 establishes the U.S. Army Medical Storekeepers; four USAMS officers appointed as medical purveyors.

2 August 1862: Letterman Plan in the Army of the Potomac puts officers detailed to the Ambulance Corps in command of ambulance units.

11 March 1864: Ambulance Corps established by law; implemented in War Department General Orders 106, 16 March 1864. The law expired in 1866.

28 July 1866: Commissioned grades authorized for USAMS officers.

23 June 1917: War Department General Orders 75 establishes the U.S. Army Ambulance Service (USAAS), which federalizes volunteer ambulance units of the American Red Cross, the Norton-Harjes Ambulance Organization, and the American Field Service.

30 June 1917: War Department General Orders 80 establishes the Sanitary Corps (SnC). Both the USAAS and SnC established based on authority for national emergency contained in the Act of 18 May 1917. Both cease to exist in the active Army after the war, but SnC continues in reserve components.

4 June 1920: National Defense Act of 1920 establishes the Medical Administrative Corps in both the Regular Army and the reserve components. Initially authorized 140 officers in the Regular Army, that number drops to 16 in 1935.

12 July 1943: Act of July 12, 1943, establishes the Pharmacy Corps as a Regular Army branch and transfers to that corps officers of the Regular Army Medical Administrative Corps.

17 June 1945: Col. Edward Reynolds, MAC, Chief, Supply Service, Office of the Surgeon General, promoted to brigadier general.

4 August 1947: National Security Act of 1947 replaces the Sanitary Corps, Pharmacy Corps, and Medical Administrative Corps with the Medical Service Corps (MSC), organized in four sections.

10 November 1966: Act of 24 September 1966 authorizes one MSC brigadier general in the Regular Army. Col. William A. Hamrick, MSC, promoted to brigadier general.

12 December 1980: Defense Officer Personnel Management Act establishes the Army general officer authorization on the basis of 75 per 10,000 Regular Army commissioned officers on the Active Duty List.

25 October 1985: Promotion of Col. Walter F. Johnson III, MSC, to brigadier general results in two Medical Service Corps general officers on active duty, Johnson and Brig. Gen. France F. Jordan.

Appendix B

First Officers Appointed in the Regular Army Medical Administrative Corps (1 July 1920 Date of Rank)

Captains

Name	Birthplace	Date of Birth
Berkowitz, Alexander	Germany	22 Nov 1872
Bice, Lonzo R.	Arkansas	28 Aug 1875
Bitterman, Theodore	Indiana	8 Oct 1873
Brown, Arthur E.	England	24 Dec 1880
Brown, Clark L.	New York	9 Jul 1876
Burkard, Oscar	Germany	21 Dec 1877
Byers, Jason D.	West Virginia	17 Jun 1874
Davis, Harry A.	Alabama	17 Mar 1875
Dawson, John H.	Pennsylvania	6 Sep 1881
Dean, Herbert N.	Ohio	7 Aug 1879
Dickson, Robert A.	New York	18 Nov 1875
Dougherty, Meyer M.	Illinois	15 Nov 1873
Eisenman, Francis J.	New York	31 May 1879
England, Thomas M.	Ohio	14 Oct 1876
Ferguson, Robert S.	Illinois	3 Aug 1878
Freebourn, William J.	Pennsylvania	8 Dec 1879
Fuller, Harry N.	Michigan	25 Dec 1874
Graner, Carl	Ohio	18 Jul 1876
Greene, Earl F.	Vermont	9 Feb 1869
Hamner, James F.	Virginia	17 Apr 1873
Harris, Samuel J.	Kentucky	8 Jan 1878
Holt, Frank	New York	1 May 1871
Irving, Robert B.	Wisconsin	24 Oct 1877
Killikelly, Henry	Ireland	15 May 1875
Kincaid, Kenneth G.	Michigan	3 Oct 1870
Leedom, Chester B.	Ohio	2 May 1877
Lothrop, James N.	Texas	2 Aug 1876
Lovelly, Edward A., Jr.	Michigan	2 Aug 1881
McFarland, William	Virginia	22 Sep 1874
McKenzie, Robert S.	District of Columbia	5 Mar 1885
Marcus, Samuel	Germany	1 Dec 1872
Morehouse, Arthur	Michigan	15 Jan 1882

Name	Birthplace	Date of Birth
Pennington, Samuel W.	Maryland	2 Jul 1877
Perry, Clifford H.	New York	8 Jun 1879
Peterson, Robert	Pennsylvania	12 Nov 1873
Phares, Walter L.	West Virginia	6 Dec 1874
Roby, Albert A.	Wisconsin	22 Sep 1875
Sands, John R.	New York	23 Jan 1877
Scull, James A.	Indiana	17 Nov 1868
Smelsey, Samuel	New York	3 Aug 1873
Stimmel, Clarence O.	Ohio	4 Jul 1879
Tandrop, Otto A.	South Dakota	11 Sep 1883
Thomas, Frederick	South Carolina	4 Mar 1871
Vass, George E.	Kentucky	22 Aug 1869
Weber, Eugene	Oregon	1 May 1880
Weinberg, Max	Germany	14 Jan 1877
Wells, Fred O.	South Carolina	30 Jan 1885
Whitmarch, Paul L.	New York	10 Sep 1872
Williams, Thomas G.	New York	11 Sep 1876
Williams, William G.	Wisconsin	29 Jul 1882
Young, George C.	Connecticut	18 Nov 1873
	First Lieutenants	
Brooks, Robert R.	New York	13 Nov 1876
Burke, Edmund	New York	13 Sep 1879
Cleave, John W.	England	13 Apr 1870
Eble, Charles F.	Kentucky	13 Feb 1877
Greene, Harry	Tennessee	10 Dec 1881
Hunter, William	Pennsylvania	11 Aug 1881
Kennedy, Robert G.	Pennsylvania	9 Sep 1877
Luse, William E.	Indiana	26 May 1876
Manning, Charles G.	Ohio	28 Feb 1873
Ogle, Pinkney L.	Tennessee	14 Jan 1882
Pollard, Louis J.	Wisconsin	14 May 1881
Simmons, Frederick S.	England	15 Oct 1874
Simons, Elmer H.	Ohio	11 Oct 1882
Sly, Charles S.	New York	19 Jul 1872
Sweeney, James	New Hampshire	19 May 1872
Sykes, Edw. D.	Massachusetts	12 Jun 1886
Tanney, Louis L.	Pennsylvania	11 Sep 1882
Tremblay, James A.	Canada	18 Sep 1879
Walker, Ravello M.	Virginia	20 Oct 1870
Williamson, William H.	Minnesota	30 Aug 1875
	Second Lieutenants	
Adams, Wardlow M.	North Carolina	19 Jun 1883
Alley, Richard M.	Massachusetts	4 Feb 1883
Barton, Willard M.	Massachusetts	5 Feb 1881

Name	Birthplace	Date of Birth
Brittain, Thomas T.	South Carolina	7 Oct 1883
Brown, John O.	Illinois	3 May 1881
Butler, John H.	Ireland	16 Mar 1878
Caterer, Horace J.	England	26 Feb 1892
Chase, George P.	Missouri	21 Feb 1877
Christensen, Jens	Denmark	2 Nov 1884
Clark, Stanley A.	Connecticut	21 Apr 1891
Coleman, William F.	New York	19 Jun 1881
Couture, Omer A.	Massachusetts	10 May 1894
Crawford, Frank A.	Kansas	13 Nov 1880
Dolby, Ralph P.	Canada	16 Mar 1882
Doray, Alexander J.	New York	30 Mar 1889
Doyle, George	Georgia	5 Sep 1889
Ekman, George A.	Illinois	18 Feb 1891
Evans, William D.	Illinois	29 Aug 1875
Fleming, Davidson M.	Pennsylvania	26 Aug 1884
Foley, John D.	Minnesota	24 Feb 1887
Fort, Manly W.	North Carolina	7 Dec 1889
Fredericks, William	Wisconsin	8 Nov 1886
Gill, Bruce D.	Georgia	3 Sep 1876
Gilmour, Frederick	Nova Scotia	25 Oct 1888
Gorton, Glen D.	New York	6 Oct 1872
Harrison, Fred A.	Kansas	17 May 1881
Hepburn, Alexander	Ireland	5 Oct 1877
Hester, Thomas G.	North Carolina	24 Apr 1886
Hicks, Maurice	Alabama	15 Mar 1891
Holland, Henry	Texas	9 Aug 1879
Houck, Alfred T.	Pennsylvania	9 Oct 1877
Huffine, Berbian	Tennessee	13 Feb 1886
Humes, Richard E.	Pennsylvania	17 Apr 1883
Jennings, Harry M.	Virginia	24 Mar 1881
Kernan, William H.	Maryland	18 Jan 1891
Kimball, Charles F.	Massachusetts	26 Oct 1886
Kinzer, Amos S.	Pennsylvania	20 Apr 1874
Linden, Robert R.	New York	7 May 1878
Luscomb, Benjamin R.	Massachusetts	27 Dec 1884
Lynch, Francis E.	Massachusetts	23 Jan 1890
McElwain, Richard H.	Missouri	20 Apr 1885
McKelvey, William T.	Ireland	19 Mar 1881
Mace, Paul A.	California	17 Nov 1889
Mael, Jesse H.	Iowa	30 Sep 1884
Miller, Leo J.	Pennsylvania	16 Sep 1884
Mims, Martin D.	Alabama	22 Oct 1881
Moore, Francis	New York	14 Sep 1882
Morgan, John L.	Pennsylvania	12 May 1877

Name	Birthplace	Date of Birth
Murphree, William M.	Tennessee	27 Apr 1888
Paxton, Homer W.	Virginia	1 Sep 1889
Prater, Nealey	Texas	25 Mar 1888
Ramsey, James A.	Tennessee	22 May 1886
Ransom, Louis	New York	18 Mar 1876
Rice, Harvey I.	Massachusetts	3 Jun 1870
Schaefer, John D.	Indiana	23 Dec 1892
Schwieger, John C.	Minnesota	28 Oct 1883
Sheffler, Fritz J.	New York	29 Nov 1889
Smith, William M.	Unknown	Unknown
Speight, Clyde A.	Tennessee	11 Feb 1880
Stein, Leslie H.	Pennsylvania	27 May 1877
Steiner, Frank	Illinois	26 Sep 1885
Stevens, Everett R.	Massachusetts	6 Jan 1888
Stockwell, Harrison L.	Ohio	28 Jan 1878
Talbot, Max V.	Iowa	2 Dec 1880
Tier, Irving E.	New Jersey	12 Apr 1881
Tobin, Walter W.	Massachusetts	22 Aug 1878
Watfield, John A.	Pennsylvania	21 Jul 1885
Weir, Samuel A.	Ireland	8 Jun 1875
Whelan, William E.	Ohio	13 Oct 1873
Wilson, Robert N.	Kentucky	9 Jan 1888

Source: War Department, *Army List and Directory, 1921* (Washington, D.C.: The Adjutant General's Office, 1921).

Appendix C

Zone of the Interior Hospital Positions Opened to Medical Administrative Corps Officers in 1941

Hospital Size (in Beds)	Adjutant	MSO	Enlisted Detachment Commander	Mess Officer	Asst. Registrar*	Asst. Adjutant	Asst. MSO	Asst. Enlisted Detachment Commander	Asst. Mess Officer
50, 75		2LT							
100, 150, 200	1LT	2LT	1LT						
250, 300, 350, 400	1LT	1LT	1LT	CPT					
450	1LT	1LT	1LT	CPT					
500, 600, 700	CPT	CPT	CPT	CPT		2LT			2LT
750, 800, 900	CPT	CPT	CPT	CPT		2LT	1LT	2LT	
1,000	CPT	CPT	CPT	**		2LT		1LT	2LT
1,500, 2,000	CPT	CPT	CPT	**	1LT	2LT	2LT	1LT	1LT

* The registrar was required to be a Medical Corps officer.

** The mess officer was required to be a Medical Corps major in hospitals of 1,000 beds or greater.

Source: Clarence M. Smith, *The Medical Department: Hospitalization and Evacuation, Zone of Interior*, volume in series United States Army in World War II (Washington, D.C.: Office of the Chief of Military History, Department of the Army, 1956), p. 132.

Appendix D

Chiefs and Assistant Chiefs of the Medical Service Corps 1947–1994

Chiefs

Col. Othmar F. Goriup	September 1947–August 1951
Col. Robert L. Black	September 1951–March 1955
Col. Bernard Aabel	April 1955–June 1959
Col. Roy D. Maxwell	July 1959–February 1963
Brig. Gen. William A. Hamrick*	March 1963–July 1969
Brig. Gen. Manley G. Morrison	August 1969–August 1973
Brig. Gen. John E. Haggerty	August 1973–September 1977
Brig. Gen. James J. Young	October 1977–September 1981
Brig. Gen. France F. Jordan	October 1981–February 1984
Brig. Gen. Walter F. Johnson III**	March 1984–October 1988
Brig. Gen. Bruce T. Miketinac	November 1988–July 1992
Brig. Gen. Jerome V. Foust	September 1992–October 1996
Brig. Gen. Mack C. Hill	November 1996–

* Promoted to brigadier general 10 November 1966
** Promoted to brigadier general 25 October 1985

Assistant Chiefs

Pharmacy, Supply, and Administration Section

Lt. Col. John J. Painter	March 1949–September 1951
Lt. Col. Henry D. Roth	September 1951–July 1955
Harlan W. Layer	July 1955–October 1955
Col. James H. MacKin	November 1955–August 1956
Col. Clarence V. Frey	August 1956–June 1959
Col. Dale E. Thompson	June 1959–June 1963
Col. Clarence V. Frey	June 1963–September 1966
Col. Frank E. Stillman, Jr.	September 1966–April 1970
Col. Andrew T. Colyer	May 1970–February 1972
Col. Leonard T. Crosby, Jr.	March 1972–March 1973
Col. Raymond E. Adams	April 1973–March 1975
Col. James J. Young	March 1975–September 1977
Col. Eugene Lail	January 1978–June 1979
Col. Fred L. Walter	January 1980–June 1983
Col. Douglas J. Silvernale	July 1983–October 1985
Col. Douglas E. Moore	November 1985–November 1988
Col. Ronald G. Newman	October 1989–January 1991

Col. Henry T. Waters	February 1991–July 1992
Col. Charles G. Stevens	September 1993–August 1995
Col. Merle J. Snyder	September 1995–

Medical Allied Sciences Section

Lt. Col. Ludwig R. Kuhn	May 1948–March 1949
Col. Charles S. Gersoni	March 1949–August 1951
Col. Monroe E. Freeman	September 1951–May 1956
Col. Roy Maxwell	May 1956–July 1959
Col. Harvey W. Coddington	August 1959–May 1964
Col. Tomas C. Jefferis	December 1964–April 1967
Col. George W. Johnston	May 1967–April 1968
Col. Ralph W. Morgan	May 1968–May 1971
Col. Donald H. Hunter	June 1971–June 1973
Col. Charles A. Thomas	July 1973–June 1974
Col. Robert M. Angel	July 1974–September 1977
Col. Dan C. Cavanaugh	January 1978–December 1980
Col. Edward L. Maillet	January 1981–April 1983
Col. James E. Spiker, Jr.	May 1983–August 1990
Col. Robert O. Pick	September 1990–March 1992
Col. George C. Southworth	April 1992–December 1994
Col. John C. O'Brien, Jr.	February 1995–

Sanitary Engineering Section

Col. Raymond J. Karpen	March 1949–April 1951
Col. Stanley J. Weidenkopf	May 1952–March 1955
Lt. Col. Floyd L. Berry	March 1955–September 1958
Lt. Col. Robert G. McCall	September 1958–June 1962
Col. Converse R. Lewis, Jr.	July 1962–October 1966
Col. John Redmond, Jr.	November 1966–June 1970
Col. Bernard L. Goldstein	July 1970–June 1973
Col. Hunter G. Taft, Jr.	July 1973–March 1975
Col. James E. Anderson	March 1975–July 1977
Col. Alfred D. Kneessy	August 1977–August 1981
Col. J. Earl Herndon, Jr.	February 1982–May 1987
Col. Kenneth W. Vorpahl	June 1987–July 1991
Col. Robert J. Fitz	February 1992–January 1995
Col. Steven J. Stone	February 1995–

Optometry Section

Col. John Sheridan	September 1951–January 1960
Col. Billy Greene	January 1960–May 1970
Col. Herbert J. Thompson	May 1970–June 1971
Col. Henry E. Maes	June 1971–January 1974
Lt. Col. Gene Bourland	April 1974–July 1975
Col. Arthur R. Giroux	August 1975–April 1983
Col. John T. Leddy	May 1983–July 1989

Col. John F. Pyle	October 1989–February 1993
Col. Jerry D. Davis	March 1993–

Appendix E

Specialties of the Medical Allied Sciences Section May 1948

Specialty	MOS*
Research Psychologist	2231
Clinical Psychologist	2232
Psychological Assistant	2239
Bacteriologist	3307
Biochemist	3309
Parasitologist	3310
Serologist	3311
Clinical Laboratory Officer	3314
Entomologist	3315
Nutrition Officer	3316
Aviation Physiologist	3327
Psychiatric Social Worker	3605

* MOS = Military Occupational Specialty

Source: Technical Manual 12–406, Officer Classification, Commissioned and Warrant, February 1946, with change 1, 4 February 1948; Special Regulation 605–105–1, Personnel Classification System, 19 May 1950, both in PL.

Appendix F

National Organizations Invited To Attend the Medical Allied Sciences Conference 27–28 May 1948

American Association for Advancement of Science
American Association of Economic Entomologists
American Association of Psychiatric Social Workers
American Chemical Society
American Institute of Biological Sciences
American Institute of Nutrition
American Physiological Society
American Psychological Association
American Public Health Association
American Society of Biological Chemists
American Society of Parasitologists
American Society of Professional Biologists
Entomological Society of America
Society of American Bacteriologists

Source: Office of the Surgeon General, Agenda for Conference on the Medical Allied Sciences Section of the Medical Service Corps, 27–28 May 1948, DASG-MS.

Appendix G

Biographies of the Chiefs of the Medical Service Corps

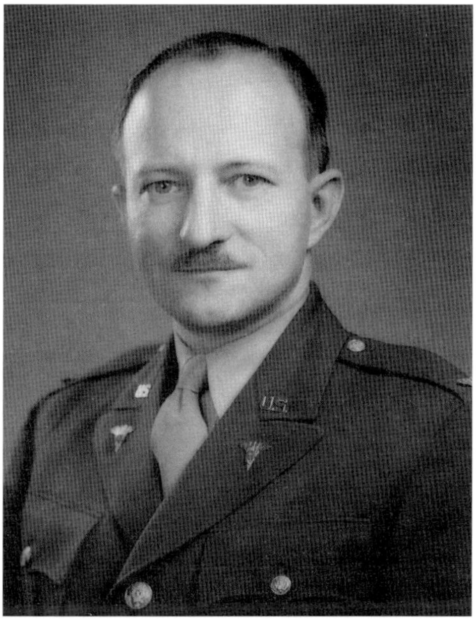

Col. Othmar F. Goriup
September 1947–August 1951

Col. Othmar F. Goriup, a graduate pharmacist and fellow of the American College of Apothecaries, was appointed the first Chief of the Medical Service Corps on 24 September 1947, serving until 1951 in that capacity. His pharmacy background was an important factor in his selection. The Surgeon General, Maj. Gen. George Armstrong, believed it was "gratifying to the pharmaceutical profession."

Born in Graz, Austria, in 1905, Goriup had come to the United States in 1915 at the age of ten. He was certified as a pharmacist upon completion of training at the University of Pittsburgh, Pennsylvania, in 1929. He received a B.S. in chemistry from St. Bonaventure College, New York, in 1939. He was commissioned in the Medical Administrative Corps Reserve in 1933 and entered active duty in 1941 as the Executive Officer of the station hospital at Langley Air Field, Virginia. This was followed by assignments as the Administrative Assistant to the Surgeon of the Air Transport Command in Washington, D.C., and as Chief of the Supply and Operations Division, Headquarters, Air Transport Command. In the latter capacity he planned and implemented the medical organization for the Air Transport Command. Goriup was serving in the Office of the Air Surgeon on the War Department Staff when selected as Chief of the Medical Service Corps. He said that when he left the air staff and moved to the Army Surgeon General's Office it was unfamiliar territory.

After his tour as Chief, MSC, he served as the Executive Officer of five Medical Department organizations: Medical Field Service School, Fort Sam Houston, Texas; Chief Surgeon's Office, Far East Command, Tokyo, Japan; Station Hospital, Camp Zama, Japan; Forest Glen Annex, Walter Reed Army Medical Center, Washington, D.C.; and The Historical Unit, Office of the Surgeon General, Washington, D.C. Colonel Goriup retired from the Army in

1960. He died in 1980 in Silver Spring, Maryland. His son, Lt. Col. Franklin J. Goriup, USA, Ret., was also an MSC. He passed away in 1989.

Source: Goriup in THU, OTSG, Rpt, sub: AEB for MSC History, 13 November 1958; THU, OTSG, biographical summary, 30 September 1960; Goriup, Standard Form 57, Application for Federal Service, 30 December 1961; Obituary, *Washington Post*, 3 August 1980; Roderick M. Engert, USACMH, biography, May 1981, all in DASG-MS; Goriup Bio File, folder 25, box 14/18, MSC-USACMH.

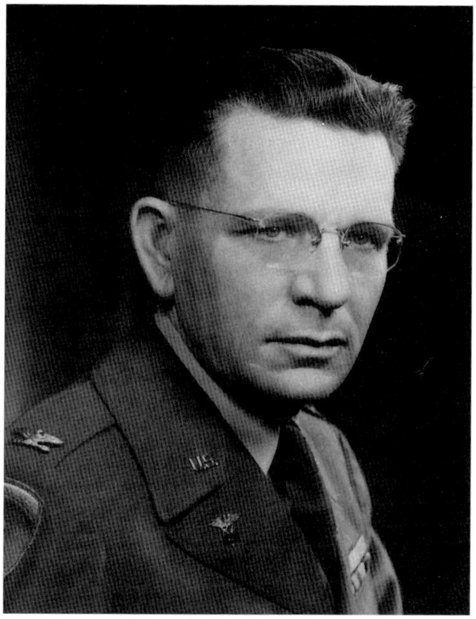

Col. Robert L. Black
September 1951–March 1955

Col. Robert L. Black replaced Col. Othmar F. Goriup as Chief of the Medical Service Corps during the first year of the Korean War. Black was born in Channing, Texas, in 1903 and enlisted in the Army in 1925 after graduation from high school and a variety of jobs including service as an ordinary sailor in the Merchant Marine. He successfully competed for one of four Medical Administrative Corps vacancies in 1928 and reported to Fitzsimons General Hospital, Denver, Colorado, as its medical supply officer. In 1929 he was assigned to the Schofield Barracks Station Hospital in Hawaii. There, as the sole Medical Administrative Corps officer, he served as medical supply officer, adjutant, mess officer, registrar, troop commander, recreation officer, and summary courts officer. Later, in 1937, he became the medical supply officer at Fort Sam Houston, Texas, where he replaced a physician.

In 1941, at the time of Pearl Harbor, Black was Chief of Finance and Supply in the Surgeon's Office, Headquarters, IX Corps Area, Presidio of San Francisco, California. He assumed command of the Medical Depot, Savannah, Georgia, followed by a move to Denver, Colorado, where he supervised construction of a medical depot and then became its first commander. He was assigned to the Supply Division, Surgeon General's Office, in 1942, with staff responsibility for operation of the twenty medical depots in the United States. In November 1944 he was reassigned as Chief of Supply, Office of the Surgeon, United Kingdom Base of the European Theater, which was initially responsible for providing 150,000 hospital beds in support of the invasion of Europe and later with closing hospital units after the defeat of Germany.

In July 1945 Black became the Chief of Supply, Surgeon's Office, European Theater. He returned to the United States in 1946 to attend the Industrial College of the Armed Forces, followed by assignment as Medical Supply Officer, General Distribution Point, San Antonio, Texas. Colonel Black returned to the Surgeon General's Office in 1948 as the Assistant Chief of the Personnel Division.

Colonel Black was a hospital administrator for eighteen years following his retirement from the Army in 1955, including employment at the United Mine Workers Hospital in Harley, Kentucky; the California Rehabilitation Center, Santa Monica, California; and the Community Hospital of Hollywood, California. He died in 1992 in Palm Springs, California.

Source: OTSG, Medical Service Corps History Project, "Panel Discussion With Former Chiefs of the Medical Service Corps," Washington, D.C., 6 May 1983, DASG-MS; Col. Robert L. Black, USA, Ret., interview with Lt. Col. Michael C. Baker, MSC, Palm Springs, California, 7 March 1984, Project 84–16, Senior Officers Oral History Program, U.S. Army Military History Institute, Carlisle Barracks, Pennsylvania; Black to Parker, 17 May 1960, MSC-USACMH; Black to Ginn, 24 December 1984, DASG-MS.

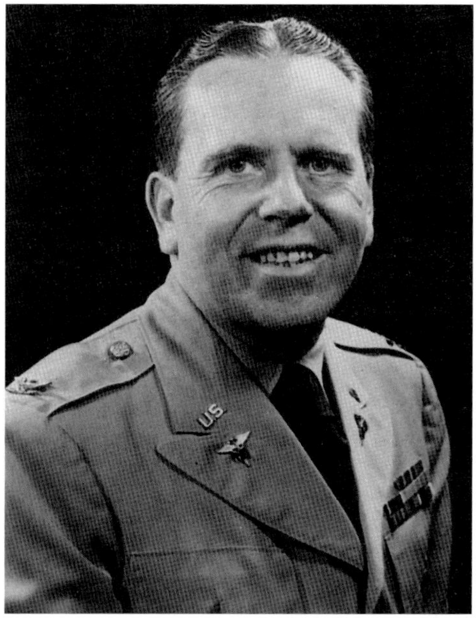

Col. Bernard Aabel
April 1955–June 1959

Col. Robert L. Black was succeeded by Col. Bernard Aabel. Aabel was born in Minneapolis, Minnesota, in 1907. He received a B.S. in pharmacy from the University of Minnesota in 1932 and entered the pharmaceutical business. He was commissioned in the Medical Administrative Corps in 1940 and entered active duty in 1941. He was a graduate of the Army War College.

Aabel landed on OMAHA Beach in 1944 as the S–2 of the 68th Medical Group and was wounded that October. His postwar assignments included Deputy Commander of the Medical Replacement Center at Camp Pickett, Virginia, and duty with the Surgeon General's Personnel Division, Washington, D.C. There, as a Pharmacy Corps major, he testified in support of formation of the Medical Service Corps. His performance was such that Senator Millard E. Tydings of Maryland recommended Aabel's appointment as chief of the new corps. In 1948 Aabel became the Assistant Military Attaché in Helsinki, Finland, following training duty with the Intelligence Division of the Army Staff. He was promoted to colonel in 1950 on the tenth anniversary of his entry on active duty and received Finland's Order of the White Rose for his attaché duty in 1951.

When selected Chief of the Medical Service Corps, Colonel Aabel was serving as Chief of the Surgeon General's Officer Procurement Branch. He continued to serve in that role, thereby starting a precedent of "dual-hatting" the Chief of the Medical Service Corps. After his term as Chief, Aabel became the Surgeon General's liaison officer to the Central Intelligence Agency. He retired from the Army in 1962.

At the time of his death in 1968 Aabel was director of the American Medical Association's International Health Department at the AMA's headquarters in Chicago. In 1972 the Secretary of the Army named the administration building of the new Academy of Health Sciences (successor to the Medical Field Service School) Aabel Hall.

Source: Norman D. Moore, biography of Aabel, THU, OTSG, May 1968, DASG-MS; DA, HQ Fort Sam Houston, Texas, GO 136, 15 November 1972, Stimson Library, AHS; U.S. Congress, House, Committee on Armed Services, Hearings on H.R. 1982 "To Establish a Permanent Medical Service Corps in the Medical Department of the Regular Army," 80th Cong., 1st sess., beginning 20 February 1947, see 12 March 1947 (Aabel biography); "Froehlke to Speak—Army Secretary," *Express and News*, San Antonio, Texas, 9 December 1972.

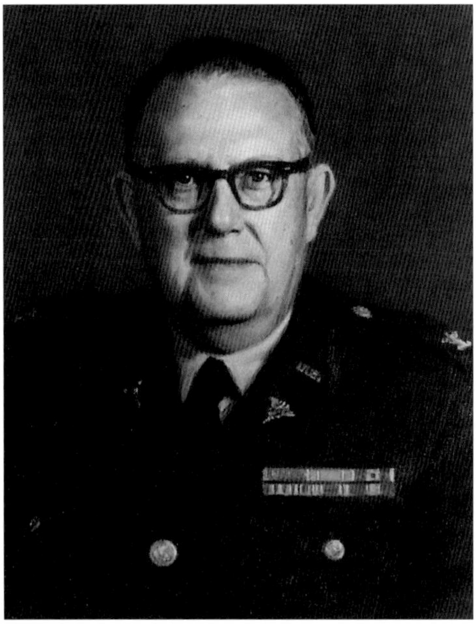

Col. Roy D. Maxwell
July 1959–February 1963

Col. Bernard Aabel was succeeded in 1959 by Col. Roy D. Maxwell, a nuclear medicine specialist and the only officer of the Medical Allied Sciences Section appointed Chief of the Medical Service Corps. Maxwell was born in 1907 in Oklahoma City, Oklahoma, and received a B.A. from Oklahoma City University in 1930. He received an M.S. and a Ph.D. in chemistry from the University of Iowa and was a chemistry professor when he was commissioned in the Sanitary Corps in 1941. He was a 1945 Command and General Staff College graduate and was the author of journal articles on organic chemistry and radiochemistry. He was a pioneer in the use of radioisotopes in biochemical studies.

Maxwell's first assignment was as Chief of the Biochemistry Section of the Fifth Service Command Laboratory at Fort Benjamin Harrison, Indiana. There he served from 1941 to 1946 as chief of the biochemistry section, as well as detachment commander, adjutant, and executive officer. After the war Maxwell was the radiological safety officer for the Bikini nuclear weapons tests. He then undertook postgraduate work in radiochemistry and biophysics at the University of California. From 1949 to 1951 he was Chief of the Department of Biophysics at the Army Medical Service Graduate School in Washington, D.C. (later the Walter Reed Army Institute of Research). He next became Chief of the Physiology and Pharmacology Division. From 1955 to 1957 he was Chief of the Fallout Study Group, Weapons Effects Division, of the Headquarters, Armed Forces Special Weapons Project.

When Colonel Maxwell was appointed Chief of the Medical Service Corps he was Special Assistant for Nuclear Warfare Instruction and Casualty Studies to the Commandant of the Army Medical Service School. While serving as Chief of the Corps, Maxwell was appointed to a special project with the Atomic Energy Commission, duties that occupied him fully beginning in August 1962. Col. Dale L. Thompson, Executive Officer of the Personnel Division, served as Acting Chief of the Corps in Maxwell's absence, beginning 7 August 1962. Maxwell retired from the Army in 1963. He died in 1993 in Grand Rapids, Michigan.

Source: Technical Liaison Division, OTSG, biography, February 1962; Maxwell, Ginn interview, Washington, D.C., 5 December 1983; OTSG, Special Orders No. 30, 7 August 1962, all in DASG-MS.

Brig. Gen. William A. Hamrick
March 1963–July 1969

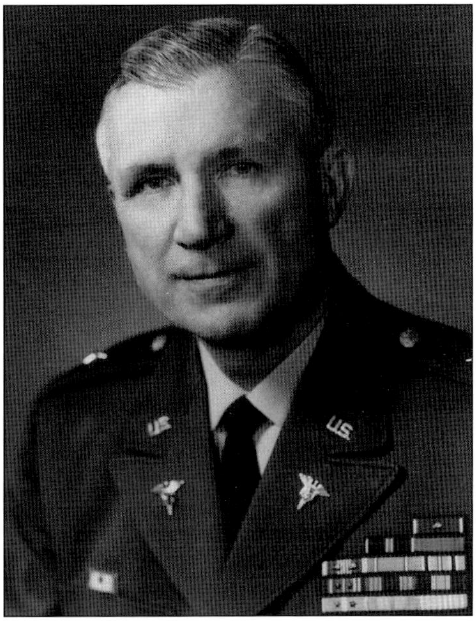

Col. William A. Hamrick was born in 1912 in Vernon, Indiana. He took office in March 1963 and served as Chief of the Medical Service Corps for the next six years, a period that included the Army buildup in Vietnam. Hamrick attended Oklahoma Military Academy from 1928 to 1932, graduating as the outstanding military cadet with a certificate that allowed commissioning as a second lieutenant when he reached the age of twenty-one. Following graduation from Oklahoma A&M College in 1934, he was commissioned in the Infantry and served on active duty with the 2d Infantry Division from 1936 to 1937. In 1940 he was recalled to active duty at Fort Sam Houston, Texas, as a classification officer at the reception center where he made initial assignments for newly enlisted soldiers. He served in a variety of assignments as an Adjutant General Corps officer. In 1946 he was accepted as a lieutenant colonel for Regular Army integration into the Medical Service Corps.

In 1950 Hamrick went to Korea as the Personnel Officer for the Eighth Army Surgeon. He returned to the United States as the Executive Officer, Fitzsimons Army Medical Center, from 1951 to 1952, followed by duty in Washington, D.C., with the Assistant Secretary of Defense for Manpower and Personnel. In 1956 he completed the Army–Baylor University Program in Hospital Administration and became the program's director, followed by a tour as the Executive Officer for the Surgeon, U.S. Army, Europe. He was a fellow of the American College of Hospital Administrators (later, the American College of Healthcare Executives). When selected as Corps Chief in 1963, Hamrick was the Executive Officer of William Beaumont General Hospital, El Paso, Texas. He became the first general officer in the Medical Service Corps on 10 November 1966. General Hamrick passed away in San Antonio, Texas, in 1995.

Source: Technical Liaison Division, OTSG, biography, 21 September 1988, DASG-MS.

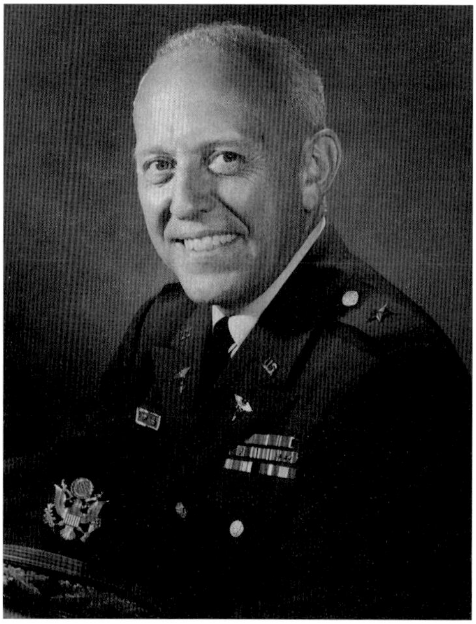

Brig. Gen. Manley G. Morrison
August 1969–August 1973

Brig. Gen. William A. Hamrick was replaced by Brig. Gen. Manley G. Morrison in 1973. He was serving as the Executive Officer for the Surgeon General's Comptroller when appointed Chief of the Medical Service Corps.

Morrison was born in Weston, West Virginia, in July 1915. When Japan attacked Pearl Harbor he was executive chief steward for the Union Pacific Railroad at Sun Valley, Idaho. The railroad had promoted him to that rank at the age of twenty-seven. His promotion to division superintendent (a position normally reached after the age of sixty) exempted him from the draft. He never ceased being very proud of a promotion which he believed was "higher than I ever attained in the military service as far as status was concerned—including Chief of the Corps."

Volunteering for military service, Morrison was assigned to Army hospital food service due to his experience in hotel and food service management. He was commissioned in the Medical Administrative Corps at Camp Barkeley, Texas, in 1942 for duty in hospital food service, but he had no connection with that field after his initial assignment in a medical battalion. Morrison found that the Army's food service system precluded the possibility of preparing food tastefully. Its sanitation rules required keeping meat absolutely frozen until served, and one of his vivid memories was watching the cooks chopping beef carcasses apart with fire axes so they could get the meat into the oven.

Morrison's career covered assignments in a wide range of administrative specialties, including logistics, plans and training, registrar, and comptroller. His World War II duty included Medical Supply Officer, 636th Clearing Company, and S–3, 430th Medical Battalion, Ninth Army. His postwar assignments included Registrar, Letterman General Hospital, San Francisco, California; Chief of Medical Statistics, Office of the Surgeon, U.S. Army, Europe; Comptroller, Walter Reed Army Medical Center; Army Staff duty in the Office of the Deputy Chief of Staff for Logistics; and Chief of the Special Projects Office of the Surgeon General's Office; followed by another tour in Europe as Executive Officer for the Surgeon, U.S. Army, Europe. He completed a B.S. in military science at the University of Maryland in 1958 and an M.A. in public administration at American University in 1960. He was a graduate of the Army Command and General Staff College regular (resident) course and of the Army War College.

Source: Technical Liaison Office, OTSG, biography, August 1969; Public Affairs Office, OTSG, official biography, September 1971; Morrison, Ginn interview, Washington, D.C., 7 May 1983, all in DASG-MS.

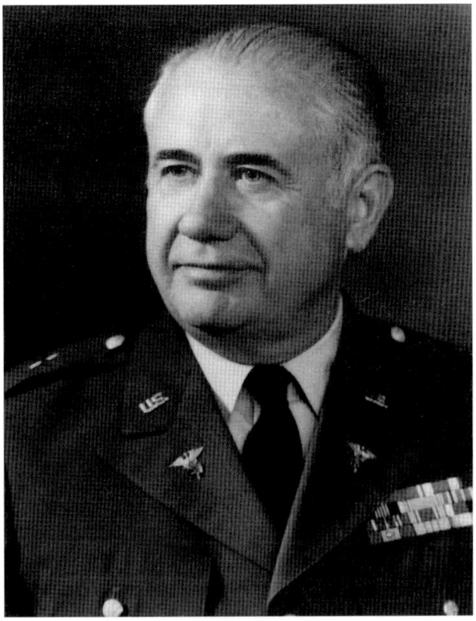

Brig. Gen. John E. Haggerty
August 1973–September 1977

Brig. Gen. Manley G. Morrison was succeeded by Brig. Gen. John E. Haggerty, who came to Washington in 1973 from Denver, Colorado, where he was serving as Director of the Office of the Civilian Health and Medical Program of the Uniformed Services (CHAMPUS). General Haggerty's concurrent appointment as the Surgeon General's Director of Resources Management, another Medical Department general officer position, returned the Medical Service Corps Chief to a "dual-hatted" position. He was commissioned in the Medical Administrative Corps (MAC) in 1942 from the Officer Candidate School, Carlisle Barracks, Pennsylvania, and was familiar to thousands of MAC officers as an OCS company commander at Camp Barkeley, Texas.

Haggerty was born in 1918 in Reading, Massachusetts. He received a B.S. from the University of Maryland and a law degree from Suffolk University Law School. His assignments included executive officer of two Army hospitals and of the U.S. Army Medical Research and Development Command. Staff duty included assignments to the Army General Staff in the Office of the Assistant Chief of Staff, G–4 (Logistics), the staff of the Surgeon, U.S. Army, Europe, and as Plans and Operations Officer on the joint staff of the Surgeon, United States Pacific Command, Hawaii. He was a graduate of the Army's Command and General Staff College regular course and of the Army War College.

When Haggerty retired in 1977 he became the administrator of the New England Primate Center, Harvard University, where he found a certain pleasure in working with monkeys. "They might bite, but they don't talk back and never ask for overtime pay." In 1978 the Association of Military Surgeons of the United States—a society of federal health agencies established in 1891 and incorporated by Congress in 1903—awarded Haggerty the Ray E. Brown Award for outstanding accomplishment in federal health care management.

Source: Resume, 30 September 1977, and Haggerty, Ginn interview, Washington, D.C., 7 May 1983, both in DASG-MS; MSC Newsletter, 1 December 1978.

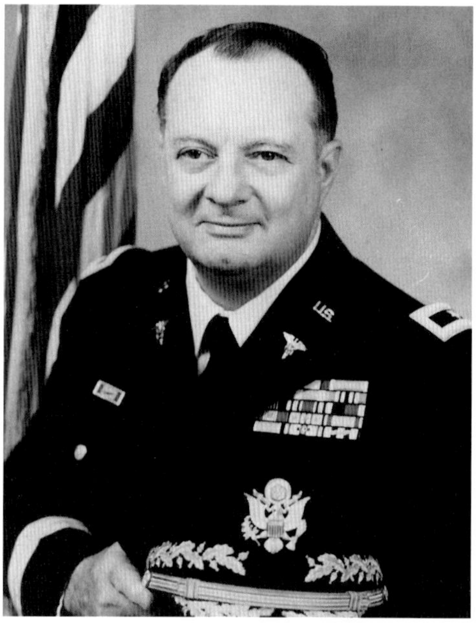

Brig. Gen. James J. Young
October 1977–September 1981

Brig. Gen. John E. Haggerty was succeeded in October 1977 by Brig. Gen. James J. Young, who was serving in the Surgeon General's Office as the Deputy Director of Resources Management. Young also replaced Haggerty as Director of Resources Management, a continuation of the practice of "dual-hatting" the Medical Service Corps Chief.

Young was born in Fort Ringgold, Texas, in 1926. He was commissioned in the Medical Administrative Corps in 1947 through the Fort Benning Infantry OCS after a short period as an enlisted artillery soldier. He later earned an M.S. in military science from the University of Maryland, an M.H.A. through the Army-Baylor Program, and a Ph.D. in health care administration from the University of Iowa. His principal assignments included staff officer duty at Department of the Army and joint staff levels; Chief of Plans and Operations for the Surgeon, Military Assistance Command, Vietnam; and Executive Officer of the U.S. Army Hospital, Fort Ord, California. From 1973 to 1975 he served as the Army representative and senior military analyst on the presidentially mandated Military Health Care Study conducted by the Department of Defense, the Department of Health, Education, and Welfare, and the Office of Management and Budget. The *Report of the Military Health Care Study*, published in 1985, was a landmark tri-service review of the military health care system.

Following his retirement, Young became Vice Chancellor for Health Affairs, State Board of Regents, West Virginia. In 1989 he became dean of the Medical School of the University of Texas at San Antonio. He was one of the few non-physician medical school deans in the United States.

Source: Resume of service career and curriculum vitae, 7 October 1981; Retirement ceremony program, 29 September 1981, The Pentagon; MSC Newsletter, 2 August 1982, all in DASG-MS.

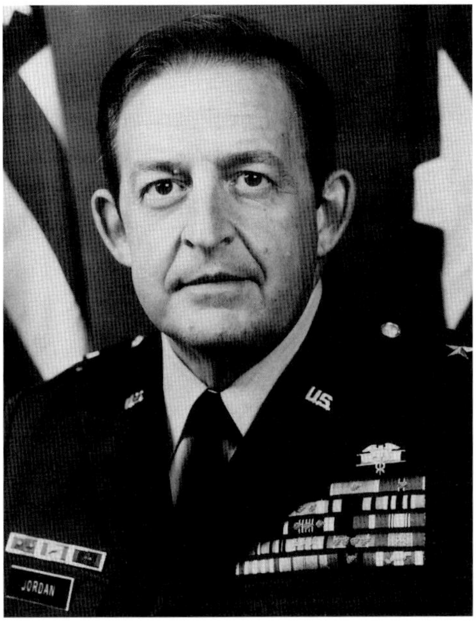

Brig. Gen. France F. Jordan
October 1981–February 1984

Brig. Gen. James J. Young was replaced in October 1981 by Brig. Gen. France F. Jordan, who was serving as Director of Personnel for the Surgeon General and Commander of the U.S. Army Medical Department Personnel Support Agency, positions he retained when appointed Chief of the Medical Service Corps.

Jordan was born in Liberty, North Carolina, in 1934. He was commissioned in 1956 from the ROTC program at Davidson College, North Carolina. He was a graduate of the U.S. Army War College and of the regular course of the Command and General Staff College. His initial assignment was as a platoon leader, followed by duty as a company commander at the Medical Training Center of Brooke Army Medical Center. In 1958 he was selected as aide-de-camp to Maj. Gen. William E. Shambora, the medical center commander.

His subsequent assignments included duty with the Army General Staff; Deputy Chief of Staff for Plans and Operations, U.S. Army Medical Command, Vietnam; Chief, Operations Division, and later Executive Officer, U.S. Army Medical Research and Development Command; Commander, 44th Medical Brigade; Deputy Director for Health Care Operations, OTSG; and Executive Officer for the Surgeon General. In May 1983, while serving as Chief of the Medical Service Corps, he was named Director of Resources Management, OTSG.

In 1984 the Association of Military Surgeons of the United States named Jordan as the first recipient of the Outstanding Federal Services Health Administrator Award. In January 1984 he was selected as the first MSC officer to fill the two-star billet of Deputy Assistant Secretary of Defense for Medical Readiness, a position from which he retired in 1987. He received the Defense Distinguished Service Medal upon his retirement, as well as the United States Public Health Service Outstanding Service Medal.

Source: Curriculum vitae in MSC Newsletter, 20 November 1981, and in Jordan to Ginn, 25 April and 2 October 1988, all in DASG-MS.

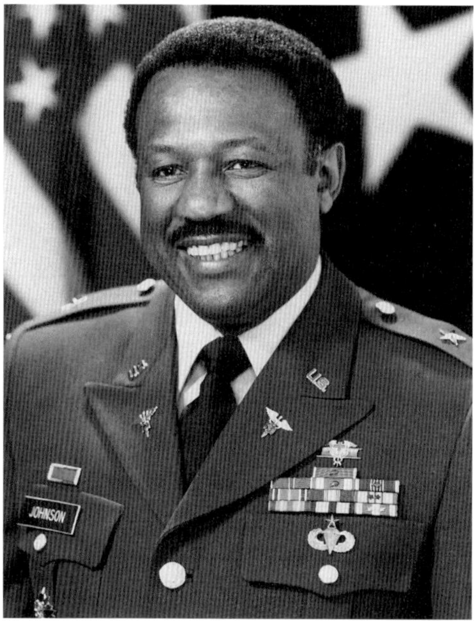

Brig. Gen. Walter F. Johnson III
March 1984–October 1988

Col. Walter F. Johnson III replaced Brig. Gen. France F. Jordan as Chief of the Medical Service Corps in March 1984. He began his tour in the rank of colonel since the Medical Service Corps star authorization was not initially augmented upon General Jordan's move to the Office of the Secretary of Defense. Johnson was promoted to brigadier general in October 1985 when a Medical Department star became available, making him the first black, the first paratrooper, and the youngest officer appointed as Chief of the Medical Service Corps. He was initially "dual-hatted" by retention in his position as Executive Officer to the Surgeon General. In October 1985 he was promoted to brigadier general and became the first Medical Service Corps officer appointed as the Surgeon General's Director of Health Care Operations.

Johnson was born in Charleston, South Carolina, in 1939. Commissioned from West Virginia State College ROTC, Johnson served his first tour as a medical platoon leader in the 82d Airborne Division. He held a master's degree in international relations from the University of Missouri. He was a graduate of the Command and General Staff College regular course and of the Industrial College of the Armed Forces.

Johnson's assignments were concentrated in the operations field and included plans officer for the 44th Medical Brigade in Vietnam; instructor at the Medical Field Service School; Chief of the Plans, Force Structure, and Mobilization Branch of the Surgeon General's Office; and commander of the 2d Medical Battalion in Korea. In 1981 he was appointed to concurrent duty as Deputy Director of Personnel and Assistant to the Chief of the Medical Service Corps (General Jordan). This was followed by his appointment as Executive Officer for the Surgeon General, the position he was holding when appointed Chief of the Corps.

In 1988 the Association of Military Surgeons of the United States recognized General Johnson with its Outstanding Federal Services Health Administrator Award. He accepted a position with the American Hospital Association upon his retirement from the Army that year and became the association's senior vice president in 1991.

Source: Curriculum vitae, 1 March 1984; Department of the Army news release, 12 March 1984, both in DASG-MS.

Brig. Gen. Bruce T. Miketinac
November 1988–July 1992

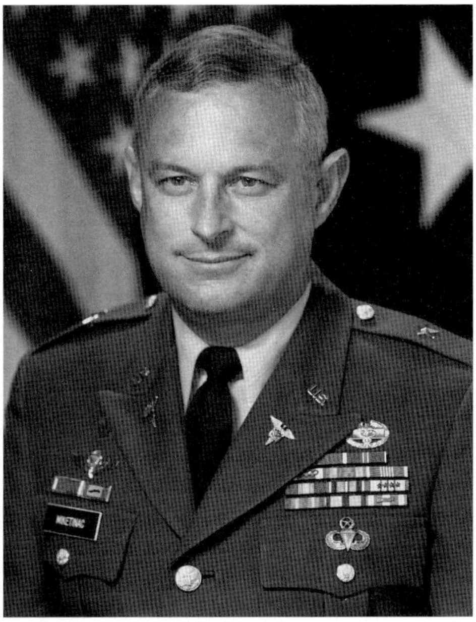

Brig. Gen. Bruce T. Miketinac replaced Brig. Gen. Walter F. Johnson as Chief of the Medical Service Corps and as the Surgeon General's Director of Health Care Operations on 1 November 1988, returning to Washington, D.C., from San Antonio, Texas, where he was the Deputy Commandant of the Academy of Health Sciences, U.S. Army. Miketinac was born in Escanaba, Michigan, in 1941 and was commissioned from the ROTC program at Saint Norbert College. He later earned a Master of Business Administration with a concentration in health care administration from the University of Notre Dame, where he also was class president. His military education included the regular course of the Army Command and General Staff College and the Army War College.

General Miketinac's first assignment upon entering active duty in 1963 was as medical operations assistant in the 2d Airborne Battle Group of the 82d Airborne Division, Fort Bragg, North Carolina, and later, as company commander in the division's 307th Medical Battalion. He also served as the battalion S–2 (intelligence), S–3 (operations), and S–4 (logistics). His Vietnam service was as administrative officer for the Division Surgeon, 1st Cavalry Division. His specialty concentration was in personnel, and assignments included S–1 (personnel) for the 7th Medical Brigade, Ludwigsburg, Germany; Chief of the Human Resources Management Branch of the Academy of Health Sciences; and Chief of the Medical Service Corps Career Activities Office, U.S. Army Medical Personnel Support Agency, Washington, D.C. Other assignments included command of the 307th Medical Battalion, 82d Airborne Division, and command of the 44th Medical Brigade, both at Fort Bragg. His awards and decorations included the Legion of Merit, the Air Medal, the Combat Medical Badge, and the Master Parachutist Badge.

Source: Department of the Army, Public Affairs Office, U.S. Army Biography, 1988, DASG-MS.

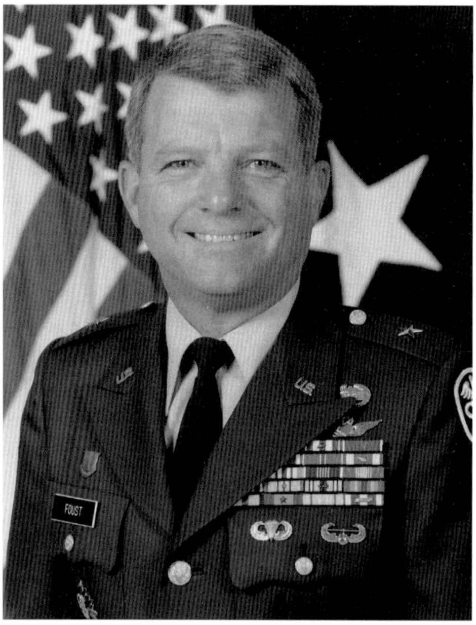

Brig. Gen. Jerome V. Foust
September 1992–October 1996

Brig. Gen. Jerome V. Foust succeeded Brig. Gen. Bruce T. Miketinac as Chief of the Medical Service Corps on 30 September 1992 and assumed the duty of Deputy Commander of the Army Medical Department Center and School the following month. In a break with tradition, he remained at Fort Sam Houston, Texas, where he had been serving as the Post Commander (and the first MSC to command the post). He had previously been assigned to the same installation as the Deputy Chief of Staff for Operations of the Health Services Command (HSC). General Foust was born in Fort Smith, Arkansas, in 1943. He was commissioned through the ROTC program at Troy State University, Alabama, in 1966, and received a master's degree from Saint Mary's University, San Antonio, Texas. He was a graduate of the U.S. Army Command and General Staff College and of the U.S. Army War College.

General Foust's primary specialty was medical aviation. He served two tours in Vietnam with the 54th Medical Detachment and the 237th Medical Detachment Dustoff units. Other tours included Army Staff duty in the Pentagon from 1980 to 1984, Chief of Mobilization and Planning at HSC, Commander of the 326th Medical Battalion of the 101st Airborne Division (Airmobile), and instructor at the Academy of Health Sciences, Fort Sam Houston. He served as Commander of the 44th Medical Brigade of the XVIII Airborne Corps from 1989 to 1991, deploying the brigade in support of combat operations in Panama in 1989 and in the Persian Gulf in 1990. The brigade's Gulf War deployment consisted of 2 medical groups; 12 evacuation, combat support, and mobile Army surgical hospitals; 4 medical battalions; and 64 company- or detachment-size units totaling over 6,500 soldiers. Foust's awards and decorations included two awards of the Silver Star, the Legion of Merit, Distinguished Flying Cross, thirty-seven awards of the Air Medal, and the Combat Medical, Master Army Aviator, Parachutist, and Air Assault Badges.

Source: Health Services Command *Mercury*, October 1992, and biography, undated, both in DASG-MS.

Brig. Gen. Mack C. Hill
November 1996–

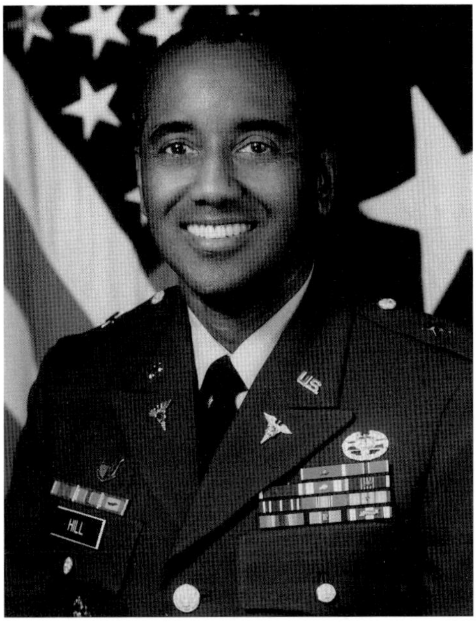

Brig. Gen. Mack C. Hill replaced Brig. Gen. Jerome V. Foust as Chief of the Medical Service Corps in November 1996. Hill was born in Tampa, Florida, in 1942. He graduated from Florida A&M University in 1965 with a major in history, and earned a Master of Arts in management from Webster University in 1977. His military education included the resident Command and General Staff College and the Industrial College of the Armed Forces.

General Hill's specialty area was logistics, and after an initial assignment as a company commander in the Medical Training Center, Fort Sam Houston, he served in Vietnam as the Medical Supply Officer for the 9th Infantry Division. This was followed by assignments as medical supply officer of the 33d Field Hospital in Wuerzburg, Germany; the Academy of Health Sciences, Fort Sam Houston; and the U.S. Army Hospital, Fort Carson, Colorado. Other positions included Chief of the Logistics Division, 130th Station Hospital, Heidelberg, Germany; Chief of the Materiel Branch, 7th Medical Command, Heidelberg; Chief of the Plans, Doctrine, and Materiel Development Branch, Office of the Surgeon General; and Chief, Logistics Division, Tripler Army Medical Center, Hawaii. General Hill commanded the 47th Medical Supply, Optical, and Maintenance Battalion, Fort Hood, Texas, from July 1986 to August 1988, and the U.S. Army Medical Materiel Agency, Fort Detrick, Maryland, from July 1990 to June 1992. He was serving as the Director of Logistics, Office of the Surgeon General, when selected as Chief of the MSC. His awards and decorations included two awards of the Legion of Merit, the Purple Heart, and the Combat Medical Badge.

Source: Resume of service career and curriculum vitae, 20 March 1996; Officer Record Brief, 16 February 1996.

Appendix H

Medical Service Corps Specialties in 1961

Active Component, 31 December 1961

MOS	Title	Actual Strength
Pharmacy, Supply, and Administration Section		3,107
Pharmacy Career Field		89
3318	Pharmacy Officer	89
Supply Career Field		448
4000	General Supply Officer	14
4010	Supply Staff Officer (G–4, S–4)	10
4310	Purchasing & Contracting Officer	8
4490	Medical Supply Officer	416
Comptroller Career Field		137
2401	Machine Records Officer	1
2402	ADPS Plans and Operations Officer	1
2610	Management Analyst	89
6000	Comptroller	41
6302	Budget & Fiscal Officer	5
Personnel Career Field		328
2110	Adjutant	60
2200	Personnel Officer	107
2210	Personnel Management Officer	16
2260	Personnel Staff Officer (G–1, S–1)	61
2334	Selective Service Officer	2
2900	Headquarters Unit Commander	70
5000	Special Services Officer	3
5505	Information Officer	9
Registrar Career Field		123
2431	Medical Registrar	123
Hospital Administration Career Field		162
3012	Hospital Administrator	162

MOS	Title	Actual Strength
Pharmacy, Supply, and Administration Section—Continued		
Medical Technical Intelligence Career Field		30
8642	Military Intelligence Officer	8
9300	Intelligence Liaison Officer	8
9301	Combat Intelligence Staff Officer (S–2, G–2)	1
9330	Translation Officer (Designated Language)	1
9340	Technical Intelligence Coordination Officer	8
9666	Intelligence Research	3
9332	Interpreter	1
Operations & Training Field		1,343
2162	Operations and Training Staff Officer	187
2520	Training Officer	123
2548	Training Aids Officer	1
2622	Training Center Unit Officer	25
3506	Field Medical Assistant	1,007
Aviation Career Field		141
1980	Fixed Wing Aviator	1
1981	Rotary Wing Aviator	133
1983	Aviation Unit Commander	7
Non-Career Field		66
0009	Special Assignment	1
2120	Administrative Officer	63
7422	Safety Engineer	1
7601	Electronic Engineer	1
Medical Students		82
0006	Student Officer (Senior Medical Students)	66
	Excess Leave—Medical School	16
Warrant Officers		158
3506	Field Medical Assistant	99
4890	Medical Equipment Repair Technician	11
4990	Medical Supply Officer	48
Medical Allied Sciences Section		472
Psychology Career Field		88
2230	Psychologist	15
2232	Clinical Psychologist	35
2239	Psychological Assistant	38
Social Work Career Field		116
3606	Social Work Officer	116

MOS	Title	Actual Strength
Medical Allied Sciences Section—Continued		
Podiatry Career Field		21
3350	Podiatrist	21
Entomology Career Field		49
3315	Entomologist	49
Nuclear Science Career Field		20
3308	Nuclear Medical Science Officer	19
7312	Physicist-Chemist	1
Laboratory Sciences Career Field		178
3307	Bacteriologist	48
3309	Biochemist	47
3310	Parasitologist	10
3311	Immunologist	12
3314	Clinical Laboratory Officer	58
3327	Physiologist	3
Sanitary Engineering Section		99
7960	Sanitary Engineer	99
Optometry Section		154
3340	Optometry Officer	147
4891	Optical Shop Officer	7
Total Medical Service Corps		3,832

Source: Director, Resources Management, OTSG, Status of Medical Service Corps, as of 31 December 1961; Maj. Ray Bateman, SF, Distribution Division, Officer Personnel Management Directorate, PERSCOM, Rpt, subj., Medical Equipment Repair, 6 Feb 1995, both in DASG-MS.

Appendix I

Principal Attempts at Writing the MSC History

1. *Early Efforts.* 1953 to 1957:

a. 1953: Col. Robert L. Black, MSC, writes 31-page draft.

b. 1954: 1st Lt. R. W. Bamberger, MSC, writes 74-page draft.

c. 1957: Maj. Gen. James P. Cooney, MC, "Some Notes on the Historical Development of the Medical Service Corps," *U.S. Armed Forces Medical Journal* 8 (February 1957): 254–63.

2. *1958 MSC History Project.* 1958 to 1964: Official Army multi-author project begun 13 November 1958 with first meeting of The Surgeon General's Advisory Editorial Board for the History of the U.S. Army Medical Service Corps, held at The Historical Unit (THU), Forest Glen, Md. THU later becomes a division of the U.S. Army Center of Military History (USACMH).

3. *1965 MSC History Project.* 1965 to 1977: Single-author project begun 11 June 1965 with meeting of the Advisory Editorial Board at THU. Maj. Joseph Israeloff, MSC, appointed as author of MSC history through World War II. Three revisions are attempted.

a. 1969: 2d Lt. Frederick W. Obermiller, MSC.

b. 1973: Mr. Dwight D. Oland.

c. 1975: Colonel Israeloff. Assigned to USACMH, he retires in 1976, taking the draft into retirement for revision.

4. *1978 MSC History Project.* 1978 to 1982: Mr. Oland is tasked to rewrite the volume on 7 July 1978. Brig. Gen. Douglas Kinnard, Chief of Military History, terminates the incomplete effort in July 1982, ending its status as an official U.S. Army project of the USACMH.

5. *1983 MSC History Project.* 1983 to 1995: Single-author project approved on 1 May 1983 as a complete restart by the Office of the Surgeon General. Maj. Richard V. N. Ginn, MSC, is designated as author and assigned to the task full-time from 1 August 1983 to May 1986 as Special Assistant to the Chief, MSC. He moves to Belgium in 1989 and takes the project with him through five subsequent assignments.

a. 1990: USACMH Panel meets on 14 November and makes recommendations for revision of the manuscript.

b. 1992: Brig. Gen. Harold W. Nelson, Chief of Military History, on 26 February approves revised manuscript for publication. CMH contracts with an editor who defaults. A contract with a new editor is let on 31 January 1994, and the edited manuscript is furnished to CMH in February 1995.

Appendix J

Carmack Medal Winners, 1958–1996

Date	Name
June 1958	1st Lt. Charles B. Counselman
December 1958	1st Lt. William G. Pfeiffer
June 1959	Capt. Bernard K. Mulrenin
December 1959	1st Lt. James M. Eubanks
June 1960	1st Lt. James C. Huff
December 1960	Capt. David E. Sullivan
June 1961	Capt. Harral A. Bigham
May 1962	Capt. David B. Willis
May 1963	Capt. Gilbert L. Jacox
May 1964	Capt. James G. Van Straten
May 1965	Capt. Rudolph Moreau, Jr.
May 1966	Capt. Thomas A. Janke
June 1967	Maj. Jon N. Harris
December 1967	Capt. Douglas R. Stutz
February 1968	Capt. Bernard A. Schiefer
June 1968	Maj. Donald G. Ebner
December 1968	Maj. Robert M. Quillin
March 1969	Capt. Jack O. Harrington
July 1969	Capt. Theodore C. Reineck, Jr.
December 1969	Capt. Joseph E. Salko
June 1970	Capt. Roger W. Wiley
December 1970	Maj. Jerry J. Stelmach
June 1971	Capt. Paul P. Brooke, Jr.
December 1971	Capt. John A. Coventry
July 1972	Capt. Milton E. Turner
December 1972	Capt. Kent G. Washburn
June 1973 (Tie)	Capt. Raymond J. Burke II
	Capt. Walter J. Skeistaitis
December 1973	Capt. Thomas M. Driskill, Jr.
June 1974	Capt. William S. Borders, Jr.
December 1974 (Tie)	Capt. Hugh M. McLear
	Capt. Arthur F. Steinberg
June 1975 (Tie)	Capt. William R. Cahill
	Capt. Harold J. Harland
December 1975	Maj. Melvin E. Modderman
June 1976	Capt. Thomas D. Murphy
December 1976	Capt. Merle J. Snyder
June 1977	Capt. Herbert A. Coley

Date	Name
December 1977	Capt. Frank W. Hillard
July 1978	Capt. Carrick T. Troutman, Jr.
December 1978	Capt. Gary S. Palmer
June 1979	Capt. Michael F. Huebner
December 1979	Capt. Tommy W. Mayes
June 1980	Capt. Robert J. Poux
December 1980	Capt. Thomas G. Fuller
June 1981	Capt. Nancy K. Raiha
December 1981	Capt. Daniel D. Remund
June 1982	Capt. Rebecca J. Mackoy
December 1982	Capt. Eric J. Rubel
June 1983	Capt. John C. Kotulak
December 1983	Capt. Theodore P. Landry
June 1984	Capt. Eric R. Abraham
December 1984	Capt. John A. Miller
May 1985 (Tie)	Capt. Robert J. Thompson
	Capt. Brett D. Walker
November 1985	Capt. David A. Pattillo
June 1986	Capt. Nancy K. Willcockson
November 1986	Capt. Francis L. McVeigh II
May 1987	Capt. Dan E. Harms
November 1987	Capt. Scott W. Gordon
February 1988	Capt. Barclay P. Butler
June 1988	Capt. Norman O. Wolfe
December 1988	Capt. John D. Quinlivan
February 1989	Capt. Randy P. Buchnowski
May 1989	Capt. Peter T. Shaul
December 1989	Capt. Gregory Gahm
May 1990	Capt. Ann Grediagan
December 1990	1st Lt. Vicki Oyadomari
May 1991	Capt. Claude Hines, Jr.
December 1991	Capt. David R. Petray
May 1992	Capt. Berthony Ladouceur
December 1992	Capt. Vovanni T. Kotoriy
May 1993	Capt. Jean D. Blando
December 1993	Capt. Patricia Darnauer
June 1994	Capt. James D. McLain
December 1994	Capt. Thomas C. Delk
June 1995	1st Lt. Mark A. Ireland
December 1995	1st Lt. Amy C. S. Brinson
May 1996	Capt. Michael A. Rivers

Source: Capt. Shirley F. Palmatier, MS, Adjutant General, Academy of Health Sciences (AHS), U.S. Army, Fort Sam Houston, Texas, Memo to Lt. Col. Richard V. N. Ginn, 16 April 1986; Maj. Jeremy L. Olson, MS, Department of Health Care Operations, AHS, 26 July 1994, Memo to Ginn; Lt. Col. Cheryl L. Silkwood, MS, MSC Branch, Health Services Division, PERSCOM, notes of telephone conversation with Ginn, 18 January 1996. All in DASG-MS.

Appendix K

Medical Service Corps Specialties in 1972

Career Fields and Military Occupational Specialties (MOS)
Active Component, 30 June 1972

Title and MOS	Actual Strength
Administrative Specialties	
Comptroller (2402, 2610, 2800)	149
Hospital Administration (3012)	76
Medical Aviation (1981, 1987, 2518, 4823)	359
Medical Technical Intelligence (9300)	6
Operations and Training (2162, 2520, 3506)	1,773
Personnel (2110, 2120, 2200, 2210, 2260, 2900, 5505)	358
Registrar (2431)	185
Supply (4010, 4490)	433
Non-Career Fields (0600, 2030, 2421, 9310)	6
Student Programs Charged to MSC (medical, dental, veterinary)	199
Medical Equipment Repair Specialist (202A) (Warrant Officers)	84
Scientific Specialties	
Audiology (3360)	25
Entomology (3315)	83
Laboratory Science (3307, 3309, 3310, 3311, 3314, 3327)	286
Military Community Oral Health Manager (3380)	6
Nuclear Science (3308)	40
Optometry (3340)	284
Pharmacy (3318)	166
Podiatry (3360)	39
Psychology (2239, 3620, 8430)	139
Sanitary Engineering (3370, 7960)	188
Social Work (3606)	260
Total Medical Service Corps	5,144

Source: Surgeon General Report, 1972, p. 110, and 1974, p. 38 (for MOS groupings); Maj. Ray Bateman, SF, Distribution Division, Officer Personnel Management Directorate, PERSCOM, Rpt, subj., Medical Equipment Repair, 6 Feb 1995, DASG-MS.

Appendix L

Medical Service Corps Specialties in 1982

Active Component, 30 June 1982

SSI*	Old MOS	Title	Actual Strength
		Administrative Specialties	
67A	3012	Health Care Administrator	131
67B	3065	Field Medical Assistant**	1,677
67C	3510	Health Services Comptroller	101
67D	3510	Biomedical Information Systems Officer	100
67E	3530	Patient Administration Officer	155
67F	3560, 2200	Health Services Personnel Manager	271
67G	3565	Health Services Manpower Control Officer	6
67H	3570, 2162	Health Services Plans, Operations, Intelligence, and Training Officer	117
67J	3581, 1980	Aeromedical Evacuation Officer	332
67K	3590, 4490	Health Services Materiel Officer	343
67L	3595	Health Facilities Planning Officer	22
670A (MOS)		Health Services Maintenance Technician (Warrant Officers)	93
		Scientific Specialties	
68A	3307	Microbiologist	56
68B	3308	Nuclear Medical Science Officer	54
68C	3309	Biochemist	81
68D	3310	Parasitologist	18
68E	3311	Immunologist	30
68F	3314	Clinical Laboratory Officer/ Laboratory Manager	92
68G	3315	Entomologist	81
68H	3318	Pharmacy Officer	215
68J	3327	Physiologist	25
68K	3340	Optometry Officer	219
68L	3350	Podiatrist	52
68M	3360	Audiologist	70
68N	3370	Environmental Science Officer	143
68P	3371	Sanitary Engineer	94
68R	3606	Social Work Officer	253
68S	3620	Psychologist	87
68T	3621	Health Services Research Psychologist	45
68U	3639	Behavioral Science Associate	31

Total Officers	4,901
Total Medical Service Corps	4,994

* SSI=Specialty skill identifier
** Includes 246 medical students

Source: DASG-PTH, Rpt, subj., Officer Strength, 1 Sep 1982; DASG-RMM, Rpt, subj., MSC, FY 1975 to FY 1981, both in DASG-MS.

Appendix M

Medical Service Corps Specialties in 1994

Commissioned Officers Arranged in Eight Medical Functional Areas
Active Component, 30 September 1994

AOC*/MOS	Title	Actual Strength
	Health Services (AOC 67A00**)	
70A67	Health Care Administration	224
70B67	Health Services Administration***	1,466
70C67	Health Services Comptroller	100
70D67	Health Services Systems Management	97
70E67	Patient Administration	98
70F67	Health Services Human Resources	200
70H67	Health Services Plans, Operations, Intelligence, Security, and Training	257
70K67	Health Services Materiel	512
670A	Health Services Maintenance Technician (Warrant Officers)	79
	Laboratory Sciences (AOC 67B00**)	
71A67	Microbiology	35
71B67	Biochemistry	73
71C67	Parasitology	8
71D67	Immunology	13
71E57	Clinical Laboratory	98
71F67	Research Psychology	28
	Preventive Medicine (AOC 67C00**)	
72A67	Nuclear Medical Science	65
72B67	Entomology	53
72C67	Audiology	44
72D67	Environmental Science	166
72E67	Sanitary Engineer	74
	Behavioral Sciences (AOC 67D00**)	
73A67	Social Work	153
73B67	Clinical Psychology	92
67E00	Pharmacy	158
67F00	Optometry	139
67G00	Podiatry	29
67J20	Aeromedical Evacuation	310

Total Medical Service Corps	4,571

* AOC=Area of concentration
** Used for coding specialty immaterial positions in documents
*** Includes 248 medical students

Source: AR 611–101, *Commissioned Officer Classification System*, change 5, 1 July 1994; TAPC-OPH, Rpt, sub: MSC Strength, 3 Oct 1994, DASG-MS.

Appendix N

Chief, Medical Service Corps, Award of Excellence 1982–1993

Name	Category
1982	
1st Lt. Duane C. Goodno	Administrative Specialties
Capt. Erik A. Henchal	Scientific Specialties
1983	
Capt. James G. Solomon	Administrative Specialties
Capt. Eric G. Daxon	Scientific Specialties
CW2 Cornelius L. Reeder	Warrant Officers
1984	
Capt. David L. Dickson	Administrative Specialties
Capt. David A. Rubenstein	Scientific Specialties
CW2 David A. Thomas	Warrant Officers
1985	
Capt. James R. Greenwood	Administrative Specialties
Capt. John W. Harbell	Scientific Specialties
CW2 David H. Lamwers	Warrant Officers
1986	
Capt. David L. Stanley	Administrative Specialties
Capt. Scott Gordon	Scientific Specialties
CW2 Juan R. Pagan	Warrant Officers
Capt. Marisa P. Parker	U.S. Army Reserve
1987	
Capt. Conrad A. Clyburn	Administrative Specialties
Capt. Noel R. Webster	Scientific Specialties
CW2 David E. Reece	Warrant Officers
Capt. Faith A. Frank	U.S. Army Reserve
1988	
Capt. Marilou D. Overla	Administrative Specialties
Capt. Beau J. Freund	Scientific Specialties
CW2 Raymond M. Sgrillo	Warrant Officers
Capt. Jane L. Meyer	U.S. Army Reserve
1989	
Capt. Stephen Wilkinson	Administrative Specialties
Capt. Thomas G. Eccles III	Scientific Specialties
CW2 William L. Adams	Warrant Officers
1st Lt. Judith A. Davenport	U.S. Army Reserve

Name	Category
1990	
Capt. George D. Trantow	Administrative Specialties
Capt. Brian J. Lukey	Scientific Specialties
CW2 Robert T. Hansen	Warrant Officers
Capt. Mary L. Ivanoff	Army National Guard
Capt. Cheryl L. Becker	U.S. Army Reserve
1991	
Capt. Randall G. Anderson	Administrative Specialties
Capt. Spencer J. Campbell	Scientific Specialties
CW2 Curtis L. Head	Warrant Officers
1st Lt. Annmarie Amaral	Army National Guard
Capt. Steven Wieneke	U.S. Army Reserve
1992	
1st Lt. Bradley A. Golden	Administrative Specialties
Capt. Carl A. Castro	Scientific Specialties
CW2 John K. Rosarius	Warrant Officers
Capt. John H. Grote, Jr.	Army National Guard
Capt. J. Michael French	U.S. Army Reserve
1993	
Capt. John F. Jessop	Administrative Specialties
1st Lt. Timothy G. Bosetti	Scientific Specialties
CW2 Curtis W. Randolph	Warrant Officers
Capt. Ronald L. Goldstein	Army National Guard
Capt. Eve A. Seibel	U.S. Army Reserve
1994	
Capt. Robert L. Goodman	Administrative Specialties
Capt. Scott C. Wright	Scientific Specialties
CW2 Kurt D. Kobashigawa	Warrant Officers
Capt. Daniel D. Darland	Army National Guard
Capt. Anne M. Guevara	U.S. Army Reserve
1994	
Capt. Steven G. Millward	Administrative Specialties
Capt. John Spain	Scientific Specialties
CW2 Michael W. Taylor	Warrant Officers
Capt. Rodney L. Walls	Army National Guard
Capt. John R. Yuen	U.S. Army Reserve

Source: MSC Newsletters, 25 March 1983, 8 October 1984, 21 June 1985, 29 September 1986, 14 August 1987, 15 December 1987, 15 November 1988, May 1990, March 1991, March 1994; February 1995, electronic mail msg, Ch, MSC, 17 October 1995; Plaque, Office of the Chief, Medical Service Corps; U.S. Army Medical Command newspaper *Mercury* (December 1994).

Bibliographical Note

Archival Collections

The author researched thousands of documents, and as much as possible the account was drawn from those primary sources. Documents cited in the notes are originals or accurate copies.

The following is a listing of the primary source holdings and their acronyms as used in the notes. These are also spelled out the first time they are used in the book.

AHA	American Hospital Association Library, Chicago, Illinois
DASG-MS	Office of the Chief, Medical Service Corps, Office of the Surgeon General, Washington, D.C. (The office relocated to the Army Medical Department Center and School, Fort Sam Houston, San Antonio, Texas, in 1994.)
DTIC	Defense Technical Information Center, Springfield, Virginia
JML	Joint Medical Library of the Army and Air Force Surgeons General, Washington, D.C.
NARA-NA	National Archives, National Archives and Records Administration, Washington, D.C.
NARA-WNRC	Washington National Records Center, National Archives and Records Administration, Suitland, Maryland
PL	Pentagon Library, The Pentagon, Washington, D.C.
SL	Stimson Library, Academy of Health Sciences, U.S. Army, Fort Sam Houston, San Antonio, Texas
USACMH	U.S. Army Center of Military History, Washington, D.C.
USAMHI	U.S. Army Military History Institute, Carlisle Barracks, Pennsylvania
USUHS	Uniformed Services University of the Health Sciences Library, Bethesda, Maryland
WRAIR	Walter Reed Army Institute of Research, Washington, D.C., now a unit of the U.S. Army Medical Research and Materiel Command

The most valuable collections were in three locations in the Washington, D.C., area.

A. *U.S. Army Center of Military History (USACMH).* The author relied heavily on USACMH holdings. A principal source was eighteen file boxes of documents accumulated during the various earlier attempts at writing the history; they are identified as MSC-USACMH in the notes. These files were especially valuable for the World War I and World War II periods. USACMH has prepared them for accession by the National Archives and Records Administration

(NARA). They were loaned to the author and will be returned to USACMH for accession by NARA when this volume is published. Storage will be in Record Group 112, The Surgeon General. USACMH prepared the files for accession after most of the research for the book was completed. Records reviewed after that preparation occurred are further identified with a box number.

1. The USACMH collection of Medical Department interviews is a must.

a. Korea. The premier portion of this collection is 139 interviews by USACMH historian Samuel Milner, conducted principally from 1966 to 1967. They are professional interviews by a trained historian and are invaluable for insight into the Medical Department's Korean War experience. Most are handwritten; none were taped. They were very useful to the author for the post–World War II period.

b. Vietnam. The Vietnam period is illuminated in interviews conducted by the 27th Military History Detachment in Vietnam. Interviews of Dustoff crews conducted by Capt. Peter Dorland, MSC, were useful in documenting the aeromedical evacuation story. Maj. Louis Drogi, MSC, conducted eighty-six interviews for a proposed monograph on the role of Special Forces in Vietnam; they are of limited value. The USACMH collection also includes a series of Lessons Learned interviews conducted in the Surgeon General's Office during the Vietnam period.

2. A particularly valuable USACMH holding is a bound collection of forty-one volumes of notes of the surgeon general's daily staff meetings from 1947 to 1969. Arlyne Fransway, the surgeon general's secretary, prepared typed summaries of those morning meetings for twenty years until her retirement in 1967. The minutes, often with relevant documents attached, were circulated daily among the surgeon general, the deputy surgeon general, and the executive officer. Entitled *Surgeon General Early Morning Conference Notes*, they are cited in this volume as SG Conference plus the date. Circulation of the minutes was confined to a small group for most of the period covered. The discussions were candid and confidential and, as General Armstrong cautioned, "many subjects should go no further."[1] Fransway's notes picked up the tenor of the meetings, as when she wrote on 9 September 1955: "Mr. Cogan threw in a bomb shell by saying that he always felt all the hospitals should be under the command of Army areas." She left a rich lode for the historian.

3. The USACMH library is also a good source. It has a variety of useful holdings, including some documentary items such as unit yearbooks. A tip to the researcher is to look at the collection of Department of Defense telephone books for an idea of the changes to military offices over the years. As a supplement to that, a collection of OTSG telephone directories was maintained from the period July 1963 through 1986 within the Directorate of Personnel, OTSG. Those directories provide greater detail than the DOD phone books, but their current location is unknown.

B. *National Archives and Records Administration (NARA).* The Washington National Records Center of NARA was a good source for documents retired by the Surgeon General's Office since World War II, and those accession and box numbers are given in the notes. Some use was made of holdings by the National

Archives (NARA) for the period prior to 1945, and those are also cited in the notes.

C. *Office of The Surgeon General (OTSG).* The files of the Office of the Chief, Medical Service Corps, were also a valuable source. Those files will be processed for accession in Record Group 112 of NARA following publication of this book. They will be labeled Medical Service Corps History files, as part of the working files of the volume. The documents principally cover the period between Korea and Vietnam. The files include the typed transcripts of thirty interviews conducted by the author and transcripts of two panel meetings of retired chiefs of the corps conducted in 1983 and 1985.

There are several other sources which deserve special mention.

The Joint Medical Library of the Army and Air Force Surgeons General (JML). This library is collocated with OTSG. It served the author well during the research phase as a means to gain access to the various collections in the Washington, D.C., area, especially the National Library of Medicine. In addition, the library has some valuable holdings for research into the Medical Department.

Medical Bulletin/AMEDD Journal. One of the holdings of the Joint Medical Library of the Army and Air Force Surgeons General is a journal/newsletter of the Medical Department published from 1919 to 1974 and resumed in 1987. Because of the multiplicity of titles it has held over the years it is referred to throughout the notes as *Medical Bulletin* until 1987 and *AMEDD Journal* from 1987 until the present. TSG initially published it as the *Medico-Military Review* from 1919 to 1921. It was retitled the *Army Medical Bulletin* from 1922 to 1943, and in 1943 the journal became the *Bulletin of the U.S. Army Medical Department.* In 1950 it was absorbed into the *United States Armed Forces Medical Journal (AFMJ)*, which unified the Army and Navy bulletins until the demise of *AFMJ* in 1960. The functions performed by the *AFMJ* were assumed by *Military Medicine*, the privately printed journal of the Association of Military Surgeons of the United States.

Despite "unification" of the journals, TSG resumed distribution of an Army newsletter with Surgeon General's Office *Notes*, 1953–54; SGO *Memos*, 1955–57; *Medical Bulletin*, 1958–59; and U.S. Army Technical Bulletins 8–1 through 8–24, entitled *The Surgeon General: Professional and Administrative Guidance Material*, 1960–69. This was followed by *Newsletter of the U.S. Army Medical Department*, 1970–73, followed by the *AMEDD Spectrum* in 1974, when publication of a departmental journal or newsletter ceased. In 1987 the surgeon general designated the *Medical Bulletin of the U.S. Army, Europe*, published by the 7th Medical Command in Heidelberg, Germany, as the new house organ. It was initially entitled the *Medical Bulletin of the U.S. Army Medical Department.* That was quickly changed to the *Journal of the U.S. Army Medical Department.* In July 1994 its editorial office was relocated to the newly formed U.S. Army Medical Command at Fort Sam Houston, San Antonio, Texas, as a result of the drawdown of U.S. forces in Europe. This also marked the end of a 25-year affiliation for its editor, Ms. Ingeborg Sosa, who began as the assistant editor in July 1969 and was promoted to editor in July 1974.

Annual Report. Another valuable source was the Surgeon General's *Annual Report.* Surgeon General Joseph Lovell inaugurated annual reports beginning with his appointment as the first head of a permanent Medical Department in 1818. It was a regularly published document during the years 1818 to 1941, 1953 to 1954, and 1954 to 1975, when it ceased as a routine publication (a final report for 1976–80 was published in 1988). Printing of the report by the Government Printing Office began during the Civil War, making it more accessible to a wider audience. The Joint Medical Library has copies of the pre–Civil War reports. Both JML and the Pentagon Library have copies of the printed reports.

During the post-Vietnam period the surgeon general terminated any department-wide bulletin, ceased publishing an annual report, and lost the department's history section. Those actions weakened the communication links essential for cohesion and made the department increasingly unable to either know or tell its history. Resumption of the *Medical Bulletin* in 1987 was a healthy sign. Its relocation to San Antonio in 1994 was another good sign since European reductions would surely have spelled its eventual demise if it had not been given a more solid footing than an overseas command in the post–Cold War era.

The Pentagon Library (PL). Located in The Pentagon, Washington, D.C., the Pentagon Library (formerly the Army Library) is an excellent general reference source. Its collection of general orders, publications, and regulations dating from 1809 to the present are especially helpful.

The American Hospital Association (AHA) Library. Located in the AHA headquarters, Chicago, Illinois, this library houses the Lewis E. Weeks Series of the Hospital Administration Oral History Collection. This is a collection of interviews with prominent figures in health care administration beginning in 1978. While of limited value to this project, it would be useful for research into the development of that specialty.

Official Histories

The Surgeon General published major historical accounts of Medical Department activities following the Civil War, World War I, and World War II. They are invaluable to the researcher and are highlighted here.

The Medical and Surgical History of the War of the Rebellion owes its being to the foresight of Brig. Gen. William A. Hammond, the surgeon general from April 1862 to May 1864. It was published in two volumes by the Surgeon General's Office as a landmark medical history.

The operations of the Medical Department in World War I were recorded by the Surgeon General's Office in *The Medical Department in the World War*, published in fifteen volumes from 1921 to 1929. This was another landmark medical history and an important contribution to the world literature. No volume is devoted to the Sanitary Corps or other predecessor organizations of the Medical Service Corps. References to those groups and their members are scattered throughout. The following volumes were referenced in this book: *Administration, American Expeditionary Forces*, *Communicable and Other Diseases*, *Field Operations*, *Finance and Supply*, *Sanitation*, *Surgery*, and *Training*.

World War II medical operations were documented in the massive *Medical Department of the United States Army in World War II*, published in forty-two volumes, the bulk of which were under the general editorship of Col. John B. Coates, MC. The history was divided into two parts, an administrative series (six volumes) and a clinical series (thirty-two volumes), the latter in five categories: internal medicine, neuropsychiatry, preventive medicine, surgery, and miscellaneous. This was also a major contribution by the Medical Department to the world literature. No volume is devoted to predecessor organizations of the Medical Service Corps. References to those groups and their members are scattered throughout. The following volumes were referenced in this book: *Blood Program in World War II*, *Communicable Diseases: Arthropodborne Diseases Other than Malaria*, *Communicable Diseases: Malaria*, *Medical Supply in World War II*, *Medical Training in World War II*, *Organization and Administration in World War II*, *Orthopedic Surgery in the Zone of Interior*, *Personnel in World War II*, and *Special Fields*.

Bibliographies and Finding Aids

Several bibliographies and finding aids were an assistance. They are listed along with their locations. Copies are also in the working files of this book.

Louise A. Arnold, Gettysburg National Military Park, report, subject, Selected Bibliography: Medicine of the Civil War, 1979, 19 pages, typewritten. Gettysburg National Park, National Park Service. Copy in DASG-MS.

Charles W. Ellsworth, Archivist, USACMH, report, subject, Preliminary Guide to the Records of the U.S. Army Medical Department on File in The Historical Unit, U.S. AMEDD, 1960–1969, May 1975, 112 pages, typewritten. This is an example of checklists and finding aids in the Medical Department files of the Center of Military History. USACMH.

OTSG, DA Forms 2172, Records Shipment Lists 135, Records Transmittal and Receipt. These are transmittal documents for Surgeon General records retired to the Washington National Records Center, NARA, for the period since World War II. NARA-WNRC.

Esther E. Rohlader, Research and Archives Branch, The Historical Unit, OTSG, report, subject, Bibliography, undated (1957), 9 pages, typewritten. This is a bibliography of Medical Service Corps articles published from 1945 to 1957 and archival sources for the same period plus World War I and the interwar period. USACMH.

George A. Scheirer, Managing Editor, *Bulletin of the U.S. Army Medical Department*, OTSG, report, subject, Army Medical Department Chronology, 1775–1947, 1 October 1947, 84 pages, typewritten. While not a listing of sources, this document is a useful aid for the researcher. USACMH.

John J. Slonaker, Research Historian, USAMHI, report, subject, The American Field Service, 7 May 1982. This lists published histories and accounts of the American Field Service (AFS) in World War I. The AFS was a private voluntary ambulance service organized in 1914 that was a predecessor organization of the U.S. Army Ambulance Service, formed in 1917. USAMHI.

John J. Slonaker, report, subject, The U.S. Army and Sanitation Service (Including Service with the Food Division), 5 September 1974. This is a listing of

U.S. Army Military History Institute holdings on the Sanitary Corps and the Food Division of the Surgeon General's Office in World War I. USAMHI.

Richard J. Sommers, Chief, Archives Branch, USAMHI, report, subject, Manuscript Holdings of the U.S. Army Military History Research Collection, Volume I, 1972; Volume II, 1975. USAMHI.

Patricia Taylor, National Archives, NARA, report, subject, Preliminary Inventory of the Textual Records of the Surgeon General (Army), (Record Group 112), 1964, 51 pages, typewritten. This is a description of Record Group 112, a collection of about 4,200 cubic feet of files accumulated since the permanent establishment of the Medical Department in 1818 through 1946. NARA-NA.

USACMH, Standard Form 135, Records Transmittal and Receipt, subject, Documents Used in Preparation of the History of the Medical Service Corps, January 1986. This is a listing of the contents of each of the eighteen boxes of documents accumulated in the attempts to write the history of the Medical Service Corps prior to 1983. The forms were prepared for accession of the files by the NARA and will be retired upon publication of this volume. They are supplemented by a report, subject, Records Locator, a detailed listing prepared by Col. Robert D. Linder, MSC, USAR, 20 October 1983. USACMH.

Secondary Sources

The author consulted over three hundred books and more than four hundred and fifty periodical articles. Those sources are documented in the notes as they are cited.

[1]SG Conference, 23 February 1951.

Illustration Credits

Illustrations, on the pages listed, appear courtesy of the following sources:

Parke-Davis/Warner-Lambert: p. 2
National Library of Medicine: pp. 7, 10, 14, 21, 23, 25, 26, 94
Library of Congress: pp. 15, 36, 39 *(top)*, 47
Cook Collection Valentine Museum: p. 18
State Historical Society of Wisconsin: p. 39 *(bottom)*
Office of the Chief, Medical Service Corps: pp. 40, 50 *(top and bottom)*, 62, 63, 69 *(top and bottom)*, 92, 146, 166, 173, 179, 196, 268, 279, 291, 312, 323, 324, 325, 326, 327, 340, 352, 354, 357, 390, 408, 430, 436 (*top left* and *bottom*), 479, 481, 482, 483, 484, 485, 486, 487, 488, 489, 490, 491
National Archives: pp. 43, 44, 71 *(top left, top right, and bottom)*, 73, 128, 134, 136, 140 *(bottom)*, 145, 163, 169, 176, 182, 211, 236, 238, 240, 245, 247, 255, 257, 284, 294
Lehigh County Historical Society: p. 46
Otis Historical Archives, National Museum of Health and Medicine: pp. 56, 140 *(top)*
National Academy of Sciences: pp. 75, 76
U.S. Army Military History Institute: p. 90
Air Force History Office, Kelly Air Force Base: p. 93
National Defense University: p. 104
George Washington University: p. 108
Armed Forces Institute of Pathology: pp. 110, 118, 165, 205, 206
E. J. Williams: p. 129
U.S. Army: pp. 130, 137, 158, 271, 278, 285, 286, 292, 328, 351, 355, 477
Department of Agriculture: p. 168
R. E. Pryor, Jr: p. 170
James T. Richards: p. 210
American Optical Association: 221
Presidio Press: p. 241
Edward H. Frick: p. 253
George Hunter: p. 256
Walter Reed Army Institute of Research: pp. 293, 316, 353
Luis P. Carranza: p. 306
John R. Howard: p. 311
Charles R. Angel: p. 318
U.S. Army Medical Department: p. 336
William C. Luehrs: p. 343
DOD Still Media Records Center: pp. 374, 393, 399, 422, 426, 441
Priscilla M. Alston: p. 380

Donald H. Triano: p. 383 (*right*)
Scott S. Beaty: p. 388
Robert F. Elliott: p. 395
National Aeronautics and Space Agency: p. 403
Arthur R. Hapner: p. 424
Harry Lee Whitlock II: pp. 431, 436 (*top right*)
Richard Kennedy: p. 436 (*middle*)
Steve Horosko III: p. 443
Dale Brown: p. 444

Index

Index

ISBN 0-16-045353-4